Critical Care Hematology

Shakti Bedanta Mishra
Editor

Critical Care Hematology

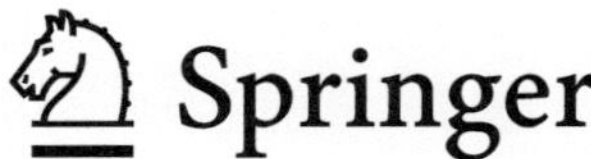

Editor
Shakti Bedanta Mishra
Department of Critical Care Medicine
IMS and SUM Hospital
Bhubaneswar, Odisha, India

ISBN 978-981-97-5567-7 ISBN 978-981-97-5565-3 (eBook)
https://doi.org/10.1007/978-981-97-5565-3

This Springer imprint is published by the registered company Springer Nature Singapore Pte Ltd.
The registered company address is: 152 Beach Road, #21-01/04 Gateway East, Singapore 189721, Singapore

Foreword

Critical Care Medicine is a subspecialty that has grown rapidly in the past three and half decades. India started late but caught up with the rest of the world soon to branch out to various subspecialty intensive care units (ICUs). Hematology, not long ago considered a laboratory specialty in almost all hospitals in India barring a handful of big teaching hospitals, is very much a clinical subspecialty now in most teaching and even in corporate hospitals dealing with certain diseases, related to hematological that are potentially life-threatening. Medical innovations and newer therapeutic options in such conditions often precipitate life-threatening complications that need intensive monitoring and care in ICUs. Certain general conditions, such as sepsis, medical, and surgical emergencies, complicate these conditions to create life-threatening complications that require critical care support. Hematology ICU is accepted by many tertiary care hospitals even in India, as a subspecialty of Intensive Care Medicine. Therefore, it is appropriate that a comprehensive monograph must be brought out on the said subspecialty.

The book starts with general core diagnostic tools essential in making a primary diagnosis in a critically ill hematology patient. It then describes common disorders such as anemia, leukocytopenia, thrombocytopenia, thrombosis, and sickle cell disease. Transfusion medicine, an important and common intervention for hematology and oncology, is appropriately included in the monograph. Oncology-related issues due to the disease and its therapy are described extensively under two subheadings (i) general hematologic issues associated with oncology and (ii) oncology-specific issues. Infections in critical care are at the core of critical care management and hematology is no exception. Infection has been addressed through opportunistic infections, febrile neutropenia, and invasive fungal infections focusing on prevention, identification, and management in immunocompromised hosts. The book also includes the management of postoperative bleeding, all-important compassionate care, and end-of-life care. The book concludes with comprehensive strategies for critical care pathways in hematology, outcome, and prognosis of the conditions.

I find the monograph handy for a critical care physician even in a general ICU. I am sure this will be an important foundational resource for post-graduates and students of critical care medicine in any subspecialty.

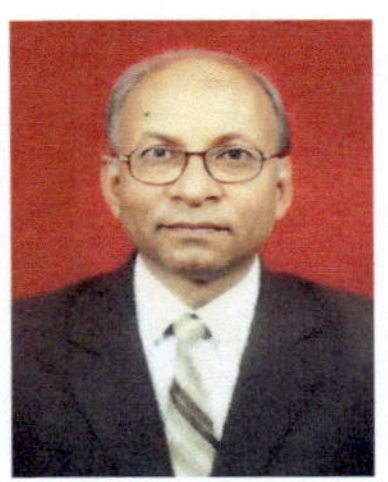

Head of Critical Care Medicine
SUM Ultimate Medicare, A Unit of SOA
Bhubaneswar, Odisha, India

Banambar Ray

Preface

In the realm of critical care, the intersection of hematology and intensive care medicine presents unique and complex challenges. This book, *Critical Care Hematology*, is designed to serve as a comprehensive guide for residents working in the ICU, providing them with a clear and structured approach to managing hematological patients.

The journey through this book is intended to be practical and user-friendly. Each chapter is meticulously crafted with algorithms, infographics, and diagrams that simplify complex decision-making processes. These visual aids will help guide the reader through critical steps, from initial assessment and diagnostic testing to the management of complications and therapeutic interventions.

Our aim is to equip ICU residents with a robust framework to navigate the intricacies of hematological conditions in critically ill patients. However, the utility of this book extends beyond its primary audience. Medicine specialists, hematologists, intensivists, and even nurses will find it to be a valuable reference, aiding them in delivering high-quality care to their patients.

The strength of this book lies in its practical approach, drawing from the collective expertise of seasoned clinicians and educators. It encapsulates years of experience and knowledge, distilled into actionable insights that can be readily applied in the high-stakes environment of the ICU.

As you delve into *Critical Care Hematology*, we hope it becomes an indispensable part of your professional toolkit, enhancing your ability to deliver compassionate, evidence-based care to some of the most vulnerable patients. This book is a testament to our commitment to education and excellence in critical care medicine.

This comprehensive guide is the result of collaboration among leading experts in the fields of critical care and hematology. The content is carefully curated to provide the latest evidence-based practices and guidelines, ensuring that readers are equipped with the most up-to-date information to make informed clinical decisions.

The book also addresses the growing need for a multidisciplinary approach in critical care settings. It emphasizes the importance of effective communication and collaboration among healthcare professionals from various specialties, ultimately aiming to improve patient outcomes and overall quality of care.

In addition to its practical utility, *Critical Care Hematology* serves as a platform for ongoing professional development. The insights and best practices shared within its pages are intended to spark discussions, inspire innovation, and contribute to the continuous advancement of critical care and hematology as dynamic fields of medicine.

We are confident that this book will serve as a valuable resource for healthcare professionals at all levels, from trainees to seasoned practitioners. Whether used as a quick reference guide or a comprehensive study tool, *Critical Care Hematology* is poised to make a meaningful impact on the delivery of care in critical care units worldwide.

Bhubaneswar, Odisha, India Shakti Bedanta Mishra

Contents

Abbreviations

2-HG	2-Hydroxyglutarate
AA	Aplastic anemia
AA	Arachidonic acid
ABG	Arterial blood gas
ABO	Blood group system (no full form; part of blood grouping terminology)
ACCP	American College of Chest Physicians
ACD	Anemia of chronic disease
ACS	Acute chest syndrome
ACS	Acute coronary syndromes
ACTH	Adrenocorticotropic hormone
ADAMTS13	A disintegrin and metalloprotease with a thrombospondin type 1 motif member 13
ADCs	Antibody-drug conjugates
ADP	Adenosine-diphosphate
ADQI	Acute Dialysis Quality Initiative
AFB	Acid-fast bacilli
aHUS	Atypical hemolytic uremic syndrome
AIDS	Acquired immunodeficiency syndrome
AIHA	Autoimmune hemolytic anemia
AKI	Acute kidney injury
AL	Amyloid light-chain
ALL	Acute lymphoblastic leukemia
allo-HSCT	Allogeneic hematopoietic stem cell transplantation
ALPS	Autoimmune lymphoproliferative syndrome
AML	Acute myeloid leukemia
ANA	Antinuclear antibody
ANC	Absolute neutrophil count
APACHE II	Acute Physiology and Chronic Health Evaluation II
APACHE	Acute Physiology and Chronic Health Evaluation
APL	Acute promyelocytic leukemia

APLA	Antip-hospholipid antibody
APML	Acute promyelocytic leukemia
APS	Antiphospholipid syndrome
aPTT	Activated partial thromboplastin time
ARDS	Acute respiratory distress syndrome
ARF	Acute respiratory failure
ASH	American Society of Hematology
ASIS	Antero-superior iliac spine
AT III	Antithrombin III
ATRA	All-trans retinoic acid
BAL	Bronchoalveolar lavage
B-ALL	B-acute lymphoblastic leukemia
BD	Twice daily
BG	Beta-D-glucans
BiPAP	Bilevel positive airway pressure
BiTEs	Bispecific T-cell engagers
BMA	Bone marrow aspirate
BME	Bone marrow examination
BMFS	Bone marrow failure syndromes
BMT	Bone marrow transplant
BNP	Brain natriuretic peptide
BSS	Bernard-Soulier syndrome
BT	Bleeding time
BUN	Blood urea nitrogen
Ca	Calcium
CAMT	Congenital amegakaryocytic thrombocytopenia
CAPS	Catastrophic antiphospholipid syndrome
CAR	Chimeric antigen receptor
CAR-T	Chimeric antigen receptor T-cell
CBC	Complete blood count
CCI	Corrected count increment
CI	Confidence interval
CLL	Chronic lymphocytic leukemia
CML	Chronic myeloid leukemia
CMML	Chronic myelomonocytic leukemia
CMV	Cytomegalovirus
CNS	Central nervous system
COPD	Chronic Obstructive Pulmonary Disease
cP	Centipoise
CPAP	Continuous positive airway pressure
CPB	Cardiopulmonary bypass
CPDA	Citrate phosphate dextrose adenine
CRS	Cytokine release syndrome
CSE	Convulsive status epilepticus
CSF	Cerebrospinal fluid

CT	Computed tomography
CTA	CT angiography
CTCL	Cutaneous T-cell lymphoma
CVC	Central Venous Catheter
CVID	Common variable immunodeficiency
CVT	Cerebral venous sinus thrombosis
DAH	Diffuse alveolar hemorrhage
DAT	Direct antibody test
DAT	Direct antiglobulin test
DC	Dyskeratosis congenita
DCR	Damage control resuscitation
DCT/ICT	Direct and indirect coombs test
DDAVP	Desmopressin
DIC	Disseminated intravascular coagulation
DIC	Disseminated intravascular coagulopathy
DI-TMA	Drug-induced thrombotic microangiopathy
DITP	Drug-induced immune thrombocytopenia
DLBCL	Diffuse large B-cell lymphoma
DLC	Differential count
DM1	Derivative of maytansine 1
DNA	Deoxyribonucleic acid
DOAC	Directly acting oral anticoagulants
DVT	Deep vein thrombosis
EACA	ε-Aminocaproic acid
EBV	Epstein-Barr virus
ECG	Electrocardiogram
ECMO	Extracorporeal membrane oxygenation
ECOG PS	Eastern Cooperative Oncology Group Performance Status
ECOG	Eastern Cooperative Oncology Group
EGFR	Epidermal growth factor receptor
ELISA	Enzyme-linked immunosorbent assay
EOLC	End-of-life care
EPI	Epinephrine
ERAS	Enhanced recovery after surgery
ERFE	Erythroferrone
ESA	Erythropoietin-stimulating agents
ESR	Erythrocyte sedimentation rate
EVLWI	Extravascular lung water index
FA	Folic acid
FAB	French-American-British (classification)
FALLS	Fluid administration limited by lung sonography
FAST	Focused assessment with sonography for trauma
FCM	Flowcytometry
FDA	Food and Drug Administration
FFP	Fresh frozen plasma

FiO_2	Fraction of inspired oxygen
FLT3-ITD	FMS-like tyrosine kinase 3—internal tandem duplication (mutation)
FN	Febrile Neutropenia
FNHTRs	Febrile nonhemolytic transfusion reactions
FSP	Fibrin split products
FUO	Fever of unknown origin
G6PD	Glucose-6-phosphate dehydrogenase
G-CSF	Granulocyte colony-stimulating factor
GDFT	Goal-directed fluid therapy
GEDVI	Global end-diastolic volume index
GI	Gastrointestinal
GISTs	Gastrointestinal stromal tumors
GMS	Grocott's methenamine silver
GPIIb/IIIa	Glycoprotein IIb/IIIa
GVHD	Graft-versus-host-disease
GVHD	Gut graft-versus-host disease
Hb	Hemoglobin
HB	Hemoglobin
HbA	Hemoglobin A
HbS	Hemoglobin S
HbSS	Hemoglobin SS
HBV	Hepatitis B virus
HCL	Hairy cell leukemia
Hct	Hematocrit
HCT	Hematopoietic cell transplantation
HCV	Hepatitis C virus
HDAC	Histone deacetylase
HELLP	Hemolysis, elevated liver enzymes, and low platelet count
HFNC	High-flow nasal cannula
HFNO	High-flow nasal oxygen
Hh	Hedgehog
HHM	Hematologic malignancies
HHM	Humoral hypercalcemia of malignancy
HIPA	Heparin-induced platelet activation
HIPEC	Hyperthermic intraperitoneal chemotherapy
HIT	Heparin-induced thrombocytopenia
HIV	Human immunodeficiency virus
HL	Hodgkin's lymphoma
HLA	Human leukocyte antigen
HLH	Hemophagocytic lymphohistiocytosis
HLH/MAS	Hemophagocytic lymphohistiocytosis/macrophage activation syndrome
HNA	Human neutrophil antigen
HPA	Human platelet antigen
HPS	Hemophagocytic syndrome

HRCT	High-resolution computed tomography
HRQOL	Health-related quality of life
HSCT	Hematopoietic stem cell transplantation
HSV	Herpes simplex virus
HUS	Hemolytic uremic syndrome
HVS	Hyperviscosity syndrome
IAT	Indirect antiglobulin test
iCa	Ionized calcium
ICAM	Intercellular adhesion molecule
ICH	Intracerebral hemorrhage
ICH	Intracranial hemorrhage
ICNARC	Intensive Care National Audit & Research Centre
ICU	Intensive care unit
ICU-VTE	Intensive care unit-venous thromboembolism
IDA	Iron deficiency anemia
IDH	Isocitrate dehydrogenase
IFD	Invasive fungal disease
IFE	Serum immuno-fixation test
IFI	Invasive fungal infection
IFN-γ	Interferon-gamma
IgA	Immunoglobulin A
IgG	Immunoglobulin G
IgM	Immunoglobulin M
IHC	Immunohistochemistry
IL-1β	Interleukin-1 beta
IL-2	Interleukin-2
IL-6	Interleukin-6
IL-8	Interleukin 8
IMV	Invasive mechanical ventilation
INR	International normalized ratio
ISTH	International Society on Thrombosis and Haemostasis
ITP	Immune thrombocytopenia
ITP	Immune thrombocytopenic purpura
IU	International units
IV	Intravenous
IVIG	Intravenous immunoglobulin
JAAM	Japanese Association for Acute Medicine
JMML	Juvenile myelomonocytic leukemia
LD	Leishman-Donovan (bodies)
LDH	Lactate dehydrogenase
LFT	Liver function test
LFTs	Liver function tests
LMWH	Low-molecular-weight heparin
LTOWB	Low-titer group O whole blood
M4	Myelomonocytic (subtype of AML)

M5	Monocytic (subtype of AML)
MA	Maximum amplitude
mAbs	Monoclonal antibodies
MAHA	Microangiopathic hemolytic anemia
MAL	Mixed acute leukemia
MASCC	Multinational Association for Supportive Care in Cancer
MCH	Mean corpuscular hemoglobin
MCHC	Mean corpuscular hemoglobin concentration
MCV	Mean corpuscular volume
MDN	Myelodysplastic neoplasm
MDS	Myelodysplastic syndromes
MGUS	Monoclonal gammopathy of undetermined significance
MLL	Mixed lineage leukemia (gene)
MM	Multiple myeloma
MMAE	Monomethyl auristatin E
MMPs	Matrix metalloproteinases
MODS	Multiple organ dysfunction syndrome
MOFS	Multiorgan failure syndrome
MPM	Mortality probability models
MPN	Myeloproliferative neoplasm
MPV	Mean platelet volume
MRA	Magnetic resonance angiography
MRI	Magnetic resonance imaging
MRSA	Methicillin-Resistant Staphylococcus Aureus
MTP	Massive transfusion protocol
NCCN	National Comprehensive Cancer Network
NCCT	Non-contrast computed tomography
NCSE	Non-convulsive status epilepticus
NGS	Next-Generation Sequencing
NHL	Non-Hodgkin lymphoma
NIV	Non-invasive ventilation
NOACs	Novel oral anticoagulants
NS	Normal saline
NSCLC	Non-small cell lung cancer
OBRI	Outpatient bleeding risk index
ONSD	Optic nerve sheath diameter
OR	Odds ratio
PAI-1	Plasminogen activator inhibitor-1
PAS	Periodic acid–Schiff
PBM	Patient blood management
PBS	Peripheral blood smear
PC	Palliative care
PCC	Prothrombin complex concentrates
PCP	Pneumocystis carinii pneumonia
PCR	Plateletcrit

PCR	Polymerase chain reaction
PCV	Packed cell volume
PDGFR	Platelet-derived growth factor receptor
PDW	Platelet distribution width
PE	Pulmonary embolism
PE38	Pseudomonas exotoxin A
PEA	PF4-dependent P-selectin expression assay
PET-CT	Positron emission tomography—computed tomography
PF4	Platelet factor 4
PFA	Platelet function analyzer
PI3K	Phosphatidylinositol 3-kinase
PICC	Inserted central catheter
PICU	Pediatric intensive care unit
PID	Primary immunodeficiency
PLASMIC	(Score predicting severe ADAMTS13 deficiency, no full form in text)
PNH	Paroxysmal nocturnal hemoglobinuria
PNS	Peripheral nervous system
POC	Point-of-care
POCUS	Point-of-care ultrasound
PPH	Postpartum hemorrhage
PRBCs	Packed red blood cells
PRES	Posterior reversible encephalopathy syndrome
PRES	Posterior reversible leukoencephalopathy syndrome
PROMMTT	Prospective observational multicenter major trauma transfusion
PROPPR	Pragmatic randomized optimal platelet and plasma ratios
PS	Peripheral smear
PSGL-1	P-selectin glycoprotein ligand 1
PSIS	Postero-superior iliac spine
PT	Prothrombin time
PTCL	Peripheral T-cell lymphoma
PTHrP	Parathyroid hormone-related protein
PTLD	Post-transplant lymphoproliferative disorder
PTP	Post-transfusion purpura
PTSD	Post-traumatic stress disorder
PTT	Partial thromboplastin time
PUO	Pyrexia of unknown origin
PVRI	Pulmonary vascular resistance index
PVT	Portal vein thrombosis
QOL	Quality of life
R/o	Rule out
RANKL	Receptor activator of nuclear factor kappa-B ligand
RBC	Red blood cell
RBC	Red blood cell count
RBCs	Red blood cells

RCT	Randomized controlled trial
RDP	Random donor platelets
RDTs	Rapid Diagnostic Tests
RDW	Red cell distribution width
RES	Reticuloendothelial system
rFVIIa	Recombinant factor VIIa
RI	Reference interval (in laboratory testing)
RiCOF	Ristocetin cofactor
ROTEM	Rotational thromboelastometry
RPI	Reticulocyte production index
RRT	Renal replacement therapy
RSV	Respiratory syncytial virus
RTA	Renal tubular acidosis
RT-PCR	Reverse transcription polymerase chain reaction
RUSH	Rapid ultrasound for shock and hypotension
S. stercoralis	*Strongyloides stercoralis*
SAPS	Simplified Acute Physiology Score
SBP	Systolic blood pressure
SCD	Sickle cell disease
SCID	Severe combined immunodeficiency
SCN	Severe congenital neutropenia
SE	Status epilepticus
SIC	Sepsis-induced coagulopathy
SINE	Selective inhibitors of nuclear export
SIRS	Systemic inflammatory response syndrome
SLE	Systemic lupus erythematosus
SMO	Smoothened
SOAP	Sepsis occurrence in acutely ill patients
SOFA	Sequential Organ Failure Assessment
SPEP	Serum protein electrophoresis
SRA	Serotonin release assay
SSG	Surviving sepsis guidelines
STEC	Shiga toxin-producing *Escherichia Coli*
STEC-HUS	Shiga toxin-producing *Escherichia coli* hemolytic uremic syndrome
STEMI	ST-elevation myocardial infarction
SVCS	Superior vena cava syndrome
SVRI	Systemic vascular resistance index
TACO	Transfusion-associated circulatory overload
TAFI	Thrombin activatable fibrinolysis inhibitor
TA-GVHD	Transfusion-associated graft-versus-host disease
TA-TMA	Transplant-associated thrombotic microangiopathy
TCR	T-cell receptors
TEG	Thromboelastography
TGA	Thrombin generation assay
Th2	T-helper 2

TILs	Tumor-infiltrating lymphocytes
TIPS	Transjugular intrahepatic portosystemic shunt
TKIs	Tyrosine kinase inhibitors
TLC	Total leukocyte count
TLS	Tumor lysis syndrome
TMA	Thrombotic microangiopathic anemias
TMA	Thrombotic microangiopathies
TMA	Thrombotic microangiopathy
TMP/SMX	Trimethoprim-sulfamethoxazole
TNF-α	Tumor necrosis factor-alpha
tPA	tissue plasminogen activator
TPE	Therapeutic plasma exchange
TPN	Total parenteral nutrition
TRALI	Transfusion-related acute lung injury
TRIM	Transfusion-related immunomodulation
tt	thrombin time
TTP	Thrombotic thrombocytopenic purpura
TXA	Tranexamic acid
UFH	Unfractionated heparin
USA	United States of America
USS	Upshaw-Schulman syndrome
UTI	Urinary tract infection
V/Q	Ventilation/perfusion
VCAM	Vascular cell adhesion molecule
VEGFRs	Vascular endothelial growth factor receptors
VKAs	Vitamin K antagonists
VOC	Vaso-occlusive crises
VTE	Venous thromboembolism
VWD	von Willebrand disease
vWF	von Willebrand factor
VZV	Varicella-Zoster virus
WAS	Wiskott-Aldrich syndrome
WBC	White blood cell
WBC	White blood cell count
WBCs	White blood cells
WHO	World Health Organization
WM	Waldenström macroglobulinemia
Xa	Factor Xa (anti-factor Xa assay)
XLT	X-linked thrombocytopenia
ZN	Ziehl-Neelsen (stain)

Part I
Diagnostic Foundations

Chapter 1
Guide to Simplified Complete Blood Count and Peripheral Smear Analysis

Shruti Mishra

Learning Points

1. Foundational Knowledge of CBC and peripheral smear (PS): Understand the essential components of the complete blood count (CBC) and peripheral smear (PS), including their roles in evaluating an individual's hematological health. Grasp the significance of each component in diagnosing and managing diseases.
2. Interpretation Skills: Develop skills to interpret CBC and PS reports accurately, understanding variations in red blood cell (RBC), white blood cell (WBC), and platelet parameters, and their implications for patient care. Learn to navigate the complexities of differential counts and morphological assessments in peripheral smears.
3. Application of Advanced Technologies: Recognize the application of emerging technologies, such as machine learning and advanced image processing, in enhancing the diagnostic accuracy of parasitic infections and abnormal cell detection in blood smears.
4. Practical Clinical Application: Equip yourself with practical knowledge and skills to apply CBC and PS analysis in clinical settings. Understand how these tests influence clinical decisions, treatment planning, and monitoring of various hematological conditions.

S. Mishra (✉)
Bone Marrow Transplantation and Stem Cell Research Centre, Institute of Medical Sciences, Banaras Hindu University, Varanasi, Uttar Pradesh, India
e-mail: drshruti.mishra@bhu.ac.in

S. B. Mishra (ed.), *Critical Care Hematology*,
https://doi.org/10.1007/978-981-97-5565-3_1

1.1 Introduction

The complete blood count (CBC) is a pivotal diagnostic test in clinical medicine, offering a comprehensive assessment of the blood's cellular components. This section will explore the components of the CBC, emphasizing its role as one of the most informative single investigations in medical diagnostics (Seo and Lee 2022).

1.2 Components of the CBC

- *Red Blood Cell Count (RBC)*: Measures the number of red blood cells, essential for oxygen transport.
- *White Blood Cell Count (WBC)*: Quantifies the white blood cells, crucial for immune response. The white blood cell count and its differential are pivotal in diagnosing and managing various diseases, including infections and hematological disorders (Choi et al. 2017).
- *Platelet Count*: Assesses the number of platelets, vital for blood clotting.
- *Hemoglobin (Hb)*: Gauges the amount of hemoglobin, the oxygen-carrying protein in red blood cells.
- *Hematocrit (Hct)*: Percentage of red blood cells in the blood, indicating the blood's capacity to carry oxygen.
- *Differential Count*: Provides a breakdown of different types of white blood cells, each playing a unique role in the immune system. Automated systems for differential count in various biological samples have been developed, offering high accuracy and replicability (Choi et al. 2017, Gulati et al. 2022).

1.3 Interpretation of CBC Reports

When interpreting the complete blood count (CBC), it is vital to consider the normal ranges for each component, as these ranges vary significantly among newborns, neonates, infants, and children. The assessment of total counts, hemoglobin, hematocrit, and cell volumes, such as mean corpuscular volume (MCV) and packed cell volume (PCV), can result in three possible findings: normal, increased, or decreased levels (Varghese et al. 2023).

Each variation in these measurements needs to be assessed both individually and in the context of the overall health and age-specific norms to derive accurate conclusions. While this chapter provides tables that outline these variations and their interpretations, it is important to note that a detailed exploration of each individual variation is beyond the scope of this book (Tables 1.1, 1.2 and 1.3). This section aims to guide the initial analysis, encouraging further investigation and consultation of specialized texts for a comprehensive understanding (de Almeida et al. 2017; Elsafty et al. 2021).

Table 1.1 RBC parameters

RBC parameters	Normal range	Abnormal values	Interpretation
Hemoglobin (Hb)	13.5–16.5gm/dl (Males) 12–16 gm/dl (Females)	>16.5 gm/dl in Males; >16 gm/dl in Females	Polycythemia
		<13.5gm/dl in Males; <12 gm/dl in Females	Anemia
Hematocrit/packed cell volume (Hct/PCV)	41–49% (Males) 36–48% (Females)	>49% in Males; >48% in Females	Polycythemia
		< 41.0% in Males; < 36.0% in Females	Anemia
RBC count	4.5–5.5 × 10^6/cumm (Males) 3.8–4.8 × 10^6/cumm (Females)	Counts lower than normal indicate anemia but higher count can be seen in hemolytic anemias as well as polycythemia	Anemia or Polycythemia is *NOT* defined as per RBC count
Mean corpuscular volume (MCV)	80– 100 fl	<80 fl	Microcytic (Small sized RBCs)
		80–100 fl	Normocytic (Normal Sized RBCs)
		>100 fl	Macrocytic (Large sized RBCs)[a]
Mean corpuscular hemoglobin (MCH)[b]	27–32 pg	Low	Hypochromic
		Normal	Normochromic
Mean corpuscular hemoglobin concentration (MCHC)	31.5–34.5 gm/dl	Low	Hypochromic
		Normal	Normochromic
		High	Hereditary Spherocytosis Severe Sickle cell anemia Autoimmune hemolytic anemia (AIHA) Xerocytosis
Red cell distribution width as coefficient of variation (RDW-CV)[c]	11.6–14%	> 14%	Varying sized RBCs (anisocytosis) are present which can be seen in: Iron deficiency anemia (IDA) Anemia of chronic disease (ACD) Megaloblastic anemia Transfused patients Sickle cell anemias Active hemolysis with increased Reticulocytes

[a]Raised MCV: Increased MCV can also be seen spuriously in conditions like:
- Auto-agglutination
- Rouleaux formation
- Increased reticulocyte count (active hemolysis or blood loss cases)

[b]MCH: This value is never more than normal

[c]RDW: Can never be less than normal

Table 1.2 WBC parameters

WBC parameters	Normal range	Abnormal values	Interpretation
Total leukocyte count (TLC)	4000–11,000/cumm	<4000/cumm	Leukopenia
		>11,000/cumm	Leukocytosis
		>50,000/cumm	Most likely Leukemia than Leukemoid Reaction
Differential count (DLC)	Neutrophils: 2000–7000/cumm (40–80%)	Neutropenia	Congenital Acquired Bone marrow failure syndromes (BMFS)/Aplastic anemia (AA) Splenomegaly Sepsis Drug induced
		Neutrophilia	Infection Trauma, stress Malignancy Metabolic disorders Corticosteroids
	Lymphocytes: 1000–3000/cumm (20–40%)[a]	Lymphopenia	Congenital immunodeficiency Acquired immunodeficiency like human immunodeficiency virus (HIV)/Acquired immunodeficiency syndrome (AIDS) Drug Induced
		Lymphocytosis	Viral Infections Lymphomas/Leukemia Drug induced Immunological disease
	Monocytes 200–1000/cumm (2–10%)	Monocytopenia	Hairy cell leukemia Corticosteroids
		Monocytosis	Mycobacterial infections Myelodysplastic neoplasm (MDN)/myeloproliferative neoplasms (MPNs) like chronic myelo-monocytic leukemia (CMML)/Juvenile myelo-monocytic leukemia (JMML) Subacute Bacterial Endocarditis
	Eosinophils: 20–500/cumm (1–6%)	Eosinopenia	Sepsis Adrenocorticotropic hormone (ACTH)
		Eosinophilia	Hypersensitivity reaction Parasitic infection Drug induced Myeloproliferative Neoplasms
	Basophils: 20–100/cumm (<1–2%)	Basophilia	Chronic myeloid leukemia (CML) Other BCR-ABL1 negative MPNs

Counts lower than normal are called *cytopenia*; while a raised counts has a suffix of *cytosis* or *philia*

[a]Lymphocyte count: Will normally be higher in neonates, infants, and young children

Table 1.3 Platelet parameters

Platelet parameters	Normal range	Abnormal values	Interpretation
Platelet count	150–450 × 10^3/cumm	<25 × 10^3/cumm	Very severe thrombocytopenia
		<50 × 10^3/cumm	Severe thrombocytopenia
		50–<75 × 10^3/cumm	Moderate thrombocytopenia
		75–<150 × 10^3/cumm	Mild thrombocytopenia
		>450 × 10^3/cumm	Thrombocytosis Reactive Neoplastic (MPNs)
Mean platelet volume (MPV)	6.5–12 fl	< 6.5 fl	Small-sized platelet (Microplatelets)
		>12 fl	Large-sized platelets (Macroplatelets)
Platelet distribution width (PDW)	9.6–15.2 fl	> 15.2 fl	Platelet anisocytosis
Plateletcrit (PCR)	0.19–0.39%	< 0.19%	Reduced platelet mass
		>0.39%	Increased platelet mass

1.3.1 Interpretation of Peripheral Smear (PS) Reports

Peripheral smear (PS) reports play a crucial role in the diagnostic process, especially in cases of cytopenias. These reports, primarily focused on morphological assessment, are instrumental in narrowing down potential diagnoses.

1.3.2 Significance of Morphological Assessment

Morphological analysis in a peripheral smear report is vital for identifying several key features:

- *Parasites*: Detection of parasites that may affect the blood. Innovative approaches, such as the use of machine learning algorithms for the detection and classification of peripheral plasmodium parasites in blood smears, have shown promising results in enhancing the accuracy of parasite detection.

- *Abnormal Cells*: Identification of unusual cells such as blasts and promyelocytes, which are indicative of various hematological disorders. The development of advanced image processing techniques has significantly improved the detection and analysis of abnormal cells, contributing to the accurate diagnosis of blood-related disorders (Tavakoli et al. 2021) (Fig. 1.1).

Table 1.4 depicts the various morphological findings found on peripheral smear reports. The algorithms give a straightforward step-by-step approach by combining CBC and PS report interpretations.

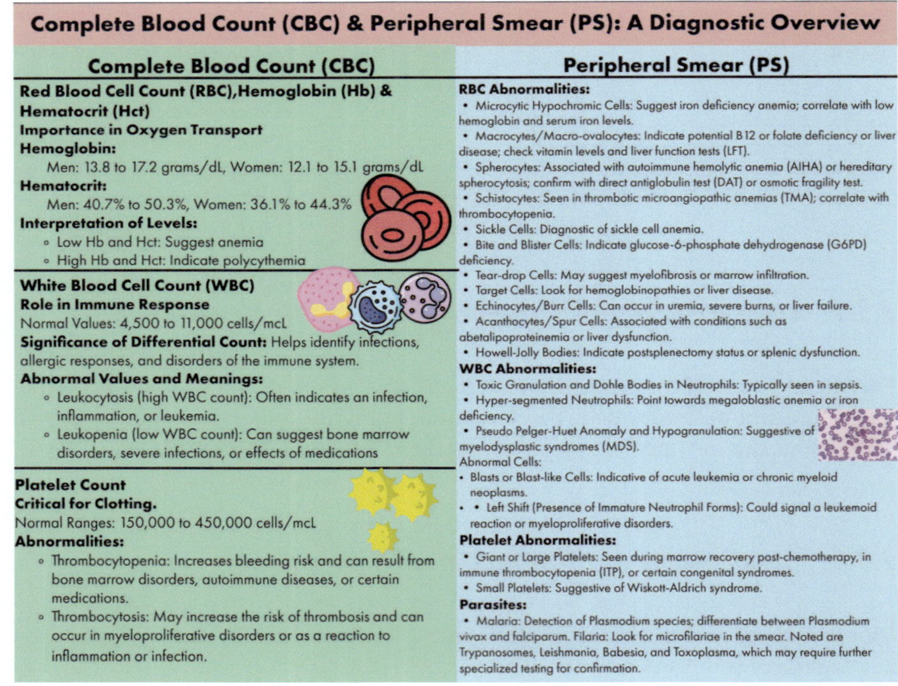

Fig. 1.1 Complete blood count (CBC) and peripheral smear (PS): a diagnostic overview

Table 1.4 Interpretation of peripheral smear findings

Parameter	Findings	Interpretation
RBCs	Microcytic hypochromic	Correlate with Hemoglobin level Serum iron studies Hb-HPLC assay if suspicious of hemoglobinopathies, and proceed accordingly
	Macrocytes, macro-ovalocytes	Correlate with Vit. B12 and folic acid (FA) levels Thyroid hormone level Liver function test (LFT)
	Spherocytes	Correlate with Direct and indirect coombs test (DCT/ICT): for AIHA Osmotic fragility test: for hereditary spherocytosis
	Schistocytes	If >1% in adults along with the presence of thrombocytopenia—Thrombotic microangiopathic anemias (TMA)
	Sickle cells	Sickle cell anemia
	Bite cells and blister cells	G6PD deficiency
	Tear-drop cells with leukoerythroblastic blood picture	Myelofibrosis Primary Secondary to any metastasis
	Target cells	To look for Hemoglobinopathies Liver disorder
	Echinocytes/Burr cells	Uremia Severe burn Liver failure
	Acanthocytes/Spur cells	Alcoholic intoxication Abetalipoproteinemia Associated with neuroacanthocytosis
	Pincer or mushroom-shaped cells	Hereditary spherocytes resulting from deficiency of band 3 Erythro-leukemia Oxidant-induced hemolysis
	Howell–Jolly bodies	Post splenectomy Splenic atrophy Coeliac disease Pernicious anemia
	Heinz bodies	G6PD deficiency Oxidative hemoglobin damage
	Cabot rings	Megaloblastic anemia
	Basophilic stippling	Lead poisoning Megaloblastic anemia MDN Hemoglobinopathies
	Auto-agglutination	AIHA Cold agglutinin
	Rouleaux formation	Myeloma Polyclonal hypergammaglobulinemia

(continued)

Parameter	Findings	Interpretation
WBC	Neutrophils with toxic granulations and vacuolations, Dohle bodies	Sepsis Pregnancy Burns
	Neutrophils with nuclear hyper-segmentation	Megaloblastic anemia (most common) Iron deficiency anemia MDN
	Pseudo Pelger–Huet anomaly	MDN
	Hypogranulation	MDN
Abnormal cells	Blasts or Blast-like cells (promyelocytes, promonocytes)	Acute leukemia (>20%) MDN/MPN
	Left shift (myelocytes, meta-myelocytes, and band cells)	CML MPNs Leukoerythroblastic blood picture[a]
	Plasma cells	Plasma cell leukemia Myeloma
Platelets	Giant or large platelets	Recovering marrow Immune thrombocytopenia (ITP) MDN Bernard soulier syndrome (BSS) Congenital in some population
	Small sized platelets	Wiskott Aldrich syndrome
Parasites	Malaria	*Plasmodium vivax* *Plasmodium falciparum* Others
	Filaria	Microfilaria
	Others	Trypanosomes Leishmania Babesia Toxoplasma

[a]Leukoerythroblastic blood picture: Myeloid left shift with nucleated RBCs

Detailed Algorithmic Approach to Various Scenarios

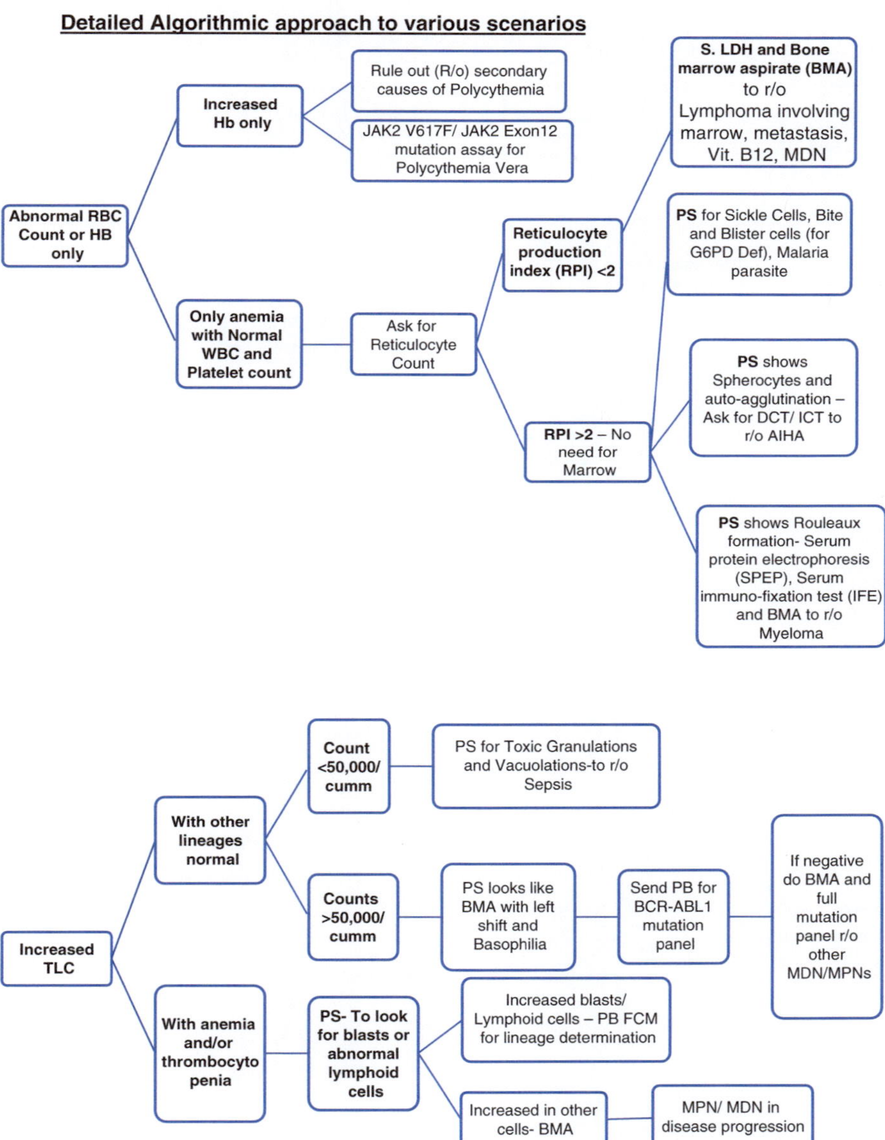

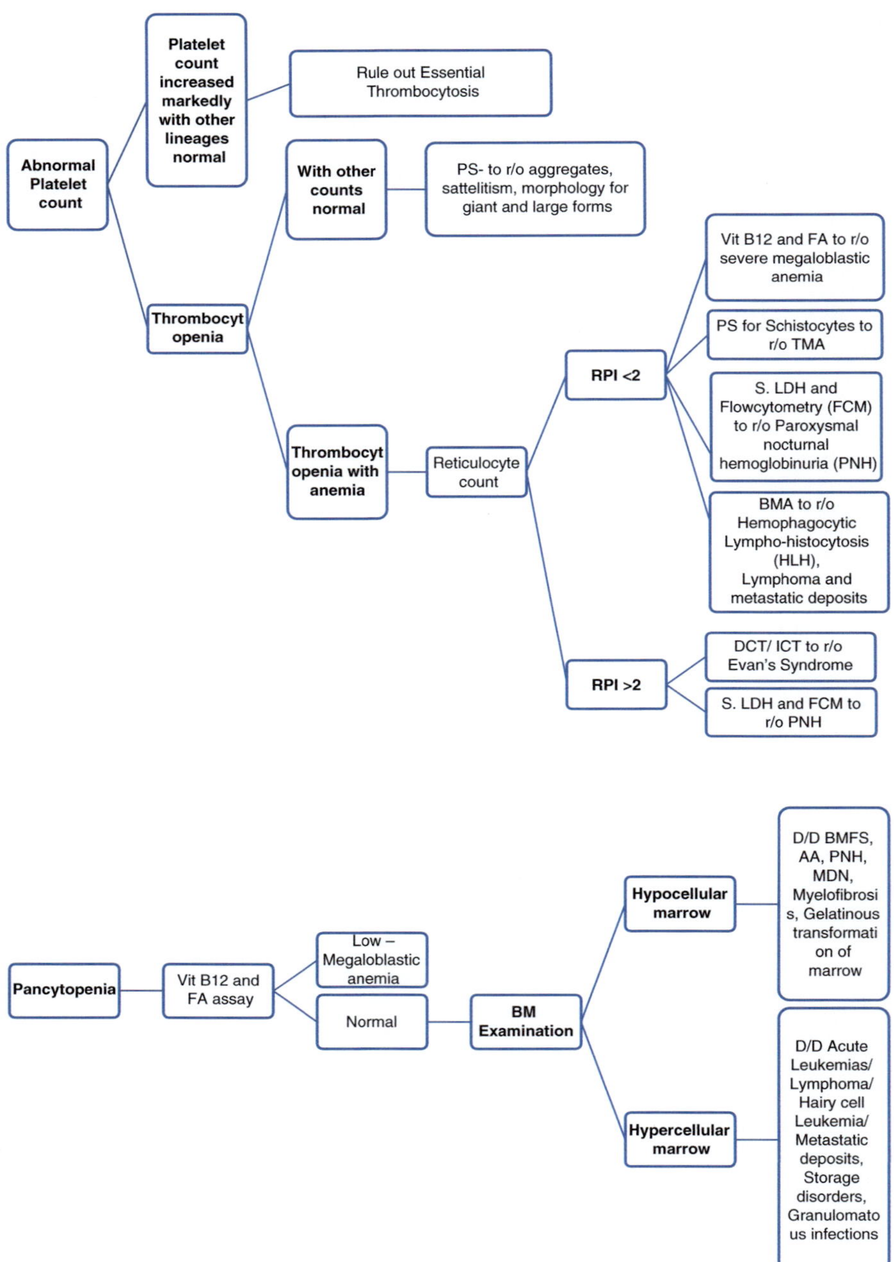
Abnormal Platelet count
Platelet count increased markedly with other lineages normal
Rule out Essential Thrombocytosis
Thrombocytopenia
With other counts normal
PS- to r/o aggregates, sattelitism, morphology for giant and large forms
Thrombocytopenia with anemia
Reticulocyte count
RPI <2
Vit B12 and FA to r/o severe megaloblastic anemia
PS for Schistocytes to r/o TMA
S. LDH and Flowcytometry (FCM) to r/o Paroxysmal nocturnal hemoglobinuria (PNH)
BMA to r/o Hemophagocytic Lympho-histocytosis (HLH), Lymphoma and metastatic deposits
RPI >2
DCT/ ICT to r/o Evan's Syndrome
S. LDH and FCM to r/o PNH
Pancytopenia
Vit B12 and FA assay
Low – Megaloblastic anemia
Normal
BM Examination
Hypocellular marrow
D/D BMFS, AA, PNH, MDN, Myelofibrosis, Gelatinous transformation of marrow
Hypercellular marrow
D/D Acute Leukemias/ Lymphoma/ Hairy cell Leukemia/ Metastatic deposits, Storage disorders, Granulomatous infections

References

Choi JW, Ku Y, Yoo BW, Kim JA, Lee DS, Chai YJ, Kim HC (2017) White blood cell differential count of maturation stages in bone marrow smear using dual-stage convolutional neural networks. PLoS One 12(12):e0189259

de Almeida BS, Alves BDCA, de Sousa Gehrke F, Adami F, Fonseca FLA (2017) Complete blood count interpretation: a survey of health professional in Brazil. Int Arch Med 10:299

Elsafty A, Ahmed Y, Soliman A, Morsy AA (2021) A novel automated hematopathologist-styled commenter for complete blood count and smear review. Am J Clin Pathol 156:S100–S100. Cary: Oxford University Press

Gulati G, Uppal G, Gong J (2022) Unreliable automated complete blood count results: causes, recognition, and resolution. Ann Lab Med 42(5):515

Seo IH, Lee YJ (2022) Usefulness of complete blood count (CBC) to assess cardiovascular and metabolic diseases in clinical settings: a comprehensive literature review. Biomedicines 10(11):2697

Tavakoli S, Ghaffari A, Kouzehkanan ZM, Hosseini R (2021) New segmentation and feature extraction algorithm for classification of white blood cells in peripheral smear images. Sci Rep 11(1):19428

Varghese RGB, Manickam N, Mohanraj A (2023) Enhancing the interpretational skills of complete blood count reports by second year medical students using competency based learning method. J Curr Res Sci Med 9(1):48–52

Chapter 2
Bone Marrow Biopsy in ICU

Sarita Pradhan

Learning Points

1. Bone marrow production and its implication in hematological conditions.
2. Indications for bone marrow aspirate and biopsy, including unexplained cytopenias and suspected malignancies.
3. Preferred biopsy sites and procedural steps, emphasizing the use of the posterosuperior iliac spine.
4. Handling and storage of samples for various assays ensuring sample integrity.
5. Precautions to avoid complications from the biopsy procedure, including site selection and management of coagulopathy.
6. Interpretation of findings, such as cellularity and lineage proliferation, for accurate diagnosis.
7. Algorithmic approach to pancytopenia for differential diagnosis and management.

2.1 Introduction

Bone marrow examination (BME) is a critical diagnostic tool in the management of various conditions encountered in critical care settings. This chapter delves into the indications for conducting a bone marrow examination, highlighting its significance in unraveling diagnoses that remain elusive through conventional testing. The rationale behind BME lies in its comprehensive ability to evaluate the hematopoietic system, offering insights into abnormalities that could explain systemic manifestations in critically ill patients (Bain et al. 2019).

S. Pradhan (✉)
Department of Pathology, IMS and Sum Hospital, Bhubaneswar, Odisha, India

S. B. Mishra (ed.), *Critical Care Hematology*,
https://doi.org/10.1007/978-981-97-5565-3_2

2.2 Indications of Bone Marrow Biopsy

- Unexplained Severe Thrombocytopenia
- Pancytopenia
- Severe Neutropenia/Agranulocytosis
- Suspected Hemophagocytic Lymphohistiocytosis (HLH)
- Unexplained Splenomegaly and Hepatomegaly
- Suspected Acute Leukemias and Lymphomas Involving Marrow
- Suspected Metastases of Nonhematopoietic Malignancies to Bone Marrow
- Pyrexia of Unknown Origin (PUO)
- Infections
- Paraproteinemias

1. *Unexplained Severe Thrombocytopenia*: Severe thrombocytopenia, particularly when not attributable to sepsis or multiorgan failure, necessitates a bone marrow examination to identify underlying hematologic disorders. Thrombocytopenia, defined as a platelet count below the normal range, may signal bone marrow suppression or increased platelet destruction, warranting further investigation (Smock and Perkins 2014).
2. *Pancytopenia*: The diagnostic complexity of new-onset pancytopenia, which can be influenced by various conditions including Fanconi anemia, dyskeratosis congenita, and other bone marrow failure syndromes, emphasizes the importance of bone marrow examination. These conditions showcase the range of marrow cellularity from normal to complete aplasia, highlighting the necessity of a comprehensive diagnostic approach including genetic testing and consideration of congenital abnormalities (Weinzierl and Arber 2013).
3. *Severe Neutropenia/Agranulocytosis*: Severe neutropenia or agranulocytosis, often presenting as an acute reduction in neutrophil count, raises concerns for marrow pathology. Acquired neutropenia is commonly caused by various infections, drugs and autoimmune diseases. Although any infection can potentially cause neutropenia, it usually occurs following viral infections. Though in most infections, the neutropenia is usually brief and self-limited, but in EBV and HIV infections neutropenia can be prolonged. BME can help, if cause of neutropenia is not apparent or does not resolve after discontinuation of drugs (to rule out Myelodysplastic syndrome, leukemias or marrow infiltration by other malignancies). Congenital neutropenias, though extremely rare, including severe congenital neutropenia (SCN), are characterized by low neutrophil counts leading to chronic, severe infections, with SCN being potentially life-threatening if not managed properly. The diagnosis and treatment have been significantly influenced by advances in understanding the genetic mutations responsible for these conditions, highlighting the importance of bone marrow examination for accurate diagnosis and management.
4. *Suspected Hemophagocytic Lymphohistiocytosis (HLH)*: HLH is addressed within the context of pancytopenia, which can manifest in various syndromes including HLH. This life-threatening syndrome is characterized by excessive

immune activation, requiring prompt diagnosis. Bone marrow examination plays a crucial role in revealing the characteristic hemophagocytosis, aiding in diagnosis and management (Weinzierl and Arber 2013).

5. *Unexplained Splenomegaly and Hepatomegaly*: Conditions like dyskeratosis congenita (DC) and Shwachman-Diamond syndrome, which can present with pancytopenia, also include hepatomegaly among their symptoms. Hairy cell Leukemias, hypersplenism, myelofibrosis, storage disorders and infections like tuberculosis and visceral leishmaniasis are other important differentials of pancytopenias and splenomegaly. These conditions underscore the complexity of diagnoses that bone marrow examination can help clarify by revealing underlying hematologic malignancies or infiltrative diseases not evident through other diagnostic modalities (Weinzierl and Arber 2013).
6. *Suspected Acute Leukemias and Lymphomas Involving Marrow*: Acute leukemias and lymphomas suspected based on peripheral blood smear and clinical presentation can indeed be confirmed through BME, which demonstrates malignant cells within the marrow. It provides bone marrow samples for additional testing like immunophenotyping, molecular studies and cytogenetics, which aid in further characterisation of leukemias and lymphomas.
7. *Suspected Metastases of Nonhematopoietic Malignancies to Bone Marrow*: The discussion on pancytopenia includes the potential for the bone marrow to reveal metastatic involvement from nonhematologic cancers, altering prognosis and treatment approach. The detailed diagnosis process through BME highlights its pivotal role (Weinzierl and Arber 2013).
8. *Pyrexia of Unknown Origin (PUO)*: In the context of PUO, BME's utility in diagnosing hidden infections, malignancies, or autoimmune diseases is critical, as PUO can sometimes be a manifestation of underlying hematologic conditions that pancytopenia and bone marrow examination can help identify.
9. *Infections*: BME's value in identifying atypical infections, especially when peripheral blood cultures fail to yield results, is part of the broader diagnostic approach to pancytopenia, which includes investigating potential infectious causes behind abnormal blood counts (Weinzierl and Arber 2013).
10. *Paraproteinemias*: In cases of suspected paraproteinemias such as multiple myeloma, BME is essential for the detection and enumeration of clonal plasma cells, providing critical diagnostic and prognostic information. This aligns with the comprehensive diagnostic process for pancytopenia, highlighting the integral role of BME in diagnosing various hematologic conditions (Weinzierl and Arber 2013).

2.3 Contraindications to Bone Marrow

- Severe Anatomical Deformities
- Sternal Aspirate Contraindications

- Severe Osteoporosis
- Coagulopathies
- Severe Hemophilias
- Disseminated Intravascular Coagulation (DIC)
- Considerations in Thrombocytopenia

1. *Severe Anatomical Deformities*

Severe anatomical deformities of potential aspiration or biopsy sites pose a significant contraindication due to the increased risk of injury or inability to accurately access the marrow space. Deformities may result from congenital conditions, trauma, or surgical alterations.

2. *Sternal Aspirate Contraindications*

Severe Osteoporosis

The risk of penetrating the sternum and causing injury to underlying structures, such as the heart or great vessels, renders sternal aspiration contraindicated in patients with severe osteoporosis. Alternative sites, like the posterior iliac crest, are preferred.

3. *Coagulopathies*

Coagulopathies, including severe hemophilias and disseminated intravascular coagulation (DIC), generally preclude bone marrow biopsy due to the heightened risk of bleeding. However, bone marrow aspirations may still be performed under specific conditions.

4. *Severe Hemophilias*

In cases of severe hemophilia, bone marrow biopsy is usually avoided. If necessary, bone marrow aspiration can be conducted with adequate hemostatic control, including the pre-procedure administration of factor replacement therapy to minimize bleeding risks.

5. *Disseminated Intravascular Coagulation (DIC)*

Similarly, in DIC, the risk of bleeding complicates the decision to perform a bone marrow biopsy. Careful risk-benefit assessment and correction of coagulopathy, when possible, are essential before considering a bone marrow procedure.

6. *Considerations in Thrombocytopenia*

Healthcare providers often weigh the potential diagnostic benefits against the bleeding risks. In some cases, treatment to increase platelet counts or other measures to manage bleeding risk may be taken prior to the procedure. This ensures that necessary diagnostic steps can be safely taken to manage the patient's condition effectively.

2.4 Bone Marrow Procedure

The bone marrow procedure, encompassing both aspiration and biopsy, is a pivotal diagnostic and therapeutic tool in hematological and oncological medicine. Its execution requires meticulous preparation, understanding of anatomical sites, patient counseling, and post-procedure management to ensure safety, accuracy, and minimal discomfort. This chapter provides a comprehensive guide to conducting bone marrow procedures.

Outline

- Selection of Anatomical Sites
- Pre-Procedural Preparation
- Procedure Steps
- Post-Procedural Care
- Types of Samples and Their Management
- Considerations Before and After the Procedure

1. Selection of Anatomical Sites
   - *Postero-Superior Iliac Spine (PSIS)*: The most preferred site due to its accessibility and lower risk of complications.
   - *Antero-Superior Iliac Spine (ASIS)*: An alternative site, albeit used less frequently.
   - *Sternum*: Reserved exclusively for aspiration due to the risk of penetrating vital organs.
   - *Tibial Tuberosity*: Only considered for aspirations in infants, with caution to avoid damage to the growth plate.
2. Pre-Procedural Preparation
   - *Patient Counseling and Informed Consent*: Essential for ethical and legal compliance.
   - *Detailed Documentation*: Including patient history, clinical findings, previous treatments, and relevant laboratory results.
   - *CBC and Peripheral Smear Preparation*: To establish baseline hematological status.
3. Procedure Steps
   - *Positioning*: The patient is placed in the left lateral position if PSIS is the chosen site.
   - *Cleaning*: The skin is cleaned with alcohol swabs.
   - *Anesthesia*: Local infiltration with 2% lignocaine ensures minimal discomfort.
   - *Aspiration and Biopsy*: Using the appropriate needle, samples are collected for various assays.
4. Post-Procedural Care
   - *Adequate Pressure Application*: To minimize bleeding.
   - *Pressure Bandage*: Ensures hemostasis and aids in healing.

5. Types of Samples and Their Management

    - *Bone Marrow Aspirate*: Includes cytology smears, samples for immuno-phenotyping (both EDTA and heparin vial can be used), molecular assays (in EDTA vial), cytogenetics (in heparin vial), and culture. Sample, if not processed immediately, should be stored at 2–8 degree.
    - *Bone Marrow Biopsy*: Imprint smears shoud be taken and the trephine biopsy itself, shoud be preserved in neutral buffered formalin for histopathological examination.

6. Considerations Before and After the Procedure

    - *Avoidance of Infected or Anomalous Sites*: To reduce the risk of complications.
    - *Osteoporosis and Myeloma*: Caution is advised against sternum procedures.
    - *Severe Coagulopathies*: Procedures should be covered with fresh frozen plasma.
    - *Infection Risks*: Adequate care is necessary to avoid rare but serious complications (Fig. 2.1)

2.5 Steps of Bone Marrow Procedure

- Patient counselling: As in all invasive procedures, the patient should be adequately counceled and informed about the indications and the possible outcome of the procedure. Informed consent should be taken from the patient or relatives prior to the procedure.
- Documentation: Relevant clinical histories, drug allergies, and co-morbities should be documented. Any pre-medications, if given, should be explained.
- A complete blood count (CBC) must be obtained prior to the procedure if not done within 48 h of the procedure.
- Preferred anatomic sites for bone marrow aspiration and biopsy: Posteriorsuperior iliac spine (PSIS). Anterior superior iliac crest can be used in the case of severely obese people where PSIS may not be localized. The medial surface of tibial tuberosity is the preferred site in infants. A sternal puncture can be used in rare circumstances to obtain bone marrow aspirates only if the patient is immobile or has received radiotherapy in the pelvis.
- Instruments for bone marrow aspiration and biopsy: Salah's bone marrow aspiration needle and Jamshidi bone marrow trephine biopsy needle (can be used for both aspiration and biopsy).
- Patient positioning: Left lateral position while collecting bone marrow from the left posterior iliac crest.
- Patient preparation and procedure: Using universal sterile precautions, the skin around the area is cleaned with 70% alcohol. The skin, subcutaneous tissue, and the periosteum overlying the PSIS are infiltrated with 6–7 ml of 2% lidocaine.

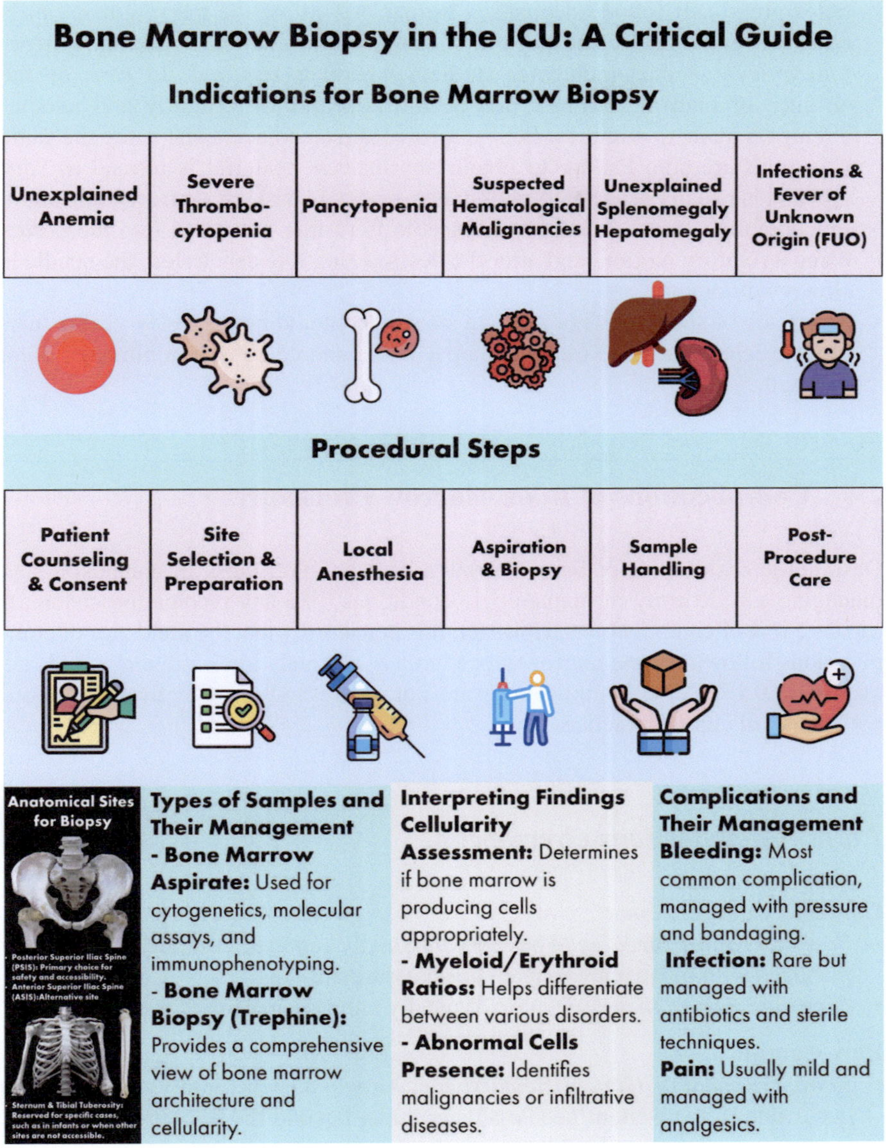

Fig. 2.1 Bone marrow biopsy in the ICU: a critical guide

After waiting for a few minutes to achieve local anesthesia, the bone marrow needle is passed perpendicularly into the iliac crest using a rotator motion, till the needle enters the cavity. After the needle is fixed, the stellate is removed, and using a 2 ml syringe, 1–2 ml of bone marrow is aspirated to make smears. The smears are checked for adequacy by checking the presence of marrow par-

ticles grossly. If found adequate, a further 4–5 ml of the marrow material is collected in an EDTA and heparin vacuatainer for additional testing (flowcytometry/cytogenetics/molecular studies) wherever required. In case of the absence of marrow particles, the needle is withdrawn slightly and another attempt is made to withdraw bone marrow from an adjacent site using the same skin puncture site. Failure to obtain any marrow material is termed as "dry tap"and is usually associated with bone marrow fibrosis or marrow infiltration. For obtaining trephine biopsy, the needle is further advanced into the cortex using a rotatory motion, and after the desired length is penetrated, the needle is slowly withdrawn.
- Adequacy of specimen: For aspirate smears, it should have grossly visible marrow particles. Adequate trephine biopsy tissue should be of a minimum 1.5 cm in length.

2.6 Complications of Bone Marrow Procedure

Despite the critical role of bone marrow aspiration and biopsy in diagnosing and managing a wide array of hematologic conditions, like any medical procedure, it carries a risk of complications. However, it is noteworthy that the incidence of complications following bone marrow procedures is relatively low, with a reported rate of around 0.1%. Most complications are not severe and are effectively managed with standard clinical practices.

2.6.1 Complications Overview

Common Complications

- *Post-procedural Bleeding*: The most frequently reported complication, usually managed with manual pressure and/or pressure dressing.
- *Persistent Pain at the Biopsy Site*: Typically requires analgesics for relief.

Rare Complications

- *Retroperitoneal or Gluteal Hemorrhage*: Although exceedingly rare, these can occur due to inadvertent needle advancement beyond the bone marrow cavity, leading to significant blood loss.
- *Sacroilitis*: Infection of the sacroiliac joint, which may arise from a direct inoculation of bacteria at the time of the procedure.
- *Cardiac Tamponade in Case of Sternal Puncture*: A critical and life-threatening complication, although extremely rare, can occur if the needle penetrates too deeply into the sternum, reaching the heart.

2.7 Management of Complications

Immediate Management

- *Bleeding*: Application of manual pressure followed by a pressure dressing. Monitoring vital signs and hemoglobin levels post-procedure is essential to detect significant blood loss.
- *Pain Management*: Administering analgesics, ensuring proper technique, and the use of local anesthetics during the procedure can minimize pain.

Management of Rare Complications

- *Retroperitoneal or Gluteal Hemorrhage*: Requires immediate imaging to confirm the diagnosis, followed by transfusion support and possibly surgical intervention or angiographic embolization.
- *Sacroilitis*: Early diagnosis through imaging and microbial cultures, followed by appropriate antibiotic therapy, is crucial for management.
- *Cardiac Tamponade*: This demands immediate recognition, echocardiography for confirmation, and pericardiocentesis to relieve the pressure on the heart.

2.8 Interpretation

1. Assessment of cellularity: Marrow aspiration smears with several fragments give a rough estimate of marrow cellularity but trephine biopsy is considered the ideal specimen to assess the cellularity of bone marrow. Assessment of cellularity on aparticulate smears may lead to interpretative errors so should be attempted only on trephine biopsy.
2. Bone marrow aspirate differential count: A differential count on at least 500 cells in an aspirate smear is done to obtain a myeloid:erythroid ratio, relative proportions of lymphocytes, plasma cells, and abnormal cells if any. Maturation patterns of erythroid and myeloid lineages along with evidences of dysplasia, if any is documented. Increased macrophages with or without evidence of hemophagocytosis, megakaryocyte numbers, morphology, and iron stores must be documented. Relevant stains like ZN stain for AFB and fungal stains must be done when required.
3. Trephine biopsy examination: It enables the assessment of bone marrow architecture, cellularity, distribution of hematopoietic elements, and enables the detection of focal involvement by lymphomas, metastatic tumors, and granulomas that are often not evident in the aspirate smears. It provides tissue for further workup like immunohistochemistry and molecular workup wherever required. Assessment of megakaryoctyic morphology, topography and fibrosis by reticulin and masson trichome stains is another advantage of trephine biopsy, especially in myeloproliferative neoplasms.

   Differential diagnosis based on examination of marrow aspirate and biopsy.

(a) Pancytopenia with Hypocellular Marrow: Aplastic anemia, PNH (paroxysmalnocturnal hemoglobinuria), and hypoplastic MDS
(b) Pancytopenia with hypercellular marrow or normocellular marrow

- Trilineage hematopoiesis: hypersplenism
- Megaloblastic erythroid hyperplasia: megaloblastic anemia
- Significant dysplasia on morphology: myelodysplastic syndrome (MDS)
- Increased blasts/atypical lymphoid cells/abnormal cells: Marrow infiltrative disorders like leukemia/lymphoma/metastases of nonhematopoietic tumors
- Increased macrophages with evidence of hemophagocytosis in conjuctuion: HLH/hemophagocytic syndrome, if the clinical and laboratory parameters (ferritin/fibrinogen/ triglyceride) are fulfilled
- Evidence of granulomas/LD bodies/malarial parasites or pigments infective etiology like tuberculosis, kala-azar, and malaria, respectively

(c) Isolated thrombocytopenia with adequate megakaryocytes in a cellular marrow: Peripheral destruction of platelets.
(d) Neutropenia/agranulocytosis with myeloid maturation arrest in the marrow.

Flowchart

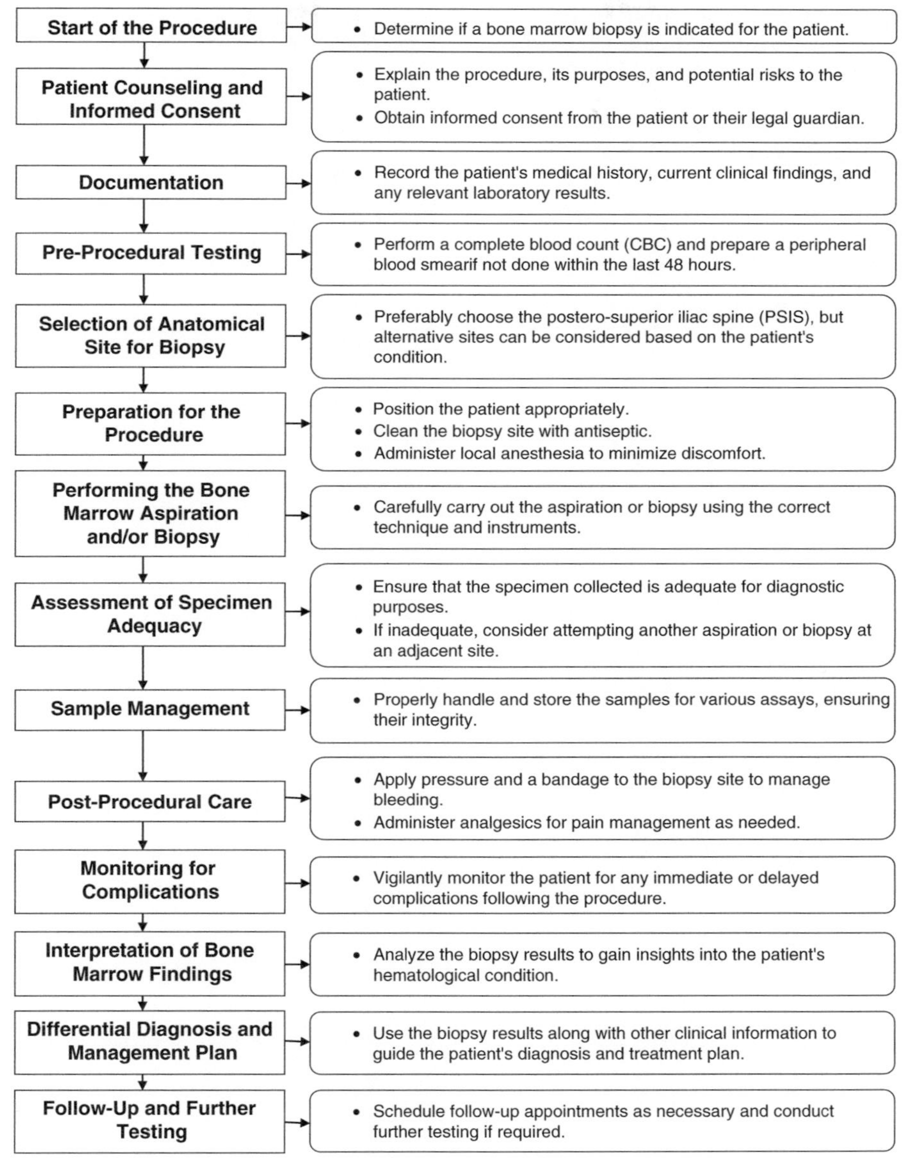

Bone Marrow Biopsy Procedure Flowchart

References

Bain BJ, Clark DM, Wilkins BS (2019) Bone marrow pathology. Wiley

Smock KJ, Perkins SL (2014) Thrombocytopenia: an update. Int J Lab Hematol 36(3):269–278

Weinzierl EP, Arber DA (2013) The differential diagnosis and bone marrow evaluation of new-onset pancytopenia. Am J Clin Pathol 139(1):9–29

Chapter 3
Abnormal Clotting Profile

Shruti Mishra

Learning Points

1. Understanding Hemostasis in the ICU: Recognize the importance of hemostasis management in the ICU to maintain the balance between preventing blood loss and avoiding thrombotic complications. This includes understanding the physiological mechanisms of clot formation and the delicate balance that must be maintained to prevent both bleeding and thrombosis.
2. Diagnostic Approach to Coagulopathy: Grasp the significance of initial diagnostic tests such as prothrombin time (PT), activated partial thromboplastin time (aPTT), fibrinogen assays, platelet count, and bleeding time (BT) for patients at risk of bleeding, as well as the use of D-dimer and lupus anticoagulant tests for assessing thrombotic disorders.
3. Management Strategies in Coagulopathies: Learn about the various management options for coagulopathies in the ICU, ranging from plasma transfusions for correcting coagulopathies, to thromboprophylaxis with unfractionated heparin (UFH) or low-molecular-weight heparin (LMWH) for deep vein thrombosis (DVT) prevention.
4. Personalized Care and Precision in Management: Emphasize the necessity of precision in diagnostic sampling and the application of individualized management strategies. This underscores the significance of specialized training for healthcare providers in tailoring treatment strategies to mitigate bleeding and thrombotic risks.

S. Mishra (✉)
Bone Marrow Transplantation and Stem Cell Research Centre, Institute of Medical Sciences, Banaras Hindu University, Varanasi, Uttar Pradesh, India
e-mail: drshruti.mishra@bhu.ac.in

S. B. Mishra (ed.), *Critical Care Hematology*,
https://doi.org/10.1007/978-981-97-5565-3_3

3.1 Introduction

Hemostasis is the process whereby the body that tries to maintain the blood in the liquid state while inside intact blood vessels, or to change it into a gel-like consistency when the continuity of vessel walls is breached. It is a very delicate balance, and any tilt toward any side yields very devastating results. As often said, coagulation is a double-edged sword—too much or too little can be dangerous. The approach toward abnormality in coagulation reports requires a basic brush upon the basics of these assays. Routine first-line assays in any patient with bleeding include prothrombin time (PT), activated partial thromboplastic time (aPTT), fibrinogen assay, platelet count, and bleeding time (BT). The remaining assays in the thrombotic panel include D-dimer and lupus anticoagulant tests with Paroxysmal Nocturnal Hemoglobinuria (PNH) clone assessment and PET-CT for occult malignancy.

3.1.1 *The Classical Coagulation Cascade*

- The classical coagulation cascade has been applied historically to serve as a model for the rationale underlying the complex course of blood coagulation. It is further divided into two pathways: the intrinsic and extrinsic merging in a common pathway. This model elaborates the activation of coagulation factors sequentially, which ultimately results in the formation of stable blood clots (Fig. 3.1).
- *Intrinsic Pathway*: This is initiated whenever blood gets exposed to a negatively charged surface, and this will lead to the activation of factor XII (Hageman factor). Factor XIIa initiates a series of reactions, which includes the activation of

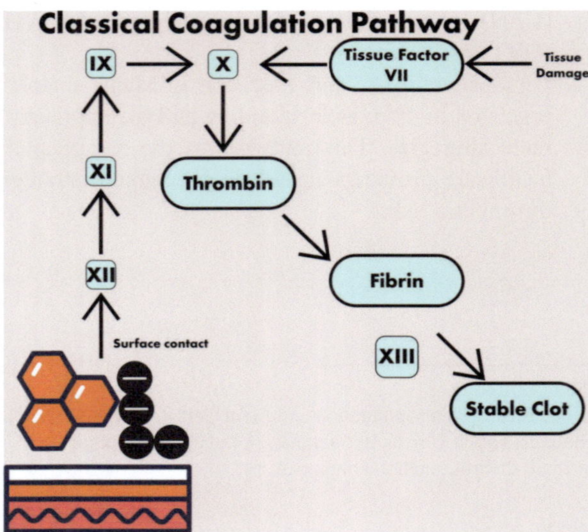

Fig. 3.1 Classical coagulation pathway

factors XI, IX, and VIII, which culminates in the final activation of factor X in the presence of calcium ions and platelet phospholipids (PF3).

- *Extrinsic Pathway*: Triggered by tissue injury, the path is mediated by thromboplastin (factor III) and activation of factor VII. Tissue thromboplastin (Tb) reacts with Ca^{2+} ions and factor VII to form a complex that activates factor X directly.
- *Common Pathway*: After the activation of factor X in both pathways, it further activates pro-thrombin to thrombin with the help of factor V, PF3, and Ca^{2+} ions. Insoluble fibrinogen is further converted into insoluble fibrin, and active factor XIII stabilizes the cross-linked fibrin clot. Indeed, this classical model of clotting has been very instructive both in understanding the disease processes that affect coagulation and in the potential development and use of novel anticoagulant therapies. However, it is somewhat simplified and does not fully account for the complexity of coagulation in vivo.

3.1.2 The Cell-Based Model of Coagulation

The cell-based model of coagulation is more elaborative in the insight of the coagulation process, whereby the main player, the cellular surfaces, takes a lead in the orchestration of clot formation. This is subcategorized into three phases: initiation, amplification, and propagation; hence, it reflects a sequence of events with more physiological accuracy (Fig. 3.2).

- *Initiation phase*: This involves tissue factor (TF)-bearing cells. The process is precipitated by vascular injury, where the sub-endothelium, which contains TF, a membrane-bound glycoprotein, gets exposed. Circulating factor VII is then activated and forms a complex with TF, activating factor X to Xa and, to a lesser extent, factor IX to IXa. Factor Xa generates a small amount of thrombin, insufficient to form a clot but enough to initiate the process.
- *Amplification Phase*: This occurs on the surface of activated platelets. The small amount of thrombin that is formed during the initiation serves to activate more platelets and factors V, VIII, IX and XI on these platelets. The activated platelets provide phospholipid surfaces that support the assembly of a number of coagulation factor complexes, which markedly increase the generation of thrombin.
- *Phase of propagation*: This phase also takes place at the surface of activated platelets, resulting in large-scale production of thrombin, and is affected by the assembled coagulation complexes. Thrombin cuts fibrinogen to yield fibrin and also activates factor XIII, which is essential in the stabilization of clots. It also activates factor XIII, a transamidase that crosslinks fibrin and further activates more platelets; this justifies the support of the clotting. The cell-based model has been able to identify the important role that cellular elements, in particular platelets and endothelial cells, play during the process of coagulation. This points to the great importance of local thrombin generation and regulation of coagulation by cellular surfaces in a manner that gives a better account of the coagulation mechanism in vivo.

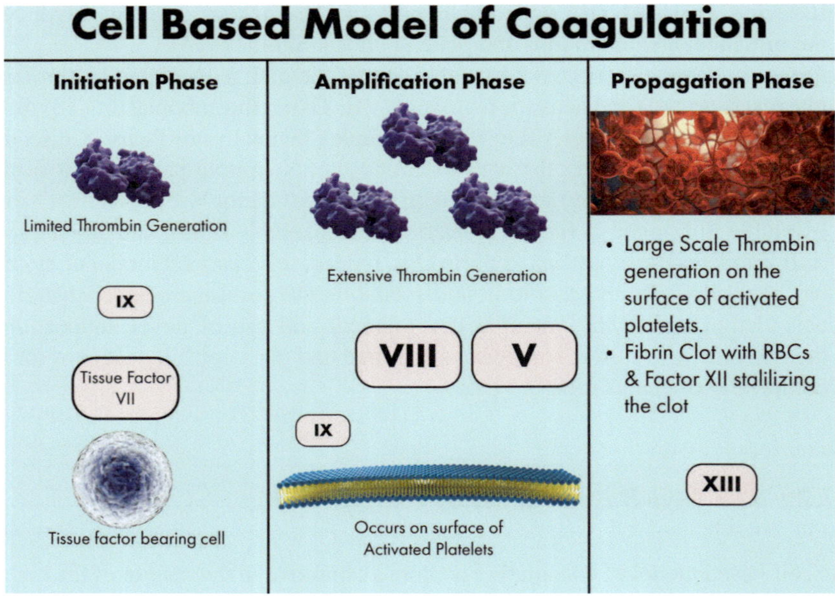

Fig. 3.2 Cell based model of coagulation

The fundamental difference between the classical coagulation cascade and the cell-based model of coagulation lies in their conceptualization of how blood clotting is initiated, propagated, and regulated.

3.1.3 Classical Coagulation Cascade

- The classical model describes coagulation as a linear sequence of enzymatic reactions, divided into intrinsic, extrinsic, and common pathways.
- It emphasizes the role of circulating coagulation factors in plasma and their sequential activation.
- This model was based on observations from clotting experiments in test tubes, leading to a simplified representation that does not fully capture the complexity of in vivo coagulation.

3.1.4 Cell-Based Model of Coagulation

- The cell-based model presents coagulation as a series of processes that occur on cell surfaces, particularly those of platelets and endothelial cells.

- It divides coagulation into three phases: initiation (on tissue factor-bearing cells), amplification (on the surface of activated platelets), and propagation (further thrombin generation on activated platelets), highlighting the dynamic and regulated nature of coagulation in the body.
- This model emphasizes the importance of cellular contributions to coagulation, including the role of membrane-bound coagulation factors and cellular interactions.

3.1.5 Clinical Significance of Knowing the Cell-Based Pathway

Improved Understanding of Hemostasis: The cell-based model offers a more accurate representation of coagulation as it occurs in the body. This understanding is crucial for clinicians to identify and treat coagulopathies effectively.

- *Targeted Therapies*: Knowledge of the cell-based pathway allows for the development of more targeted therapeutic interventions. By understanding the specific roles of cells and membrane-bound factors in coagulation, clinicians can tailor treatments to address the underlying mechanisms of clotting disorders.
- *Management of Bleeding Disorders*: The cell-based model provides insights into the complex interactions between platelets, endothelial cells, and coagulation factors. This is particularly relevant in managing conditions like hemophilia and von Willebrand disease, where the interaction between clotting factors and the vascular endothelium can influence disease severity and treatment response.
- *Thrombosis Prevention*: Recognizing the significance of tissue factor and cell surfaces in initiating coagulation helps in the prevention and management of thrombotic events. Anticoagulants that target specific factors or cellular interactions can be used more effectively to prevent clot formation in high-risk patients.
- *Diagnostic Approaches*: The cell-based model underscores the limitations of traditional coagulation tests, which may not fully capture the complexity of in vivo hemostasis. This awareness encourages the use of more sophisticated diagnostic tools, such as thromboelastography, that can provide a more comprehensive assessment of clotting function.

3.1.6 Bleeding Events

Bleeding risks are higher in patients in ICU. There are various iatrogenic causes that have be taken into consideration. One of the crucial aspects is proper training of staffs in ICU so that sampling errors can be avoided. An abnormal coagulation profile in a hemostatically stable patient should raise a query regarding sampling errors first. Sampling from channels requires attention. Sampling should not be done from the channel when fluids are being transfused; also heparin flushed channels should be used with caution (Retter and Barrett 2015).

In critically ill patients with coagulation issues, obtaining a medical history can be difficult. Diagnosis relies on abnormal coagulation test results, even if the profile appears normal. Platelet and coagulation disorders show distinct bleeding patterns: platelet-related issues cause immediate bleeding post-injury, while coagulation problems lead to delayed bleeding. Petechiae, small bleeding spots due to venous pressure, are common in platelet disorders. Ecchymoses, soft tissue hematomas without trauma history, occur in patients with severe coagulation problems (Retter and Barrett 2015).

3.1.7 Thrombotic Events

Thrombotic events are frequently seen in ICU patients both during and after ICU stay. Pulmonary embolism and deep vein thrombosis are the most common forms found. Padua Prediction Score is used for predicting thrombotic events in ICU patients. The ICU-VTE score for ICU patients includes six risk indicators: central venous catheter use, immobility for 4+ days, past VTE, mechanical ventilation, hemoglobin ≥ 9 g/dL, and platelet count >250,000/μL at admission. Guidelines recommend giving prophylactic antithrombotic coverage to patients admitted in the ICU. Contraindications includes intracranial or any other life-threatening bleeding, history of any recent major trauma or surgical procedures and marked thrombocytopenia, and platelet count $<30 \times 10^9$/L (Neuenfeldt et al. 2021).

3.1.8 Risk Factors for Bleeding: The HEMORR2HAGES Score

The HEMORR$_2$HAGES score, highlighted by Retter and Barrett, provides a valuable tool for assessing the risk factors for bleeding in ICU patients. This scoring system takes into account various patient-specific factors, including

- hepatic or renal disease
- ethanol abuse
- Malignancy
- older age
- reduced platelet count or function
- re-bleeding risk
- hypertension (uncontrolled)
- anemia
- genetic factors
- excessive fall risk
- stroke history.

By evaluating patients according to these criteria, clinicians can quantify the bleeding risk, guiding the decision-making process regarding anticoagulation therapy and other interventions. This structured approach enhances patient assessment and enables targeted, personalized care for those at an increased risk of bleeding.

3.1.9 Workup for Coagulopathy in ICU Patients

Accurate diagnosis of coagulopathy in the intensive care unit (ICU) is paramount for the effective management of critically ill patients. Coagulopathy, a condition where the blood's ability to coagulate (form clots) is impaired, can lead to either an increased risk of bleeding or thrombosis. In the ICU setting, where patients often present with complex medical histories and critical illnesses, identifying coagulopathy is crucial for guiding therapeutic decisions, preventing further complications, and improving patient outcomes. The complexity of hemostasis, influenced by various factors including liver function, medication, and the underlying disease process, necessitates a comprehensive approach to diagnosis and management.

3.1.10 Initial Clinical Assessment

Patient History: The first step in evaluating a patient with suspected coagulopathy involves a detailed patient history. Key aspects include the following:

- *Bleeding or Thrombotic Events*: A history of unusual bleeding (e.g., from gums, nosebleeds, in the stool or urine, or excessive menstrual bleeding) or thrombotic events (such as deep vein thrombosis or pulmonary embolism) could indicate an underlying coagulopathy.
- *Medication History*: Many medications can influence coagulation. It is essential to obtain a detailed history of medication use, including over-the-counter drugs, herbal supplements, anticoagulants (warfarin, heparin, and direct oral anticoagulants), and antiplatelet agents, and any recent changes to medication regimens.
- *Underlying Health Conditions*: Conditions such as liver disease, renal dysfunction, malignancies, and inherited coagulation disorders can contribute to coagulopathy. A history of alcohol use, viral hepatitis, or symptoms suggestive of liver disease (jaundice and ascites) is particularly relevant, as liver dysfunction plays a critical role in hemostasis.
- *Physical Examination*: A thorough physical examination is crucial and should focus on the following:
  - *Signs of Bleeding*: Look for petechiae, purpura, hematomas, and active bleeding sites. Mucosal bleeding, such as epistaxis or gum bleeding should also be noted.

- *Thrombosis Indicators*: Check for signs of deep vein thrombosis, such as swelling, redness, and tenderness in the extremities. Examination of the chest may reveal signs suggestive of pulmonary embolism, like tachypnea and pleuritic chest pain.
- *Liver Dysfunction Signs*: Features of liver disease, including jaundice, spider angiomas, palmar erythema, and ascites, can indicate a hepatic contribution to coagulopathy. Enlargement of the liver or spleen should also be documented.

The initial clinical assessment forms the foundation of the diagnostic process for coagulopathy in the ICU, guiding further investigations and management decisions. This step is vital for distinguishing between different causes of coagulopathy and tailoring treatment to address the underlying pathology effectively.

3.2 Laboratory Tests

3.2.1 Initial Screening Tests

The evaluation of coagulopathy in ICU patients requires an array of laboratory tests that provide insights into the coagulation pathway's function. These tests are pivotal for diagnosing coagulopathy, understanding its etiology, monitoring the effectiveness of treatment, and guiding clinical management.

3.2.1.1 Prothrombin Time (PT) and International Normalized Ratio (INR)

PT measures the time it takes for blood to clot, focusing on the extrinsic and common pathways of the coagulation cascade. It is particularly sensitive to changes in the levels of clotting factors I (fibrinogen), II (prothrombin), V, VII, and X. The INR is a standardized way of expressing PT, accounting for variations in test performance between different laboratories. PT/INR is crucial for patients on anticoagulant therapy with warfarin and for assessing liver function, as many clotting factors are produced in the liver.

3.2.1.2 Activated Partial Thromboplastin Time (aPTT)

aPTT assesses the integrity of the intrinsic and common coagulation pathways, including factors VIII, IX, XI, XII, X, V, II (prothrombin), and I (fibrinogen). It is utilized to screen for deficiencies or inhibitors of these factors and to monitor heparin therapy. aPTT serves as a pivotal test for evaluating the coagulation system's overall health and identifying potential defects within the intrinsic pathway.

3.2.1.3 Platelet Count

This test quantifies the blood's platelet numbers, crucial for blood clot formation and wound healing. Thrombocytopenia, a condition marked by a low platelet count, may lead to bleeding complications, while thrombocytosis, a high platelet count, can elevate the risk of thrombosis. Platelet count is an essential measure in assessing bleeding risk, particularly significant in patients with liver disease, where platelet counts may be influenced by splenic sequestration or diminished production.

3.2.1.4 Mixing Studies

These specialized laboratory tests distinguish between a factor deficiency and the presence of an inhibitor in the coagulation system, frequent causes of prolonged prothrombin time (PT) and activated partial thromboplastin time (aPTT) in patients with coagulopathies. The fundamental approach involves combining the patient's plasma with normal plasma (often referred to as pooled normal plasma) and reassessing the clotting time.

Here's how to interpret the results of mixing studies:

Interpretations of Mixing Studies

1. Correction of Clotting Time:

   Interpretation: Indicates a factor deficiency.
   Mechanism: The addition of normal plasma provides the deficient factor(s) in the patient's plasma, correcting the prolonged clotting time.
   Further Steps: Quantitative assays for individual coagulation factors should be performed to identify the specific factor deficiency.

2. No Correction of Clotting Time (Partial or No Improvement):

   Interpretation: Suggests the presence of an inhibitor.
   Mechanism: Inhibitors, such as autoantibodies against coagulation factors (e.g., factor VIII) in acquired hemophilia, or nonspecific inhibitors like lupus anticoagulant, interfere with the clotting process. Even after the addition of normal plasma, the inhibitor's presence prevents the normalization of clotting time.
   Further Steps: Specific assays to identify the type of inhibitor, such as lupus anticoagulant testing, Bethesda assay (for factor VIII inhibitors), or platelet neutralization assays, may be required.
   Immediate vs. Delayed Correction: Some inhibitors may show a temporary correction of clotting times immediately after mixing but revert to prolonged clotting times after incubation at 37 °C for 1–2 h (incubation correction test). This phenomenon is particularly characteristic of specific factor inhibitors and necessitates further testing to confirm the type and strength of the inhibitor.
   Specific Considerations: Factor VIII Inhibitors: In cases of acquired hemophilia, the Bethesda assay is used to quantify the inhibitor's strength.

Lupus Anticoagulant: The presence of Lupus anticoagulant can cause prolonged aPTT (depending on the sensitivity of the reagent), that does not correct with mixing studies, prompting specific assays.
Nonspecific Inhibitors: Certain conditions, such as antiphospholipid syndrome, can present with inhibitors that affect multiple coagulation factors, leading to complex coagulopathies.
Clinical Relevance: Understanding the results of mixing studies is crucial for diagnosing the underlying cause of a coagulopathy. It directs the subsequent management, whether it involves replacing the deficient factor(s) in cases of factor deficiency or managing the inhibitor's effects. In the case of inhibitors, treatment strategies may include immunosuppression, bypassing agents, or immunomodulatory therapies depending on the type and severity of the inhibitor present.

3.2.1.5 Fibrinogen Level

Fibrinogen, a soluble plasma protein, is converted into fibrin during clot formation. The fibrinogen level test measures the amount of fibrinogen in the blood, providing information on the body's capacity to form clots. Abnormally low levels may indicate a bleeding risk or disseminated intravascular coagulation (DIC), while high levels can be associated with an increased risk of thrombosis.

3.2.1.6 Bleeding Time (BT)

Although less commonly performed today due to its variability and dependence on operator technique, BT measures the time it takes for a standardized skin incision to stop bleeding. It assesses vascular integrity and platelet function, offering a functional assessment of the initial phase of hemostasis. Despite its limitations, BT can provide useful adjunctive information in certain clinical contexts.

These initial screening tests are essential for establishing the presence and nature of coagulopathy in ICU patients. They offer valuable insights into the coagulation status, guiding further diagnostic evaluations and informing therapeutic decisions.

3.2.2 Additional Diagnostic Tests

Beyond the initial screening tests, a suite of additional diagnostic tests provides deeper insights into the complex mechanisms underlying coagulopathy. These tests can pinpoint specific deficiencies or dysfunctions within the coagulation system, aiding in the formulation of targeted treatment strategies.

3.2.2.1 D-Dimer

This test measures the amount of fibrin degradation product present in the blood, indicative of active blood clot formation and breakdown. Elevated D-dimer levels can be found in conditions such as disseminated intravascular coagulation (DIC), deep vein thrombosis (DVT), pulmonary embolism (PE), and recent surgery or trauma. It is particularly useful in the ICU for assessing patients with suspected thrombotic disorders and for monitoring the efficacy of anticoagulant therapy.

3.2.2.2 Lupus Anticoagulant (LA)

LA testing is crucial for identifying antiphospholipid syndrome (APS), an autoimmune disorder that predisposes to thrombosis. LA can paradoxically prolong clotting times in vitro (e.g., aPTT) while promoting thrombosis in vivo. Detecting LA involves a series of tests to demonstrate prolonged phospholipid-dependent clotting, which is not corrected by mixing with normal plasma, and confirmation that the inhibitor is specific to phospholipids.

Coagulation Factor Assays: These assays measure the activity of individual coagulation factors to identify specific deficiencies or excesses. They are essential for diagnosing conditions like hemophilia A and B (factor VIII and IX deficiencies, respectively), von Willebrand disease, and other rare factor deficiencies. Factor assays are pivotal for patients with unexplained bleeding or thrombosis where initial screening tests suggest a specific pathway defect.

3.2.2.3 Antithrombin III (AT III)

AT III is a natural anticoagulant that inhibits several enzymes in the coagulation cascade, primarily thrombin and factor Xa. Reduced levels of AT III can increase the risk of thrombosis. Assessing AT III levels is important in patients with unexplained thrombotic episodes and in monitoring the effectiveness of heparin therapy, as heparin's anticoagulant effect is mediated through AT III.

3.2.2.4 Protein C and Protein S

Both are vitamin K-dependent proteins that play a crucial role in regulating coagulation by inactivating factors Va and VIIIa. Deficiencies in protein C or protein S can lead to an increased risk of thrombosis and are evaluated in patients with a personal or family history of venous thromboembolism. These tests are often performed following an initial finding of LA to differentiate between thrombotic risk factors.

3.2.2.5 Von Willebrand factor (vWF) Activity

vWF is a crucial protein in hemostasis, mediating platelet adhesion to the subendothelial matrix and carrying factor VIII in the circulation. Assessing vWF activity, along with antigen levels and multimer analysis, is key to diagnosing von Willebrand disease, the most common inherited bleeding disorder. This test is especially relevant in patients with mucocutaneous bleeding patterns and normal platelet counts.

3.3 Advanced Diagnostics

In addition to standard and additional diagnostic tests, advanced diagnostic tools like thromboelastography (TEG) or rotational thromboelastometry (ROTEM) and thrombin generation assays (TGAs) offer a dynamic and comprehensive assessment of the coagulation status. These tools provide insights into the functionality of the coagulation system beyond what is possible with traditional tests, enabling a more nuanced approach to managing complex coagulopathies in the ICU.

3.3.1 Thromboelastography (TEG) and Rotational Thromboelastometry (ROTEM)

TEG and ROTEM are point-of-care testing modalities that assess the viscoelastic properties of blood as it clots under low shear conditions, simulating sluggish venous flow. These tests provide a real-time, dynamic picture of clot formation, stabilization, and dissolution, offering valuable information on all phases of hemostasis, from coagulation factor activation and fibrin formation to clot retraction and fibrinolysis. They are particularly useful in complex clinical scenarios such as liver transplantation, cardiac surgery, trauma, and DIC, where traditional tests may not fully capture the patient's coagulation status.

TEG and ROTEM can guide transfusion therapy by identifying specific deficits in the coagulation cascade, allowing for targeted replacement of coagulation factors, fibrinogen, platelets, or the use of antifibrinolytic agents. These advanced diagnostics have been shown to reduce unnecessary transfusions, thereby minimizing the risk of transfusion-related complications and improving patient outcomes.

3.3.2 Thrombin Generation Assays (TGAs)

TGAs measure the ability of plasma to generate thrombin, the key enzyme in the coagulation cascade that converts fibrinogen to fibrin, forming a stable clot. Unlike traditional coagulation tests that provide a static snapshot of the coagulation potential, TGAs offer a dynamic and comprehensive evaluation of thrombin generation and decay over time, reflecting the net effect of procoagulant and anticoagulant forces in the plasma.

TGAs are particularly useful for assessing the risk of thrombosis or bleeding in patients with complex coagulopathies, including those with liver disease, hemophilia, and antiphospholipid syndrome. By measuring parameters such as the lag time to thrombin generation, peak thrombin, and the endogenous thrombin potential, TGAs can help tailor anticoagulant therapy, predict the risk of thrombosis, and monitor the efficacy of interventions designed to restore hemostatic balance.

3.4 Imaging Studies

Imaging studies play a crucial role in the assessment and management of thrombotic complications in critically ill patients. These modalities complement laboratory tests by providing direct visualization of thrombi and assessing their impact on the vascular system and surrounding tissues. Imaging is essential for confirming the diagnosis, understanding the extent of thrombosis, guiding therapeutic interventions, and monitoring response to treatment.

3.4.1 Doppler Ultrasound

Deep Vein Thrombosis (DVT): Doppler ultrasound is the first-line imaging modality for the diagnosis of DVT. It combines traditional ultrasound imaging to visualize the vein's structure with Doppler techniques to assess blood flow. This noninvasive, widely available, and cost-effective method allows for the direct observation of thrombi within the deep veins, usually of the legs or pelvis. It can detect flow abnormalities indicative of a clot, such as the absence of flow, reduced flow, or lack of compressibility of the vein.

Portal Vein Thrombosis (PVT): Doppler ultrasound is also invaluable in diagnosing PVT, a significant complication in patients with liver disease, particularly cirrhosis. It can visualize thrombosis in the portal vein and assess its hemodynamic effects, including portal hypertension and the development of collateral circulation. Doppler ultrasound provides essential information for the management of patients with liver disease and suspected PVT, guiding decisions on anticoagulation therapy and liver transplantation.

3.4.2 CT and MRI

Advanced Imaging Needs: When Doppler ultrasound is inconclusive, or when detailed anatomical information is required, computed tomography (CT) and magnetic resonance imaging (MRI) offer more advanced imaging capabilities. Both modalities are particularly useful for visualizing thrombosis in the abdomen, chest, and cerebral venous system.

CT Angiography (CTA): CTA is highly effective for diagnosing thrombosis in the pulmonary arteries (pulmonary embolism), aorta, and cerebral arteries. It provides high-resolution images that can detect clots, assess the extent of thrombosis, and identify complications such as pulmonary infarction or aneurysm formation. CTA is fast and widely available, making it an essential tool for urgent evaluation of thrombotic events.

Magnetic Resonance Angiography (MRA): MRA offers a nonionizing radiation alternative to CTA, with excellent soft tissue contrast. It is particularly useful for imaging venous thrombosis in the brain, neck, and abdomen. MRA can assess the age of a thrombus, distinguish between acute and chronic thrombosis, and evaluate the surrounding venous structures for collateral formation or compression.

Imaging studies are integral to the multidisciplinary approach required for managing thrombotic complications in critically ill patients. They provide crucial diagnostic and prognostic information that guides therapy, from anticoagulation to interventional procedures, ensuring optimal patient outcomes.

3.5 Special Considerations

Liver Dysfunction: Liver failure significantly impacts the workup for coagulopathy due to the liver's central role in producing most coagulation factors, inhibitors, and fibrinolytic proteins. This multifaceted impact necessitates a careful interpretation of coagulation tests and may require the use of more specialized assessments to understand the complete hemostatic picture:

Coagulation Tests Interpretation: Standard coagulation tests like PT/INR and aPTT can be prolonged in liver dysfunction, reflecting a decrease in the synthesis of vitamin K-dependent clotting factors (II, VII, IX, and X) and proteins C and S. However, these tests only provide a partial view of the coagulation status. Liver failure also leads to a reduction in the production of natural anticoagulants and an impaired clearance of activated clotting factors and fibrinolytic proteins, which can rebalance or even tilt the hemostatic system toward hypercoagulability or a bleeding tendency.

Thrombocytopenia: Thrombocytopenia, common in liver disease due to splenic sequestration or decreased thrombopoietin production, affects the interpretation of bleeding risk. However, increased levels of von Willebrand factor and decreased levels of its cleaving protease, ADAMTS13, can partially compensate for reduced platelet numbers, impacting the assessment of bleeding risk.

Advanced Diagnostics: Tools like TEG or ROTEM and TGAs become particularly valuable in patients with liver dysfunction. They provide a more comprehensive view of clot formation and dissolution, offering insights into the patient's overall hemostatic profile beyond what standard tests can reveal.

Renal Dysfunction: Renal failure also influences coagulation and the workup for coagulopathy, primarily through effects on platelet function and the accumulation of uremic toxins that can interfere with various components of hemostasis.

Platelet Dysfunction: Although platelet counts may remain within the normal range in patients with renal dysfunction, platelet function is often impaired, leading to a bleeding tendency. This dysfunction is not detected by standard coagulation tests like PT/INR or aPTT, highlighting the need for platelet function tests or bleeding time, despite its limitations.

Accumulation of Uremic Toxins: These toxins can interfere with multiple hemostatic pathways, including platelet-vessel wall interactions, platelet aggregation, and the coagulation cascade, complicating the assessment of bleeding risk and thrombotic tendencies.

Use of Heparin in Hemodialysis: Patients with renal failure often undergo hemodialysis, which requires anticoagulation, usually with heparin, to prevent clotting in the dialysis circuit. This necessitates careful monitoring of coagulation status to balance the risk of bleeding with the need for effective anticoagulation.

Adjustments in Diagnostic Approach: Given the impacts on platelet function and the risk of heparin-induced thrombocytopenia (HIT) in this patient population, additional tests such as heparin-platelet factor 4 antibodies may be warranted. Moreover, assessing for uremia-induced platelet dysfunction may involve specific platelet function assays.

3.6 Management

Abnormal coagulation profile can be seen as follows:

1. Bleeding Time: If prolonged, this can be due to:
   (a) platelet deficiency
   (b) platelet dysfunction—can be tested with platelet function assay (PFA), platelet aggregometry, and platelet flowcytometry
   (c) vWF deficiency—further tested by vWF antigen assay and Ristocetin Co-factor Assay (RiCOF)
   (d) blood vessel-related disorders like Henoch Schonlein Purpura
2. Thrombocytopenia confirmed on peripheral smears

3. Prolonged PT and aPTT—when prolonged, ask for mixing studies where 50:50 patient plasma is mixed with pooled normal plasma and re-assayed. If corrected, then it indicates factor deficiency, and if still prolonged, then it indicates the presence of inhibitors or anticoagulants.
4. Fibrinogen deficiency
5. Increased D-dimer—Indicates clot formation. With thrombocytopenia and schistocytes, the presence of D-dimer indicates microangiopathic hemolytic anemia (MAHA), which includes thrombotic thrombocytopenic purpura (TTP)/ Henoch Schonlein Purpura (Hus)/Disseminated Intravascular Coagulopathy (DIC).

3.7 Coagulation Abnormalities

The most important thing in management of coagulopathies in patients is to curate the treatment as per individual needs and not treat the lab parameters alone. Abnormal parameters in a stable patient should warrant a caution. Repeat from a fresh site and preferably not a vein where channels are present. Further workup should be done only if abnormal parameters are seen twice.

Mostly replacements are done in bleeding patients, and prophylactic factor replacements are usually not recommended strongly.

Plasma transfusion is beneficial for patients needing volume resuscitation and coagulopathy correction, particularly trauma or massive bleeding cases. Key parameters to maintain include temperature >35 °C, ionized calcium >1.1 mmol/L, and pH >7.25. A systematic transfusion therapy with a local massive transfusion protocol is used to enhance blood product delivery, including packed red blood cells, FFP, platelets, and cryoprecipitate if fibrinogen is <2.0 g/L. Tranexamic acid is administered at 1 g followed by an 8-h infusion of another gram (Singh 2019).

Risks of FFP transfusion include TRALI, transfusion-related circulatory overload, allergic reactions, and rare transmission of infections, febrile reactions, hemolytic reactions, and RBC alloimmunization.

Factor concentrate therapy guided by viscoelastic testing (TEG or ROTEM) can also be done.

3.7.1 Thrombocytopenia

Thrombocytopenia occurs in 13–50% of ICU admissions, with platelet transfusions primarily utilized for trauma-related bleeding, hemorrhage prevention in cases of low counts, and for individuals with platelet dysfunction. Transfusion decisions often hinge on platelet counts, expecting a 30–50 × 10^9/L increase per pooled unit transfused. Unresponsive cases may indicate antiplatelet antibodies, bleeding, thrombosis, or other factors. The British Society of Haematology suggests keeping platelet counts above 75 × 10^9/L for those bleeding, although 55% of transfusions are prophylactic, particularly in non-bleeding patients. The efficacy of such prophylactic measures in the critically ill remains under-researched, with some studies showing no direct correlation between thrombocytopenia and post-procedure bleeding, such as after liver transplants. Hematological malignancy patients may need counts over 100 × 10^9/L to prevent spontaneous bleeding, while sepsis patients might require a threshold of 20 × 10^9/L. Establishing an ideal platelet count threshold in critical care is essential, which is currently aimed at >20 × 10^9/L.

3.7.2 Thrombosis Management

For thrombosis management, deep vein thrombosis (DVT) and pulmonary embolism (PE) significantly impact ICU patients. Thromboprophylaxis has proven to lower mortality, with three RCTs showing reduced DVT incidences in treated groups. Guidelines endorse unfractionated heparin (UFH) or low-molecular-weight heparin (LMWH) for DVT prevention in these settings. The PROTECT trial explores these thromboprophylaxis approaches further. The American College of Chest Physicians recommends routine VTE risk assessment and prophylaxis in critical care, using LMWH or low-dose UFH for moderate risk patients and mechanical methods for those with a higher bleeding risk, transitioning to pharmacologic measures as the risk diminishes (Ejaz et al. 2018).

Flowchart

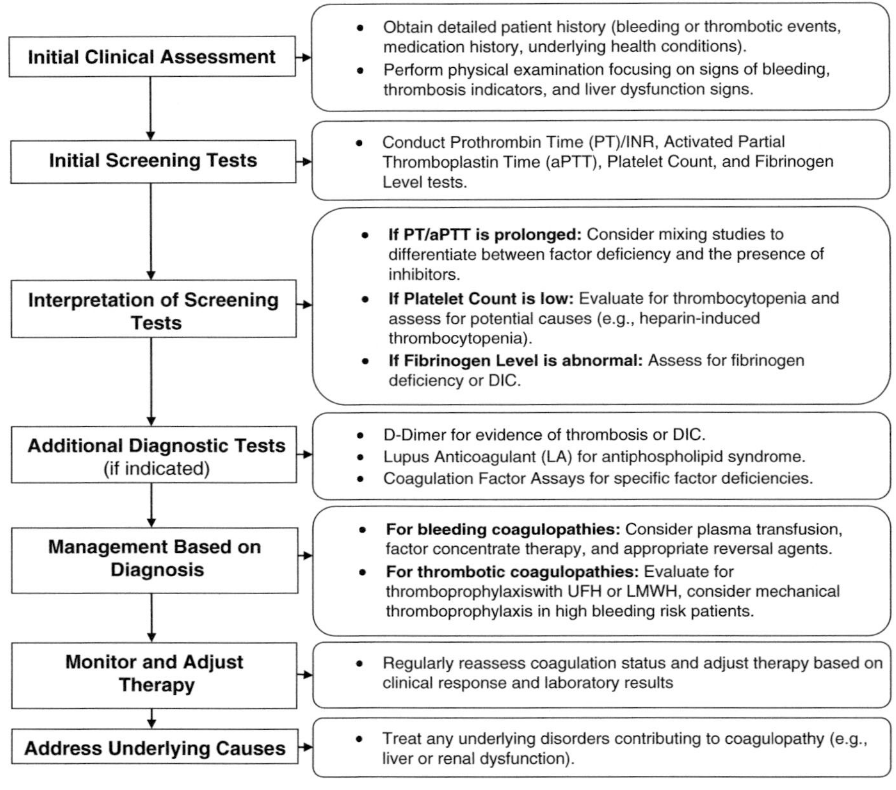

Abnormal Clotting Profile Flowchart

References

Ejaz A, Ahmed MM, Tasleem A, Niazi MRK, Ahsraf MF, Ahmad I et al (2018) Thromboprophylaxis in intensive care unit patients: a literature review. Cureus 10(9):e3341

Neuenfeldt FS, Weigand MA, Fischer D (2021) Coagulopathies in intensive care medicine: balancing act between thrombosis and bleeding. J Clin Med 10(22):5369

Retter A, Barrett NA (2015) The management of abnormal haemostasis in the ICU. Anaesthesia 70:121–e41

Singh MY (2019) Approach to the coagulopathic patient in the intensive care unit. Indian J Crit Care Med 23(Suppl 3):S215

Part II
Hematological Abnormalities and Management in ICU

Chapter 4
Approach to Anemia in ICU

Nilesh Kumar and Abhishek Borkotoky

Learning Points

1. Understanding the Multifactorial Etiology of Anemia in ICU Patients: Anemia in ICU settings is often the result of a complex interplay of factors.
2. The Impact of Anemia on ICU Patient Outcomes: Anemia in critically ill patients is associated with adverse outcomes, including increased mortality, prolonged hospital stays, and a higher incidence of complications.
3. Evidence-Based Strategies for Anemia Management in the ICU: The workup for anemia is provided. The transition from liberal to restrictive transfusion practices highlights the importance of evidence-based approaches in managing anemia.
4. The Role of Patient Blood Management (PBM) in Critical Care: PBM is a multidisciplinary, evidence-based approach to optimizing the care of patients who might need transfusion.

4.1 Introduction

Anemia is a prevalent condition among patients admitted to the intensive care unit (ICU), with approximately 50% of ICU patients developing anemia during their stay, often necessitating red blood cell (RBC) transfusions (Goldhill 2012). Research indicates that between 30% and 50% of ICU patients undergo RBC transfusions, with an average of 5 units transfused during their ICU admission (Goldhill 2012). The World Health Organization (WHO) defines anemia as a hemoglobin level below

N. Kumar (✉)
IMS, Banaras Hindu University, Varanasi, Uttar Pradesh, India

A. Borkotoky (✉)
Department of Internal Medicine, IMS BHU, Benaras, Uttar Pradesh, India

S. B. Mishra (ed.), *Critical Care Hematology*,
https://doi.org/10.1007/978-981-97-5565-3_4

13 g/dL in men and below 12 g/dL in women (Borgert et al. 2016). Anemia in critically ill patients is linked to adverse outcomes, such as an increased risk of mortality (Hayden et al. 2012).

Recent advancements in critical care have prompted a transition from liberal to restrictive transfusion practices, underscoring the importance of comprehending the pathophysiology and management of anemia in ICU patients (Goldhill 2012). Anemia in ICU patients can stem from various causes, often necessitating a thorough evaluation and care plan (Vincent et al. 2002). Distinguishing whether adverse outcomes are attributable to anemia itself or RBC transfusions is challenging, emphasizing the necessity for evidence-based strategies in managing anemia in critically ill patients (Goldhill 2012).

Studies have revealed that a substantial proportion of ICU patients remain anemic even after discharge, with 50% of mechanically ventilated patients still being anemic 6 months post-ICU discharge (Siegal et al. 2023). Furthermore, the quantity of blood drawn for laboratory testing is correlated with an increased probability of RBC transfusion in non-bleeding patients, highlighting the significance of minimizing unnecessary blood loss in ICU settings.

4.2 Etiopathogenesis

Understanding the multifactorial etiology of anemia in patients involves a comprehensive approach that includes a thorough history taking, clinical examination, and appropriate laboratory investigations to identify treatable causes (Camaschella and Silvestri 2011). The complex web of causation can be categorized into two main subclasses: blood loss and bone marrow production insufficiency (Camaschella and Silvestri 2011). Primary mechanisms contributing to anemia include the loss of red blood cells due to various factors such as phlebotomy, bleeding from different sources, and decreased production of red blood cells secondary to bone marrow suppression (Camaschella and Silvestri 2011). Additionally, nutritional deficiencies and increased destruction of red blood cells or their precursors are significant contributors to anemia (Camaschella and Silvestri 2011).

Anemia is a common concern in patients with chronic heart failure, where it has been associated with adverse clinical outcomes, including increased risks of death and hospitalization (Anand et al. 2004). In patients with heart failure, anemia remains a significant predictor of adverse outcomes, emphasizing the importance of addressing anemia in this population (Anand et al. 2004). Furthermore, the relationship between anemia and heart failure is complex, involving factors such as inflammatory cytokine activation and erythropoietin resistance (Felker et al. 2004).

In individuals with kidney dysfunction, anemia is prevalent, with studies confirming the association between kidney function and hemoglobin levels (Astor et al. 2002). Chronic kidney disease and heart failure share common mechanisms that contribute to renal dysfunction and anemia, highlighting the intricate interplay between these conditions (Dobre et al. 2012). Moreover, renal dysfunction can impact the efficacy of treatment regimens in patients with chronic conditions such as hepatitis C virus infection (Nakashima et al. 2019).

4.3 Primary Mechanisms Include

(a) Loss of red blood cells (RBCs) due to phlebotomy and bleeding from a surgical site, trauma, venous access site, or gastrointestinal bleeding.
(b) Decreased production of RBCs due to suppression of bone marrow secondary to inflammatory cytokines, drugs, functional or absolute erythropoietin deficiency due to renal dysfunction.
(c) Nutritional (iron, folic acid, vitamin B12) deficiency.
(d) Increased destruction of RBCs (hemolysis) or RBC precursors in the bone marrow due to toxins and drugs.

- *Blood Loss*: The management of blood loss in the intensive care unit (ICU) is crucial for patient care. Excessive phlebotomy can lead to anemia and necessitate red blood cell (RBC) transfusions (Coene et al. 2015). Studies have shown that the daily blood drawn for lab investigations in the ICU can amount to 40–70 ml, with an average loss of about 1 unit of blood per week, contributing to anemia (Coene et al. 2015). Prolonged ICU admissions exceeding 21 days often result in multiple RBC transfusions, correlating with the volume of daily phlebotomy and further predisposing patients to anemia (Coene et al. 2015). Advances in phlebotomy techniques, such as using small-volume collection tubes, have significantly reduced blood loss related to diagnostic investigations during ICU stays (Siegal et al. 2023).
- *Bleeding*: Bleeding complications in ICUs are not only limited to surgical units but can also occur in medical settings, with active bleeding accounting for a significant portion of blood transfusions in critical care (Chant et al. 2006). Stress-induced ulcers and coagulation abnormalities are common preventable causes of bleeding in critically ill patients (Chant et al. 2006). Coagulation defects leading to consumptive coagulopathy and thrombocytopenia can exacerbate bleeding episodes in ICU patients (Chant et al. 2006).

Efforts to minimize blood loss and optimize transfusion practices in ICUs are crucial for improving patient outcomes and reducing the risks associated with anemia and excessive transfusions. Implementing strategies such as using small-volume phlebotomy tubes, adopting restrictive transfusion protocols, and addressing preventable causes of bleeding can help mitigate the impact of blood loss on patient care in the ICU.

4.4 Iron and Erythropoietin Interplay

Anemia in ICU patients is a multifactorial condition primarily driven by three significant abnormalities related to the host inflammatory response. First, the dysregulation of iron homeostasis occurs due to increased hepcidin concentrations (Riessen et al. 2015). Hepcidin, as the master regulator of iron homeostasis, reduces iron availability through mechanisms such as internalization and destruction of ferroportin, leading to iron retention in macrophages and decreased iron absorption in the gastrointestinal tract (Czempik et al. 2022a, b). This results in functional iron deficiency. Second, impaired proliferation of erythroid progenitor cells contributes to anemia in critical care settings. Last, a blunted erythropoietin response further exacerbates the condition (Riessen et al. 2015).

Recent advancements have identified erythroferrone (ERFE) as a hormone that suppresses hepcidin, allowing increased iron absorption and mobilization from iron stores (Riessen et al. 2015). Additionally, newer derivatives of erythropoietin and its congeners are being explored in trials for managing anemia in critical care (Riessen et al. 2015). Anemia is prevalent in ICU patients, with nearly all critically ill individuals becoming anemic within days of admission. It is crucial to recognize anemia early, as it is associated with adverse outcomes in acutely ill patients.

Furthermore, anemia in the ICU is often a consequence of acute systemic inflammation, known as systemic inflammatory response syndrome (SIRS) (Czempik and Krzych 2022). While anemia can be influenced by various factors like trauma, surgery, and bleeding, it can also occur in critically ill patients without evident bleeding (Juárez-Vela et al. 2022). The presence of anemia should be consistently monitored in ICU patients, as it is highly prevalent and linked to red blood cell transfusions (Czempik et al. 2022a, b). Anemia at ICU admission has been identified as an independent predictor of hospital mortality (Prin et al. 2021).

Anemia in ICU patients is a complex condition influenced by dysregulation of iron homeostasis, impaired erythropoiesis, and blunted erythropoietin response. Understanding these mechanisms and advancements in managing anemia, such as hepcidin modulation and erythropoietin derivatives, is crucial for improving outcomes in critically ill individuals.

4.5 Nutritional Deficiency

Among the causes of anemia in critical care, it is essential to consider ruling out nutritional deficiencies such as iron, B12, and folate deficiencies. Nutritional causes contribute to 9% for iron deficiency, 2% for B12 deficiency, and 2% for folate deficiency (Baker et al. 2010). Iron deficiency without anemia can have long-term adverse effects on neurodevelopment and behavior, emphasizing the importance of addressing these deficiencies promptly (Jáuregui-Lobera 2014). New approaches are necessary to effectively manage patient populations with iron-deficiency anemia (Alleyne et al. 2008).

Anemia of critical illness, resembling chronic anemia but with a sudden onset, is a commonly encountered clinical scenario (Asare 2008). Monitoring clinical indicators like low plasma ferritin, decreased plasma iron, and transferrin saturation, along with low hemoglobin content in red blood cells, can aid in the assessment of anemia (Handelman and Levin 2008). Iron supplementation during pregnancy remains a topic of interest due to its potential impact on adverse pregnancy outcomes (Müngen 2003).

Iron deficiency is a critical consideration in various populations, including postpartum women (Petraro et al. 2013), adolescent school girls (Limbu et al. 2017), and hemodialysis patients (Amjad et al. 2021). Additionally, iron deficiency anemia can manifest in extreme cases, as seen in pediatric patients with very low hemoglobin levels (Shalby et al. 2022). Furthermore, iron deficiency can be indicative of disease severity in conditions like COVID-19 (Kilercik et al. 2022).

4.6 Drug Reactions

Anemia in critical care can be attributed to various classes of drugs that induce bone marrow suppression or cause immune-mediated hemolysis. Monitoring hematocrit levels and the timing of drug initiation can help establish a temporal relationship between drug administration and the onset of anemia, along with other laboratory parameters (Northrop and Agarwal 2015). Drug-induced hemolytic anemia can occur through mechanisms such as drug adsorption, red cell membrane modification, immune complex formation, or antibody production (Mintzer et al. 2009).

Prompt recognition of drug-induced immune hemolytic anemia is crucial due to the potentially life-threatening nature of brisk hemolysis (Pecker et al. 2016). Drugs like ceftriaxone have been associated with immune hemolytic anemia, emphasizing the importance of understanding and managing these drug reactions in critical care settings (Leicht et al. 2018). Antibiotics, antineoplastic agents, and nonsteroidal anti-inflammatory drugs are common culprits in drug-induced red blood cell disorders, highlighting the need for vigilance in medication management (Walter and Carraretto 2015).

In addition to drug-induced hemolytic anemia, drugs can also lead to other hematologic syndromes through various mechanisms (Maheshwari et al. 2004). Understanding the pathogenesis and clinical aspects of drug-induced aplastic anemia is essential for effective management in clinical practice (Salama et al. 2002). Furthermore, rare occurrences of drug-induced autoimmune hemolytic anemia, such as those induced by quetiapine, underscore the importance of monitoring and recognizing adverse drug reactions in vulnerable patient populations (Joshi et al. 2014).

4.7 Anemia the Vicious Cycle

The complex issue of anemia in critical care settings is a significant concern due to its association with increased patient morbidity. Anemia reduces the oxygen-carrying capacity, leading to compensatory mechanisms such as increased heart rate to elevate cardiac output, resulting in a state of hyperdynamic circulation. Studies have shown that anemia in critical care is linked to adverse outcomes, including increased rates of intubation, prolonged mechanical ventilation, and challenges in weaning, particularly in the elderly population (Vincent et al. 2002; Leicht et al. 2018).

Patients with chronic heart conditions, chronic kidney injury, and acute myocardial infarction in critical care settings experience unfavorable outcomes when anemic (Packman 2015). Anemia in critically ill patients presents challenges, as the implications of blood transfusions are heightened in this population (Hesdorffer and Longo 2015). Moreover, drug-induced anemia and other red cell disorders are prevalent in the era of polypharmacy, necessitating a comprehensive approach to diagnosis and management (Spinelli and Bartlett 2016).

Anemia is a prevalent nutritional deficiency disorder globally, affecting pregnant, lactating, and nonpregnant nonlactating women, with significant implications for health and well-being (Walter and Carraretto 2015). Untreated cases of nutritional iron deficiency anemia can result in significantly low hemoglobin levels, underscoring the importance of early detection and intervention (Northrop and Agarwal 2015). The occurrence of anemia in inflammatory bowel diseases underscores the multifactorial nature of anemia and its association with chronic conditions (Shander et al. 2011).

4.8 Hemolysis

Hemolytic anemias encompass a range of disorders characterized by the premature destruction of red blood cells (RBCs), leading to various clinical manifestations (Brocklebank et al. 2018). The diagnosis of hemolytic anemias involves a comprehensive algorithmic approach integrating clinical signs, laboratory tests, and specific diagnostic procedures (Brocklebank et al. 2018). The initial diagnostic step often involves the Direct Coombs Test, which provides valuable insights based on its outcomes (Brocklebank et al. 2018). Depending on the results, the algorithm branches into different pathways tailored to the specific condition suspected (Brocklebank et al. 2018).

For instance, conditions like Paroxysmal Nocturnal Hemoglobinuria (PNH) require specific tests examining both RBCs and white blood cells (Brocklebank et al. 2018). In cases of suspected pregnancy-related hemolysis, the HELLP syndrome is a specific consideration (Brocklebank et al. 2018). Moreover, the algorithm accounts for special conditions like Lead Poisoning, where a venous blood test for lead levels is warranted (Brocklebank et al. 2018). Additionally, the algorithm considers congenital conditions like Congenital Dyserythropoietic Anemia, leading to specific tests such as RBC Band 3 Protein Reduction and Osmotic Fragility Erythrocyte (Brocklebank et al. 2018).

The final considerations of the algorithm emphasize the importance of morphological analysis and further testing for autoimmune hemolytic anemia or specific abnormalities, directing toward RBC enzyme deficiencies, hemoglobinopathies, and RBC membrane disorders (Brocklebank et al. 2018). Molecular testing, such as the Hereditary Hemolytic Anemia Panel Sequencing, may be considered in cases where specific genetic anomalies are suspected (Brocklebank et al. 2018).

As we have explored the multifaceted causes of anemia in critically ill patients, a systematic approach to diagnosis is crucial for effective management. The following section presents a diagnostic algorithm tailored to the unique challenges of the ICU environment, guiding clinicians from clinical assessment to specific diagnostic tests.

4.9 Diagnostic Algorithm for Anemia in ICU

Following the exploration of anemia's multifaceted etiologies within the ICU environment, it becomes imperative to adopt a systematic and precise approach to its diagnosis. Recognizing the critical need for timely and accurate identification of the underlying causes of anemia, we introduce a tailored diagnostic algorithm designed to navigate the complexities of critical care.

This algorithm begins with a comprehensive clinical assessment, incorporating patient history, symptom review, and physical examination findings, which are pivotal in the initial suspicion and categorization of anemia. Essential to this process is the consideration of common symptoms such as pallor, fatigue, and dyspnea, alongside the ICU-specific contexts that may exacerbate or mask these signs.

Subsequently, the algorithm advances to detailed laboratory testing, which forms the backbone of our diagnostic approach. Initial tests include a complete blood count (CBC), reticulocyte count, and a peripheral blood smear, accompanied by a basic metabolic panel to provide a broad overview of the patient's hematological status and to identify any immediate red flags indicative of anemia's origin.

Special attention is given to the differentiation between anemia caused by increased destruction of red blood cells, such as hemolytic anemia, versus that arising from decreased production or significant blood loss. This distinction is crucial, as it directs subsequent diagnostic pathways and therapeutic strategies. For instance, in cases of suspected hemolytic anemia, further tests like the Direct Coombs Test, lactate dehydrogenase (LDH) levels, and haptoglobin measurements are recommended.

Moreover, the algorithm incorporates steps for the investigation of less common but equally significant causes of anemia in ICU patients, such as iron deficiency, vitamin B12 and folate levels, and bone marrow function assessment. These are particularly relevant in the context of nutritional deficiencies or chronic disease states that may influence anemia's presentation and progression.

In closing, our diagnostic algorithm is a dynamic tool, adaptable to the evolving clinical picture of an ICU patient. It underscores the importance of a methodical approach to the diagnosis of anemia, guiding clinicians from initial suspicion to specific diagnostic tests and, ultimately, to the most appropriate and effective management strategies. By integrating this algorithm into the broader framework of anemia management in the ICU, we aim to enhance patient care through precision, efficiency, and a deepened understanding of this complex condition.

4.10 Management of Anemia in Critical Care

4.10.1 Preventive Measures

With a clear understanding of the specific type and cause of anemia through our diagnostic algorithm, we can now proceed to discuss targeted management strategies. Tailored treatment plans begin with a precise diagnosis, setting the stage for the most effective interventions for anemia in the ICU.

Strategies to prevent anemia in ICU patients involve reducing phlebotomy procedures, utilizing low-volume blood sampling tubes, and employing enclosed blood conservation devices (Lasocki et al. 2020; Leicht et al. 2018; Limbu et al. 2017). These preventive measures are crucial in minimizing the risk of anemia and reducing the need for red blood cell transfusions in critically ill patients. Patient Blood Management programs play a significant role in screening, diagnosing, and treating anemia, and coagulopathies, and minimizing bleeding in critical care settings (Leicht et al. 2018).

Anemia management in critical care is a multifaceted challenge, with ongoing research and controversies surrounding optimal management strategies (Leicht et al. 2018). Preventing anemia in critically ill patients is essential to mitigate the associated risks and complications, particularly in patients with chronic heart conditions, chronic kidney injury, and acute myocardial infarction (Leicht et al. 2018). Anemia in critical care can lead to adverse outcomes, emphasizing the importance of proactive management and preventive measures (Leicht et al. 2018).

Implementing preventive strategies such as reducing phlebotomy, utilizing blood conservation devices, and following Patient Blood Management programs are essential in managing and preventing anemia in critical care settings. These measures can help optimize patient outcomes and reduce the need for red blood cell transfusions, ultimately improving the quality of care provided to critically ill patients.

4.10.2 Anemia Treatment

Treatment options for anemia in critical care encompass a range of interventions, from utilizing erythropoietin-stimulating agents (ESA) to red blood cell (RBC) transfusion. ESAs are typically reserved for managing anemia in chronic kidney disease to address the imbalance caused by hepcidin downregulation and disrupted iron metabolism (López et al. 2009). However, the use of ESA in critically ill patients with anemia has not shown significant reductions in transfusion rates (Macdougall et al. 2014; Mikhail et al. 2017). Iron therapies have demonstrated limited impact on hemoglobin levels, RBC transfusion rates, or infection rates in critical care settings (Park et al. 2022).

In the Trauma ICU setting, contrasting outcomes were observed with ESA use, showing a significant reduction in survival without a corresponding increase in lower limb deep vein thrombosis rates (Kei et al. 2019). Nutritional and vitamin supplementation is recommended to address uncommon causes of anemia in critical care patients. The concept of anemia in critical care has evolved with the adoption of a "Restrictive RBC transfusion" strategy, particularly in general critical care, sepsis, and cardiac disease categories, with evidence supporting higher hemoglobin triggers in specific populations such as acute coronary syndrome or cardiac surgery (Tsubakihara et al. 2010).

The management of anemia in critical care involves a nuanced approach, considering the efficacy and safety of treatment options such as ESA, RBC transfusion, iron therapies, and nutritional supplementation. Understanding the implications of different interventions and tailoring treatment strategies to individual patient needs are essential in optimizing outcomes for critically ill individuals.

4.10.3 Patient Blood Management

Patient Blood Management (PBM) is a comprehensive approach that involves the timely application of evidence-based medical and surgical concepts to maintain hemoglobin concentration, optimize hemostasis, and minimize blood loss in order to improve patient outcomes (Spahn 2010). This strategy focuses on managing and conserving a patient's own blood to enhance patient safety and clinical results (Shander et al. 2022). PBM interventions aim to reduce the necessity for allogeneic blood transfusions and improve patient care by preserving the patient's own blood (Warner et al. 2023).

The concept of PBM has gained recognition as a patient-centered approach that surpasses transfusion-centered practices to enhance healthcare quality and outcomes (Ozawa et al. 2024). Healthcare facilities can enhance patient safety, decrease unnecessary transfusions, and control healthcare costs by implementing PBM strategies (Isbister 2015). PBM programs have been proven to enhance clinical outcomes, lower risks, and decrease the need for allogeneic blood transfusions (Hofmann et al. 2011).

Patient Blood Management signifies a shift in transfusion practice toward a patient-centered approach that strives to optimize patient outcomes, minimize blood loss, and enhance patient safety through evidence-based interventions.

Flowchart

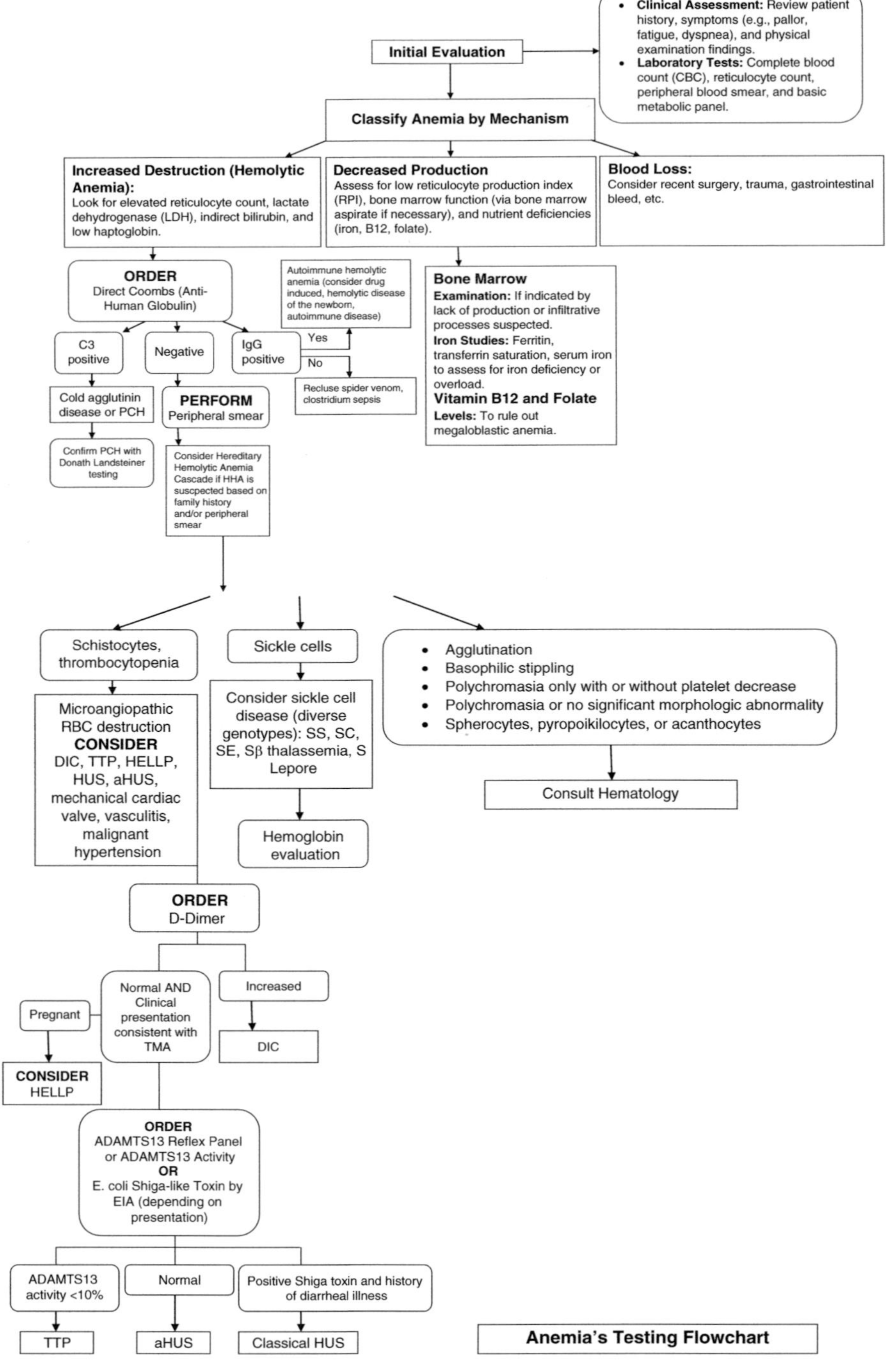
Initial Evaluation
Clinical Assessment: Review patient history, symptoms (e.g., pallor, fatigue, dyspnea), and physical examination findings.
Laboratory Tests: Complete blood count (CBC), reticulocyte count, peripheral blood smear, and basic metabolic panel.
Classify Anemia by Mechanism
Increased Destruction (Hemolytic Anemia): Look for elevated reticulocyte count, lactate dehydrogenase (LDH), indirect bilirubin, and low haptoglobin.
Decreased Production Assess for low reticulocyte production index (RPI), bone marrow function (via bone marrow aspirate if necessary), and nutrient deficiencies (iron, B12, folate).
Blood Loss: Consider recent surgery, trauma, gastrointestinal bleed, etc.
ORDER Direct Coombs (Anti-Human Globulin)
Autoimmune hemolytic anemia (consider drug induced, hemolytic disease of the newborn, autoimmune disease)
Bone Marrow Examination: If indicated by lack of production or infiltrative processes suspected.
Iron Studies: Ferritin, transferrin saturation, serum iron to assess for iron deficiency or overload.
Vitamin B12 and Folate Levels: To rule out megaloblastic anemia.
C3 positive
Negative
IgG positive
Yes
No
Recluse spider venom, clostridium sepsis
Cold agglutinin disease or PCH
PERFORM Peripheral smear
Confirm PCH with Donath Landsteiner testing
Consider Hereditary Hemolytic Anemia Cascade if HHA is suscpected based on family history and/or peripheral smear
Schistocytes, thrombocytopenia
Sickle cells
Agglutination
Basophilic stippling
Polychromasia only with or without platelet decrease
Polychromasia or no significant morphologic abnormality
Spherocytes, pyropoikilocytes, or acanthocytes
Microangiopathic RBC destruction CONSIDER DIC, TTP, HELLP, HUS, aHUS, mechanical cardiac valve, vasculitis, malignant hypertension
Consider sickle cell disease (diverse genotypes): SS, SC, SE, Sβ thalassemia, S Lepore
Consult Hematology
Hemoglobin evaluation
ORDER D-Dimer
Pregnant
Normal AND Clinical presentation consistent with TMA
Increased
DIC
CONSIDER HELLP
ORDER ADAMTS13 Reflex Panel or ADAMTS13 Activity OR E. coli Shiga-like Toxin by EIA (depending on presentation)
ADAMTS13 activity <10%
Normal
Positive Shiga toxin and history of diarrheal illness
TTP
aHUS
Classical HUS
Anemia's Testing Flowchart

References

Alleyne M, Horne MK, Miller JL (2008) Individualized treatment for iron-deficiency anemia in adults. Am J Med 121(11):943–948

Amjad AWAIS, Usmani S, Pasha HH, Khan WA, Qamar MA, Mustafa Z et al (2021) Prevalence of iron deficiency anemia in hemodialysis patients at NIKD. Pak J Med Health Sci 15(6):1192–1194

Anand I, McMurray JJ, Whitmore J, Warren M, Pham A, McCamish MA, Burton PB (2004) Anemia and its relationship to clinical outcome in heart failure. Circulation 110(2):149–154

Asare K (2008) Anemia of critical illness. Pharmacotherapy: the journal of human pharmacology and drug. Therapy 28(10):1267–1282

Astor BC, Muntner P, Levin A, Eustace JA, Coresh J (2002) Association of kidney function with anemia: the third National Health and nutrition examination survey (1988–1994). Arch Intern Med 162(12):1401–1408

Baker RD, Greer FR, Bhatia JJ, Abrams SA, Daniels SR, Schneider MB et al (2010) Clinical report-diagnosis and prevention of iron deficiency and iron-deficiency anemia in infants and young children (0–3 years of age). Pediatrics 126(5):1040–1050

Borgert M, Binnekade J, Paulus F, Vroom M, Vlaar A, Goossens A, Dongelmans D (2016) Implementation of a transfusion bundle reduces inappropriate red blood cell transfusions in intensive care–a before and after study. Transfus Med 26(6):432–439

Brocklebank V, Wood KM, Kavanagh D (2018) Thrombotic microangiopathy and the kidney. Clin J Am Soc Nephrol 13(2):300–317

Camaschella C, Silvestri L (2011) Molecular mechanisms regulating hepcidin revealed by hepcidin disorders. Sci World J 11:1357–1366

Chant C, Wilson G, Friedrich JO (2006) Anemia, transfusion, and phlebotomy practices in critically ill patients with prolonged ICU length of stay: a cohort study. Crit Care 10:1–9

Coene KLM, Roos AN, Scharnhorst V (2015) Iatrogenic anemia/twenty-five million liters of blood into the sewer: comment. J Thromb Haemost 13(6):1160–1161

Czempik PF, Krzych ŁJ (2022) Anemia of critical illness: a narrative review. Acta Haematol Pol 53(4):249–257

Czempik PF, Pluta MP, Krzych ŁJ (2022a) Hemoglobin determination using pulse co-oximetry and reduced-volume blood gas analysis in the critically Ill: a prospective cohort study. Diagnostics 12(12):2908

Czempik PF, Wilczek D, Herzyk J, Krzych ŁJ (2022b) Hospital-acquired anemia in patients hospitalized in the intensive care unit: a retrospective cohort study. J Clin Med 11(14):3939

Dobre D, Rossignol P, Metra M, Zannad F (2012) Can we prevent or treat renal dysfunction in chronic heart failure? Heart Fail Rev 17:283–290

Felker GM, Adams KF, Gattis WA, O'Connor CM (2004) Anemia as a risk factor and therapeutic target in heart failure. J Am Coll Cardiol 44(5):959–966

Goldhill D (2012) Evidence-based medicine in critical care. J Intensive Care Soc 13(1):14–16

Handelman GJ, Levin NW (2008) Iron and anemia in human biology: a review of mechanisms. Heart Fail Rev 13:393–404

Hayden SJ, Albert TJ, Watkins TR, Swenson ER (2012) Anemia in critical illness: insights into etiology, consequences, and management. Am J Respir Crit Care Med 185(10):1049–1057

Hesdorffer CS, Longo DL (2015) Drug-induced megaloblastic anemia. N Engl J Med 373(17):1649–1658

Hofmann A, Farmer S, Shander A (2011) Five drivers shifting the paradigm from product-focused transfusion practice to patient blood management. Oncologist 16(S3):3–11

Isbister JP (2015) The three-pillar matrix of patient blood management. ISBT Sci Ser 10(S1):286–294

Jáuregui-Lobera I (2014) Iron deficiency and cognitive functions. Neuropsychiatr Dis Treat 10:2087–2095

Joshi HM, Joshi JM, Patel KP, Shah KN, Patel VJ (2014) Morbidity and drug utilization pattern among admitted pregnant anaemic women and to find out rationality of drug by using Indian guidelines. Int J Basic Clin Pharmacol 3:947–953

Juárez-Vela R, Andrés-Esteban EM, Gea-Caballero V, Sánchez-González JL, Marcos-Neira P, Serrano-Lázaro A et al (2022) Related factors of anemia in critically ill patients: a prospective multicenter study. J Clin Med 11(4):1031

Kei T, Mistry N, Curley G, Pavenski K, Shehata N, Tanzini RM et al (2019) Efficacité et innocuité d'un traitement d'érythropoïétine et de fer pour réduire la transfusion de culots sanguins chez les patients chirurgicaux: une revue systématique et méta-analyse. Can J Anesth/J Can Anesth 66:716–731

Kilercik M, Ucal Y, Serdar M, Serteser M, Ozpinar A, Schweigert FJ (2022) Zinc protoporphyrin levels in COVID-19 are indicative of iron deficiency and potential predictor of disease severity. PLoS One 17(2):e0262487

Lasocki S, Pène F, Ait-Oufella H, Aubron C, Ausset S, Buffet P et al (2020) Management and prevention of anemia (acute bleeding excluded) in adult critical care patients. Ann Intensive Care 10:1–12

Leicht HB, Weinig E, Mayer B, Viebahn J, Geier A, Rau M (2018) Ceftriaxone-induced hemolytic anemia with severe renal failure: a case report and review of literature. BMC Pharmacol Toxicol 19:1–7

Limbu N, Thakur D, Das BKL, Choudhary LB, Pradhan A, Baral D (2017) Prevalence of anemia and iron deficiency in adolescent school girls of Dharan, Nepal. Asian J Med Sci 8(5):22–26

López RM, Aladrén BS, García FG (2009) Use of agents stimulating erythropoiesis in digestive diseases. World J Gastroenterol: WJG 15(37):4675

Macdougall IC, Bock AH, Carrera F, Eckardt KU, Gaillard C, Van Wyck D et al (2014) FIND-CKD: a randomized trial of intravenous ferric carboxymaltose versus oral iron in patients with chronic kidney disease and iron deficiency anaemia. Nephrol Dial Transplantat 29(11):2075–2084

Maheshwari A, Mishra R, Thuluvath PJ (2004) Post-liver-transplant anemia: etiology and management. Liver Transpl 10(2):165–173

Mikhail A, Brown C, Williams JA, Mathrani V, Shrivastava R, Evans J et al (2017) Renal association clinical practice guideline on Anaemia of chronic kidney disease. BMC Nephrol 18:1–29

Mintzer DM, Billet SN, Chmielewski L (2009) Drug-induced hematologic syndromes. Adv Hematol 2009:495863

Müngen E (2003) Iron supplementation in pregnancy, vol 31

Nakashima M, Toyoda H, Tada T, Mizuno K, Iio E, Tanaka Y et al (2019) Influence of renal dysfunction on dose reduction and virologic efficacy of regimens combining ribavirin and all-oral direct acting antivirals in patients with chronic hepatitis C virus infection. Hepatol Res 49(5):512–520

Northrop MS, Agarwal HS (2015) Ceftriaxone-induced hemolytic anemia: case report and review of literature. J Pediatr Hematol Oncol 37(1):e63–e66

Ozawa S, Ozawa-Morriello J, Rock R, Sromoski M, Walbolt S, Hall T, Pearse BL (2024) Patient blood management as an emerging concept in quality: the role of nurses. J Nurs Care Qual 39(2):129–135

Packman CH (2015) The clinical pictures of autoimmune hemolytic anemia. Transfus Med Hemother 42(5):317–324

Park H, Desai R, Liu X, Smith SM, Hincapie-Castillo J, Henry L et al (2022) Medicare bundled payment policy on anemia care, major adverse cardiovascular events, and mortality among adults undergoing hemodialysis. Clin J Am Soc Nephrol 17(6):851–860

Pecker LH, Timsar A, Pary PP, Denomme GA, Criss VR, Luban NL et al (2016) Unusual serological findings associated with ceftriaxone-induced immune hemolytic anemia in a child with disseminated low-grade glioma. Pediatr Blood Cancer 63(10):1852–1855

Petraro P, Duggan C, Urassa W, Msamanga G, Makubi A, Spiegelman D, Fawzi WW (2013) Determinants of anemia in postpartum HIV-negative women in Dar es Salaam, Tanzania. Eur J Clin Nutr 67(7):708–717

Prin M, Rui S, Pan S, Kadyaudzu C, Mehta PS, Li G, Charles A (2021) Anemia at intensive care unit admission and hospital mortality among patients at a referral Hospital in Malawi. Am Surg 87(8):1334–1340

Riessen R, Behmenburg M, Blumenstock G, Guenon D, Enkel S, Schäfer R, Haap M (2015) A simple "blood-saving bundle" reduces diagnostic blood loss and the transfusion rate in mechanically ventilated patients. PLoS One 10(9):e0138879

Salama A, Ahrens N, Kiesewetter H (2002) Serological and clinical aspects of autoimmune hemolytic anemias. Transfus Med Hemother 29(4):206–217

Shalby KY, Alradhi AY, Holdar SJ, Alghamdi AS, Alduilej SA, Albuainain S et al (2022) Extremes of anemia: the lowest hemoglobin values probably ever reported in the pediatric literature attributed to iron deficiency anemia. Am J Case Rep 23:e936252–e936251

Shander A, Javidroozi M, Ashton E (2011) Drug-induced anemia and other red cell disorders: a guide in the age of polypharmacy. Curr Clin Pharmacol 6(4):295–303

Shander A, Hardy JF, Ozawa S, Farmer SL, Hofmann A, Frank SM et al (2022) A global definition of patient blood management. Anesth Analg 135(3):476–488

Siegal DM, Belley-Côté EP, Lee SF, Hill S, D'Aragon F, Zarychanski R et al (2023) Small-volume blood collection tubes to reduce transfusions in intensive care: the STRATUS randomized clinical trial. JAMA 330(19):1872–1881

Spahn DR (2010) Anemia and patient blood management in hip and knee surgery: a systematic review of the literature. J Am Soc Anesthesiol 113(2):482–495

Spinelli E, Bartlett RH (2016) Anemia and transfusion in critical care: physiology and management. J Intensive Care Med 31(5):295–306

Tsubakihara Y, Nishi S, Akiba T, Hirakata H, Iseki K, Kubota M et al (2010) 2008 Japanese Society for Dialysis Therapy: guidelines for renal anemia in chronic kidney disease. Ther Apher Dial 14(3):240–275

Vincent JL, Baron JF, Reinhart K, Gattinoni L, Thijs L, Webb A et al (2002) Anemia and blood transfusion in critically ill patients. JAMA 288(12):1499–1507

Walter E, Carraretto M (2015) Drug-induced hyperthermia in critical care. J Intensive Care Soc 16(4):306–311

Warner MA, Shore-Lesserson L, Burns C (2023) From product to patient—transfusion and patient blood management. JAMA 330(19):1837–1838

Chapter 5
Leukopenia in ICU

Kaushik Paul

Learning Points

- *Neutropenia Classification*: Understanding the classification based on absolute neutrophil count (ANC) is critical for assessing infection risk and guiding management.
- *Causes of Leukopenia*: Identifying the broad spectrum of leukopenia causes, from drug reactions to bone marrow disorders, is essential for effective diagnosis and treatment.
- *Management Strategies*: Implementing appropriate management strategies, including G-CSF administration and strict infection prevention, can significantly improve outcomes.
- *Diagnosis and Treatment*: A thorough diagnostic approach, coupled with targeted treatment based on the underlying cause, is key to managing leukopenia in the ICU setting effectively.

5.1 Introduction

Leukopenia, recognized by diminished levels of white blood cells, plays a pivotal role as an indicator in intensive care units (ICUs) due to its correlation with heightened infection risks and adverse patient outcomes (Mark et al. 2023). A specific subset, neutropenia, defined by lower than normal neutrophil counts, stands out for its clinical significance in ICUs. Neutrophils are essential for combating infections, and their deficiency, stratified by absolute neutrophil count, heralds the potential for swift patient deterioration and complications such as sepsis (Weinkove et al. 2015).

K. Paul (✉)
Hemato-oncology and BMT, Saroj Gupta Cancer Centre and Research Institute, Kolkata, West Bengal, India

S. B. Mishra (ed.), *Critical Care Hematology*,
https://doi.org/10.1007/978-981-97-5565-3_5

Neutropenia not only presents a model for leukopenia management but also sheds light on individualized approaches for treating different white blood cell anomalies in critically ill patients (Martins and Maasdorp 2023).

The origins of neutropenia in the ICU cover a broad spectrum, from drug reactions to bone marrow infiltration by cancer. The management of neutropenia includes the application of granulocyte colony-stimulating factor (G-CSF) and strict infection prevention measures, adaptable for managing other leukopenia forms (Ostermann et al. 2013). Neutropenia has been identified as an independent risk factor for mortality in ICU patients with cancer, emphasizing the importance of understanding and managing this condition to improve patient care and outcomes in the ICU (Azoulay et al. 2015).

5.2 Etiology and Classification of Leucopenia

Leucopenia, characterized by a decreased number of white blood cells (leukocytes) in the blood, can significantly impact patient outcomes, especially in the intensive care unit (ICU) setting. Understanding the etiology and classification of leucopenia, particularly neutropenia, is essential for effective diagnosis and management. (Burton et al. 2006).

5.3 Classification of Neutropenia

Neutropenia, a common form of leucopenia, is primarily classified based on the absolute neutrophil count (ANC) in the blood, reflecting the body's capacity to combat infections. The classification integrates the widely accepted cutoff levels based on age, ethnic origin, and specific situations, emphasizing the importance of considering these factors in clinical practice.

- *Mild Neutropenia*: ANC ranging from 1000 to 1500/μL (1.0–1.5 × 10^9/L). Patients might not exhibit significant infection risks but require monitoring for potential decline in neutrophil count. For Caucasian adults, the threshold is extended up to 1.8 × 10^9/L according to the World Health Organization and the MDS/AML expert groups.
- *Moderate Neutropenia*: ANC between 500 and 1000/μL (0.5–1.0 × 10^9/L). In this range, the risk of infection increases, necessitating closer surveillance and sometimes prophylactic measures.
- *Severe Neutropenia*: ANC less than 500/μL (<0.5 × 10^9/L). Patients are at a high risk of serious infections, often requiring hospitalization, aggressive infection surveillance, and treatment strategies. The term "agranulocytosis" is reserved for severe neutropenias with ANC <0.2 × 10^9/L, associated with a high risk of severe, life-threatening infections.

5.4 Causes of Leucopenia

Leucopenia can arise from a myriad of causes, broadly categorized into congenital, acquired, immune-mediated, and infection-related origins (Khalil et al. 2018).

- *Congenital Causes*: Inherent genetic mutations can lead to conditions such as severe congenital neutropenia (Kostmann syndrome) or cyclic neutropenia, where neutropenia is present from birth and fluctuates over time, respectively.
- *Acquired Causes*: Factors such as chemotherapy, radiation therapy, and exposure to certain medications (e.g., antithyroid drugs, antipsychotics) can lead to acquired neutropenia. Nutritional deficiencies, particularly in B12, folate, and copper, also contribute to this category.
- *Drug-Induced Causes*: A variety of medications can cause neutropenia as a side effect. These include chemotherapeutic agents, anticonvulsants, and antibiotics like penicillin. Drug-induced neutropenia can result from direct bone marrow suppression or immune mechanisms leading to increased destruction of neutrophils.
- *Immune-Mediated Causes*: Autoimmune disorders, such as systemic lupus erythematosus (SLE) and rheumatoid arthritis, can lead to the development of autoantibodies against neutrophils, causing their destruction (Chamnanchanunt et al. 2021).
- *Infection-Related Causes*: Certain viral, bacterial, and parasitic infections can transiently or persistently reduce leukocyte counts through the direct infection of bone marrow cells or immune-mediated destruction. Common culprits include HIV, hepatitis viruses, and malaria (Scelfo et al. 2021).

5.5 Pathophysiology of Neutropenia

Neutropenia, a subset of leucopenia, involves a decrease in the absolute number of neutrophils in the blood, affecting the body's primary defense against infections (Gogri et al. 2023) Understanding the role of neutrophils in infection and immunity, along with the mechanisms leading to neutropenia, is crucial for comprehending its clinical implications.

Role of Neutrophils in Infection and Immunity

Neutrophils are pivotal components of the innate immune system, acting as the first line of defense against invading pathogens. They are capable of ingesting and killing microbes through various mechanisms, including phagocytosis, degranulation, and the formation of neutrophil extracellular traps (NETs). Neutrophils also modulate the immune response by producing cytokines and chemokines, which recruit and activate other immune cells. The efficiency of these processes determines the effectiveness of the body's response to infections (Roberts and Huang 2017).

Mechanisms Leading to Neutropenia

The development of neutropenia can be attributed to three primary mechanisms: reduced production, increased destruction, and abnormal distribution of neutrophils. Each mechanism has distinct pathophysiological underpinnings and clinical implications (Skokowa et al. 2017).

- *Reduced Production*: This occurs when the bone marrow fails to produce an adequate number of neutrophils. Causes can be intrinsic, such as genetic disorders affecting neutrophil production (e.g., severe congenital neutropenia), or extrinsic, such as chemotherapy or radiation therapy, which damages the bone marrow. Nutritional deficiencies and certain medications can also impair neutrophil production (Kyritsi et al. 2015).
- *Increased Destruction*: Autoimmune processes, drug reactions, and severe infections can lead to the premature destruction of neutrophils. In autoimmune neutropenia, the body produces antibodies against neutrophils, targeting them for destruction. Drug-induced neutropenia often involves immune mechanisms where drug-bound neutrophils are recognized as foreign and destroyed. Severe infections can consume neutrophils at a rate that outpaces the bone marrow's capacity to produce them (Diez-Feijóo et al. 2022; Gulino et al. 2004).
- *Abnormal Distribution*: Neutropenia can result from an abnormal sequestration or distribution of neutrophils within the body. For example, in conditions like hypersplenism, an enlarged spleen traps neutrophils, reducing their numbers in peripheral blood. This distribution issue can also be seen in certain infections or inflammatory states where neutrophils are marginated along the vascular endothelium, away from the circulating blood pool.

5.6 Clinical Manifestations of Neutropenia

Neutropenia, particularly when severe, can lead to various clinical manifestations primarily due to the compromised ability of the immune system to fight infections. The nature and severity of these manifestations can be influenced significantly by underlying diseases or conditions (Lee and Lee 2020).

Common Infections and Complications Associated with Severe Neutropenia

- *Bacterial Infections*: Patients with severe neutropenia are at a high risk for bacterial infections. These can manifest as skin infections, pneumonia, bacteremia, and sepsis. Common pathogens include *Staphylococcus aureus*, *Pseudomonas aeruginosa*, and various Gram-negative bacilli (Andrès et al. 2019).
- *Fungal Infections*: The risk for fungal infections increases, especially in persistently neutropenic patients. Invasive aspergillosis, candidiasis, and other fungal infections can present as serious complications, often challenging to diagnose and treat.

- *Oral Ulcerations and Gingivitis*: Neutropenic patients frequently suffer from oral complications, including painful ulcers, gingivitis, and periodontitis, which can lead to significant discomfort and secondary infections (Gomes et al. 2023).
- *Fever of Unknown Origin (FUO)*: Neutropenic fever, characterized by an elevated temperature without an immediately identifiable source, is a common and potentially serious condition, warranting prompt investigation and treatment.

Impact of Underlying Diseases and Conditions on Leucopenia Severity

- *Bone Marrow Disorders*: Conditions such as aplastic anemia, myelodysplastic syndromes, and leukemia directly affect the bone marrow's capacity to produce neutrophils, often leading to severe neutropenia and an increased risk of infections and complications.
- *Autoimmune Diseases*: Disorders like systemic lupus erythematosus (SLE) and rheumatoid arthritis can cause autoimmune neutropenia, where the severity of neutropenia can fluctuate with disease activity.
- *Chemotherapy and Radiation Therapy*: Cancer treatments can cause cytotoxic damage to the bone marrow, leading to acute or chronic neutropenia. The severity often correlates with the treatment's intensity and duration.
- *Nutritional Deficiencies*: Deficiencies in vitamins and minerals crucial for neutrophil production, such as vitamin B12, folate, and copper, can lead to varying degrees of neutropenia, compounded by the underlying nutritional status.
- *Infections*: Certain viral infections, notably HIV and hepatitis, can directly suppress bone marrow or cause immune-mediated destruction of neutrophils, influencing the severity and clinical course of neutropenia (Fig. 5.1).

5.7 Diagnosis of Neutropenia

The diagnostic framework for neutropenia integrates comprehensive assessment strategies aimed at elucidating the root causes, evaluating the severity, and shaping the management plan. This approach is grounded in an initial evaluation that combines detailed clinical history and physical examination with fundamental laboratory assessments. Subsequent diagnostic measures are tailored based on these preliminary insights to accurately diagnose specific causes of neutropenia (Adapted from Fioredda et al. 2023).

5.8 Initial Evaluation Strategy

5.8.1 Clinical History

A meticulously obtained clinical history is pivotal, offering essential insights into potential causes of neutropenia. This history should encompass inquiries regarding:

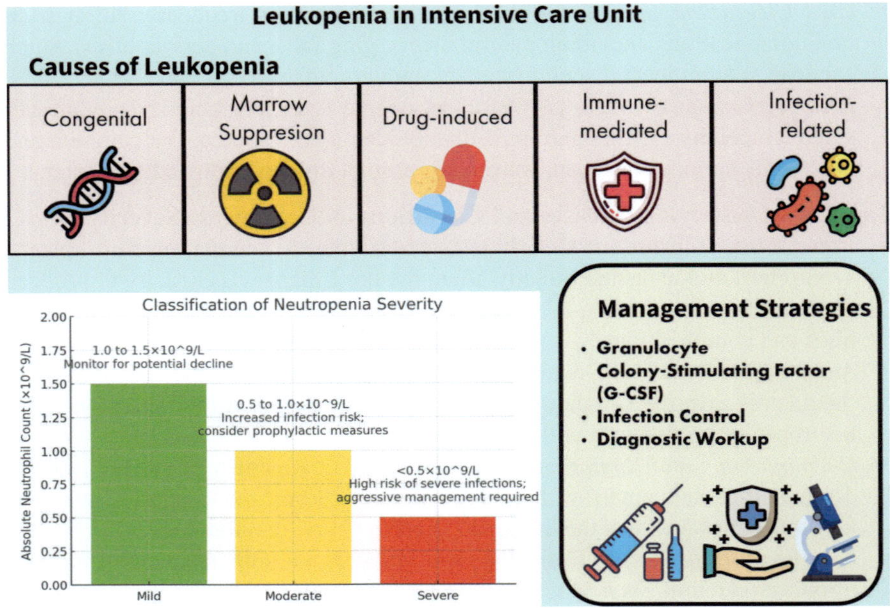

Fig. 5.1 Leukopenia in intensive care unit

- Recent infections or drug exposures, inclusive of chemotherapy, that could precipitate neutropenia.
- Familial instances of hematological conditions, which may suggest a genetic predisposition.
- Symptoms that could hint at autoimmune disorders or ongoing infections, contributing to neutropenia.

5.8.2 Physical Examination

The physical examination is crucial for detecting:

- Signs indicative of infection (e.g., oral ulcers, skin lesions), which could be related to or exacerbate neutropenia.
- Splenomegaly, a possible sign of hypersplenism contributing to neutropenia.
- Physical anomalies suggestive of congenital syndromes (e.g., stature discrepancies, developmental delays), which may be associated with neutropenia.

5.8.3 Laboratory Tests

Essential initial laboratory evaluations include:

- *Complete Blood Count (CBC) with Differential*: To calculate the absolute neutrophil count (ANC) and identify any associated hematologic abnormalities, such as anemia or thrombocytopenia.
- *Peripheral Blood Smear*: This test is instrumental in evaluating neutrophil morphology and detecting the presence of immature cells or dysplastic signs.
- *Basic Metabolic Panel*: Provides a general health overview and identifies potential contributors to neutropenia, such as liver or kidney dysfunction.

5.8.4 Advanced Diagnostics

Bone Marrow Evaluation

- *Bone Marrow Aspiration and Biopsy*: A critical step for assessing bone marrow functionality and structure. This diagnostic tool aids in distinguishing between neutrophil production deficits and increased destruction scenarios and may uncover marrow infiltration by malignancies or marrow failure syndromes.

Genetic Testing

- *Targeted Gene Panels*: Indispensable for the identification of congenital neutropenia forms. These panels are designed to detect mutations in specific genes like ELANE, G6PC3, or HAX1, associated with various forms of neutropenia.

Immune Assays

- *Direct Antiglobulin Test (DAT)*: Evaluates for the presence of antibodies directly bound to neutrophils, indicative of autoimmune neutropenia.
- *Indirect Antiglobulin Test*: Identifies antibodies against neutrophils circulating in plasma, significant for diagnosing autoimmune and drug-induced neutropenia.

Infectious Disease Screening

- *Focused Testing*: Based on clinical judgment and patient history, screening for HIV, hepatitis, and other pertinent infections is crucial for identifying infectious etiologies of neutropenia.

Nutritional Evaluations

- *Nutrient Level Assessments*: Evaluating levels of critical nutrients such as vitamin B12, folate, and copper can reveal nutritional deficiencies that might lead to neutropenia.

5.9 Treatment Approaches for Leucopenia in the ICU

Management of leucopenia, especially in the intensive care unit (ICU), requires a nuanced approach that addresses the underlying cause, prevents infections, and mitigates the risk of complications. Treatment strategies vary based on the etiology of leucopenia and the severity of neutropenia (Fioredda et al. 2023).

5.9.1 *General Management Strategies*

- *Infection Prevention and Control*: Implement strict infection control practices, including hand hygiene, use of protective barriers, and prophylactic antibiotics in cases of severe neutropenia or high infection risk.
- *Monitoring*: Close monitoring of complete blood count (CBC) and signs of infection. This includes regular temperature checks and surveillance for new or worsening symptoms.
- *Supportive Care*: Ensure adequate nutrition and hydration, manage comorbidities, and provide supportive treatment for any complications, such as transfusions for anemia or thrombocytopenia if needed.
- *Fever Management*: Immediate empirical antibiotic therapy is recommended for neutropenic patients with fever, as delays can lead to rapid deterioration.

5.9.2 *Specific Therapies Based on Underlying Cause*

- *Granulocyte Colony-Stimulating Factor (G-CSF)*: For neutropenia due to bone marrow suppression or congenital production defects, G-CSF stimulates the production of neutrophils and can reduce the duration of neutropenia. Examples include filgrastim and pegfilgrastim.
- *Withdrawal of Causative Agents*: If neutropenia is drug-induced, identifying and discontinuing the offending medication is crucial. Supportive care is provided while monitoring the recovery of neutrophil counts.
- *Treatment of Underlying Disease*: Addressing the root cause of neutropenia is fundamental.
  - For autoimmune neutropenia, treatments may include corticosteroids or immunosuppressants.
  - In cases of nutritional deficiencies, supplementation of the deficient nutrient (e.g., vitamin B12, folate) is necessary.
  - For infection-induced neutropenia, targeted antimicrobial therapy is essential.

- *Bone Marrow Transplant*: Considered for severe congenital neutropenias or cases where other treatments have failed, particularly if there is a progression to bone marrow failure syndromes or leukemia.
- *Genetic Therapies*: Emerging treatments for specific genetic causes of neutropenia, such as gene therapy, are under investigation and hold promise for the future.

5.9.3 Considerations in ICU Settings

In the ICU, where patients are at high risk for infections and complications, the approach to managing leucopenia must be aggressive and proactive. Collaboration among a multidisciplinary team including hematologists, infectious disease specialists, and ICU physicians is vital to ensure comprehensive care.

5.10 Prognosis and Complications of Leucopenia

Leucopenia, particularly in critical care settings such as the ICU, presents unique challenges in patient management, with the prognosis heavily influenced by the underlying cause, severity of the leukopenia, and the presence of comorbid conditions. Understanding the risk factors for adverse outcomes and vigilant monitoring for potential complications are key components of care (Vallot et al. 2003).

5.10.1 Risk Factors for Adverse Outcomes in Leucopenic Patients

- *Severity of Neutropenia*: Severe neutropenia (ANC < 500/μL) significantly increases the risk of infections, which can lead to sepsis and increased mortality.
- *Duration of Neutropenia*: Prolonged neutropenia poses a higher risk of developing serious infections, including fungal infections, which are harder to treat and can lead to worse outcomes.
- *Underlying Hematologic Disorders*: Patients with underlying bone marrow dysfunction or hematologic malignancies have a poorer prognosis due to the disease process itself and the complications of potential treatments.
- *Comorbid Conditions*: Existing comorbidities, such as diabetes, chronic renal failure, or chronic lung disease, can exacerbate the risk of infections and complicate the management of neutropenic patients.
- *Hospital-Acquired Infections*: ICU patients are at a higher risk for hospital-acquired infections, including multidrug-resistant organisms, which can significantly worsen the prognosis.

5.10.2 Monitoring for Transformation to More Severe Conditions

- *Myelodysplastic Syndromes (MDS) and Acute Myeloid Leukemia (AML)*: Patients with chronic neutropenia, especially those with congenital forms or associated with hematologic disorders, should be closely monitored for signs of transformation to MDS or AML. This includes regular complete blood counts (CBCs) and periodic bone marrow evaluations.
- *Morphological Changes in Blood and Bone Marrow*: Changes in cell morphology, appearance of blasts in peripheral blood, or evidence of dysplasia in the bone marrow warrant further investigation to rule out transformation.
- *Genetic and Molecular Monitoring*: Emerging technologies allow for the detection of molecular markers and genetic mutations that may predict the transformation to more severe conditions. Regular monitoring using these tools can provide early warning signs.

5.10.3 Complications

- *Infections*: The most immediate and serious complication of leucopenia is the increased susceptibility to bacterial, viral, and fungal infections. These infections can rapidly progress to sepsis and septic shock in neutropenic patients.
- *Drug Toxicity*: Treatment for leucopenia and its underlying causes can sometimes lead to drug toxicity, requiring careful monitoring and dose adjustments.
- *Graft-versus-Host Disease (GVHD)*: In cases where stem cell transplantation is used as treatment, GVHD is a potential complication that can affect various organs and tissues.
- *Quality of Life Impairments*: Chronic management of leucopenia, fear of infections, and hospital admissions can significantly impact patients' quality of life.

5.11 Conclusion

Managing leucopenia in the ICU setting is a complex challenge that necessitates a comprehensive and multifaceted approach. The key to effective management lies in early identification, understanding the underlying causes, and implementing appropriate therapeutic strategies while being vigilant for complications.

5.11.1 Future Directions in Research and Treatment

- *Genetic and Molecular Insights*: Advancements in genetic and molecular diagnostics hold promise for identifying individuals at risk of leucopenia and its complications, enabling targeted interventions and personalized medicine approaches.
- *Novel Therapeutics*: Research into new therapeutic agents and strategies, including immunomodulatory drugs and targeted therapies, is crucial for improving outcomes in patients with leucopenia. This includes exploring the role of stem cell therapy and gene editing technologies in congenital forms of neutropenia.
- *Improving Infection Control*: Ongoing research into vaccine development, antimicrobial stewardship, and infection prevention practices will play a critical role in safeguarding leucopenic patients from infectious complications.
- *Quality of Life Studies*: As treatments improve and patients live longer, research focusing on the quality of life, psychosocial impacts, and long-term outcomes of leucopenia patients will become increasingly important.

Flowchart

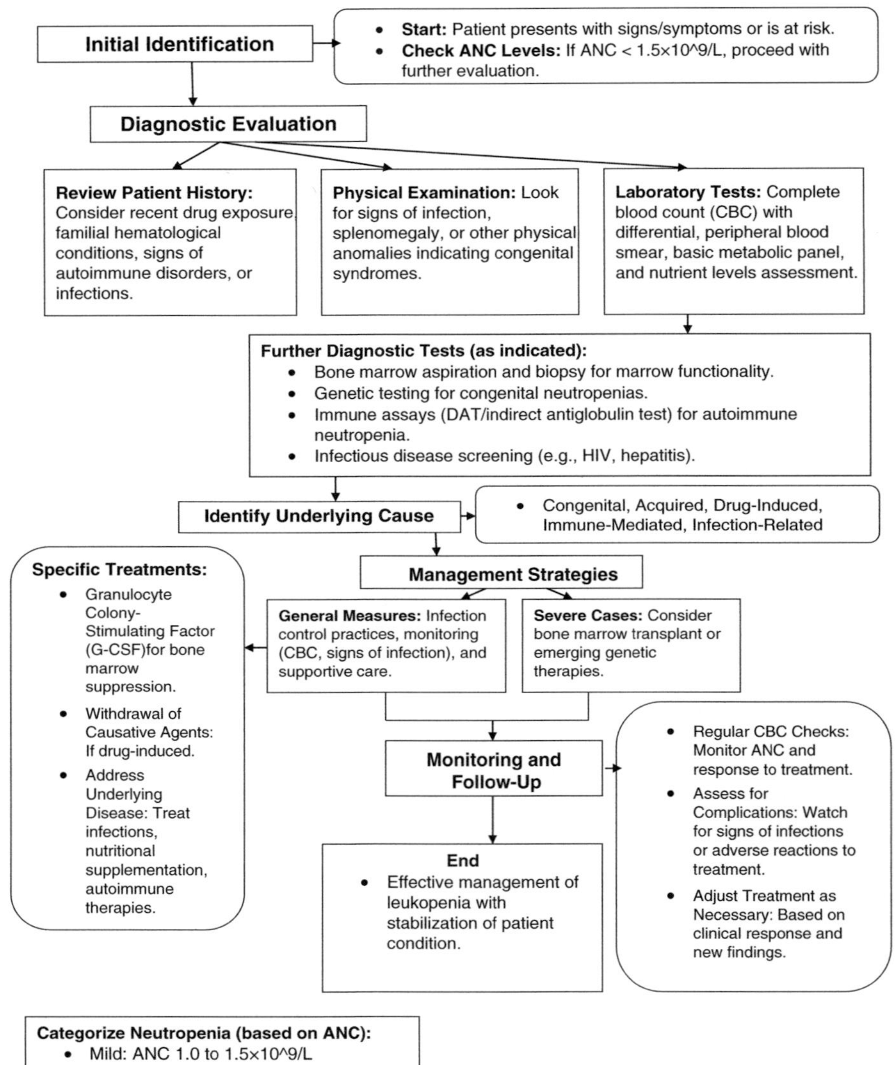
Initial Identification
Start: Patient presents with signs/symptoms or is at risk.
Check ANC Levels: If ANC < 1.5×10^9/L, proceed with further evaluation.
Diagnostic Evaluation
Review Patient History: Consider recent drug exposure, familial hematological conditions, signs of autoimmune disorders, or infections.
Physical Examination: Look for signs of infection, splenomegaly, or other physical anomalies indicating congenital syndromes.
Laboratory Tests: Complete blood count (CBC) with differential, peripheral blood smear, basic metabolic panel, and nutrient levels assessment.
Further Diagnostic Tests (as indicated):
Bone marrow aspiration and biopsy for marrow functionality.
Genetic testing for congenital neutropenias.
Immune assays (DAT/indirect antiglobulin test) for autoimmune neutropenia.
Infectious disease screening (e.g., HIV, hepatitis).
Identify Underlying Cause
Congenital, Acquired, Drug-Induced, Immune-Mediated, Infection-Related
Specific Treatments:
Granulocyte Colony-Stimulating Factor (G-CSF)for bone marrow suppression.
Withdrawal of Causative Agents: If drug-induced.
Address Underlying Disease: Treat infections, nutritional supplementation, autoimmune therapies.
Management Strategies
General Measures: Infection control practices, monitoring (CBC, signs of infection), and supportive care.
Severe Cases: Consider bone marrow transplant or emerging genetic therapies.
Monitoring and Follow-Up
Regular CBC Checks: Monitor ANC and response to treatment.
Assess for Complications: Watch for signs of infections or adverse reactions to treatment.
Adjust Treatment as Necessary: Based on clinical response and new findings.
End
Effective management of leukopenia with stabilization of patient condition.
Categorize Neutropenia (based on ANC):
Mild: ANC 1.0 to 1.5×10^9/L
Moderate: ANC 0.5 to 1.0×10^9/L
Severe: ANC < 0.5×10^9/L
Approach to Leukopenia in ICU Flowchart

References

Andrès E, Lorenzo Villalba N, Zulfiqar AA, Serraj K, Mourot-Cottet R, Gottenberg JE (2019) State of art of idiosyncratic drug-induced neutropenia or agranulocytosis, with a focus on biotherapies. J Clin Med 8(9):1351

Azoulay E, Pène F, Darmon M, Lengliné E, Benoit D, Soares M et al (2015) Managing critically ill hematology patients: time to think differently. Blood Rev 29(6):359–367

Burton CM, Andersen CB, Jensen AS, Iversen M, Milman N, Boesgaard S et al (2006) The incidence of acute cellular rejection after lung transplantation: a comparative study of anti-thymocyte globulin and daclizumab. J Heart Lung Transplant 25(6):638–647

Chamnanchanunt S, Thungthong P, Abdulkanan A, Nakhakes C (2021) False-positive nonstructural protein 1 antigen in a patient with philadelphia chromosome-positive acute lymphoblastic leukemia: A case report with literature review. Am J Case Rep 22:e928865–e928861

Diez-Feijóo R, Rodríguez-Sevilla JJ, Fernández-Rodríguez C, Colomo L (2022) Case Report: High Doses of Intravenous Immunoglobulins as a Successful Treatment for Late Onset Immune Agranulocytosis After Rituximab Plus Bendamustine. Front Immunol 12:798251

Fioredda F, Skokowa J, Tamary H, Spanoudakis M, Farruggia P, Almeida A et al (2023) The European guidelines on diagnosis and management of neutropenia in adults and children: a consensus between the European Hematology Association and the EuNet-INNOCHRON COST Action. Hemasphere 7(4):e872

Gogri H, Parihar M, Kulkarni S, Madkaikar M, Sharma J, Gorakshakar A (2023) Phenotyping and genotyping of HNA: prevalence, risk of alloimmunization, and HNA incompatibilities in Indians. Transfus Med Hemother 50(1):30–38

Gomes RFT, Klein M, Castelo EF, Carrard VC (2023) Generalized gingival necrosis in a patient under methimazole use. Spec Care Dentist 43(4):475–480

Gulino AV, Moratto D, Sozzani S, Cavadini P, Otero K, Tassone L et al (2004) Altered leukocyte response to CXCL12 in patients with warts hypogammaglobulinemia, infections, myelokathexis (WHIM) syndrome. Blood 104(2):444–452

Khalil MAM, Khalil MAU, Khan TFT, Tan J (2018) Drug-induced hematological cytopenia in kidney transplantation and the challenges it poses for kidney transplant physicians. J Transplant 2018:2018

Kyritsi EMA, Yiakoumis X, Pangalis GA, Pontikoglou C, Pyrovolaki K, Kalpadakis C et al (2015) High frequency of thyroid disorders in patients presenting with neutropenia to an outpatient hematology clinic STROBE-compliant article. Medicine 94(23):e886

Lee N, Lee BC (2020) Incidence of severe chronic neutropenia in South Korea and related clinical manifestations: a National Health Insurance Database Study. Medicina 56(6):262

Mark C, Gibson P, Lafay-Cousin L, Martin G, Oberoi S, Pecheux L et al (2023) Outcomes of coronavirus disease 2019 infection in children and adolescents with cancer in Canada: population-based study and systematic review. J Pediatr Hematol Oncol 45(6):e689–e694

Martins CDS, Maasdorp SD (2023) Outcomes of patients with haematological malignancies and febrile neutropenia at the Universitas Academic Hospital multidisciplinary intensive care unit, Free State Province, South Africa. Afr J Thorac Crit Care Med 29(1):18–23

Ostermann M, Raimundo M, Williams A, Whiteley C, Beale R (2013) Retrospective analysis of outcome of women with breast or gynaecological cancer in the intensive care unit. JRSM Short Rep 4(1):1–5

Roberts AW, Huang DCS (2017) Targeting BCL2 with BH3 mimetics: basic science and clinical application of venetoclax in chronic lymphocytic leukemia and related B cell malignancies. Clin Pharmacol Ther 101(1):89–98

Scelfo C, Menzella F, Fontana M, Ghidoni G, Galeone C, Facciolongo NC (2021) Pneumonia and invasive pneumococcal diseases: the role of pneumococcal conjugate vaccine in the era of multi-drug resistance. Vaccine 9(5):420

Skokowa J, Dale DC, Touw IP, Zeidler C, Welte K (2017) Severe congenital neutropenias. Nat Rev Dis Prim 3(1):1–18

Vallot F, Paesmans M, Berghmans T, Sculier JP (2003) Leucopenia is an independent predictor in cancer patients requiring invasive mechanical ventilation: a prognostic factor analysis in a series of 168 patients. Support Care Cancer 11:236–241

Weinkove R, Bailey M, Bellomo R, Saxena MK, Tam CS, Pilcher DV et al (2015) Association between early peak temperature and mortality in neutropenic sepsis. Ann Hematol 94:857–864

Chapter 6
Approach to Thrombocytopenia in ICU

Kalyani Rajesh Patil and Rajesh Bhagavan Patil

Learning Points

1. Diverse Causes and Mechanisms: Thrombocytopenia in the ICU setting arises from a complex interplay of factors, including pseudothrombocytopenia, dilutional effects, increased consumption, decreased production, and immune-mediated destruction of platelets.
2. Critical Role of Timely and Targeted Laboratory Investigations: Laboratory tests such as complete blood counts (CBC), peripheral smear examinations, and specific assays (e.g., for diagnosing HIT) are pivotal in confirming the cause of thrombocytopenia.
3. Association with Thrombosis: Despite being primarily associated with an increased risk of bleeding, thrombocytopenia can paradoxically coexist with or signal the presence of thrombotic conditions.
4. Algorithmic Approach to Diagnosis and Management: The chapter outlines a structured algorithm for approaching thrombocytopenia in ICU patients.

6.1 Introduction

Thrombocytopenia, often identified when platelet counts fall below 150 × 10^9/L, is a frequently observed blood disorder among patients in the intensive care unit (ICU). The initial prevalence of thrombocytopenia upon ICU admission in adults

---

K. R. Patil
Department of Pathology, Rajiv Gandhi Medical College & CSMH,
Thane, Maharashtra, India

R. B. Patil (✉)
Department of Bone Marrow Transplant, MCGM- CTC, PHO and BMT Center,
Mumbai, Maharashtra, India

S. B. Mishra (ed.), *Critical Care Hematology*,
https://doi.org/10.1007/978-981-97-5565-3_6

varies significantly, reported between 8.3% and 67.6%, depending on various factors. During their stay in the ICU, 14–44% of patients may develop thrombocytopenia. Such variability in figures can be attributed to the diverse patient demographics, the nature of the ICU (be it medical, surgical, or cardiac), and differing criteria for defining thrombocytopenia in numerous studies (Zarychanski and Houston 2017). Even though severe thrombocytopenia (with platelet counts ≤20 × 10^9/L) is linked to increased bleeding risk, even a moderate reduction in platelet count is associated with organ dysfunction and negative outcomes. The causes behind thrombocytopenia in ICU settings are typically complex, and addressing a single factor may not suffice to restore normal platelet levels (Thachil and Warkentin 2017). Pinpointing the precise cause is crucial for tailoring treatment strategies for each patient. Whereas platelet transfusions may benefit patients suffering from reduced platelet production or heightened destruction, they might prove harmful in cases involving augmented platelet activation within blood vessels (Greinacher and Selleng 2016).

6.2 Mechanisms of Thrombocytopenia (Thachil and Warkentin 2017; Greinacher and Selleng 2016)

Thrombocytopenia, a reduction in the platelet count below the normal range, has multiple mechanisms and associated causes. Pseudothrombocytopenia, a laboratory artifact often caused by the anticoagulant EDTA, can mimic true thrombocytopenia. Platelet counts may also be affected by hemodilution after massive blood transfusions. Actual consumption of platelets is a critical factor seen in various clinical conditions, including massive trauma, disseminated intravascular coagulation (DIC), sepsis, and hemophagocytic syndrome (HLH), as well as in patients undergoing extracorporeal circulation. Platelet sequestration, primarily in conditions of hepatosplenomegaly due to portal hypertension and hypersplenism, can also lower the circulating platelet count. Impaired production of platelets is another significant concern, occurring due to intoxicants like alcohol and drugs, infections (including HIV, HCV, EBV, CMV), nutritional deficiencies (B12, folate), bone marrow suppression from infiltrative diseases (leukemia, tumors), and treatment-related effects from radiotherapy and chemotherapy. Moreover, direct destruction of platelets is involved in immune-mediated conditions such as immune thrombocytopenia (ITP), drug-induced thrombocytopenia (from agents like ranitidine, beta-lactam antibiotics, vancomycin, and linezolid), heparin-induced thrombocytopenia (HIT), thrombotic microangiopathies including thrombotic thrombocytopenic purpura (TTP), hemolytic uremic syndrome (HUS), HELLP syndrome, and post-transfusion purpura (PTP).

DITP, Drug-induced immune thrombocytopenia; HIT, Heparin-induced thrombocytopenia; TMA, Thrombotic microangiopathy; TTP, Thrombotic thrombocytopenic purpura; HUS, Hemolytic uremic syndrome; HELLP, Hemolysis, Elevated liver enzymes, Low platelet count; PTP, Post transfusion purpura

6.3 Cause of Thrombocytopenia in ICU (Zarychanski and Houston 2017)

Clinical assessment of thrombocytopenia should systematically categorize causes based on their prevalence and the imperative of their recognition. Common causes like sepsis and DIC often have a well-established link with platelet depletion. Thrombocytopenia ensuing from platelet consumption is frequently observed in trauma, particularly with cardiopulmonary bypass as a complication of mechanical circulatory support devices like intra-aortic balloon pumps. Dilutional thrombocytopenia follows massive transfusions, while myelosuppressive chemotherapy typically leads to a decreased production of platelets. On the other side of the spectrum, less common but clinically significant causes such as HIT, HLH, and various thrombotic microangiopathies (TTP, HUS, HELLP syndrome), as well as conditions like post-transfusion purpura, demand vigilant consideration due to their potential severity. These less common causes can often be distinguished through careful clinical and laboratory evaluation, ensuring that they are not erroneously missed when more frequent etiologies are also present.

6.4 Approach to Thrombocytopenia in ICU

Identifying the root causes of thrombocytopenia is essential in the management of critically ill patients, given that treatment strategies vary greatly based on the specific condition at hand. Platelet transfusions may be beneficial for patients experiencing decreased platelet production or heightened platelet usage or destruction. However, such interventions could pose risks in cases of heparin-induced thrombocytopenia (HIT) or thrombotic thrombocytopenic purpura (TTP), and might also be contraindicated in certain thrombogenic variants of disseminated intravascular coagulation (DIC) (Greinacher and Selleng 2016).

Pointers to consider when evaluating thrombocytopenia are as follows: (Zarychanski and Houston 2017; Thachil and Warkentin 2017)

- Temporal pattern of thrombocytopenia
- Association with thrombosis
- Value of absolute platelet count
- If thrombocytopenia is associated with abnormal coagulation profile

1. *Time Frame for Development of Thrombocytopenia*: While evaluating thrombocytopenia in ICU, there are three time frames to consider (Zarychanski and Houston 2017).

    - *Past* (Zarychanski and Houston 2017).

    - The etiological investigation of thrombocytopenia in a critical care setting requires a thorough exploration of the patient's medical history. The framework for this assessment considers three primary facets: the context of ICU admission, any pre-existing conditions, and the patient's platelet counts before ICU admission. For example, the reason for ICU admission may offer clues, such as whether it was precipitated by catastrophic illnesses like TTP or HLH, or if it followed a major surgery or trauma accompanied by massive transfusion. Understanding pre-existing conditions—such as malignancies, liver disease, pregnancy, ITP, aplastic anemia, and leukemia—provides essential context that may explain the current platelet levels. Furthermore, knowledge of the baseline platelet counts before ICU admission can offer critical insights into the chronicity or acuity of the thrombocytopenia, influencing the direction of subsequent diagnostics and management.

- *Present* (Zarychanski and Houston 2017)
- The trajectory of a patient's platelet count during the ICU stay allows inferences about likely causes. Several distinct trajectories may be recognized.
- The clinical trajectory of thrombocytopenia can often be discerned by observing the pattern of platelet count changes over time, which may hint at underlying causes. A continuous low platelet count from the onset of critical illness suggests an independent cause of thrombocytopenia, such as marrow failure or hypersplenism. If the platelet count drops precipitously following an event like major surgery or a massive transfusion but then quickly recovers, the cause is likely dilutional or consumption-related. In contrast, a gradual decline following the initial days of ICU admission, with recovery only as the critical illness improves points toward secondary causes like sepsis or multisystem inflammatory illnesses. Should platelets decline and persist at low levels despite recovery from the primary condition, this could indicate a more insidious cause such as an iatrogenic factor. Lastly, a scenario where platelets fall within the first few days and remain low, in the context of persistent multiorgan failure, suggests a complex interplay of factors including sepsis, DIC, and potentially, hemophagocytic syndrome (HPS). Recognizing these temporal patterns is key in differentiating the etiologies of thrombocytopenia, thereby guiding appropriate and timely interventions.
- The usual time frame for the development of thrombocytopenia *in HIT is between 5 and 14 days* after the initiation of heparin therapy. For DITP, thrombocytopenia develops *7–14 days* after the new drug has been initiated. A rare but life-threatening cause for sudden onset thrombocytopenia and bleeding is PTP which develops *7–10* days following blood transfusion in some multiparous women (Greinacher and Selleng 2016)
- *Future Trajectory* (Zarychanski and Houston 2017)
- Determining the cause of thrombocytopenia enables the prediction of platelet count trends. When the platelet count aligns with the expected recovery trajectory, it can eliminate the need for further testing. On the other hand, if the count diverges from the forecasted path, prompt diagnostic and therapeutic measures can be strategically implemented.

2. *Association with Thrombosis* (Zarychanski and Houston 2017; Thachil and Warkentin 2017)

   Thrombocytopenia, although typically associated with bleeding risk, can paradoxically be associated with thrombosis in several pathological conditions. One well-documented instance is heparin-induced thrombocytopenia (HIT), wherein an immunologic response to heparin leads to a prothrombotic state despite decreased platelet counts. Catastrophic antiphospholipid syndrome (CAPS), another critical condition, is characterized by the presence of antiphospholipid antibodies that predispose patients to thrombosis, which can be venous or arterial, and often occurs concurrently with thrombocytopenia. In the setting of malignancies, a prothrombotic variant of disseminated intravascular coagulation (DIC) can arise, characterized by prominent clotting rather than bleeding, compounded by the malignancy's intrinsic hypercoagulable state.

   Ischemic liver injury is another context where thrombocytopenia coexists with thrombosis; the hepatic pathology often leads to both a reduced platelet count and a predisposition to clot formation. Additionally, massive clot thrombocytopenia, as seen in cases of pulmonary embolism, illustrates a state where major thrombotic events result in significant platelet consumption, leading to thrombocytopenia. The understanding of these associations is crucial, as the presence of thrombocytopenia in these disorders does not preclude thrombosis, and in fact, may be a marker of its occurrence, necessitating a nuanced approach to clinical management that balances the risks of bleeding with those of clotting.
3. *Severity of Thrombocytopenia* (Zarychanski and Houston 2017; Thachil and Warkentin 2017; Greinacher and Selleng 2016)

   - *Severe thrombocytopenia (< 20 × 10 ⁹/L)*

   - Severe thrombocytopenia, defined as a platelet count below 20 × 10^9/L, can be indicative of a variety of underlying conditions, each necessitating a different clinical approach. Immune thrombocytopenia (ITP) is an autoimmune disorder where antibodies target platelets, leading to their destruction and a consequent drop in platelet count. Drug-induced immune thrombocytopenia (DITP) shares a similar pathophysiology to ITP but is triggered by medication, resulting in the production of drug-dependent antibodies that cause platelet destruction. Post-transfusion purpura (PTP) is a rare but severe reaction following a transfusion, where an immune response against transfused platelets causes a rapid decline in the patient's platelet count.

   - Another condition associated with severe thrombocytopenia is hemophagocytic syndrome (HLH), a life-threatening immunological disorder characterized by the overactivation of immune cells, leading to phagocytosis of platelets among other blood cells. Furthermore, overt disseminated intravascular coagulation (DIC), typically secondary to an underlying condition such as sepsis or malignancy, can result in extensive platelet consumption due to the activation of the coagulation cascade. Marrow failure, whether due to the toxic effects of chemotherapy or infiltration by aggressive hematological neoplasms, also leads to a profound decrease in platelet production, causing severe thrombocytopenia. These conditions not only underline the complexity of differential diagnosis in thrombocytopenia but also highlight the need for urgent investigation and tailored treatment strategies to address the underlying cause and mitigate the risk of hemorrhage.

- In cases of heparin-induced thrombocytopenia (HIT), a notable reduction in platelet count by 50%, typically reaching a nadir of 20–80 × 10^9/L, is commonly observed. Conversely, in thrombotic microangiopathies (TMA), characteristics include hemolysis, a negative direct Coombs test, the presence of fragmented red cells on the blood smear, and a typical platelet count nadir of 10–30 × 10^9/L. TMAs are also associated with thrombotic complications alongside neurological symptoms (as seen in thrombotic thrombocytopenic purpura, TTP) or renal symptoms (as observed in hemolytic uremic syndrome, HUS), complications during pregnancy (like in HELLP syndrome), and elevated levels of lactate dehydrogenase (Greinacher and Selleng 2016).

Importance of Laboratory Investigations: Advising timely and appropriate laboratory investigations help confirm the underlying cause of thrombocytopenia.

1. *Complete Blood Counts (CBC)*

Thrombocytopenia with anemia is seen in hemolyticanemia like TMA, underlying bone marrow disorder like myelodysplasia and aplastic anemia.

Associated leucocytosis usually seen in sepsis, although in a few cases with sepsis, leucopenia is observed due to bone marrow suppression or hemophagocytosis. Leucocytosis with abnormal cells can be seen in leukemia.

2. *Peripheral Smear*

The utility of peripheral smear cannot be more emphasized than its role in arriving at the underlying diagnosis of thrombocytopenia. *Pseudo thrombocytopenia* should be ruled out in every patient by observing the peripheral smear for any platelet clumps or platelet satellitism. Also in all cases of thrombocytopenia, the estimation of manual platelet count on smear should be done as cell counters may sometimes show low count in cases of giant or large platelets. A careful review of the smear should be done for the presence of schistocytes to help diagnose clinicians with conditions like TTP and HUS. *Serial monitoring by quantifying schistocytes also needs to be done in these cases to assess the efficacy of treatment*. ICSH has given separate guidelines for the identification and quantification of schistocytes (Zini et al. 2012).

3. *Bone Marrow Examination*

Bone marrow examination is usually indicated wherein the underlying hematological condition is suspected. Bone marrow examination can also prove useful in the diagnosis of hemophagocytic syndrome.

4. *Diagnosis of Heparin-Induced Thrombocytopenia*

The diagnosis of HIT is primarily clinical as there is no test that can be performed with sufficient speed, sensitivity, and specificity. The laboratory tests should be performed after consideration of the clinical likelihood or pre-test probability for which a 4 T scoring system has been devised. There are antibody tests that lack sensitivity and specificity. For confirmation, either functional assay wherein platelet activation is detected or immunological tests which detect the presence of PF4-heparin dependent antibodies are detected can be performed (Laffan and Manning 2006).

6.5 Conclusion

In summary, understanding the context of the ICU admission, a detailed medical and drug history, careful physical examination, timing of onset of thrombocytopenia, and its association with thrombosis are crucial pointers for arriving at the underlying cause of thrombocytopenia. This information however has to be supported by appropriate laboratory tests like CBC, peripheral smear examination, coagulation studies, and cultures to confirm the diagnosis. Several different etiologies like sepsis and DIC need to be kept in mind when trying to establish the cause including not so common causes like HIT, HPS, DITP, and PTP. Pseudothrombocytopenia must be ruled out in every ICU patient having thrombocytopenia by a careful assessment of peripheral smear thus avoiding unnecessary interventions or platelet transfusions (Fig. 6.1).

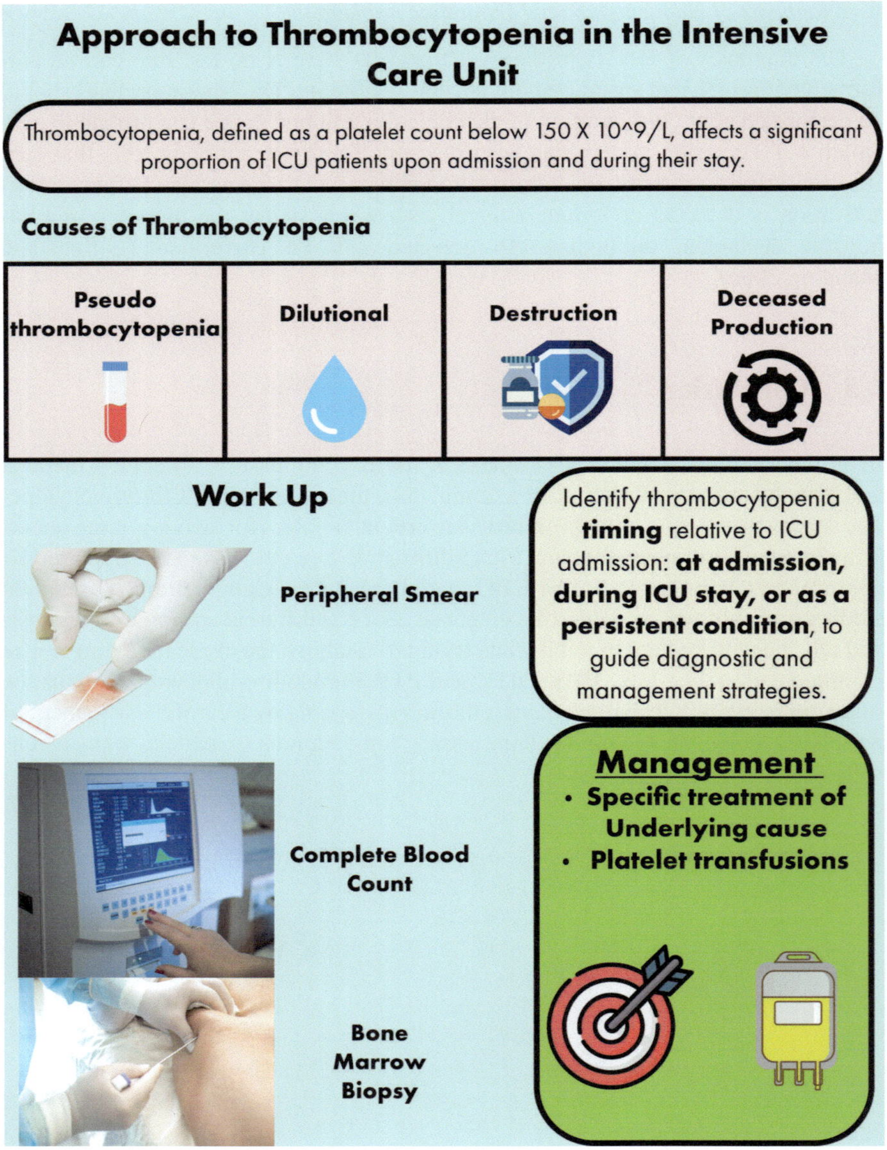

Approach to Thrombocytopenia in the Intensive Care Unit

Thrombocytopenia, defined as a platelet count below 150 X 10^9/L, affects a significant proportion of ICU patients upon admission and during their stay.

Causes of Thrombocytopenia

Pseudo thrombocytopenia	Dilutional	Destruction	Deceased Production

Work Up

Peripheral Smear

Complete Blood Count

Bone Marrow Biopsy

Identify thrombocytopenia **timing** relative to ICU admission: **at admission, during ICU stay, or as a persistent condition**, to guide diagnostic and management strategies.

Management

- **Specific treatment of Underlying cause**
- **Platelet transfusions**

Fig. 6.1 Approach to thrombocytopenia in the intensive care unit

Flowchart

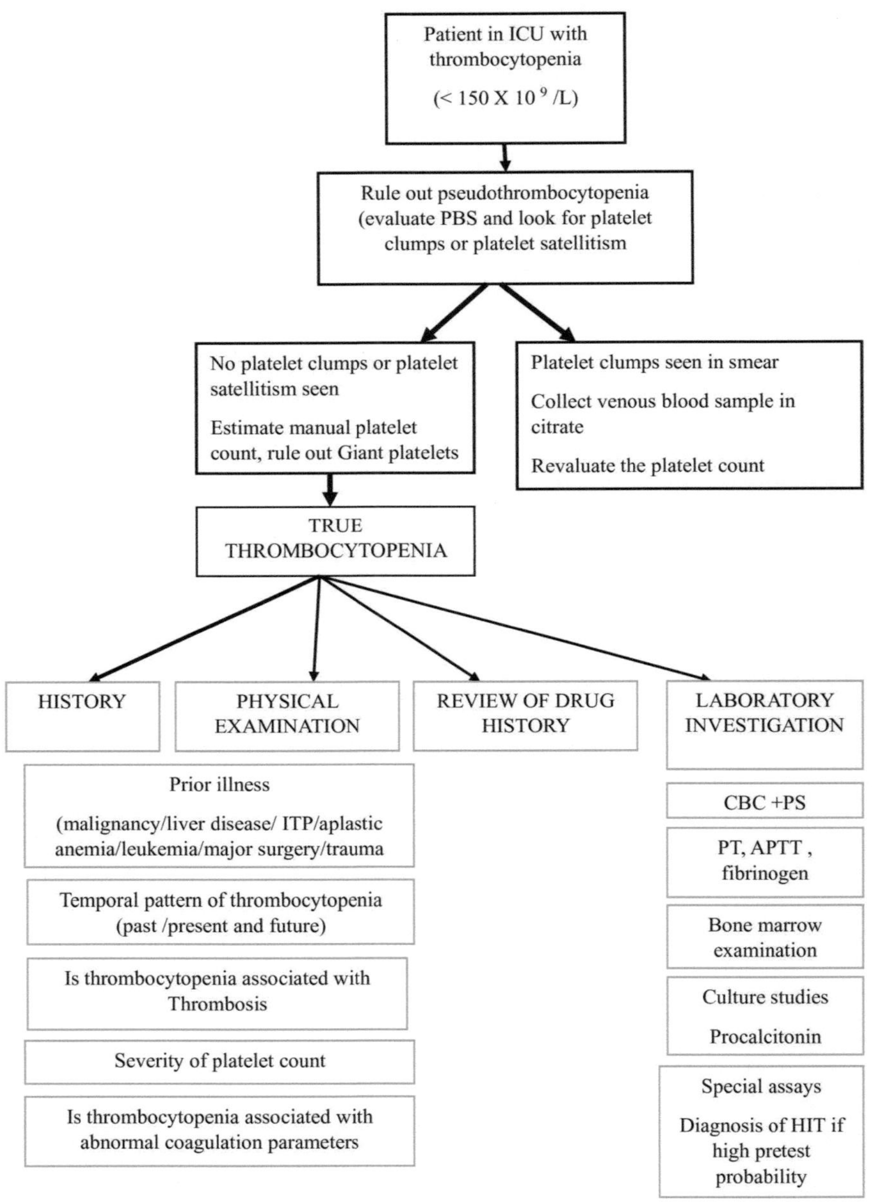
ALGORITHM FOR APPROACH TO THROMBOCYTOPENIA IN ICU
Patient in ICU with thrombocytopenia
(< 150 X 10 9 /L)
Rule out pseudothrombocytopenia (evaluate PBS and look for platelet clumps or platelet satellitism
No platelet clumps or platelet satellitism seen
Estimate manual platelet count, rule out Giant platelets
Platelet clumps seen in smear
Collect venous blood sample in citrate
Revaluate the platelet count
TRUE THROMBOCYTOPENIA
HISTORY
PHYSICAL EXAMINATION
REVIEW OF DRUG HISTORY
LABORATORY INVESTIGATION
Prior illness
(malignancy/liver disease/ ITP/aplastic anemia/leukemia/major surgery/trauma
Temporal pattern of thrombocytopenia (past /present and future)
Is thrombocytopenia associated with Thrombosis
Severity of platelet count
Is thrombocytopenia associated with abnormal coagulation parameters
CBC +PS
PT, APTT , fibrinogen
Bone marrow examination
Culture studies
Procalcitonin
Special assays
Diagnosis of HIT if high pretest probability

References

Greinacher A, Selleng S (2016) How I evaluate and treat thrombocytopenia in the intensive care unit patient. Blood 128(26):3032–3042

Laffan M, Manning R (2006) Chapter 18: Laboratory control of anticoagulant, thrombolytic, and antiplatelet therapy. In: Dacie and Lewis practical haematology, p 465

Thachil J, Warkentin TE (2017) How do we approach thrombocytopenia in critically ill patients? Br J Haematol 177(1):27–38

Zarychanski R, Houston DS (2017) Assessing thrombocytopenia in the intensive care unit: the past, present, and future. Hematology Am Soc Hematol Educ Program 2017(1):660–666

Zini G, d'Onofrio G, Briggs C, Erber W, Jou JM, Lee SH et al (2012) ICSH recommendations for identification, diagnostic value, and quantitation of schistocytes. Int J Lab Hematol 34(2):107–116

Chapter 7
Pediatric Hemolysis

Annapoorani Ramasamy and Anitha Veerachamy

Learning Points

1. Understanding Hemolysis Types and Diagnosis: Gain insight into the distinction between intravascular and extravascular hemolysis, the significance of laboratory values like reticulocyte count and indirect bilirubin, and the diagnostic criteria used to identify different types of hemolytic anemia in children.
2. Management of Autoimmune Hemolytic Anemia (AIHA): Learn about the approaches to managing AIHA, including using steroids, immunoglobulins, and plasmapheresis, and the importance of recognizing and treating this condition early to avoid severe complications.
3. Role of G6PD Deficiency in Pediatric Hemolysis: Understand how G6PD deficiency triggers hemolysis, the environmental and pharmacological factors that can exacerbate this condition, and safe practices for managing affected individuals.
4. Thrombotic Microangiopathy (TMA) in Pediatrics: Explore the pathophysiology, diagnostic criteria, and treatment strategies for TMA, including the critical roles of plasmapheresis and renal replacement therapy in severe cases.

7.1 Introduction

Hemolysis is the premature destruction of red blood cells (RBC) resulting in anemia, high indirect bilirubin, and high reticulocytes due to increased erythropoiesis secondary to anemia (Hill and Hill 2018). It can be either extravascular or intravascular (Table 7.1).

A. Ramasamy (✉) · A. Veerachamy
Department of Pediatric Hematology and Oncology, Meenakshi Mission Hospital and Research Centre, Madurai, Tamil Nadu, India

S. B. Mishra (ed.), *Critical Care Hematology*,
https://doi.org/10.1007/978-981-97-5565-3_7

Table 7.1 Distinction of intravascular and extravascular RBC destruction

	Extravascular hemolysis	Intravascular hemolysis
Site of destruction	Macrophages in the liver and spleen	Complement mediated intravascular
Presentation	Subacute and chronic	Acute episodic
Organomegaly	Likely	Less likely
Lab evidence		
Plasma/serum		
Plasma-free hemoglobin	Absent	High
Serum haptoglobin	Normal	Low/absent
Serum hemopexin	Normal	Low/absent
Methemoglobin	Normal	High
Unconjugated bilirubin	High	High
LDH	High	Very high
Reticulocytes	High	High
Urine		
Hemoglobinuria (urine dipstick positive for blood but no RBCs in microscopy)	Absent	Present
Hemosiderin	Normal	High
Urobilinogen	High	High

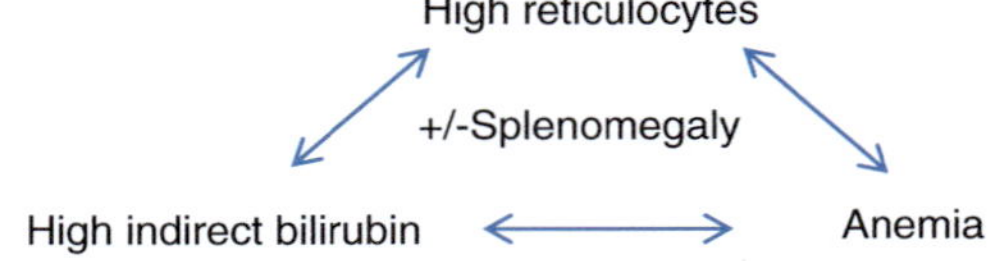

- Spurious leukocytosis in a patient with hemolysis and high reticulocytes

$$\text{Corrected WBC} = \text{Total WBC X100} / (\text{nRBC per 100 WBC} + 100)$$

- Absolute reticulocyte count (50000–1 lakh) = reticulocyte % x RBC count (10^6/mm^3)
- Reticulocytopenia in AIHA
  - During the early week of presentation
  - associated Parvo virus B19 infection
  - Vitamin B12 deficiency
  - Marrow infiltrative disease
- Normal or high haptoglobin in AIHA during acute phase reaction
- Haptoglobin can be low in severe liver disease and H° variant of haptoglobin

Various causes of hemolytic anemia are listed in Table 7.2.

Table 7.2 Causes of hemolytic anemia (common causes are highlighted) (Voulgaridou and Kalfa 2021)

I. Intrinsic RBC defect	
1. Red cell membrane disorders	**Hereditary spherocytosis** Hereditary elliptocytosis, pyropoikilocytosis, and related disorders Stomatocytosis syndromes Xerostomia Hydrocytosis Rh null syndrome GLUT1 deficiency Tangier disease Abetalipoproteinemia Phytosterolemia
2. Red cell enzymopathies	Deficiency of **Glucose 6 phosphate dehydrogenase (G6PD)** **Pyruvate kinase (PK)** Hexokinase, glucose phosphate isomerase Phosphofructokinase Triosephosphate kinase Phosphoglycerate kinase Aldolase Glutathione metabolism 5′ Nucleotidase
3. Hemoglobinopathies	Alpha thalassaemias **Beta thalassaemias** **Sickle cell disease** Unstable hemoglobins or hemoglobin variants
II. Immune hemolysis	**Autoimmune hemolytic anemia** (primary and secondary) Alloimmune hemolytic anemia

(continued)

Table 7.2 (continued)

III. Nonimmune hemolysis	Primary thrombotic microangiopathy (TMA) Infections Complicated malaria Clostridia *Haemophilus influenza* B Babesiosis Severe sepsis and DIC Envenomation—spider and snake venoms Toxins—arsenic, lead, and copper Drugs Congenital dyserythropoietic anemia Systemic disorders HELLP syndrome Malignancy (lymphoma) Malignant hypertension Burns End stage liver disease PNH Capillary hemangioma Kassabach Merit syndrome, renal artery stenosis, severe aortic coarctation, large vessel thrombus, vasculitis, TIPS, dysfunctional cardiac valves, or cardiac assist devices Others Drowning, March hemoglobinuria, ECMO, cardiac bypass

PNH Paroxysmal Nocturnal Hemoglobinuria, *HELLP* Hemolysis Elevated Liver enzymes and Low platelets, *DIC* disseminated intravascular hemolysis, *ECMO* Extracorporeal Membrane Oxygenation, *TIPS* Transjugular Intrahepatic portosystemic Shunt, *APLA* AntiPhosphoLipid Antibody

7.2 G6PD Deficiency

X-linked deficiency affects >400 million people worldwide. The global distribution of G6PD deficiency disorder parallels that of malaria. Over 140 mutations have been described in the gene responsible for the synthesis of the G6PD protein in the X chromosome. Hence, the clinical picture in females is a rare exception in the case of the Lyon Beutler hypothesis of inactivation of the X chromosome.

7.2.1 *Clinical Picture*

Most individuals with G6PD deficiency are asymptomatic, unless triggered. Infection, stress, and oxidants (drugs, toxins, and food) increase oxidant damage to G6PD-deficient RBCs producing intracellular heme precipitates (Heinz bodies) that cause damage to the RBC membrane and intravascular hemolysis. The degree of hemolysis varies with the inciting agent, amount ingested, and severity of the enzyme deficiency. The list of drugs and chemicals upon ingestion that can lead to oxidant damage and hemolysis in G6PD individuals are mentioned in Table 7.3 (Voulgaridou and Kalfa 2021).

1. Pathological neonatal jaundice and kernicterus
2. Asymptomatic unless triggered
3. Acute intravascular hemolysis within 24–48 h of exposure to oxidant trigger—sudden onset fatigue, pallor, jaundice, abdomen pain and vomiting, dark urine
4. Chronic nonspherocytic hemolytic anemia

7.2.2 Diagnosis

1. Evidence of acute intravascular hemolysis
2. Peripheral smear (Fig. 7.1): Bite cells and polychromatic reticulocytes. Unstained or supravital preparations of RBCs reveal Heinz bodies
3. G6PD enzyme activity or enzyme level
4. G6PD enzyme variants are identified by electrophoretic and molecular analysis

The defect is accentuated in the G6PD A variant as the RBCs age. The age-labile enzyme is abundant and more stable in younger RBCs. Hence, G6PD enzyme activity or level can be normal during acute episodes. On high suspicion, G6PD level has to be repeated after recovery from illness (Voulgaridou and Kalfa 2021).

Table 7.3 Common medications that predispose hemolysis and hence to be avoided or used with caution in patients with G6PD deficiency

Antibacterials	**Chemicals**
Sulfonamides Trimethoprim-sulfamethoxazole Dapsone Quinolones Nitrofurantoin Nalidixic acid Chloramphenicol	Phenylhydrazine Benzene Naphthalene (moth balls) 2,4,6-trinitrotoluene
Antimalarial	Others
Primaquine Pamaquine Chloroquine Quinacrine	Acetaminophen Acetanilide Vitamin K analogs Methylene blue, toluidine blue Probenecid Dimercaprol Acetylsalicylic acid Phenazopyridine Rasburicase L DOPA Glyburide Diphenhydramine Colchicine
Anthelminthics	
Beta naphthol Stibophen Niridazole	

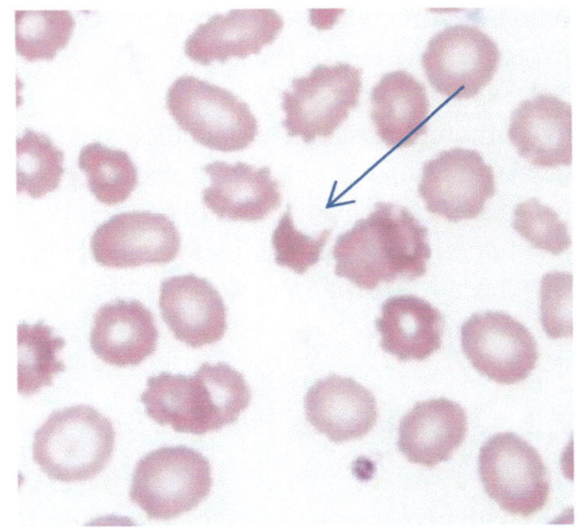

Fig. 7.1 Peripheral smear in G6PD-deficient hemolysis. Note the fragmented cell (blue arrow) that has been amputated, leaving a straight border with sharp angulated edges. These are also called "bite cells" as the semi-circular indent on the edge of their membrane gives the appearance of a bite being taken out of the cell

7.2.3 Treatment

If severe, supportive therapy may require blood transfusions, although recovery is the rule when the oxidant agent is discontinued.

7.2.4 Differential Diagnosis

- Hemolytic disease of the newborn
- Autoimmune hemolytic anemia
- Unstable hemoglobins
- Pyruvate kinase deficiency

7.3 Autoimmune Hemolytic Anemia (AIHA)

AIHA is the premature destruction of RBCs secondary to autoantibodies against red cell antigens. It is usually associated with the positive Direct Antibody Test (DAT). Evans syndrome is seen in about 30% of AIHA, wherein there is concurrent immune cytopenia of at least two cell lineages either autoimmune neutropenia (AIN) or immune thrombocytopenia (ITP). The first episode of AIHA generally presents as an acute fulminant and life-threatening event with <5% mortality. Patients present with symptoms of acute onset, rapid progressing, and severe anemia. Dark urine is common. Arterial and venous thrombosis are seen in up to 25% of patients, especially with acute severe intravascular hemolysis.

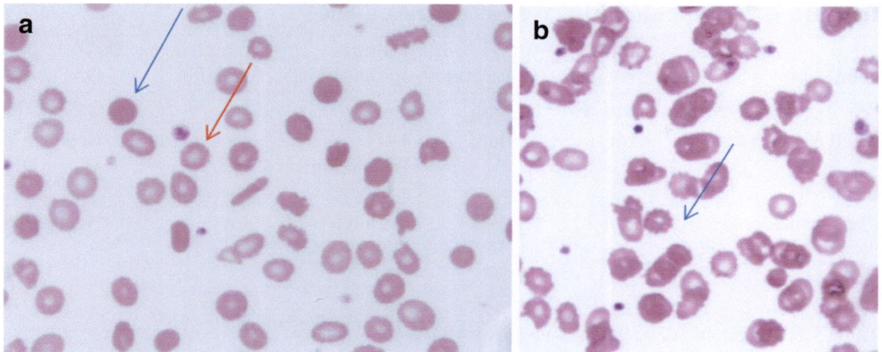

Fig. 7.2 Peripheral smear in AIHA. (**a**) Spherocytes are spherical RBCs without central pallor (blue arrow). Note that they are smaller than normal red blood cells (red arrow). (**b**) Agglutination of blood cells is evidenced by variable-sized clumps of RBCs (blue arrow)

7.3.1 Pathophysiology

The antibodies bind to RBC membrane antigens at 37 °C and are typically IgG; IgA and monomeric IgM are rare. The antibody-coated RBCs are phagocytosed by splenic macrophages via Fcγ receptors. When the antibodies binding the RBCs have a high affinity for complement, they trigger the complement cascade and they are phagocytosed by the liver macrophages via C3 receptors. Complement activation can result in intravascular hemolysis via membrane attack complex (C5b–C9). Peripheral smear (Fig. 7.2) has spherocytes and agglutination (Loirat et al. 2016).

7.3.2 Various Forms of AIHA

Once DAT is positive with polyspecific sera, then proceed with monospecific reagents to identify IgG or C3d. Laboratory features of various forms of AIHA are noted in Table 7.4.

DAT can be negative in 10% of AIHA. The "Extended Coomb's test," available in reference laboratories, provides a higher DAT positivity rate, in case of negative DAT and high clinical suspicion of AIHA. Further work-up for DAT-negative AIHA is shown in Table 7.5.

wAIHA being the common variant, other forms of AIHA also need mention in their presentation and management as shown in Table 7.6.

About 40% of AIHA is primary or idiopathic. Hence, a majority of the patients can have underlying disorders predisposing to AIHA as listed in Table 7.7.

Table 7.4 Laboratory characteristics of various forms of AIHA

Clinical form	Antibody specificity	Ig class	Thermal optimum (°C)	Complement activation	DAT
Warm AIHA (wAIHA)	Anti-rh	IgG	34–37	−/+	IgG ± C3d
Cold AIHA (CAD/ CAS)	Anti-I/i	IgM	4–27 Wide thermal amplitude	+++	Neg or c3d +
Paroxysmal cold hemoglobinuria (PCH)	Anti-P	IgG Biphasic	Fixation 4–27 Lysis 34–37	+++	Neg or c3d +

Table 7.5 Further workup for DAT-negative AIHA

	Test	Titer	Diagnosis
Negative DAT	Monospecific DAT for IgM, IgG, IgA, and c3d		Based on Ig subclass
DAT c3d ± IgG	DAggT Saline-suspended red cells with patient serum incubated at room temperature for 30–60 min	>64 at 4 °C <64	CAD Insignificant CAD
DAT c3d ± IgG DAggT negative Insignificant CAD	Donath Landsteiner antibody		PCH

Table 7.6 Clinical characteristics of various forms of AIHA

Clinical form and frequency	Site of hemolysis	Onset of illness	Etiology	Course	Treatment
wAIHA 60–70%	Extravascular	Acute fulminant	Idiopathic	Can be life threatening; Response to medications	Immunosuppressants
CAS/ CAD 20–25%	Extra and intravascular	Subacute	Post infectious, Lymphoproliferative disease	Symptoms of cold exposure; Self-limiting illness	Supportive Antimicrobials Avoid cold exposure
PCH 5–10%	Intravascular	Acute Fulminant	Post infectious	Transient	Supportive Antimicrobials Avoid cold exposure
Mixed AIHA < 5%	Extra and intravascular	Acute	Idiopathic Post infectious	Acute fulminant	Immunosuppressants

Table 7.7 Causes for secondary AIHA

Immune-mediated disease	Systemic lupus erythematosus
Inborn error of immunity (IEI)	Common variable Immunodeficiency (CVID) Severe combined ImmunoDeficiency (SCID) Wiskott Aldrich syndrome (WAS) Autoimmune lymphoproliferative syndrome (ALPS) and ALPS like disorders
Infections	**Viral** HIV, hepatitis A, B, and C EBV, CMV, and herpes viruses Parvo virus, rubella, and measles Influenza and SARS COV2 **Bacterial** *Mycoplasma, Hemophilus influenza, Brucella, Clostridium difficile* **Parasites**—visceral Leishmaniasis
Malignancy	Lymphoma, leukemia, myelodysplasia
Hematopoietic stem cell transplantation recipients	Lymphocyte passenger syndrome ABO incompatibility Viral infections EBV-related lymphoproliferative disease
Drug induced Indirect coombs positive Antibody in RBC eluate	**Antimicrobials** Penicillins, Cephalosporins, Chlorambucil, Etarnecept **Chemotherapy** Purine nucleoside analogs: Fludarabine, Cladarabine, Pentostatin Bendamustine, Lenalidomide **Monoclonal antibody** Eculizumab, Efazulimab **Check point inhibitors** **Others** Acetaminophen, ibuprofen, α methyl DOPA, interferon α

7.3.3 Differential Diagnosis

1. TMA
2. Post transfusion-related acute or delayed hemolytic reactions
3. Paroxysmal nocturnal hemoglobinuria (PNH)

7.3.4 Management

It requires prompt diagnosis, initiation of treatment, and close monitoring. Primary and secondary sets of investigations are listed in Table 7.8 (Loirat et al. 2016).

Table 7.8 Investigations

Emergency set of investigations	1. Complete hemogram, peripheral smear (spherocytes, polychromasia, and agglutination) 2. Reticulocyte count[a], LDH, liver, and renal function test 3. Direct and indirect Coombs test 4. Blood grouping, typing, and cross matching
Second set of investigations	Serum haptoglobin and hemopexin Urine hemoglobin and hemosiderin Viral markers: HIV, HBV, HCV
Based on suspicion of underlying disorders	ANA profile Immunoglobulin levels Lymphocyte subset analysis Double negative T-cell subset ALPS or PID gene panel

[a]Reticulocytes can be low in case of an immune attack on late erythroid precursors and reflect a severe form of the disease

7.3.5 *Treatment*

The main goal of treatment is to improve the hemoglobin level by reducing hemolysis and hence prevent cardiac compromise (Loirat et al. 2016).

1. Patient has to be supported with oxygen and strict bed rest.
2. Continuous hemodynamic and fluid monitoring in a pediatric intensive care unit.
3. Steroids.

   Methylprednisolone is the emergent drug of choice in wAIHA. The dose range of 2– 6 mg/kg/day in 8–12 hourly is given. Megadose of up to 30 mg/kg/day has been used. The response is apparent in 24–72 h of steroid initiation in up to 80% of cases. After 3–5 days of a pulse course of steroids and once the general condition is better, oral prednisolone is initiated at a dose of 1 mg/kg/day.
4. Blood transfusion.

   Warranted only in symptomatic, rapid progressing, and life-threatening anemia. Close interaction between the hematologist and blood bank technicians is required. Packed red cell transfusion has to be given under close hemodynamic monitoring.

   (i) In case of emergency transfusion—provide O-negative blood group
   (ii) With limited possible time—provide ABO, Rh(CDE), and K matched (if possible JK and FY matching)
   (iii) In case of IAT positive—do autoadsorption or alloadsorption (previously transfused) techniques and then provide ABO and Rh-compatible blood (JK, FY matching if possible)

5. In case of nonresponse to steroids and requiring multiple transfusions even after 48–72 h of initiation of steroids, immunoglobulin (IVIg) at 1gm/kg/day for 2 days is recommended.
6. Plasmapheresis is the case of inadequate response to the above measures.
7. Rituximab (anti-CD20 chimeric antibody), second-line immunosuppressive agents, and splenectomy are further therapy options in case of steroid-refractory or steroid-dependent AIHA.

7.4 Thrombotic Microangiopathies (TMA)

TMA includes features of MicroAngiopathic hemolytic anemia (MAHA), thrombocytopenia, and microvascular thrombosis resulting in end organ damage, especially acute kidney injury. Laboratory confirmation of TMA includes the evidence of intravascular hemolysis (high reticulocyte, high LDH, low serum haptoglobin, hemoglobinuria), indirect hyperbilirubinemia, and schistocytes in peripheral smear (Fig. 7.3) with negative DAT. TMA can be due to genetic mutations in various genes or secondary to multiple systemic disorders as listed in Table 7.9.

Upon diagnosis of TMA, while investigating for the cause, immediate plasmapheresis is warranted. Renal replacement therapy is required in case of acute renal failure and oliguria. Rule out associated infections, disease (autoimmune, malignancy, post transplantation status), and drugs causing TMA. aHUS is likely when

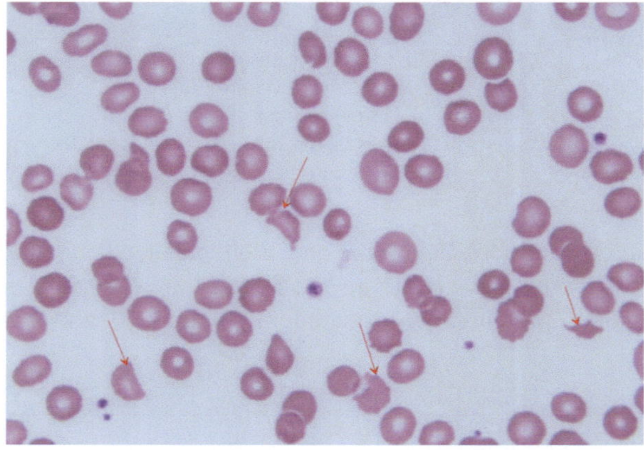

Fig. 7.3 Peripheral smear in TMA. Schistocytes (red arrow) are fragmented red blood cells suggesting red blood cell injury from damaged endothelium and is a characteristic feature of microangiopathichemolyticanemia

Table 7.9 Various causes of TMA

Thrombotic thrombocytopenic purpura (TTP) ADAMTS13 < 10%	1. Congenital ADAMTS13 deficiency cTTP 2. Auto-immune ADAMTS13 deficiency iTTP
Hemolytic uremic syndromes (HUS)	1. Infection associated Shiga toxin producing *E.* Coli—STEC HUS *Shigella dysenteriae* *Strep. pneumonia* Clostridia, *H. influenza*, Babesiosis Viral infections—Influenza, HIV, EBV, etc. 2. Cobalamin C defect 3. Atypical HUS–aHUS (i) DGKε defect (ii) THBD, PLG gene defect iii) Complement-mediated HUS Complement gene mutation in CFH, CFI, CFB, MCP,C3, CD46, etc. anti-CFH antibody (iv) HUS without identified complement or DGKε defect
TMA associated with coexisting disease/condition	Autoimmune disease—SLE, APLA syndrome, vasculitis syndromes, scleroderma renal crisis Sepsis/DIC Hepatitis B post vaccination status Malignancy Bone marrow or solid organ transplantation Drugs Chemotherapy Calcineurin inhibitor mTOR inhibitor Ticlopidine, quinine Malignant hypertension Kasabach Meritt syndrome Renal artery stenosis Large vessel thrombi HELLP syndrome

there is high creatinine (>2.26 mg/dl) and high platelet count (>30 x10^9/L) as opposed to TTP, wherein low creatinine and platelets are observed. Further workup and treatment for TMA are consolidated in Table 7.10 and Fig. 7.4 (Loirat et al. 2016).

Table 7.10 Workup and management

	Etiology	Investigations	Management
1.	STEC HUS	Stool or rectal swab culture RT PCR for STX genes Serum anti-lipopolysaccharides antibodies	Supportive care Renal replacement therapy ± Plasma exchange
2.	*S. pneumoniae* HUS	Bacterial culture (blood, pleural fluid or CSF) *S. pneumoniae* soluble polysaccharide antigen (urine/CSF) 16 s ribosomal RNA (PCR) (pleural fluid /CSF)	
3.	Influenza	Influenza A culture, antigen detection, PCR (nasopharyngeal swab) or serology	
4.	Cobalamine defect	Megaloblastic anemia Plasma:High homocysteine, low methionine levels Plasma/urine: High methyl-malonic acid. Diagnosis confirmed by gene sequencing	Parenteral hydroxocobalamin, betaine, carnitine supplements, and leucovorin calcium
5.	TTP	Plasma ADAMTS13 activity Anti-ADAMTS13 antibodies Gene sequencing	cTTP Plasma therapy rADAMTS13 replacement Immune TTP Plasma exchange Immunosuppressants
6.	aHUS	Serum Complement levels Anti CFH antibodies Gene sequencing and MLPA	Plasma exchange until diagnosis established Immunosuppressants Anti-C5 therapy (Eculizumab) Anti-CD20 therapy (Rituximab) Antibiotic prophylaxis Vaccination Liver transplantation

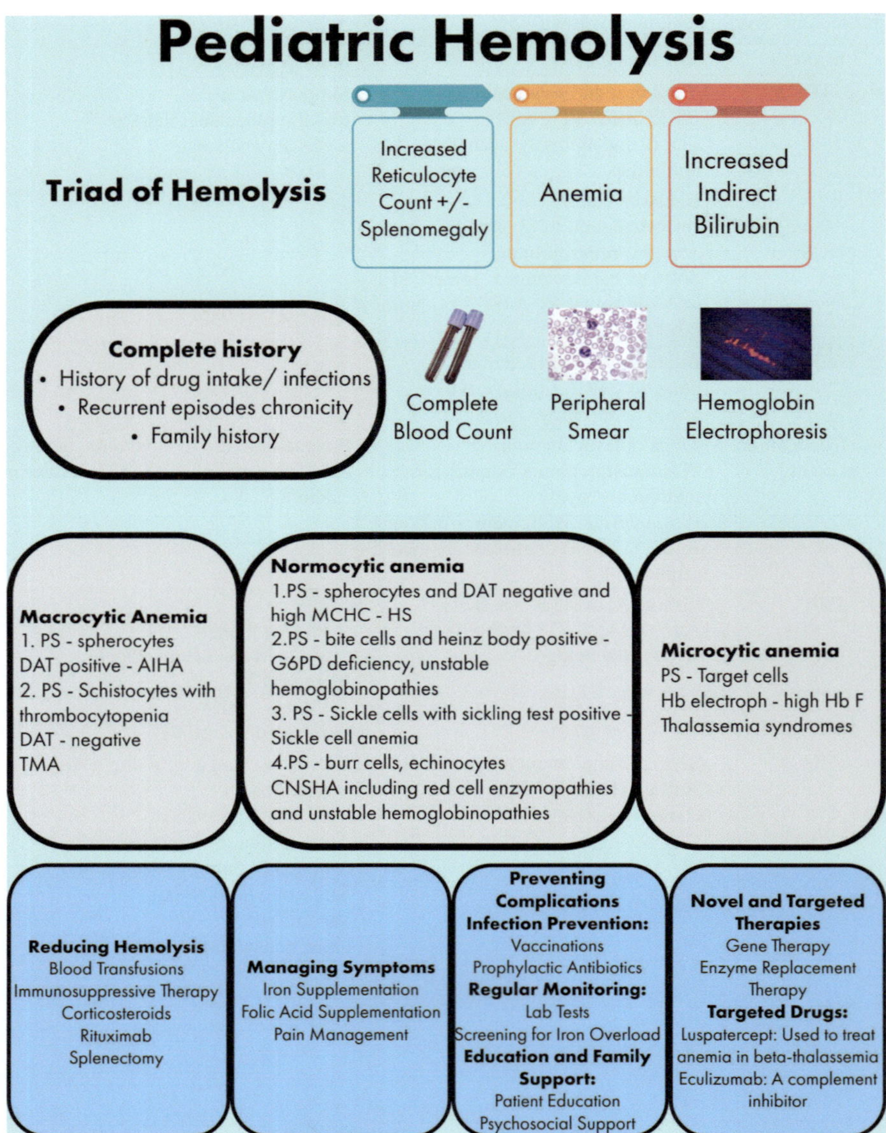

Fig. 7.4 A simple approach to the cause of hemolytic anemia

References

Hill A, Hill QA (2018) Autoimmune hemolytic anemia. Hematology Am Soc Hematol Educ Program 2018(1):382–389

Loirat C, Fakhouri F, Ariceta G, Besbas N, Bitzan M, Bjerre A et al (2016) An international consensus approach to the management of atypical hemolytic uremic syndrome in children. Pediatr Nephrol 31:15–39

Voulgaridou A, Kalfa TA (2021) Autoimmune hemolytic anemia in the pediatric setting. J Clin Med 10(2):216

Chapter 8
Approach to Thrombocytopenia (Pediatric Patients)

Amit Jain and Rajesh Patil

Learning Points

1. Categorization and Severity Assessment: Thrombocytopenia is categorized based on platelet counts, with different thresholds delineating mild, moderate, and severe conditions.
2. Diagnostic Evaluation Strategy: The initial diagnostic approach for pediatric thrombocytopenia involves a thorough clinical history and physical examination, complemented by a complete blood count and peripheral smear analysis.
3. Management Approaches Based on Underlying Causes: Management strategies should be tailored according to the identified underlying causes of thrombocytopenia.
4. Importance of Monitoring and Supportive Care: In the PICU setting, continuous monitoring of platelet counts and general health are crucial due to the potential rapid change in the patient's condition.

8.1 Introduction

- Thrombocytopenia is defined as a platelet count less than 150×10^9/L and is the commonest cause of faulty primary hemostasis.
- Manifestation may range from no bleeding to life-threatening bleeding and/or thrombosis.

A. Jain (✉)
Pediatric Hematology – Oncology & BMT, MCGM—Comprehensive Thalassemia Care, Pediatric Hematology—Oncology & BMT, Mumbai, Maharashtra, India

R. Patil
Department of Bone Marrow Transplant, MCGM—Comprehensive Thalassemia Care, Pediatric Hematology—Oncology & BMT, Mumbai, Maharashtra, India

S. B. Mishra (ed.), *Critical Care Hematology*,
https://doi.org/10.1007/978-981-97-5565-3_8

- The relationship between the risk of bleeding and the severity of thrombocytopenia is undetermined.
- The risk of spontaneous bleeding is higher when the platelet count is less than 10,000/microliter.

The prevalence of thrombocytopenia varies from 12% to 60% in PICU (Yilmaz et al. 2013; Patki et al. 2014). The delay in normalization of platelet count in these patients is an indicator of a guarded prognosis based on the available literature (Yilmaz et al. 2013; Patki et al. 2014). Thrombocytopenia can be further characterized as mild, moderate, and severe.

Thrombocytopenia, a condition characterized by an abnormally low number of platelets in the blood, is classified into four categories based on the platelet count measured in units of 10^9 per liter (L). A normal platelet count exceeds 150 × 10^9/L. The condition is deemed mild when the count falls between 100 × 10^9/L and 149 × 10^9/L. It is classified as moderate when the platelet count is within the range of 50 × 10^9/L–99 × 10^9/L. A count below 50 × 10^9/L is considered severe, indicating a critical decrease in platelet numbers. This classification is crucial for diagnosing the severity of thrombocytopenia and determining the appropriate medical response.

The causes of thrombocytopenia can be broadly categorized into two groups: those leading to increased destruction of platelets and those resulting from decreased production of platelets. For increased destruction, immune-mediated factors are significant, including immune thrombocytopenia and drug-induced thrombocytopenia, as well as autoimmune disorders. Microangiopathic disorders are also implicated in the elevated breakdown of platelets. On the other side, decreased production can be due to infections and sepsis, certain drugs, bone marrow failure, and bone marrow infiltration. Genetic factors can result in inherited forms of thrombocytopenia, and nutritional deficiencies are also known to reduce platelet production. Identifying the underlying cause is vital for the effective management of the condition.

8.2 Approach to Thrombocytopenia

The initial approach to the child with thrombocytopenia involves clinical history, physical examination, complete blood count, and peripheral smear analysis. The velocity of further testing depends on the clinical presentation of the child (Fig. 8.1).

Bleeding manifestations in children with thrombocytopenia range from mild cutaneous bleeding to life-threatening intracranial hemorrhage (ICH) (Table 8.1). Severe life-threatening bleeding usually occurs when the platelet count falls $<10 \times 10^9$/L.

A detailed history (Table 8.2) and thorough physical examination (Table 8.3) followed by appropriate investigation (Tables 8.4 and 8.5) help in identifying the etiology of thrombocytopenia and expedite diagnosis.

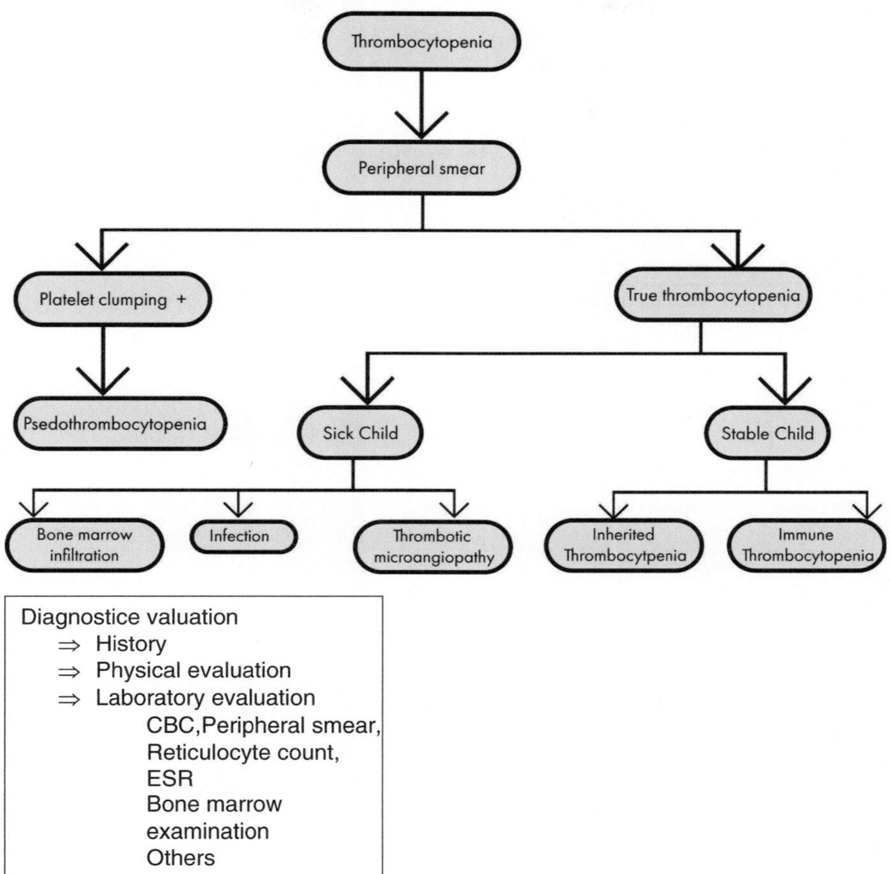

Fig. 8.1 Approach to thrombocytopenia

Table 8.1 Bleeding manifestations

Type	Cutaneous	Mucosal	Life-threatening
	Superficial skin bleed Petechiae—1–3 mm Purpura—3–10 mm Ecchymois— >10 mm	Epistaxis Gingival bleeding Wet purpura	Intra-cranial bleed Gastro-intestinal bleed Pulmonary bleed

Table 8.2 History taking

Points to enquire in history taking	Rationale
History of bleeding manifestation (cutaneous, mucosal or life-threatening) including onset, frequency, and severity of present	Estimation of blood loss
History of fever or prodromal symptoms	Acute febrile illness
History of fever or prodromal symptoms in the recent past	Immune-mediated destruction
History of vaccination in the recent past	Immune-mediated destruction
History of exposure to new medication	Drug-induced thrombocytopenia
Past history of any kind of bleeding manifestation	Chronicity of thrombocytopenia
Family history of bleeding or low platelet count	Inherited thrombocytopenia
Detail dietary evaluation	Nutritional thrombocytopenia

Table 8.3 Physical examination

General condition	Well child	Immune-mediated, inherited thrombocytopenia
	Sick child	Infection, sepsis, DIC, TMA
Growth and development		Inherited thrombocytopenia
Dysmorphism		Inherited thrombocytopenia
Auditory or hearing assessment		Inherited thrombocytopenia
Ophthalmological evaluation		Inherited thrombocytopenia
Lymph nodes		Bone marrow infiltration
Splenomegaly		Sequestration
Hepato-splenomegaly		Bone marrow infiltration
Renal failure (oliguria, hypertension)		TMA
Focal neurological deficit		Intracranial bleed

DIC Disseminated intravascular coagulation, *TMA* Thrombotic microangiopathy

Table 8.4 Complete blood count and peripheral smear

Anemia and thrombocytopenia		Infections, DIC, sepsis, thrombotic microangiopathy, Evans syndrome
Leucocytosis and thrombocytopenia		Infection, malignancy, chronic inflammation
Pancytopenia		Bone marrow failure, bone marrow infiltration, sequestration, vitamin B12 deficiency
Mild thrombocytopenia with lymphopenia		Acute viral infection
Mild to moderate thrombocytopenia with neutrophilia		Bacterial infections, sepsis
Fragmented cells (schistocytes)		TMA
Size of platelets/MPV	**Small**	WAS, XLT
	Normal	DITP, CAMT
	Large	Increased destruction, BSS, MYH9

BSS Bernold Soulier Syndrome, *CAMT* Congenital Amegakaryocytic Thrombocytopenia, *DITP* Drug-induced thrombocytopenia, *TMA* Thrombotic microangiopathy, *WAS* Wiskott Aldrich Syndrome, *XLT* X-linked Thrombocytopenia

Table 8.5 Other tests

Reticulocyte count, Coombs test	Evan syndrome
HIV, HbSAg, Anti HCV	Immune thrombocytopenia
Complete bleeding profile including fibrinogen	DIC
ADAMTS-13 activity	DIC, TTP
ANA, dSDNA	Collagen vascular diseases
Vitamin B12, ferritin	Nutritional
Electron microscopy of platelets	Structural platelet defects, inherited thrombocytopenia
Next generation sequencing	Inherited thrombocytopenia

DIC Disseminated intravascular coagulation, *TTP* Thrombotic thrombocytopenia

8.3 Diagnostic Evaluation

8.3.1 Complete Blood Count

- Hb with RBC indices
- WBC with differential blood count
- Platelet count and MPV

8.3.2 Peripheral Blood Smear

- Platelet count on smear
- Platelet size and morphology
- Platelet clumping
- Associated white and/or red blood cell abnormalities

8.4 Bone Marrow Examination

8.4.1 Indications

1. Systemic symptoms (e.g., fever, weight loss, night sweats, bone pain)
2. Involvement of other blood cell lines (anemia, leukopenia) without explanation
3. Presence of abnormal cells on peripheral blood smear
4. Some cases of inherited thrombocytopenia

8.5 Review

8.5.1 Increased Destruction

1. *Immune-mediated destruction*

A. *Immune Thrombocytopenia (ITP)* (Neunert et al. 2019): An acquired hematological condition can manifest when auto-antibodies are produced against platelets, leading to their decreased count, a state known as thrombocytopenia. This condition arises independently, not as a result of other known causes of thrombocytopenia such as drug reactions, infections, cancer, or other autoimmune diseases. It has an estimated occurrence rate of 4.0–5.3 cases per 100,000 individuals. In pediatric cases, the frequency of severe bleeding episodes, excluding intracranial hemorrhage (ICH), has been observed to vary, with reported rates ranging between 3% and 20%. Furthermore, the risk of ICH in this demographic is about 0.5%, indicating a relatively low but significant risk associated with the disorder. The International Working Group on ITP classifies ITP into the following clinical phases (Table 8.6).

The first-line treatments for newly diagnosed ITP include steroids, intravenous immunoglobulin (IVIg), and anti-RhD immunoglobulin (Table 8.7).

B. *Drug-Induced Thrombocytopenia* (Bakchoul and Marini 2018)

- Typically occurs suddenly
- Is often severe
- Can cause life-threatening bleeding and/or thrombosis

Figure 8.2 provides an approach to the diagnosis of cases with suspected DITP.

Table 8.6 Clinical phases of ITP

Definition	Duration
Newly diagnosed	<3 months
Persistent	3–12 months
Chronic	>12 months

Table 8.7 First-line therapy for acute ITP

Drug	Dose	Duration	Time to response	Response rate	Adverse event
Prednisolone	2–4 mg/kg/day	5–7 days	2–7 days	50–77%	Hyperglycemia, hypertension
IVIg	0.8–2gm/kg	Single dose	24–48 h	>80%	Infusion reactions, renal failure
Anti D	0.75mcg/kg	Single dose	24–48 h	~75%	Hemolysis

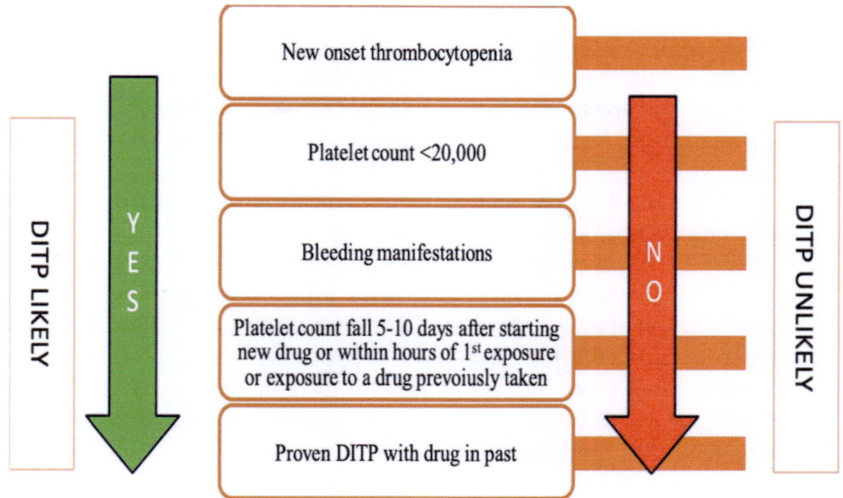

Fig. 8.2 Drug-induced thrombocytopenia

2. *Thrombotic Microangiopathy (TMA)* (Abou-Ismail et al. 2022)

Clinical-pathological diagnosis, characterized by microangiopathic hemolytic anemia, thrombocytopenia, and end-organ involvement.

The commonest cause is Disseminated Intravascular Coagulation, often triggered by multiple pathologies associated with acidosis, hypoxia. and/or shock.

8.6 Management

1. Supportive care:
   - Monitoring of renal functions and management of hypertension, fluid, and electrolyte
   - Renal replacement therapy (RRT), if required
   - Hematinics to support erythropoiesis (folic acid and erythropoietin analog)
   - Packed red cell transfusion as and when indicated
   - Platelet transfusion may be indicated for life-threatening bleeding
   - Plasma exchange esp. in immune TTP can be considered in other cases
   - Discontinuation of the drug (in drug-induced TMA)
   - Identify and treat potential triggers in TA-TMA
2. Steroids in immune TTP
3. Rituximab
4. Eculizumab: An anti-C5 monoclonal antibody that inhibits terminal complement activation has been approved to treat TMA

3. *Splenic Sequestration*

   Splenomegaly causes sequestering of 90% of the total platelet mass leading to a decrease in circulating platelets causing thrombocytopenia.

   Conditions commonly associated with splenic sequestration-induced thrombocytopenia include portal hypertension, storage disorder, leukemias, lymphomas, etc.

   Treatment of the primary etiology helps in the improvement of thrombocytopenia. In rare circumstances, splenectomy might help.
4. *Mechanical Destruction*: The employment of extracorporeal therapies such as extracorporeal membrane oxygenation (ECMO), cardiopulmonary bypass, hemodialysis, and apheresis has been linked to the development of thrombocytopenia due to the mechanical breakdown of platelets. Interestingly, the length of time a patient undergoes ECMO appears to have no significant effect on the degree of thrombocytopenia experienced. The reasons behind this are complex, involving multiple factors. Despite the advancements in medical technology, the comprehension of the precise mechanisms and the management of thrombocytopenia in the context of these extracorporeal treatments remain somewhat limited. Further research and clinical studies are needed to enhance understanding and improve therapeutic approaches for this complication.

8.7 Decreased Production

8.7.1 Infections

Thrombocytopenia frequently arises in conjunction with a range of viral infections, a phenomenon primarily due to the increased utilization of platelets in response to inflammation-triggered coagulation, their removal from general circulation, and the suppression of platelet synthesis. A characteristic pattern of mild thrombocytopenia accompanied by a reduction in lymphocytes is often seen in acute viral infections; however, these signs are not exclusively indicative of viral pathogens and cannot reliably differentiate between viral, bacterial, fungal, or parasitic infections. Notable viral culprits linked with thrombocytopenia include Epstein–Barr virus, cytomegalovirus, parvovirus, and the varicella virus. Although the associated thrombocytopenia is typically short-lived and harmless, resolving within a week, there are instances where it can progress, leading to multiorgan dysfunction that necessitates intensive care and is linked to increased rates of complications and mortality. In bacterial infections, particularly among those with weakened immune systems, thrombocytopenia can present alongside sepsis and potentially with disseminated intravascular coagulation, and some patients may develop further complications like hemophagocytic lymphohistiocytosis. Additionally, thrombocytopenia is a common complication in patients with human immunodeficiency virus (HIV), where it results from both the destruction of platelets and a decrease in their production, with management typically involving antiretroviral therapy.

8.7.1.1 Septicemia

In Pediatric Intensive Care Units (PICU), sepsis stands out as a leading cause of thrombocytopenia and represents a significant risk factor due to its association with a high mortality rate. This condition stems from a severe and misdirected immune reaction to an infection, leading to potential organ failure. Thrombocytopenia has been identified as an independent marker signaling worse prognosis in these young patients, correlating with increased death rates and prolonged hospital admissions.

It has been observed that thrombocytopenia affects 25–49% of patients in Neonatal Intensive Care Units (NICU) or PICU. The persistence or lack of resolution of thrombocytopenia is often linked with unfavorable clinical outcomes. Platelets are implicated in the formation of micro-thrombi and are considered a contributing factor to the onset of disseminated intravascular coagulation (DIC) during sepsis. The causes of thrombocytopenia in the context of sepsis are complex, including reduced platelet production, heightened consumption of platelets, increased sequestration within the microvasculature, and destruction mediated by the immune system.

Treatment strategies primarily involve the administration of antibiotics and supportive care. The criteria for platelet transfusion in these scenarios are subject to detailed consideration and are typically addressed in later discussions.

8.7.2 Bone Marrow Failure

Bone marrow failure disorders are characterized by pancytopenia and hypocellular bone marrow.

They can be either acquired or inherited.

Acquired cases are due to autoimmune attacks of marrow stem and progenitor cells leading to pancytopenia.

Thrombocytopenia in bone marrow failure can lead to varying degrees of bleeding manifestation.

The main treatment for thrombocytopenia secondary to bone marrow failure is platelet transfusion while awaiting curative treatment, viz., immunosuppressive therapy or hematopoietic stem cell transplant.

8.7.3 Bone Marrow Infiltration

Thrombocytopenia can arise from the encroachment of disease within the bone marrow cavity, progressively replacing healthy marrow with abnormal cells or tissue. This condition is relatively rare, and its causes are diverse, ranging from malignancies and metastases to myelofibrosis, hemophagocytic lymphohistiocytosis, storage disorders, Langerhans cell histiocytosis, to osteopetrosis among others.

Addressing the root disease is central to the treatment strategy for this type of thrombocytopenia.

Nutritional deficiencies: Nutritional deficits linked to thrombocytopenia primarily involve a lack of vitamin B12 or folate and, on rarer occasions, iron deficiency. These deficiencies contribute to the depletion of platelet production in the bone marrow.

Inherited thrombocytopenia (ITs): Inherited thrombocytopenia, though not as common as the acquired form, constitutes a rare and diverse collection of disorders presenting with low platelet counts, which can lead to varying degrees of bleeding. Such disorders are often associated with additional health abnormalities, including immunodeficiency, renal disease, sensorineural hearing loss, and an elevated risk of developing cancer. Platelet transfusions, and occasionally recombinant factor VII, are generally the initial treatment options for these patients. Hematopoietic stem cell transplant has shown effectiveness in certain inherited conditions, such as Wiskott–Aldrich syndrome (WAS) and Congenital Amegakaryocytic Thrombocytopenia (CAMT), and remains under investigation for others.

8.7.3.1 Platelet Transfusion

Turning to platelet transfusions, these are typically administered to prevent or manage bleeding in patients with thrombocytopenia or dysfunctional platelets. However, the correlation between severe thrombocytopenia and bleeding onset is not straightforward, as the severity of thrombocytopenia is not a reliable indicator of bleeding risk.

For the dosing of platelet transfusions, the standard is one random donor platelet unit per 10 kg body weight, up to a maximum of six units, or 5–10 ml/kg from a single donor. The preference for ABO-compatible platelets over cross-matched transfusions is not strongly guided by consensus.

The effectiveness of a platelet transfusion is measured by the Corrected Count Increment (CCI), calculated by the difference in platelet count post- and pre-transfusion, adjusted for body surface area and the number of platelets transfused. A successful platelet response is indicated by a CCI above 20% of the initial count shortly after transfusion, and over 10% after 24 h (Kahn et al. 2020).

Corrected Count Increment (CCI)

$$\frac{\left(\text{Post} - \text{transfusion platelet count}\left\langle /\mu L\right\rangle\right) - \left(\text{pre} - \text{transfusion platelet count}\left\langle /\mu L\right\rangle\right)] \times \left(\text{body surface area}\left\langle \text{m2}\right\rangle\right)}{\text{Number of platelets transfused} < \times 1011/\mu L}$$

If transfusions do not yield an adequate response, indicating platelet refractoriness, management focuses on the underlying condition, especially for nonimmune causes. For immune-mediated cases, trials of ABO-matched platelets and, if unsuccessful, HLA-matched or compatible platelets may be pursued.

Platelet refractoriness, which refers to the lack of expected increase in platelet count following a transfusion, can be caused by immune and nonimmune factors. Immune causes include alloimmune reactions, such as the presence of antibodies against Human Leukocyte Antigens (HLA) and Human Platelet Antigens (HPA), as well as autoimmune responses where the body's immune system attacks its own platelets. Nonimmune causes may involve systemic conditions like fever or sepsis, including disseminated intravascular coagulation (DIC), or adverse reactions to certain medications, for example, the antifungal drug amphotericin. Understanding these causes is critical for addressing platelet transfusion challenges in affected patients.

8.8 Summary

- Thrombocytopenia commonly presents in patients within Pediatric Intensive Care Units (PICU).
- The presence of severe thrombocytopenia over an extended period often correlates with higher instances of complications and risk of death.
- Various factors may lead to a reduction in platelet counts in children admitted to the PICU. Pinpointing the specific cause is crucial for effective treatment.
- An in-depth patient history and thorough examination are fundamental in pinpointing the precise diagnosis, which is further corroborated by selected laboratory tests and their interpretation in relation to the patient's overall health status.
- In cases where there is a notable decrease in platelets or an elevated rate of platelet consumption, platelet transfusions can be beneficial. However, these transfusions may be counterproductive in patients who are experiencing heightened platelet activation within blood vessels.
- The determination of the most effective platelet transfusion protocols for the prevention or management of hemorrhagic episodes in ICU patients with low platelet counts is still an ongoing process.

References

Abou-Ismail MY, Kapoor S, Citla Sridhar D, Nayak L, Ahuja S (2022) Thrombotic microangiopathies: an illustrated review. Res Pract Thromb Haemost 6(3):e12708

Bakchoul T, Marini I (2018) Drug-associated thrombocytopenia. Hematology Am Soc Hematol Educ Program 2018(1):576–583

Kahn S, Chegondi M, Nellis ME, Karam O (2020) Overview of plasma and platelet transfusions in critically ill children. Front Pediatr 8:601659

Neunert C, Terrell DR, Arnold DM, Buchanan G, Cines DB, Cooper N et al (2019) American Society of Hematology 2019 guidelines for immune thrombocytopenia. Blood Adv 3(23):3829–3866
Patki VK, Birru FD, Patki VV (2014) Decline in platelet count as a prognostic marker in critically ill children. J Pediatr Crit Care 1(2):13–21
Yilmaz S, Yildizdas D, Acipayam C, Bayram I, Ozcan N, Horoz OO, Tanyeli A (2013) The effect of thrombocytopenia on outcome in critically ill children. Crit Care Shock 16(2):48–57

Chapter 9
Heparin-Induced Thrombocytopenia

Sagarika Panda and Haritha Indulekha

Learning Points

1. Types and Epidemiology of HIT: This section covers the distinctions between HIT Type I and II, their prevalence, and pathophysiology. It also explores how factors like heparin type and patient characteristics influence HIT's likelihood and severity.
2. Pathophysiology of HIT: The chapter delves into the immune response in HIT, focusing on the role of platelet factor 4 (PF4) and heparin complexes in platelet activation and thrombocytopenia.
3. Diagnosing HIT: Key diagnostic strategies for HIT are discussed, including clinical evaluation and laboratory tests like the 4T's scoring system and immunoassays. Their effectiveness and limitations in confirming HIT are highlighted.
4. Managing HIT: This part explains the essential management steps for HIT, including stopping heparin and choosing alternative anticoagulants like Argatroban and Bivalirudin. It also addresses the re-exposure to heparin and new potential treatments.

S. Panda (✉)
Critical Care Medicine, IMS & SUM Hospital, Bhubaneswar, Odisha, India

H. Indulekha
Anaesthesiology and Critical Care Medicine, SGT Medical College, Gurugram, Haryana, India

S. B. Mishra (ed.), *Critical Care Hematology*,
https://doi.org/10.1007/978-981-97-5565-3_9

9.1 Introduction

Heparin, a sulphated polysaccharide with anticoagulant properties, was discovered by Dr. Henry Howell over a century ago. Its association with thrombocytopenia in animals and humans was identified in the 1940s, with the immune-related heparin-induced thrombocytopenia (HIT) first reported in 1958. HIT prevalence in adults on heparin ranges from 0.2% to 5.0%, with challenges in accurate diagnosis. In ICU settings, HIT incidence is usually below 2%, influenced by various factors (Hirsh et al. 2001; Kanaan and Al-Homsi 2009).

9.1.1 Epidemiology and Risk Factors

Thromboembolic complications occur in about 50% of HIT patients. The risk is influenced by heparin type and exposure duration, with low-molecular-weight heparin (LMWH) having a lower HIT incidence than unfractionated heparin (UFH). Bovine UFH is a more frequent HIT trigger, and higher doses escalate antibody formation risk. Patient factors like age, gender, and surgical type affect HIT likelihood, with higher incidence in older, female (excluding pregnancy), and postoperative patients, especially in cardiac surgery. Anti-PF4/heparin antibody prevalence varies by patient group, being higher in orthopaedic and cardiac surgery patients. Notably, a study found inflammation might increase HIT risk in trauma patients (Wardrop and Keeling 2008).

9.1.2 Pathophysiology

In the case of Heparin-Induced Thrombocytopenia (HIT), the administration of heparin leads to an immune reaction that targets complexes of platelet factor 4 (PF4) and heparin. PF4, a cationic protein, interacts with the anionic heparin to form complexes that are highly antigenic. These complexes, when bound to IgG antibodies, activate platelets, a process mediated by FcγRIIA receptors and tyrosine kinase pathways. This activation results in the production of thrombin and the formation of thrombi composed of platelets and fibrin, which ultimately leads to a reduction in platelet count. Additionally, the pathogenesis of HIT involves other cellular elements like endothelial cells, monocytes, and potentially T cells and neutrophil extracellular traps (NETs). At least 12 saccharides are necessary to form ultra large complexes, therefore the large-molecular-weight fragments of unfractionated heparin have greater immunogenicity than low-molecular-weight heparins. The concentration of heparin as small as 0.1–1 U/ml can cause HIT (Amiral et al. 1996) (Fig. 9.1).

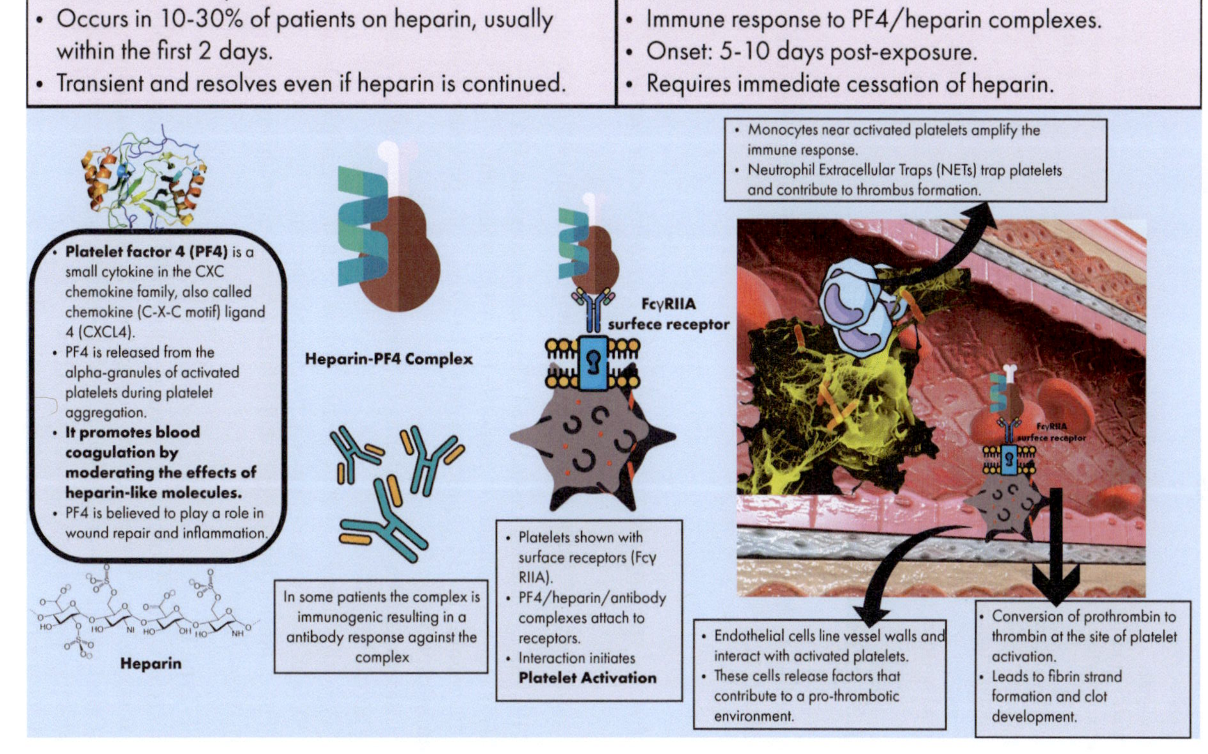

Fig. 9.1 Heparin-induced thrombocytopenia and pathophysiology

Table 9.1 Phases of HIT

Phase	Platelet count	Functional assay	Immunoassay	Anticoagulation strategy
Acute heparin-induced thrombocytopenia	Decreased	+	++	Bivalirudin
Sub-acute heparin-induced thrombocytopenia A	Normal	+	++	Heparin + Peri-operative plasmapheresis OR anti-platelet agent
Sub-acute heparin-induced thrombocytopenia B	Normal	_	+	Heparin
Remote heparin-induced thrombocytopenia	Normal	_	_	Heparin

9.1.3 Phases of HIT

According to American Society of Hematology HIT is described under four phases (Table 9.1).

9.1.4 Types of Heparin-Induced Thrombocytopenia

Heparin-Induced Thrombocytopenia is categorized into two distinct types:

HIT Type I (Heparin-Associated Thrombocytopenia, HAT)

This is a non-immunologic response to heparin treatment.

It manifests in approximately 10–30% of patients following heparin administration.

Characterized by mild thrombocytopenia, with platelet counts generally remaining above 100,000/mm^3.

Typically emerges within the first 2 days of initiating heparin treatment.

Results from direct platelet activation by heparin.

The condition is transient, with platelet counts normalizing even if heparin therapy is continued.

HIT-Type II

This type is immunologically mediated and can lead to serious complications.

It necessitates the immediate cessation of heparin upon suspicion.

Onset usually occurs 5–10 days after starting heparin therapy and is associated with more pronounced thrombocytopenia.

Characterized by the formation of antibodies against PF4/heparin complexes, increasing the risk of thrombosis.

Variations of HIT Type II Include

- Delayed Onset HIT: Emerges days to week's post-heparin discontinuation, often after surgery or infection. It involves antibodies that cross-react with PF4-glycosaminoglycan (GAG) complexes.
- Spontaneous HIT: Occurs in the absence of heparin exposure, possibly due to the activation of anti-PF4-heparin antibodies by GAGs or other polyanions. This variant shows positive results in functional assays even without prior heparin exposure.

9.2 Clinical Features

Heparin-Induced Thrombocytopenia predominantly presents as thrombocytopenia, occasionally accompanied by thrombosis. The defining feature of HIT is a significant reduction in platelet count, generally noted 4 days or more following heparin exposure. This decline typically happens between the 5th- and 14th-day post-exposure, affecting about 95% of patients. The platelet count usually drops by over 50% from the baseline, often falling below 150,000/mm^3 and averaging around 55,000/mm3. Most patients exhibit platelet counts within the range of 40,000–80,000/mm3. However, in 5–10% of cases, the count may plummet below 20,000/mm3, necessitating the consideration of alternative causes for thrombocytopenia. Rapid-onset thrombocytopenia occurring within hours of heparin administration is usually seen in individuals with preformed HIT antibodies, often due to prior heparin use within the last 100 days. In some cases, thrombocytopenia may be the sole manifestation of HIT.

9.2.1 Thrombosis and Bleeding Complications in HIT

The most critical and hazardous complication of HIT is thrombosis, which can occur in any blood vessel, inducing a state of hypercoagulability. Thromboembolic events are observed in roughly one-third to half of the patients, with venous thromboses being more prevalent than arterial. Common thrombotic events include deep vein thrombosis (DVT) and pulmonary embolism, with catheter insertion sites also being at risk. The likelihood of thrombosis correlates with the severity of thrombocytopenia. HIT can precipitate severe cardiovascular events, such as myocardial infarction, stroke, limb ischemia, sinus vein thrombosis, and mesenteric venous or arterial occlusion. Patients with thrombotic complications are at an elevated risk of major bleeding and mortality, although the overall bleeding risk in HIT patients remains relatively low, even when platelet counts are below 20,000/mm^3. In certain instances, HIT may lead to disseminated intravascular coagulation (DIC), characterized by widespread microthrombosis, decreased fibrinogen levels, and elevated fibrin degradation products (GR 1973).

9.2.2 Uncommon Clinical Outcomes of HIT

While less frequent, HIT can lead to specific atypical outcomes. Approximately 10–20% of patients with HIT develop skin lesions, such as erythematous nodules or necrotic plaques, typically around 8 days after starting heparin. These lesions can arise regardless of whether the patient is on unfractionated heparin (UFH) or low-molecular-weight heparin (LMWH). Rare manifestations of HIT include adrenal failure due to adrenal vein thrombosis and complications related to flap failure.

9.3 Diagnosis of HIT

Diagnosing HIT involves identifying thrombocytopenia and/or thrombosis that occurs in conjunction with heparin therapy while ruling out other potential causes of thrombocytopenia. Clinical assessment is crucial for estimating the likelihood of HIT before confirmation through laboratory testing. Suspicion of HIT arises with both absolute thrombocytopenia (platelet count below 150,000/mm^3) and relative thrombocytopenia (a decrease of at least 50% from the baseline). Given the diverse presentations of thrombocytopenia and its many potential causes, especially in high-risk groups, HIT may often be overlooked. Clinical scoring systems such as the 4T's have been developed to assist clinicians in evaluating the probability of HIT. While this system has demonstrated high sensitivity, its positive predictive value and inter-observer reliability remain moderate. The American Society of Hematology (ASH) endorses the use of the 4T's model. Another model, the HEP score, shows promise in increasing specificity, particularly in ICU settings, but it still requires further validation and is not widely recommended for routine clinical application (Marchetti et al. 2021).

9.3.1 Pretest probability—Clinical Scoring Systems

Understanding the 4Ts Scoring System in HIT Diagnosis
The 4Ts score is a crucial tool for evaluating the likelihood of Heparin-Induced Thrombocytopenia (HIT). It encompasses four key elements: the degree of thrombocytopenia, the timing of the platelet count drop, the presence of thrombosis or related complications, and the likelihood of other causes of thrombocytopenia. Patients are classified into three risk categories based on their total score: low (0–3), intermediate (4–5), and high (6–8). Those in the high-risk category, with scores between 6 and 8, have over an 80% chance of developing HIT, necessitating vigilant monitoring and intervention. The 4Ts score is highly effective, boasting a 99.8% negative predictive value for those in the low-risk category. However, its positive predictive value is more modest, at 14% for the intermediate group and 64% for the high-risk group.

9.3.2 The HEP Score

The HIT Expert Probability (HEP) score, a more recent diagnostic approach, has shown diagnostic accuracy comparable to the 4Ts system. This score, detailed in various studies, evaluates the probability of HIT with similar efficacy to the 4Ts.

9.3.3 Alternative Scoring for Postcardiac Surgery Patients

Specific to post-cardiopulmonary bypass (CPB) patients, a model developed by Lillo-Le Louët et al. in 2004 focuses on distinct risk factors, including biphasic platelet count changes, the time interval from CPB to suspected HIT onset, and CPB duration. The model assigns scores to these factors, with a total score of 2 or more indicating a high likelihood of HIT. This scoring system has demonstrated a positive predictive value of 62% and a negative predictive value of 97%. However, independent validation of this model is still pending. Other studies, such as Selleng et al.'s, have identified specific thrombocytopenia patterns post-surgery as indicative of HIT.

9.3.4 Laboratory Testing for HIT

The diagnosis of HIT primarily utilizes two types of laboratory assays: immunoassays and functional assays.

- *Immunoassays*: These tests detect antibodies against PF4-heparin complexes. Varieties include the PF4/heparin ELISA, particle gel immunoassay, lateral flow assays, automated latex-based assays, and chemiluminescence assays. While immunoassays are highly sensitive and offer quick results, their specificity can be as low as 30–80%, leading to potential over diagnosis. A negative result on these tests, however, can effectively rule out HIT due to their high negative predictive value.
- *Functional Assays*: These are recommended particularly for patients with a moderate to high clinical suspicion of HIT (4T score > 3) and positive immunoassay results. The serotonin release assay (SRA) is the gold standard among functional assays. Other methods include the heparin-induced platelet activation (HIPA) assay, light transmission aggregometry, the platelet viability assay, PF4-dependent P-selectin expression assay (PEA), and flow cytometry. Functional assays are more complex and require specialized laboratory conditions. A high 4T score combined with strong immunoassay positivity might suggest HIT, even if functional assays yield negative results.

9.4 Management

The management of HIT focuses on two primary strategies. (Cuker et al. 2018)

- *Immediate Cessation of Heparin*
- Heparin must be discontinued immediately upon HIT suspicion. Alternative anticoagulation should be started promptly, without delay for thrombocytopenia or confirmatory lab testing.
- *Choice of Alternative Anticoagulant*
- Selection depends on several factors including planned procedures and patient-specific considerations like liver or kidney function. Therapeutic-dose anticoagulation is necessary, as prophylactic doses are insufficient. Bilateral lower extremity compression ultrasonography is recommended for all HIT patients (Marchetti et al. 2021).

Argatroban: This synthetic L-arginine derivative acts as a direct thrombin inhibitor and is particularly useful in patients with renal impairment, as it is metabolized in the liver. However, it is contraindicated in hepatic impairment due to the increased risk of bleeding. Argatroban's anticoagulant effect is monitored via activated partial thromboplastin time (aPTT) and requires careful dosing adjustments based on aPTT results.

Bivalirudin: As a direct thrombin inhibitor, Bivalirudin is often recommended for patients with acute or subacute HIT undergoing urgent cardiac procedures. It is excreted by the kidneys, necessitating dose adjustments in patients with renal impairment. Bivalirudin offers the advantage of a short half-life, allowing for rapid normalization of coagulation status post-surgery.

Lepirudin: Derived from yeast, Lepirudin is a recombinant form of hirudin, a natural thrombin inhibitor. Its dosing needs adjustment in patients with renal insufficiency, as it is predominantly excreted via the kidneys. Lepirudin is effective in HIT patients, particularly when monitored and adjusted based on therapeutic aPTT levels.

Desirudin: Primarily used for thromboprophylaxis in hip replacement surgery, Desirudin has shown potential in managing HIT in limited studies. It is a direct thrombin inhibitor with a low risk of cross-reactivity in HIT patients. Its use in HIT requires careful monitoring due to the risk of bleeding.

Fondaparinux: This synthetic pentasaccharide is frequently used off-label for HIT. Fondaparinux acts by enhancing antithrombin III activity and selectively inhibiting factor Xa. Caution is advised in patients with end-stage renal disease due to its renal excretion and potential accumulation.

Danaparoid: A low molecular weight heparinoid, Danaparoid indirectly inhibits factor Xa. It is used in HIT due to its minimal cross-reactivity with HIT antibodies. Monitoring anti-factor Xa levels is crucial, especially in renal impairment, to ensure therapeutic efficacy and minimize bleeding risks.

Vitamin K Antagonists: Warfarin and other vitamin K antagonists are used in long-term management of HIT but should be initiated cautiously. They are typically started only after platelet counts have recovered, to avoid complications such as warfarin-induced skin necrosis.

Direct Oral Anticoagulants (DOACs): DOACs like rivaroxaban and apixaban are increasingly being used off-label for HIT. These agents offer the ease of oral administration and do not require routine laboratory monitoring. However, their use in HIT is based on limited data and clinical experience.

Therapeutic Plasma Exchange (TPE): TPE is employed in emergent situations like surgery, major bleeding, or refractory HIT. It works by removing circulating antibodies, including anti-PF4/heparin antibodies, and can be a life-saving intervention in severe cases.

Intravenous Immunoglobulin (IVIG): IVIG is used for severe or refractory HIT, potentially working by blocking Fc receptors on platelets. It can be an adjunct to anticoagulation in patients not responding to standard therapy, though it carries a risk of thrombosis.

Prophylactic Platelet Transfusion: Generally not recommended in HIT due to the risk of exacerbating thrombosis. However, it may be considered in cases of severe thrombocytopenia with active bleeding or before a surgical procedure with a high risk of bleeding.

Emerging Therapies: Research is ongoing into novel treatments for HIT, including bacterial proteases that degrade IgG, Syk inhibitors, tyrosine kinase inhibitors, and PF4 tetramerization inhibitors. These therapies hold promise for future HIT management but are currently experimental.

Re-exposure to Heparin: Typically avoided in HIT patients, re-exposure to heparin may be considered under specific conditions, such as when anti-PF4/heparin antibodies are no longer present. This approach requires careful risk-benefit analysis and close monitoring.

Flowchart

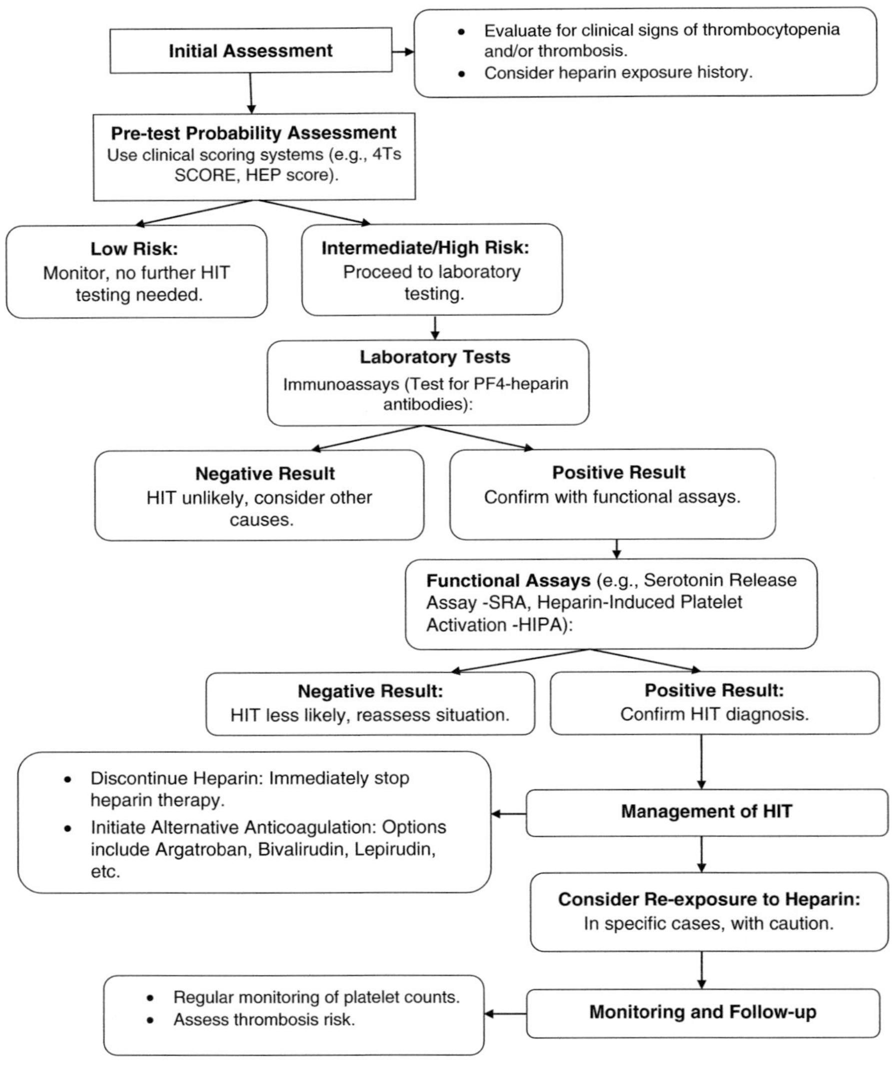
Initial Assessment
Evaluate for clinical signs of thrombocytopenia and/or thrombosis.
Consider heparin exposure history.
Pre-test Probability Assessment
Use clinical scoring systems (e.g., 4Ts SCORE, HEP score).
Low Risk:
Monitor, no further HIT testing needed.
Intermediate/High Risk:
Proceed to laboratory testing.
Laboratory Tests
Immunoassays (Test for PF4-heparin antibodies):
Negative Result
HIT unlikely, consider other causes.
Positive Result
Confirm with functional assays.
Functional Assays (e.g., Serotonin Release Assay -SRA, Heparin-Induced Platelet Activation -HIPA):
Negative Result:
HIT less likely, reassess situation.
Positive Result:
Confirm HIT diagnosis.
Management of HIT
Discontinue Heparin: Immediately stop heparin therapy.
Initiate Alternative Anticoagulation: Options include Argatroban, Bivalirudin, Lepirudin, etc.
Consider Re-exposure to Heparin:
In specific cases, with caution.
Monitoring and Follow-up
Regular monitoring of platelet counts.
Assess thrombosis risk.

References

Amiral J, Peynaud-Debayle E, Wolf M, Bridey F, Vissac AM, Meyer D (1996) Generation of antibodies to heparin-PF4 complexes without thrombocytopenia in patients treated with unfractionated or low-molecular-weight heparin. Am J Hematol 52(2):90–95

Cuker A, Arepally GM, Chong BH, Cines DB, Greinacher A, Gruel Y et al (2018) American Society of Hematology 2018 guidelines for management of venous thromboembolism: heparin-induced thrombocytopenia. Blood Adv 2(22):3360–3392

GR R (1973) Heparin induced thrombocytopenia with thrombotic and hemorrhagic manifestations. Surg Gynecol Obstet 136:409–416

Hirsh J, Anand SS, Halperin JL, Fuster V (2001) Mechanism of action and pharmacology of unfractionated heparin. Arterioscler Thromb Vasc Biol 21(7):1094–1096

Kanaan AO, Al-Homsi AS (2009) Heparin-induced thrombocytopenia: pathophysiology, diagnosis, and review of pharmacotherapy. J Pharm Pract 22(2):149–157

Marchetti M, Zermatten MG, Bertaggia Calderara D, Aliotta A, Alberio L (2021) Heparin-induced thrombocytopenia: a review of new concepts in pathogenesis, diagnosis, and management. J Clin Med 10(4):683

Wardrop D, Keeling D (2008) The story of the discovery of heparin and warfarin. Br J Haematol 141(6):757–763

Chapter 10
Patients on Anticoagulants

Shiva Kumar

Learning Point

1. Advantages and Limitations of NOACs: Novel oral anticoagulants (NOACs) offer several advantages over traditional vitamin K antagonists, such as Warfarin.
2. Assessment and Management of Bleeding Risks: Various risk scores such as the Outpatient Bleeding Risk Index (OBRI), modified OBRI, and HAS BLED index help predict bleeding risks in patients on oral anticoagulants.
3. Laboratory Testing and Monitoring: In the event of bleeding, initial tests should include hemoglobin levels, complete blood counts, and coagulation profiles like PT, aPTT, and INR. The effectiveness of these tests varies depending on whether the patient is on a vitamin K antagonist or a NOAC.
4. Reversal of Anticoagulation: The management of major bleeding in patients on NOACs may involve the use of specific reversal agents such as Idarucizumab for Dabigatran or Andexanet Alfa for factor Xa inhibitors.

10.1 Introduction

Patients will need to be started on oral anticoagulants due to varied indications like atrial fibrillation, stroke, prosthetic heart valves, venous thrombosis, chronic pulmonary embolism, etc. Traditionally vitamin K antagonists (warfarin, coumadin) were being used for the indications mentioned above. With the advent of NOACs, it is not uncommon to encounter a patient admitted to the intensive care unit on these NOACs. The advantages of these NOACs compared to vitamin K antagonists are a shorter half-life, predictable pharmacokinetics, fewer food interactions, lower rates of bleeding, and avoids the need for laboratory monitoring tests (Lazo-Langner

S. Kumar (✉)
Critical Care Medicine, Narayana Health City Bangalore, Bangalore, Karnataka, India

S. B. Mishra (ed.), *Critical Care Hematology*,
https://doi.org/10.1007/978-981-97-5565-3_10

et al. 2013). The main limitations of these NOACs are the difficulties in managing a bleeding patient as reversal of anticoagulation is not as easy as vitamin K antagonists. Reversal agents are limitedly available and expensive in resource-limited settings. This chapter focuses on the management of these bleeding patients with respect to laboratory testing and the use of reversal agents in the critical care setting.

10.1.1 Oral Anticoagulants: Vitamin K Antagonist and NOACs

10.2 Bleeding Complications in Patients on Anticoagulants

The risk of severe bleeding complications was lesser with NOACs compared to vitamin K antagonists in various studies (Loewen and Dahri 2011). There were various risk factors that were studied that puts these patients to present with severe bleeding. Various risk scores are developed which can be assessed when the patient is started on these oral NOACs. The Outpatient Bleeding Risk Index (OBRI), modified OBRI index, HAS BLED index, etc. are various scores that include various points like increased age, abnormal renal function tests, labile INR, and ethanol use which can predict the risk of bleeding in patients (Shoeb and Fang 2013; Loewen and Dahri 2011; Wallvik et al. 2021). In the critical care setting, the most common situation is a bleeding patient on these oral anticoagulants and these prediction scores are of limited use (Table 10.1).

Bleeding severity assessment in these patients is important as management is guided according to the severity. Bleeding is defined as major when one of the following is present (Tomaselli et al. 2020).

1. Bleeding at a critical site (intracranial, pericardial, pleural, intraabdominal, intraarticular, retroperitoneal, intramuscular)
2. Presence of hemodynamic instability
3. Hemoglobin decrease ≥2 g/dl or administration of ≥2 units of RBCs

If the bleeding is not major, then management is just supportive with monitoring and stopping the oral anticoagulants. The management also depends on the site of the bleeding and specific management guided to specific areas. For example, if the site of bleeding is pericardial, placement of the pericardial drain will be indicated. Stopping the anticoagulation may also put the patient at risk of thrombosis and risk of cardiac and or cerebral complications. Hence, the risk of reversal of anticoagulation must be assessed in each patient carefully (Levi 2016).

Table 10.1 Pharmacological properties of the commonly used oral anticoagulants (Zirlik and Bode 2017)

Oral anticoagulants	Mechanism of action	Oral bioavailability in %	Half-life in hours	Protein binding in %	Renal clearance in %	Food interactions	Need of coagulation monitoring	Commonly used dosage
Warfarin	Inhibits factors II, VII, IX, and X, protein C and S	100	21–43	99	80	Yes	Yes	2–5 mg
Dabigatran	Direct thrombin inhibitor (factor II)	3–7	12–17	34–35	80	No	No	150 mg BD
Apixaban	Direct factor Xa inhibitor	50	8–12	87	27	No	No	5 mg BD
Rivaroxaban	Direct factor Xa inhibitor	80–100	5–13	92–95	33	No	No	20 mg OD
Edoxaban	Direct factor Xa inhibitor	62	10–14	55	50	No	No	60 mg OD

10.3 Laboratory Measurements in a Bleeding Patient on Anticoagulants

When a bleeding patient is encountered, routine initial blood testing must include hemoglobin, total blood counts, base deficit, lactate levels, PT (prothrombin time), aPTT (activated partial thromboplastin time), and INR (international normalized ratio). INR and PT will be prolonged in patients on vitamin K antagonists, however in patients on NOACs the utility of aPTT and PT is limited (Fig. 10.1). The coagulation test must give information on any residual anticoagulant effect, which becomes important in managing these bleeding patients and when any intervention is planned (Tomaselli et al. 2020; Levi 2016). PT and APTT may be prolonged in bleeding patients on NOACs but normal values do not exclude residual anticoagulant activity. Fibrinogen levels may be falsely low in patients on dabigatran making the interpretation of fibrinogen levels difficult (Lazo-Langner et al. 2013). Thrombin time (TT) can be useful in patients on dabigatran and is sensitive to very low drug levels. Hence if TT is normal it excludes residual dabigatran activity, but if TT is elevated it is difficult to discriminate between clinically significant and insignificant drug concentrations (Tomaselli et al. 2020). The gold standard laboratory test is drug level measurement by liquid chromatography tandem mass spectrometry; however, its availability is limited. Ecarin clotting time can also be used for patients on dabigatran. For patients on factor Xa inhibitors antifactor Xa assay can also be done if

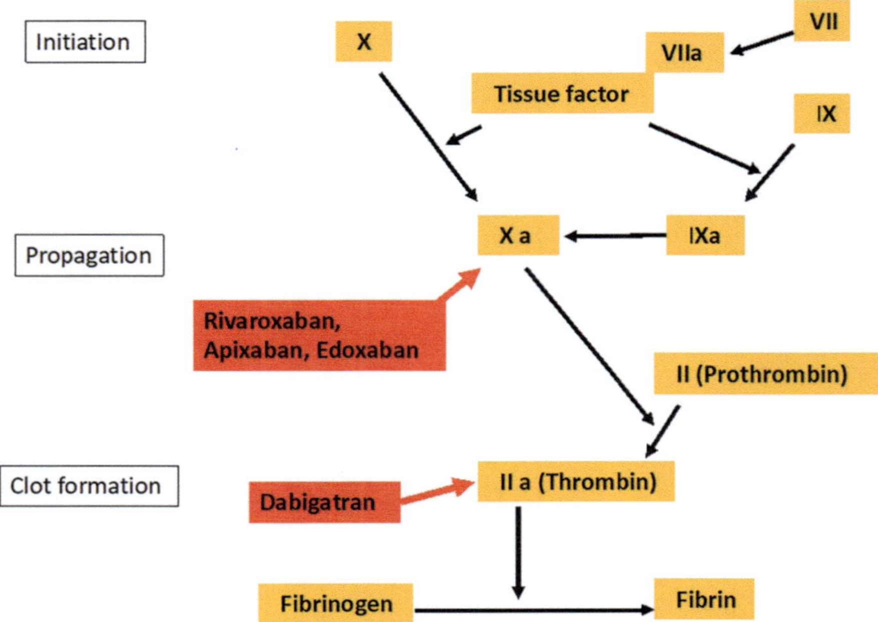

Fig. 10.1 Summarizes the site of action of the oral anticoagulants in the coagulation pathway

available (Tomaselli et al. 2020). Viscoelastic testing (TEG and ROTEM) can also be done in these patients if available. Data on the use of viscoelastic testing in patients with NOACs are limited. There is prolonged CT (clotting time) and reaction time (R) in these tests. There was a strong correlation between prolonged CT and R time with drug levels. However, viscoelastic studies can be normal even with the residual anticoagulant activity present in these patients which makes interpretation difficult (Sahli et al. 2022) (Table 10.2).

10.4 Management of Major Bleeding Patients on Oral Anticoagulants (Tomaselli et al. 2020; Lazo-Langner et al. 2013; Marras et al. 2012)

When a patient has major bleeding, the management includes—general supportive measures, resuscitation with blood products and crystalloids, identification of the bleeding site and stopping the bleeding if amenable, the use of hemostatic agents, and the use of specific antidotes.

It is important to ascertain the time of the last dose and the name of the NOACs, as most of these NOACs have a half-life of about 12 h. If the last dose is taken within 2–4 h, oral-activated charcoal can be used to reduce absorption. History of renal disease must be asked as in these patients the half-life of the drug will be prolonged. Point of care ultrasound (POCUS) must be used to assess the site of bleeding—pleural, pericardial, and abdominal. Mechanical compression can be done in cases of surface site bleeding, gastrointestinal bleeding may need endoscopy and bleeding site localization and intervention. Intervention radiology services may be utilized when the site of bleeding is localized and amenable to the same. Surgical intervention must also be planned if the site of bleeding is not amenable to intervention radiology procedures. Fluid resuscitation in the early stages of hemorrhagic shock with balanced crystalloids must be done. Colloids have no benefit in the resuscitation of these patients. Packed cell transfusion must be used early with a hemoglobin target of 7 g/dl and a target of 8 g/dl in patients with acute coronary

Table 10.2 Laboratory testing in patients on NOACs (Tomaselli et al. 2020)

NOACs	Suggested tests
Vitamin K antagonist	PT, INR
Dabigatran	Liquid chromatography tandem mass spectrometry (drug levels) Thrombin time (TT) Ecarin clotting time aPTT, PT—if above is not available
Rivaroxaban, edoxaban, Apixaban	Liquid chromatography tandem mass spectrometry (drug levels) Antifactor Xa levels PT—if the above tests are not available

syndrome. Platelets must be transfused if the platelet count is less than 50×10^9/L, the cryoprecipitate must be transfused if fibrinogen levels are <100 mg/dl. Fresh frozen plasma has no role in these patients. If the patient was on dabigatran, hemodialysis can be considered, however, hemodialysis is not effective in other NOACs as they are highly protein bound. Hypothermia and metabolic acidosis must be treated in these patients. Specific hemostatic agents can be used as mentioned in Table 10.3. In a patient with major bleeding the treatment of choice is a specific reversal agent but in situations of no availabilities hemostatic can be given. Most of the data are from healthy human volunteers and major randomized trials for the use of hemostatics are lacking. The hemostatic with the highest benefit was aPCC, if not available PCC may be used (Tomaselli et al. 2020).

The various hemostatics are summarized in Table 10.3. These hemostatic agents carry a risk of thrombotic complications and must only be used in major bleeding complications and those who require emergency surgery.

10.4.1 Reversal Agents in Bleeding Patients on NOACs (Siegal and Cuker 2013; De Marco et al. 2023)

Reversal agents can be used when a patient on a known NOAC presents with major bleeding and the reversal agent is available in the clinical setup. Reversal agents must be used in conjunction with supportive measures including resuscitation. The summary of the common reversal agents used is presented in Table 10.4. Dabigatran was the first NOAC to have a reversal agent available. Idarucizumab is a Fab fragment monoclonal antibody that binds dabigatran. In the REVERSE AD trial, Idarucizumab was found to reduce the bleeding complication and had an effective

Table 10.3 Role of hemostatic medication in bleeding patients on NOACs (Ruff et al. 2016)

Hemostatic agent	Comments
PCC (Prothrombin Complex Concentrates)	Contains factors II, IX, VII, and X, given at a dose of 50 U per kg, evidence is limited, can be used in patients on vitamin K antagonist, dabigatran, or factor Xa inhibitors
aPCC (Activated Prothrombin Complex Concentrates)	Contains factors II, IX, and X, given at a dose of 50 U per kg, achieved the best correction of coagulation factors. Evidence is limited, but can be used in patients on vitamin K antagonist, dabigatran, or factor Xa inhibitors
Recombinant factor 7	Used at a dose of 90 U/kg, evidence for use is limited, can be used in patients on dabigatran or factor Xa inhibitors
Vitamin K	Can be used in patients on vitamin K antagonists, but no role in patients on NOACs
Fresh frozen plasma	Can be used in patients on vitamin K antagonists, but has no role in patients on NOACs
Tranexamic acid	1000 mg loading dose, evidence for use is limited
Desmopressin	At a dose of 0.3 μg/kg, evidence for use is limited

Table 10.4 Summary of reversal agents used (Ruff et al. 2016)

Reversal agents	Chemical structure	Binding mechanism	Onset of action	Anticoagulants reversed	Dosage
Idarucizumab	Humanized monoclonal antibody fragment	Noncompetitive binding to dabigatran	< 5 min	Dabigatran	5 grams given as 2 doses of 2.5 g over 10 min
Andexanet Alfa	Recombinant human factor Xa	Competitive binding to direct factor Xa inhibitors	2 min	Factor Xa inhibitors	400–800 mg IV bolus followed by infusion of 4–8 mg/min
Ciraparantag	Synthetic cationic molecule	Covalent hydrogen bonding	5 min	Dabigatran and factor Xa inhibitors	100–300 mg bolus

reversal of dabigatran with minimal complications (Tomaselli et al. 2020). These reversal agents have a very minimal risk of thrombotic complications. Andexanet Alfa is a reversal agent used in patients with factor Xa inhibitors. It is a modified human recombinant FXa decoy protein. It binds the factor Xa inhibitors and intrinsic factor Xa activity is restored thus reversal of anticoagulation. In the ANNEXA-4 trial which evaluated Andexanet Alfa in bleeding patients on factor Xa inhibitors, Andexanet Alfa reduced the anti-factor Xa activity and was found to be safe (Connolly et al. 2019). Ciraparantag is a reversal agent still in the phase 2 trials stage. It can be a reversal agent against dabigatran and factor Xa inhibitors. Animal studies have found promising results and results of clinical studies are awaited. Availability and cost limit the usage of reversal agents in resource-limited settings.

10.5 Summary and Conclusion

In patients on oral anticoagulants, the most serious complication is bleeding. When a bleeding patient who is on anticoagulants presents, first ascertain the severity of bleeding as major or nonmajor bleeding. In major bleeding, initial assessment and resuscitation must begin along with the use of reversal agents if available. Hemostatic agents can be used in major bleeding including aPCC, and PCC if reversal agents are not available. There is no role of FFP in patients on NOACs. Identification of sites of bleeding and the use of intervention radiology or surgery can also be an option. Laboratory testing includes routine use of PT, a PTT, and drug assay if available. Thrombin time is sensitive for patients on dabigatran. Antifactor Xa levels can be used in patients with factor Xa inhibitors. Limited availability of reversal agents and cost limit the usage of reversal agents.

Flowchart

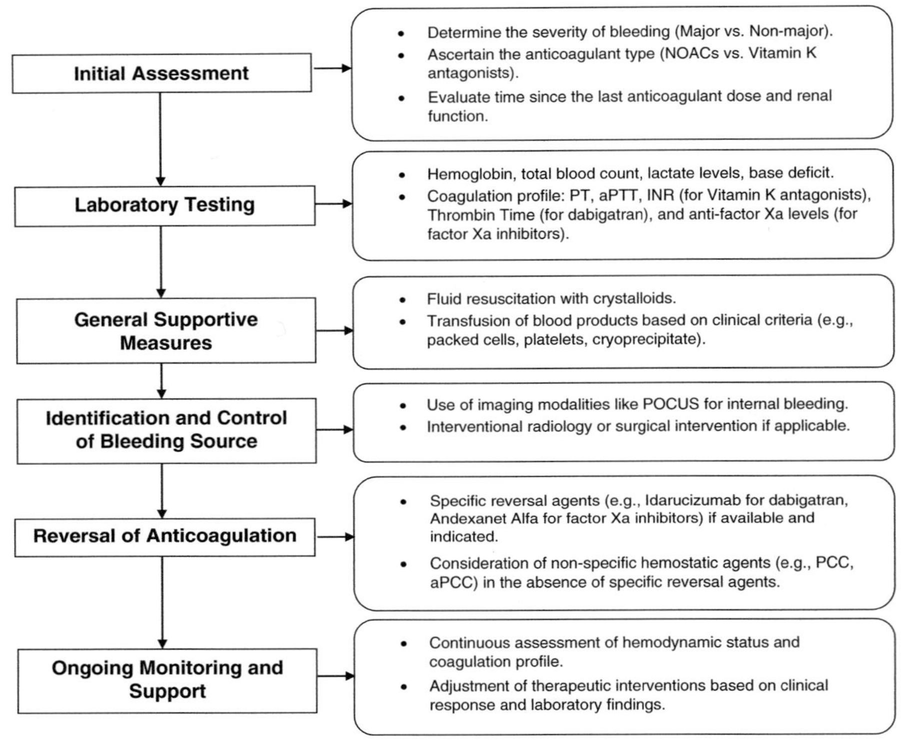

References

Connolly SJ, Crowther M, Eikelboom JW, Gibson CM, Curnutte JT, Lawrence JH et al (2019) Full study report of andexanet alfa for bleeding associated with factor Xa inhibitors. N Engl J Med 380(14):1326–1335

De Marco F, Valli G, Ancona C, Ruggieri MP (2023) Management of bleeding in patients on direct oral anticoagulants in emergency department: where we are and where we are going. Eur Heart J Suppl 25(Supplement_C):C15–C19

Lazo-Langner A, Lang ES, Douketis J (2013) Clinical review: clinical management of new oral anticoagulants: a structured review with emphasis on the reversal of bleeding complications. Crit Care 17:1–12

Levi M (2016) Management of bleeding in patients treated with direct oral anticoagulants. Crit Care 20:1–6

Loewen P, Dahri K (2011) Risk of bleeding with oral anticoagulants: an updated systematic review and performance analysis of clinical prediction rules. Ann Hematol 90(10):1191–1200

Marras E, Lo Nigro L, Berlot G (2012) Anticoagulation therapy in ICU patients. In: Hemocoagulative problems in the critically Ill patient, pp 37–60

Ruff CT, Giugliano RP, Antman EM (2016) Management of bleeding with non–vitamin K antagonist oral anticoagulants in the era of specific reversal agents. Circulation 134(3):248–261

Sahli SD, Castellucci C, Roche TR, Rössler J, Spahn DR, Kaserer A (2022) The impact of direct oral anticoagulants on viscoelastic testing–A systematic review. Front Cardiovasc Med 9:991675

Shoeb M, Fang MC (2013) Assessing bleeding risk in patients taking anticoagulants. J Thromb Thrombolysis 35:312–319

Siegal DM, Cuker A (2013) Reversal of novel oral anticoagulants in patients with major bleeding. J Thromb Thrombolysis 35(3):391–398

Tomaselli GF, Mahaffey KW, Cuker A, Dobesh PP, Doherty JU, Eikelboom JW et al (2020) 2020 ACC expert consensus decision pathway on management of bleeding in patients on oral anticoagulants: a report of the American College of Cardiology Solution Set Oversight Committee. J Am Coll Cardiol 76(5):594–622

Wallvik N, Renlund H, Själander A (2021) Bleeding risk in patients with venous thromboembolic events treated with new oral anticoagulants. J Thromb Thrombolysis 52:315–323

Zirlik A, Bode C (2017) Vitamin K antagonists: relative strengths and weaknesses vs. direct oral anticoagulants for stroke prevention in patients with atrial fibrillation. J Thromb Thrombolysis 43(3):365–379

Chapter 11
Arterial and Venous Thrombosis Patient

Alok Narasimha

Learning Point

1. Understanding Etiopathogenesis: Gain a thorough understanding of the distinct pathways involved in the initiation and progression of arterial and venous thrombosis, providing a foundation for targeted diagnostic and therapeutic strategies.
2. Diagnostic Modalities: Explore the various modalities used to evaluate arterial and venous thrombosis, including the importance of assessing risk factors for recurrent thrombotic events to guide long-term treatment planning.
3. Treatment Options: Review current treatment approaches for thrombosis, including the use of anticoagulants and antiplatelet drugs, and the decision-making process for their long-term application based on individual patient risk assessment.
4. Impact on Global Health: Discuss the significant burden of arterial and venous thrombosis on healthcare systems worldwide, highlighting the need for improved reporting and management strategies to reduce the prevalence and mortality associated with these conditions.

11.1 Introduction

Arterial and venous thrombosis is the formation of clots in the vascular system leading to impaired perfusion of tissues and cell death. These can affect any organ in the body leading to varied clinical presentation requiring differing modalities of evaluation and treatment. The decision to treat such patients with long-term anticoagulation and antiplatelet drugs depends on the assessment of risk factors for recurrent events.

A. Narasimha (✉)
Critical Care Medicine, Lyell McEwin Hospital, Elizabeth Vale, Australia

S. B. Mishra (ed.), *Critical Care Hematology*,
https://doi.org/10.1007/978-981-97-5565-3_11

The burden of arterial and venous thrombosis on healthcare systems across the world is tremendous. It is predicted that the prevalence of Ischemic Heart Disease might increase to more than 1845 per 1000,000 by the year 2030 globally. The Global burden of pulmonary embolism-related deaths is underestimated due to heterogeneous reporting and is estimated to be 24 per 100,000 population years (Barco et al. 2021). Arterial and venous thrombosis have varied and dissimilar etiologies with differing pathways for their formation. This chapter explains the pathways of formation of thrombi in these systems, with a focus on evaluation and management of the same.

11.2 Physiology of Clot Formation in the Vascular System

Blood flows without clotting in the vascular system, due to the complex interplay between blood cells (including platelets), plasma proteins, coagulation factors, inflammatory factors and cytokines, and the endothelial lining within the lumen of arteries and veins. Disturbance in one or more of these elements causes blood to clot, which prevents life-threatening hemorrhage in the presence of tissue trauma (Fig. 11.1).

Rudolf Virchow, in 1856, proposed "Virchow's triad." These are factors which predispose to the formation of thrombi and include (1) damage to the endothelial lining of the vessel wall; (2) a hypercoagulable state; and (3) arterial or venous blood stasis.

Arterial thrombi, however, are often formed as a response to rupture of atherosclerotic plaque and exposure to thrombogenic subendothelial material which triggers platelet aggregation and fibrin formation, resulting in the generation of a platelet-rich thrombus that temporarily or permanently occludes blood flow.

Venous thrombosis develops in response to sluggish blood flow causing impaired oxygen delivery to the endothelium, triggering expression of adhesion molecules on its surface, platelet aggregation, and activation of coagulation factors. This coupled with impaired clearance of activated coagulation factors by sluggish blood flow, propagates further formation of clots.

Venous thrombosis is primarily caused by abnormality in coagulation factors (hypercoagulable states) and blood stasis in contrast to arterial thrombus which is caused due to injury to the vessel wall and platelet aggregation (Table 11.1).

Although venous and arterial thrombi appear to have distinct etiopathogenesis for their formation, it was theorized that they are triggered by the same biological stimuli that activate coagulation and inflammatory pathways (Prandoni 2017).

In homeostasis, the procoagulant and anticoagulant factors work in synchrony to prevent formation of blood clots in circulation in the absence of tissue injury.

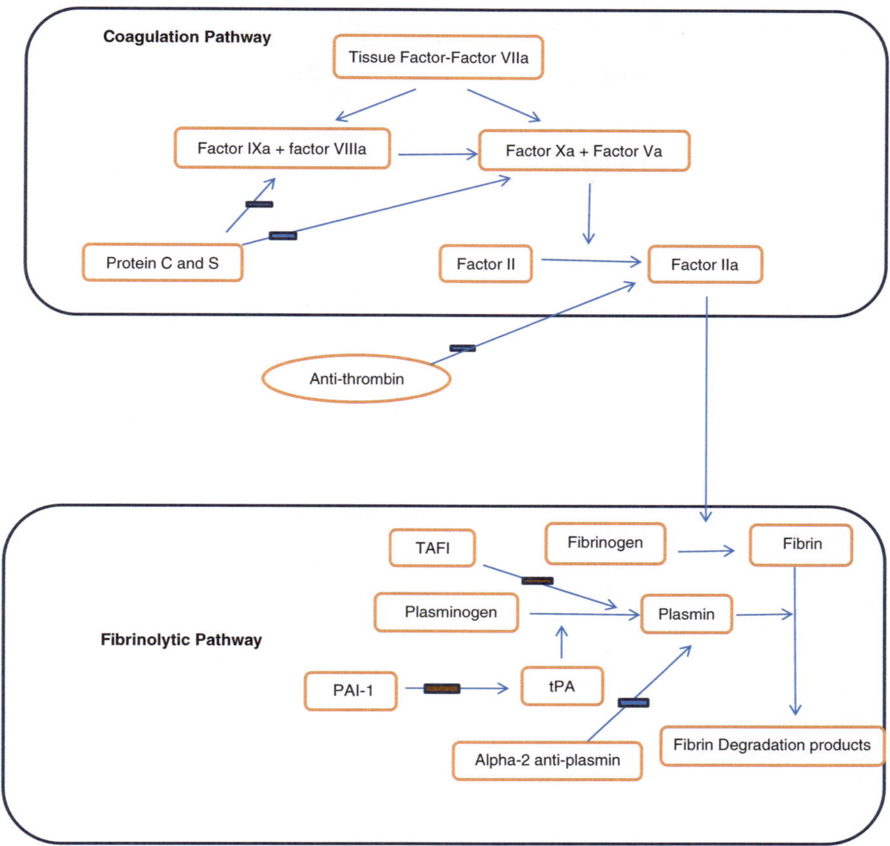

Fig. 11.1 Flow Chart describes the coagulation pathway along with the fibrinolytic pathway. Negative sign indicates factors which have an inhibitory effect on the pathway. Factors that inhibit fibrin formation include antithrombin, protein C, and protein S. Factors that inhibit fibrinolysis are Plasminogen Activator Inhibitor 1 (PAI 1), TAFI, and alpha-2 antiplasmin. (Chapin and Hajjar 2015)

Table 11.1 Following table illustrates various factors involved in clot formation and lysis. Imbalance in these factors will lead to bleeding or clotting based on the underlying pathology

Factors which promote clot formation	Factor II (thrombin), factor V, factor VII, factor VIII, factor IX, factor X, platelet activation and aggregation, VWF
Factors which inhibit clot formation	Protein C, protein S, antithrombin
Factors which lyse already formed clots	Plasmin, tissue plasminogen activator
Factors which prevent clot lysis	Alpha-2 antiplasmin, PAI1, TAFI

11.3 Etiology of Thrombosis

- *Hypercoagulable States Causing Venous Thrombosis*:
- *Hypercoagulable States Which Cause Both Arterial and Venous Thrombosis:* Acquired antiphospholipid syndrome and Heparin-induced thrombocytopenia & thrombosis (HITT).
- *Malignancies* cause prothrombogenic state, as tumor cells produce a large amount of procoagulant factors.
- *Atherosclerosis* is the accumulation of lipid plaques in the arterial wall, provokes chronic inflammatory cells and platelet activation leading to arterial thrombosis (Table 11.2).

11.4 Clinical Features and Evaluation

Thrombosis can affect any part of the vascular tree in the body causing organ-specific symptoms and signs. Arterial thrombosis, causing macrovascular thrombi leads to an ischemic cerebrovascular accident, coronary artery disease, peripheral vascular disease, and acute limb ischemia and mesenteric ischemia.

Ischemic cerebrovascular accident presents with focal neurological signs and leads to permanent disability if not treated immediately. It can also be catastrophic if the basilar artery or proximal branches of the anterior circulation in the circle of Wills get occluded. Evaluation includes emergent neuroimaging and is coupled with reestablishing perfusion by means of thrombolysis and thrombectomy. Stroke in Young (< 45–49 years) needs evaluation for predisposing factors for thrombosis in this population (Herpich and Rincon 2020).

Acute Coronary Syndromes (ACS) include ST elevation myocardial infarction (STEMI), Non-ST Elevation myocardial infarction, and Unstable Angina. These patients present with anginal chest pain, breathlessness, and perspiration. They may progress to develop shock and cardiac arrest within a short time. Evaluation includes electrocardiograph (ECG), and cardiac biomarkers like Troponin. Management focuses on reestablishing perfusion to the myocardium via thrombolysis and endovascular treatment.

Acute mesenteric ischemia presents with features of acute abdomen and is evaluated with CT angiography of the abdomen. Acute limb ischemia presents with

Table 11.2 Hypercoagulable states causing venous thrombosis

Inherited	Antithrombin III deficiency, protein C and S deficiencies, factor V Leiden (activated protein C resistance), or prothrombin gene mutations
Acquired (more common)	Medications (e.g., oral contraceptives, estrogen or other hormonal replacement), recent inflammatory conditions such as pregnancy, surgery, trauma, or infection, and chronic inflammatory conditions (e.g., morbid obesity, rheumatologic disease, ulcerative colitis, heavy smoking)

absent peripheral pulses and impaired perfusion to the limb. This is also evaluated with arterial doppler and angiography, and requires consult with a vascular surgeon for further management (Olinic et al. 2019).

Venous thrombosis leads to cerebral venous sinus thrombosis, deep vein thrombosis (DVT), and pulmonary thromboembolism (PE).

Cerebral venous sinus thrombosis (CVT) presents with headaches, seizures, and focal deficits in at-risk individuals. Evaluation includes CT and MRI venography.

Deep vein thrombosis causes pain, tenderness, fever, and swelling of the affected limb. Pulmonary embolism causes breathlessness, fever, and hypotension and may lead to cardiac arrest. When DVT or PE is suspected based on history and physical examination, a probability scoring system like Well's or Geneva scoring system should be used to decide on further evaluation of the patient. If the patient has a low probability of the diagnosis, a negative D-Dimer test effectively rules out DVT/PE. If the probability of the disease is high, these patients should undergo CT—pulmonary angiography or V/Q scan to diagnose PE and lower limb venous Doppler to diagnose DVT.

Diseases like Heparin-induced thrombocytopenia (HIT) and antiphospholipid antibody syndrome (APLA) cause both arterial and venous thrombosis. When HIT is suspected, a 4 T score should be done to assess the probability of the illness and if the probability is high, patients should be tested for PF4/H antibodies (Lee and Arepally 2013).

APLA syndrome presents with recurrent pregnancy loss in the background of a connective tissue disorder like systemic lupus erythematosus. These patients should be evaluated after discussion with a hematologist and immunologist.

Efforts should be made to elicit relevant personal and family history suggestive of inherited or acquired thrombophilias. In patients who have had a stroke at young (<45–49 years), CVT, unprovoked DVT or pulmonary embolism, and recurrent pregnancy losses, careful selection of tests to evaluate for procoagulant state, should be undertaken, whilst discussion with a hematologist. It must be remembered that initiation of anticoagulant treatment interferes with most of these tests (Table 11.3).

11.5 Treatment

Disease-specific treatment should be done in liaison with respective specialty consultations like cardiology, hematology, neurology, intervention radiology, and vascular surgeon.

Treatment of venous thrombosis involves initiation of intravenous unfractionated heparin (UFH) or low molecular weight heparin (LMWH) which is subsequently transitioned to Directly Acting Oral Anticoagulants (DOCA). Depending on the risk for recurrent thrombosis, anticoagulation may have to be continued for 3–6 months.

Table 11.3 Difference between arterial and venous thrombosis

Arterial thrombus	Venous thrombus
Step 1: Atherosclerotic plaque rupture Step 2: Exposure of thrombogenic material Step 3: Platelet aggregation Step 4: Activation of coagulation cascade Step 5: Thrombus formation	Step 1: Blood stasis Step 2: Hypercoagulable state Step 3: Endothelial damage Step 4: Activation of coagulation Step 5: Thrombus propagation
Diagnostic modalities: ECG (Electrocardiogram)—primarily used in the assessment of heart rhythm and function, which can indirectly indicate the effects of arterial clots CT angiography—offers a detailed image of both arteries and veins, used to detect blockages or clots	**Diagnostic modalities:** Venography—specifically used for visualizing venous clots, particularly deep vein thrombosis Doppler ultrasound studies—used to evaluate blood flow and detect disruptions typical of thrombosis Well's score and D-dimer testing—well's score assesses the probability of DVT/PE based on clinical criteria. D-dimer testing measures a fibrin degradation product, used to exclude DVT/PE in low-risk patients
Treatment options: **Arterial thrombosis:** **Thrombolysis**—administering medication to dissolve clots, typically used in acute settings like myocardial infarction or stroke **Antiplatelet therapy**—medications like aspirin or clopidogrel are used to prevent further platelet aggregation **Surgical interventions**—such as angioplasty or stenting to restore blood flow in affected arteries	**Treatment options:** **Venous thrombosis:** **Anticoagulation therapy**—starts with heparin (either unfractionated or low molecular weight heparin) followed by a transition to oral anticoagulants such as warfarin or DOAC's (direct oral anticoagulants) **Long-term therapy considerations**—based on risk assessment for recurrent thrombosis, which might require extended or even lifetime anticoagulation in high-risk patients

The mainstay of arterial thrombosis is reestablishing perfusion to the affected organ as soon as possible, and subsequent treatment with single or dual antiplatelets.

11.6 Summary and Conclusion

Arterial and venous thrombosis leads to diseases which cause death and severe disability, with enormous healthcare costs. Management of such patients requires basic knowledge of the functioning of hemostatic, coagulation, and fibrinolytic systems. Imbalance in these systems along with preexisting genetic and environmental risk factors causes thrombus to form. Treatment should be disease-specific and interdisciplinary to achieve optimal patient outcomes.

Flowchart

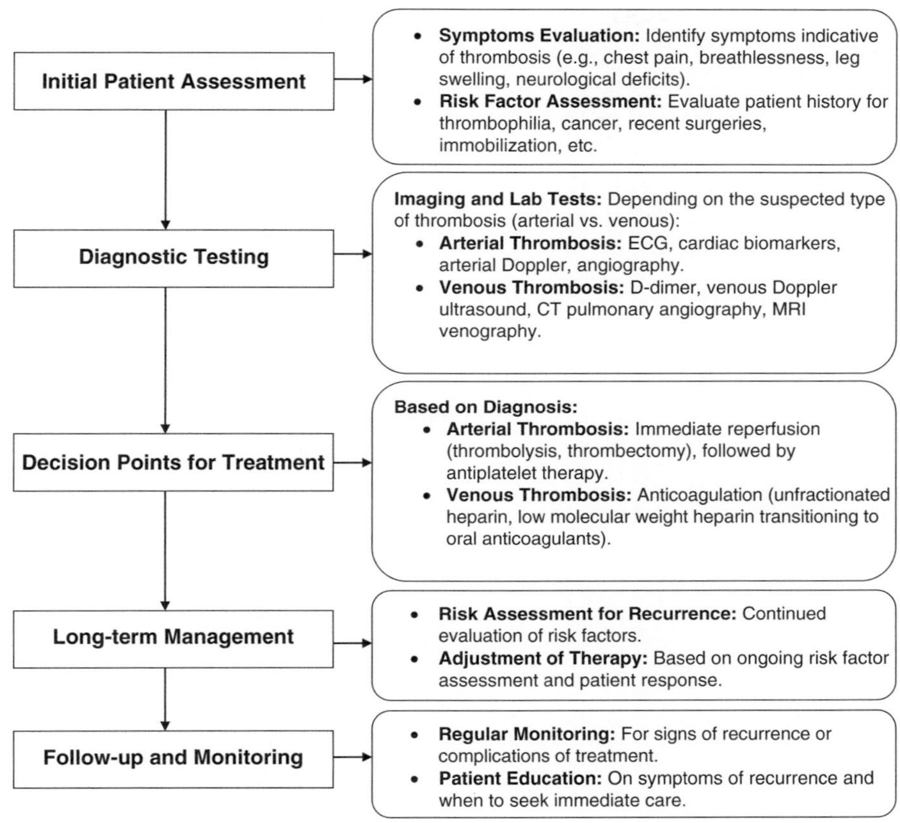

References

Barco S, Valerio L, Gallo A, Turatti G, Mahmoudpour SH, Ageno W et al (2021) Global reporting of pulmonary embolism-related deaths in the World Health Organization mortality database: vital registration data from 123 countries. Res Pract Thromb Haemost 5(5):e12520

Chapin JC, Hajjar KA (2015) Fibrinolysis and the control of blood coagulation. Blood Rev 29(1):17–24

Herpich F, Rincon F (2020) Management of acute ischemic stroke. Crit Care Med 48(11):1654–1663

Lee GM, Arepally GM (2013) Heparin-induced thrombocytopenia. Hematology Am Soc Hematol Educ Program 2013(1):668–674

Olinic DM, Stanek A, Tătaru DA, Homorodean C, Olinic M (2019) Acute limb ischemia: an update on diagnosis and management. J Clin Med 8(8):1215

Prandoni P (2017) Venous and arterial thrombosis: is there a link? In: Thrombosis and embolism: from research to clinical practice: volume 1, pp 273–283

Chapter 12
Sickle Cell Crisis

Shruti Mishra

Learning Points

1. Vaso-occlusive crises (VOC) are central to the pathology of SCD, leading to multiorgan complications.
2. Comprehensive management of acute complications in SCD requires a multidisciplinary approach. This includes hydration, pain management, prophylactic antibiotics, and transfusion therapies.
3. Preventive strategies are crucial, including penicillin prophylaxis and regular screening (e.g., transcranial Doppler for stroke risk).
4. The management of SCD in the ICU should be tailored to individual patient needs, considering the type of crisis, the affected organ systems, and the patient's baseline health status.

12.1 Introduction

Sickle cell anemia is a genetically inherited hemoglobin disorder marked by a single-nucleotide polymorphism in the beta-globin gene (Finch et al. 1973). This mutation alters the amino acid sequence, substituting glutamic acid with valine at the sixth position, producing abnormal hemoglobin S (HbS) instead of normal hemoglobin A (HbA). The manifestation of sickle cell disease can be either homozygous, where two copies of the mutated gene are present, or heterozygous, with only one affected gene (Laurentino et al. 2014).

S. Mishra (✉)
Bone Marrow Transplantation and Stem Cell Research Centre, Institute of Medical Sciences, Banaras Hindu University, Varanasi, Uttar Pradesh, India
e-mail: drshruti.mishra@bhu.ac.in

S. B. Mishra (ed.), *Critical Care Hematology*,
https://doi.org/10.1007/978-981-97-5565-3_12

There is a higher incidence of compound heterozygosity in areas where thalassemia and other hemoglobin variants are expected (Monus and Howell 2019). Patients with double heterozygous states may exhibit clinical presentations akin to those with homozygous sickle cell anemia. Globally, individuals with two copies of the HbS gene are diagnosed with Sickle Cell Anemia, while those carrying a single copy are identified as having the Sickle Cell Trait (Leavell 1954).

The clinical hallmark of Sickle Cell Anemia is the occurrence of vaso-occlusive crises, primarily caused by the obstruction of microcirculation by rigid, sickle-shaped erythrocytes (Ashraf et al. 2019). Under deoxygenated conditions, the absence of the hydrophilic glutamic acid—replaced by the hydrophobic valine—facilitates the polymerization of deoxyHbS, forcing the red blood cells (RBCs) into a sickle shape. This sickling process, which is initially reversible, becomes permanent over time as the cells lose their elasticity, leading to recurrent vaso-occlusive episodes and resultant complications like auto-splenectomy (Akinsheye and Klings 2010).

Patients may also experience other types of crises characteristic of hemolytic anemias, including:

- *Aplastic Crisis*: Characterized by a profound decrease in RBC production, often triggered by viral infections.
- *Megaloblastic Crisis*: Stemming from a deficiency in folic acid, producing abnormally large RBCs.
- *Hemolytic Crisis*: Marked by an accelerated rate of RBC destruction, resulting in anemia and jaundice.

12.2 Pulmonary Acute Chest Syndrome (ACS) in Sickle Cell Disease (SCD)

Pulmonary Acute Chest Syndrome (ACS) stands as a critical complication in Sickle Cell Disease (SCD), defined by lung injury that either complicates an acute vaso-occlusive crisis or occurs spontaneously (Belveyre et al. 2019). This condition is notably associated with a substantial risk of respiratory failure, estimated at 13%, and mortality rates reaching up to 9% in adult SCD patients (De et al. 2023). The impact of ACS extends beyond immediate health concerns, as it is linked with prolonged hospital stays, diminished long-term survival prospects, and an elevated likelihood of developing chronic pulmonary diseases (Block et al. 2021).

12.2.1 Clinical Presentation

ACS often presents with symptoms mirroring those of pneumonia, including fever, dyspnea, reduced oxygen saturation levels, and significant chest pain. Radiographic analysis typically reveals multilobar lung involvement, underscoring the severity of the condition. The etiology of ACS is multifactorial, encompassing infection, fat embolization from necrotic bone marrow, severe hemolysis, hypoventilation, and in situ pulmonary thrombosis (Field and DeBaun 2009).

12.2.2 Mechanisms Underpinning ACS

The pathogenesis of ACS is complex, with about 80% of cases following a vaso-occlusive crisis (Belveyre et al. 2019). This sequence results in RBC sickling, enhanced RBC adhesion to the endothelium, pronounced hemolysis, and vaso-occlusion, typically manifesting approximately 2.5 days posthospitalization for a vaso-occlusive episode. Key factors include:

- *Fat Embolization*: Leading to acute lung injury.
- *Pulmonary Infection*: Serving as both a trigger and exacerbating factor.
- *Pulmonary Infarction and Hypoventilation*: Contributing to localized lung damage.
- *In Situ Pulmonary Thrombosis*: Aggravating vascular occlusion within the lungs.
- The pathophysiology also involves significant ventilation-perfusion mismatches and shunting, culminating in hypoxemia.

12.2.3 Treatment Strategies for ACS

Effective management of ACS requires a multifaceted approach to address infection and mitigate vaso-occlusion. Protocols include:

- *Broad-Spectrum Antibiotics*: Administered to all patients to target potential infectious agents.
- *RBC Transfusions*: In severe cases, exchange transfusions might be necessary to enhance oxygen delivery and decrease the proportion of hemoglobin S (HbS).
- *Systemic Corticosteroids*: Proposed to aid in the prevention and resolution of ACS-induced acute respiratory distress syndrome, though their use remains contentious due to potential complications.
- *Hydroxyurea*: Demonstrated efficacy in reducing the frequency of ACS episodes.
- *Additional Therapeutics*: Including L-glutamine, Crizanlizumab, and Voxelotor, all of which have received FDA approval for managing SCD crises in adults, showing promise in the context of ACS treatment.

12.3 Multiorgan Failure Syndrome (MOFS) in Sickle Cell Disease (SCD)

Multiorgan Failure Syndrome (MOFS) is one of the most severe complications associated with Sickle Cell Disease (SCD), often precipitated by vaso-occlusive crises (Louie et al. 2018). MOFS is characterized by the acute failure of multiple organ systems, which significantly escalates the risk of mortality among affected individuals. A hallmark of patients developing MOFS is brisk hemolysis, indicating rapid destruction of red blood cells that contributes to the systemic severity of the condition (Demagny et al. 2021).

12.3.1 Pathophysiology and Complications

The onset of MOFS in the context of SCD is complex, involving a cascade of pathophysiological events:

- *Brisk Hemolysis*: This leads to the release of free hemoglobin into the circulation, scavenging nitric oxide and contributing to vascular dysfunction, inflammation, and further vaso-occlusion.
- *Fat Embolism Syndrome*: The release of fat droplets from necrotic bone marrow into the bloodstream can lead to embolism and subsequent respiratory and neurological manifestations.
- *Acute Respiratory Distress Syndrome (ARDS)*: Severe lung injury resulting from various triggers, including fat embolism and infection, can precipitate ARDS, exacerbating respiratory failure and complicating the clinical management of MOFS (Fig. 12.1).

12.3.2 Management Strategies for MOFS

Prompt and effective management is critical, given the high mortality rate associated with MOFS. The cornerstone of treatment lies in supportive care aimed at stabilizing vital functions (Trivedi et al. 2022) and mitigating the impact of organ failures:

- *Supportive Care*: Involves meticulous monitoring and management of fluid balance, oxygenation, and hemodynamic stability, along with renal replacement therapy as needed for renal failure and mechanical ventilation for respiratory failure (Siddiqui et al. 2021).
- *Systemic Corticosteroids* may be employed to reduce systemic inflammation and mitigate the severity of ARDS, though their use must be carefully weighed against potential side effects.

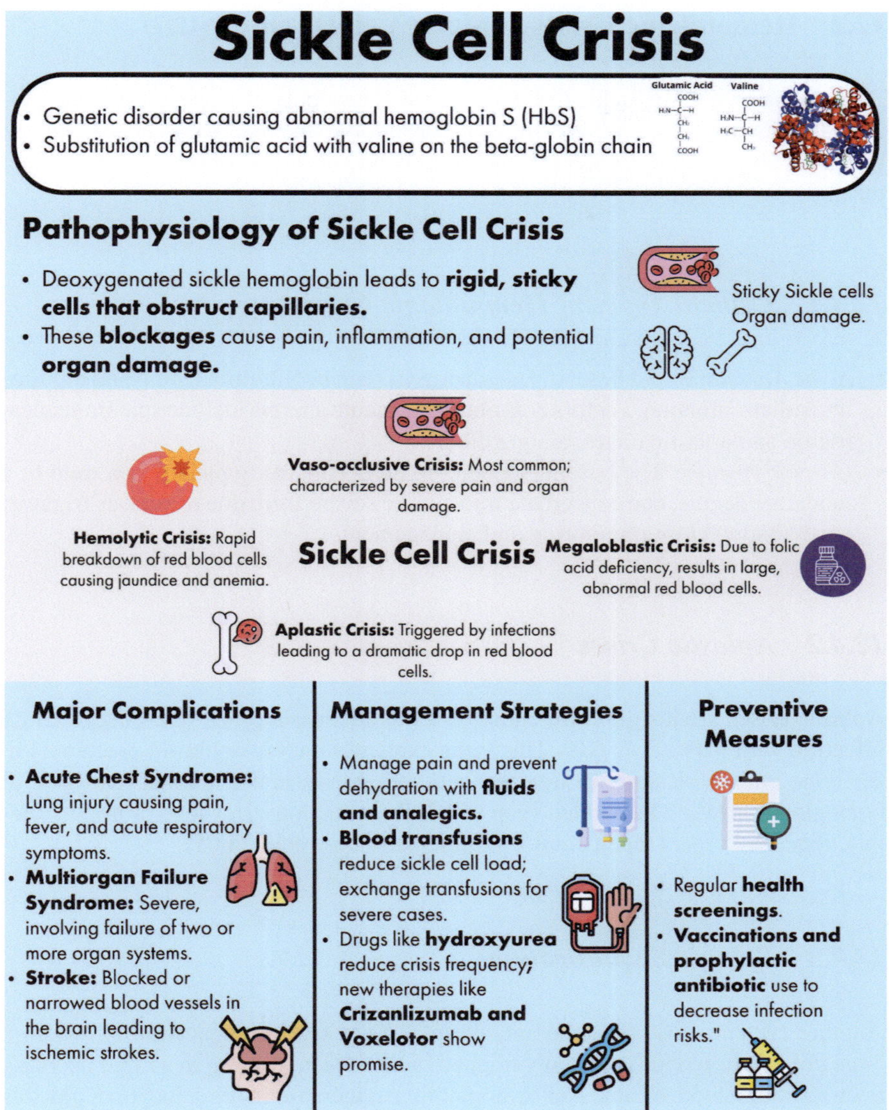

Fig. 12.1 Sickle cell crisis

- *Plasma Exchange* has been proposed as a therapeutic option to remove circulating free hemoglobin, fat globules, and inflammatory cytokines, potentially interrupting the pathophysiological processes driving MOFS (Majjiga et al. 2010).

12.4 Hematologic Crises in Sickle Cell Disease (SCD)

Hematologic Crises in Sickle Cell Disease (SCD) encompass a spectrum of complications primarily characterized by acute or chronic anemia. These crises warrant thorough investigation to identify the underlying cause and to initiate appropriate management strategies promptly (Snyder et al. (2017).

12.4.1 Critical Types of Hematologic Crises

- *Acute Anemia*: Rapid onset of anemia in SCD can be life-threatening and requires immediate attention. Factors contributing to acute anemia include splenic sequestration and aplastic crises, among others.
- *Chronic Anemia*: The baseline anemia in SCD patients, typically of a mild to a moderate degree, can exacerbate into a more severe form due to various triggers, necessitating close monitoring and management.

12.4.2 Aplastic Crises

Aplastic crises are a significant cause of acute anemia in SCD, often triggered by infection with parvovirus B19. This virus explicitly targets erythroid precursors in the bone marrow, leading to transient red cell aplasia and a marked reduction in hemoglobin levels. The sudden drop in RBC production can cause profound anemia, requiring urgent medical intervention (Moschovi et al. 2001).

12.4.3 Splenic Sequestration

Another critical cause of acute anemia in SCD is splenic sequestration, where a large volume of blood is suddenly trapped in the spleen, leading to a rapid decrease in circulating blood volume and hemoglobin. An increase in reticulocyte marks this condition count as the body attempts to compensate for the loss of red blood cells. Splenic sequestration crises can be acute and life-threatening, particularly in young children.

12.4.4 *Management of Severe Anemia in SCD*

The management of severe anemia in SCD is multifaceted, with transfusion therapy serving as the cornerstone of treatment:

- *Transfusion Therapy*: Blood transfusions are pivotal in managing severe anemia in SCD patients. They aim to promptly restore hemoglobin levels to stabilize the patient's condition. Transfusions can be either simple or exchange, depending on the anemia's severity and the presence of complications.
- *Supportive Care*: Besides transfusion, supportive care measures, including hydration and pain management, are crucial in managing hematologic crises in SCD.
- *Monitoring and Prevention*: Regular monitoring for early signs of anemia and proactive measures, such as immunizations and antibiotic prophylaxis, are essential in preventing aplastic crises and managing splenic sequestration.

12.5 Venous-Thromboembolism (VTE) Treatment Overview

The management of Venous Thromboembolism (VTE), which encompasses both deep vein thrombosis (DVT) and pulmonary embolism (PE), adheres to evidence-based guidelines established by the American College of Chest Physicians (ACCP) in 2016 (Barnes et al. 2015). These guidelines advocate for a balanced approach that weighs the efficacy of thromboprophylaxis against potential bleeding risks, emphasizing individualized patient care.

Initial and Long-Term Anticoagulation

Full-Dose Anticoagulation: Initial treatment involves full-dose anticoagulation therapy to mitigate the risk of clot propagation and embolization. The choice of anticoagulant—Heparin, Direct Oral Anticoagulants (DOACs), or Vitamin K Antagonists (VKAs)—is influenced by patient-specific factors, including renal function, potential for drug interactions, and the need for rapid reversibility of anticoagulation (Kearon and Akl 2014).

- *Heparin*: Unfractionated heparin (UFH) is often used for initial in-hospital management due to its rapid onset and ease of reversibility. Low-molecular-weight heparin (LMWH) is preferred for its predictable pharmacokinetics and lower risk of heparin-induced thrombocytopenia (HIT).
- *Direct Oral Anticoagulants (DOACs)*: Include agents such as rivaroxaban, apixaban, dabigatran, and edoxaban, offering the convenience of oral administration and reduced need for laboratory monitoring (Weitz 2006).
- *Vitamin K Antagonists (VKAs)*: Warfarin remains a mainstay for long-term anticoagulation, requiring careful monitoring of the International Normalized Ratio (INR) to maintain therapeutic efficacy while minimizing bleeding risk (Le Gal and Mottier 2012).

Duration of Anticoagulation: Anticoagulation is recommended for at least 3 months for the first unprovoked VTE event. The decision to extend anticoagulation beyond this period should consider the balance between the risk of recurrent VTE and the potential for bleeding complications (Khan et al. 2021). Extended anticoagulation is recommended for patients with low bleeding risk, mainly if the initial VTE event was provoked by a transient risk factor such as hospitalization for medical illness (Kearon 2007).

12.5.1 Special Considerations

- *Extended Anticoagulation*: In patients with low bleeding risk, extending anticoagulation beyond the initial 3-month period may be beneficial, even if a transient factor precipitated the VTE event. This approach aims to reduce the risk of recurrent VTE (Di Minno et al. 2013), (Kearon 2007).
- *Catheter-Associated Upper-Extremity Thrombosis*: Anticoagulation should be continued for thrombosis associated with central venous catheters until the catheter is removed. This strategy helps to prevent further thrombus extension and reduces the risk of embolic complications (Klok et al. 2019).

12.6 Neurological Crises in Sickle Cell Disease (SCD): Focus on Ischemic Stroke

Neurological complications, including ischemic stroke, represent a significant morbidity risk in patients with Sickle Cell Disease (SCD). The pathophysiology of stroke in SCD is complex, involving chronic hemolytic anemia, vascular inflammation, and the prothrombotic state characteristic of the disease (Riebel et al. 2003).

12.6.1 Ischemic Stroke Prevention

Preventative strategies have yielded success, particularly in pediatric SCD populations:

- *Screening*: Regular transcranial Doppler (TCD) ultrasound screening identifies children at high risk for stroke by measuring cerebral blood flow velocity. Elevated flow velocities indicate increased stroke risk (Charlotte et al. 2021).
- *Prophylactic Transfusions*: Regular red blood cell transfusions have been demonstrated to significantly reduce the risk of first stroke in children identified as high risk by TCD screening. This approach aims to decrease the hemoglobin S

(HbS) proportion to below 30% to mitigate sickling and vaso-occlusion (Herbst et al. 2020).

12.6.2 Risk of Acute Territorial Ischemia

Patients with SCD, particularly those with compromised cerebral vascular anatomy or previous infarcts, are at heightened risk of acute territorial ischemia under conditions of acute stress, dehydration, or infection (Maduakor et al. 2021). These factors can precipitate a vaso-occlusive crisis, leading to further ischemia and stroke.

12.6.3 Treatment of Acute Ischemic Stroke

- *Prompt Transfusion*: The immediate management of acute ischemic stroke in SCD involves rapid red blood cell transfusion to improve anemia, increase oxygenation, and dilute the concentration of HbS. Exchange transfusion is often employed to reduce HbS levels while avoiding volume overload quickly (Oliveira et al. 2008).
- *Oxygen Therapy*: Supplemental oxygen is administered to alleviate hypoxia, a critical precipitant of sickling in cerebral vessels (Miraulle et al. 2021).
- *Limited Evidence for Thrombolytic Use*: The application of thrombolytic therapy in SCD-associated stroke is controversial, with limited evidence supporting its use. Caution is advised, particularly in patients with HbSC disease, due to the increased risk of hemorrhagic conversion and other complications (Kato et al. 2006).

12.7 Hepatic Crises in Sickle Cell Disease (SCD)

Hepatic involvement in Sickle Cell Disease (SCD) during acute vaso-occlusive crises (VOCs) presents a spectrum of manifestations, ranging from mild hepatic enzyme elevations to severe hepatic syndromes. These complications reflect the heterogeneity of SCD and its impact on liver function and structure (Aslan et al. 2003).

12.7.1 Spectrum of Liver VOC

The liver, a highly vascular organ, is particularly susceptible to the vaso-occlusive processes of SCD, resulting in a range of clinical presentations:

- *Mild Elevations in Liver Enzymes*: Often the most minimal sign of hepatic VOC, reflecting transient ischemic insults to hepatocytes.
- *Hepatic Sequestration* is characterized by the sudden, painful enlargement of the liver due to the trapping of sickled red blood cells within the hepatic circulation, leading to rapid onset liver dysfunction and potentially life-threatening anemia.
- *Acute Intrahepatic Cholesterolasis*: Results from severe sickling within the intrahepatic bile ducts, causing obstruction and marked elevation in bilirubin levels, alongside jaundice and pruritus. This condition represents one of the more severe manifestations of liver VOC (Akaba et al. 2019).

12.7.2 Treatment Modalities for Hepatic Crises

The management of hepatic crises in SCD aims to address the underlying vaso-occlusion, restore liver function, and prevent complications:

- *Volume Expansion*: Adequate hydration is crucial to reduce blood viscosity and promote microcirculatory flow, thus mitigating the risk of further vaso-occlusion. This approach serves as a supportive measure across the spectrum of liver VOC.
- *Exchange Transfusion*: Exchange transfusion is employed for severe cases, particularly those involving hepatic sequestration or acute intrahepatic cholestasis with significant liver dysfunction. This technique rapidly reduces the proportion of sickled cells, decreases blood viscosity, and improves oxygen delivery to hepatic tissue.

12.7.3 Infectious Complications in Sickle Cell Disease (SCD)

Infectious complications constitute a significant aspect of the morbidity and mortality associated with Sickle Cell Disease (SCD). Due to the inherent immunocompromised state conferred by SCD, coupled with the complications arising from treatment modalities, patients are at an elevated risk of infection (Obaro 2009). Implementing preventive measures, understanding the impact of therapeutic interventions, and recognizing specific infection risks are paramount in managing SCD (Hardie et al. 2009).

12.8 Penicillin Prophylaxis and Sepsis Incidence

- *Penicillin Prophylaxis*: Routine penicillin prophylaxis, starting in early childhood, has markedly reduced the incidence of sepsis, particularly pneumococcal sepsis, in individuals with SCD. This approach leverages the antibiotic's effectiveness in preventing infections from encapsulated bacteria, to which SCD patients are especially vulnerable.

- *Venous Catheter Contamination*: Venous catheters, often used for long-term treatments in SCD, represent a common source of bacterial contamination and subsequent infection. Meticulous catheter care and monitoring are crucial to mitigate this risk (Miller et al. 2005).

12.9 Red Blood Cell (RBC) Alloimmunization

RBC alloimmunization, a response to foreign antigens on transfused red blood cells, can lead to delayed hemolytic transfusion reactions. These reactions pose immediate risks and complicate future transfusion efforts by limiting compatible blood availability (Teach et al. 1998).

Impact of Hydroxyurea and Iron Chelation on Infection Susceptibility

- *Hydroxyurea*: While hydroxyurea is a cornerstone in SCD management, reducing the frequency of pain crises and acute chest syndrome, its immunomodulatory effects may slightly alter infection susceptibility. The benefits of hydroxyurea, however, often outweigh potential risks, and its use is carefully monitored (Grosse et al. 2012).
- *Iron Chelation*: Iron overload, a consequence of frequent blood transfusions, necessitates chelation therapy to prevent organ damage. Iron chelation therapy can influence immune function and infection risk, necessitating vigilant monitoring for signs of infection (Alboog et al. 2015).

12.10 Malarial Parasitemia Risk in SCD

For SCD patients exposed to malaria, the risk of malarial parasitemia and consequent mortality is significantly increased. Despite the protective effect of the sickle cell trait against malaria, individuals with SCD are more susceptible to severe malarial infections. Preventive measures, including prophylactic antimalarials and mosquito avoidance strategies, are critical for SCD patients living in or traveling to endemic areas.

12.11 Conclusion

Sickle Cell Disease (SCD) is a complex hemoglobinopathy with a broad spectrum of clinical manifestations, ranging from mild anemia to life-threatening complications such as multiorgan failure syndrome (MOFS) and acute chest syndrome

(ACS). Effective management of sickle cell crisis, especially in the intensive care unit (ICU), requires understanding the disease’s pathophysiology, early recognition of symptoms, and a comprehensive, multidisciplinary approach to treatment. Advances in screening, prophylaxis, and therapeutic interventions have significantly improved the prognosis for individuals with SCD, though challenges remain in managing acute crises and preventing complications.

Flowchart

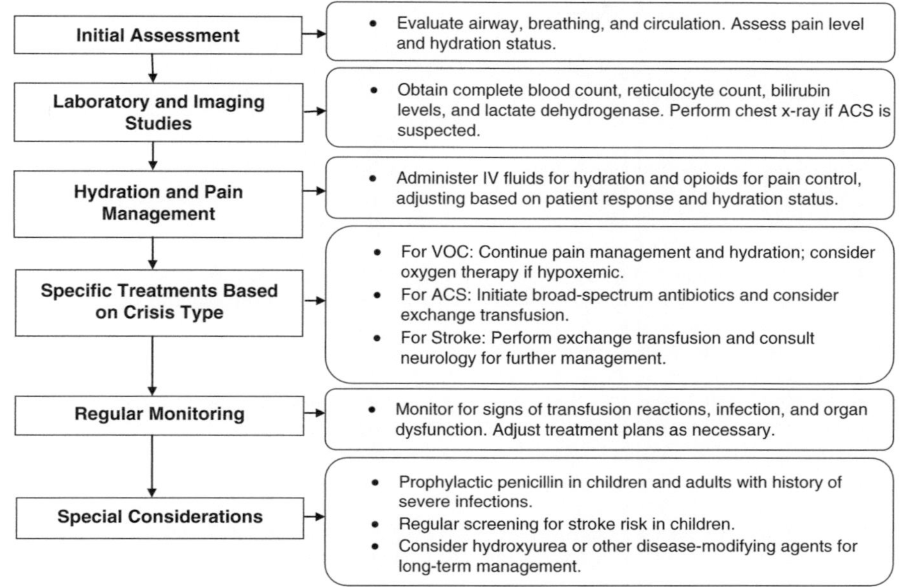

Approach to a patient with Sickle Cell Crisis in ICU Flowchart

References

Akaba K, Ofem E, Bassey OB, Oluwakorede B, Riman O (2019) Biochemical assessment of the liver in SCD in a tertiary hospital in South-South, Nigeria. J Adv Med Med Res 29:1–6

Akinsheye I, Klings ES (2010) Sickle cell anemia and vascular dysfunction: the nitric oxide connection. J Cell Physiol 224(3):620–625

Alboog A, Tayeb T, Alsager M, Alnajjar S, Damanhouri G, Jarullah J, Hindawi SI (2015) Red blood cell alloimmunization in sickle cell disease patients in Jeddah, Saudi Arabia: a pilot study. JKAU Med Sci 22(3):35–40

Ashraf F, Kancharla P, Goldfinger M (2019) Management of Hodgkin lymphoma in a sickle cell patient: a case report. Case Rep Oncol 12(1):224–227

Aslan M, Ryan TM, Townes TM, Coward L, Kirk MC, Barnes S et al (2003) Nitric oxide-dependent generation of reactive species in sickle cell disease: actin tyrosine nitration induces defective cytoskeletal polymerization. J Biol Chem 278(6):4194–4204

Barnes GD, Kanthi Y, Froehlich JB (2015) Venous thromboembolism: predicting recurrence and the need for extended anticoagulation. Vasc Med 20(2):143–152

Belveyre T, Auchet T, Levy B (2019) Spontaneous breathing during extracorporeal membrane oxygenation treatment of sickle cell disease acute chest syndrome. Respir Med Case Rep 28:100924

Block I, Günter C, Duarte Rodrigues A, Paasch S, Hesemann P, Taubert A (2021) Carbon adsorbents from spent coffee for removal of methylene blue and methyl orange from water. Materials 14(14):3996

Charlotte EE, Nicole AYA, Ingrid EK, Edgar MML, Eleonore NLE, Ritha M et al (2021) Risk factors and outcome of overt stroke in sickle cell patients admitted in two reference hospitals in Yaounde and Douala. Open J Pediatr 11(3):503–516

De A, Williams S, Yao Y, Jin Z, Brittenham GM, Kattan M et al (2023) Acute chest syndrome, airway inflammation and lung function in sickle cell disease. PLoS One 18(3):e0283349

Demagny J, Driss A, Stepanian A, Anguel N, Affo L, Roux D et al (2021) ADAMTS13 and von Willebrand factor assessment in steady state and acute vaso-occlusive crisis of sickle cell disease. Research Pract Thromb Haemost 5(1):197–203

Di Minno MND, Dentali F, Veglia F, Russolillo A, Tremoli E, Ageno W (2013) Antithrombin levels and the risk of a first episode of venous thromboembolism. A case-control study. Thromb Haemost 109(01):167–169

Field JJ, DeBaun MR (2009) Asthma and sickle cell disease: two distinct diseases or part of the same process? ASH Educ Program Book 2009(1):45–53

Finch JT, Perutz MF, Bertles JF, Döbler J (1973) Structure of sickled erythrocytes and of sickle-cell hemoglobin fibers. Proc Natl Acad Sci 70(3):718–722

Grosse SD, Atrash HK, Odame I, Amendah D, Piel FB, Williams TN (2012) The Jamaican historical experience of the impact of educational interventions on sickle cell disease child mortality. Am J Prev Med 42(6):e101–e103

Hardie R, King L, Fraser R, Reid M (2009) Prevalence of pneumococcal polysaccharide vaccine administration and incidence of invasive pneumococcal disease in children in Jamaica aged over 4 years with sickle cell disease diagnosed by newborn screening. Ann Trop Paediatr 29(3):197–202

Herbst J, Crissinger T, Baldwin K (2020) Diffuse ischemic strokes and sickle cell crisis induced by disseminated Anaplasmosis: A case report. Case Rep Neurol 11(3):271–276

Kato GJ, Hsieh M, Machado R, Taylor J, Little J, Butman JA et al (2006) Cerebrovascular disease associated with sickle cell pulmonary hypertension. Am J Hematol 81(7):503–510

Kearon C (2007) Indefinite anticoagulation after a first episode of unprovoked venous thromboembolism: yes. J Thromb Haemost 5(12):2330–2335

Kearon C, Akl EA (2014) Duration of anticoagulant therapy for deep vein thrombosis and pulmonary embolism. Blood J Am Soc Hematol 123(12):1794–1801

Khan F, Tritschler T, Kimpton M, Wells PS, Kearon C, Weitz JI et al (2021) Long-term risk of recurrent venous thromboembolism among patients receiving extended oral anticoagulant therapy for first unprovoked venous thromboembolism: A systematic review and meta-analysis. J Thromb Haemost 19(11):2801–2813

Klok FA, Presles E, Tromeur C, Barco S, Konstantinides SV, Sanchez O et al (2019) Evaluation of the predictive value of the bleeding prediction score VTE-BLEED for recurrent venous thromboembolism. Res Pract Thromb Haemost 3(3):364–371

Laurentino MR, Maia Filho PA, Barbosa MC, Bandeira ICJ, Rocha LBDS, Gonçalves RP (2014) Influence of βS-globin haplotypes and hydroxyurea on tumor necrosis factor-alpha levels in sickle cell anemia. Rev Bras Hematol Hemoter 36:121–125

Le Gal G, Mottier D (2012) New anticoagulants in the treatment of VTE. In: Seminars in respiratory and critical care medicine, vol 33, No. 02. Thieme Medical Publishers, pp 191–198

Leavell BS (1954) Treatment of sickle cell anemia. AMA Arch Intern Med 94(5):801–805

Louie JE, Anderson CJ, Fayaz M, Fomani K, Henry A, Killeen T, Mohandas N et al (2018) Case series supporting heme detoxification via therapeutic plasma exchange in acute multiorgan failure syndrome resistant to red blood cell exchange in sickle cell disease. Transfusion 58(2):470–479

Maduakor C, Alakbarzade V, Sammaraiee Y, Vakrinou A, Corobana A, Sikorska J et al (2021) The epidemiology of neurological complications in adults with sickle cell disease: a retrospective cohort study. Front Neurol 12:744118

Majjiga VS, Tripathy AK, Viswanathan K, Shukla M (2010) Thrombotic thrombocytopenic purpura and multiorgan system failure in a child with sickle cell-hemoglobin C disease. Clin Pediatr 49(10):992–996

Miller ML, Obert CA, Gao G, Daw NC, Flynn P, Tuomanen E (2005) Cephalosporin-resistant pneumococci and sickle cell disease. Emerg Infect Dis 11(8):1192

Miraulle TYS, Synèse BJ, D'assise MN, Charles RE, Clément A, Rabarijaona M, Willy R (2021) A rare complications of sickle cell disease: empyema and chronic subdural hematoma. Eur J Clin Med 2(1):23–25

Monus T, Howell CM (2019) Current and emerging treatments for sickle cell disease. JAAPA 32(9):1–5

Moschovi M, Psychou F, Menegas D, Tsangaris GT, Tzortzatou-Stathopoulou F, Nikolaidou P (2001) Hodgkin's disease in a child with sickle cell disease treated with hydroxyurea. Pediatr Hematol Oncol 18(6):371–376

Obaro S (2009) Pneumococcal infections and sickle cell disease in Africa: does absence of evidence imply evidence of absence? Arch Dis Child 94(9):713–716

Oliveira CCD, Ciasca SM, Moura-Ribeiro M (2008) Stroke in patients with sickle cell disease: clinical and neurological aspects. Arq Neuropsiquiatr 66:30–33

Riebel T, Kebelmann-Betzing C, Götze R, Overberg U (2003) Transcranial Doppler ultrasonography in neurologically asymptomatic children and young adults with sickle cell disease. Eur Radiol 13:563–570

Siddiqui RS, Ferman DA, Shi PA (2021) Further evidence for the benefit of therapeutic plasma exchange for acute multi-organ failure syndrome refractory to red cell exchange in sickle cell disease. J Clin Apher 36(5):777–779

Snyder AB, Lane PA, Zhou M, Paulukonis ST, Hulihan MM (2017) The accuracy of hospital ICD-9-CM codes for determining sickle cell disease genotype. J Rare Dis Res Treat 2(4):39

Teach SJ, Lillis KA, Grossi M (1998) Compliance with penicillin prophylaxis in patients with sickle cell disease. Arch Pediatr Adolesc Med 152(3):274–278

Trivedi K, Abbas A, Kazmi R, Shaaban H, Miller R (2022) Hyperhemolytic crisis following transfusion in sickle cell disease with acute hepatic crisis: a case report. Cureus 14(8):e27844

Weitz JI (2006) Emerging anticoagulants for the treatment of venous thromboembolism. Thromb Haemost 96(09):274–284

Part III
Transfusion Medicine in ICU

Chapter 13
Blood Components and Their Contents

Pragya Kafley and Soonam John

Learning Points

- Blood Component Separation and Preparation: Understanding the methods of blood component separation, including centrifugation and apheresis, and the general principles underlying the preparation of PRBCs, platelet concentrates, FFP, and cryoprecipitate for transfusion.
- Clinical Applications and Indications: Learning the specific clinical indications for each blood component, including the management of anemia with PRBCs, coagulopathies with FFP, thrombocytopenia with platelet concentrates, and factor deficiencies with cryoprecipitate.
- Quality Control and Donor Selection: Emphasizing the importance of stringent guidelines for donor selection, component preparation, and quality control to ensure the safety, efficacy, and ethical considerations of blood transfusions.
- Controversies and Clinical Judgment: Navigating the controversies surrounding transfusion thresholds and the decision-making process in clinical practice, encouraging a critical approach to patient care based on current evidence and guidelines.

13.1 Introduction

Blood transfusion is a critical component of modern medicine, playing a crucial role in various clinical scenarios. Understanding and managing blood components such as red blood cells, white blood cells, plasma, and platelets are essential for

P. Kafley
Medical Genetics, SGPGI, Lucknow, Uttar Pradesh, India

S. John (✉)
Transfusion Medicine, Government Medical College, Parippally, Kollam, Kerala, India

S. B. Mishra (ed.), *Critical Care Hematology*,
https://doi.org/10.1007/978-981-97-5565-3_13

successful outcomes in transfusion medicine. The chapter focuses on elucidating the characteristics, preparation methods, and clinical applications of these main blood components, providing a foundational knowledge base for healthcare professionals. Emphasizing the therapeutic potential of each component, the chapter delves into the intricacies of blood component separation, the technologies utilized, and the critical considerations in their utilization. It acknowledges the significance of evidence-based practice by adhering to the latest guidelines and research in the field, equipping practitioners to make informed decisions in patient care.

In the field of blood transfusion, several studies have been conducted to evaluate and enhance transfusion practices. For example, research by Hartley et al. (2017) focuses on interventions embedded within the UK National Comparative Audit of Blood Transfusion to improve feedback and reduce unnecessary blood transfusions. Marshall (2004) discusses a Canadian initiative aimed at defining patterns of blood transfusion in critical illness. Pine et al. (2017) highlight wide variations in blood product transfusion practices among providers caring for patients with acute leukemia in the United States. Murphy (2013) compares health outcomes in recipients of blood transfusion between observational studies and randomized clinical trials. Soliman and Elhapashy (2021) emphasizes the importance of nurses' competence in safe blood transfusion through training modules.

Furthermore, Secher et al. (2013) address the challenges of transfusion in critically ill children, emphasizing the necessity of transfusion in clinical settings. Kipkulei et al. (2019) stresses the importance of documentation in clinical blood transfusion practice to ensure safe and effective transfusions. Additionally, Murphy et al. (2005) and Murphy et al. (2003) survey the implementation of recommendations in Health Service Circulars related to better blood transfusion practices. These references collectively underscore the significance of evidence-based guidelines, training, and documentation in optimizing blood transfusion practices and ensuring patient safety.

Blood is composed of four main components: red blood cells, white blood cells, plasma, and platelets. These components can be separated through centrifugation and used for therapeutic purposes. Commonly used products for transfusion include packed red blood cells (PRBC), platelet-rich plasma, fresh frozen plasma (FFP), cryoprecipitate, and platelet concentrate. Plasma fractionation products are typically prepared by pharmaceutical companies (Burnouf 2012).

The preparation of blood components can be achieved through two main methods: whole blood donation or apheresis technique. Whole blood is collected in blood bags with an anticoagulant and an additive solution, followed by a two-step centrifugation process. Apheresis involves collecting specific components using an automated device and returning the remaining components to the donor (Cohn et al. 1944).

Strict guidelines are in place for donor selection, component preparation, and quality control of blood and blood products in transfusion services. Whole blood is centrifuged to produce various components due to the limited indications for whole blood transfusion, resulting in most collected whole blood being processed into components (Radosevich and Burnouf 2010).

13.2 General Principle of Component Preparation

This can be done in two ways either by whole blood donation or by apheresis technique (Fig. 13.1).

Whole Blood Whole blood is collected as 350 ml or 450 ml in blood bags containing an anticoagulant (CPDA-1) and an additive solution. While every transfusion service will have their own validated procedure, it mainly involves two-step centrifugation, the heavy and the light spin.

Apheresis Technique Apheresis in simple words means a collection of a single or more than one component using an automated device and returning the rest of the component to the donor. It requires an apheresis machine, the underlying principle of which may be centrifugation or filtration.

Before we proceed any further, it would be worthwhile to remember that there are stringent guidelines laid down for donor selection, component preparation, and quality control of the blood and blood products that are followed by the transfusion services.

One unit of WB when collected measures approximately 500 mL, this includes 63 mL of citrate anticoagulant/preservative solution. Each unit of whole blood is then centrifuged to make various components. There are not many indications of

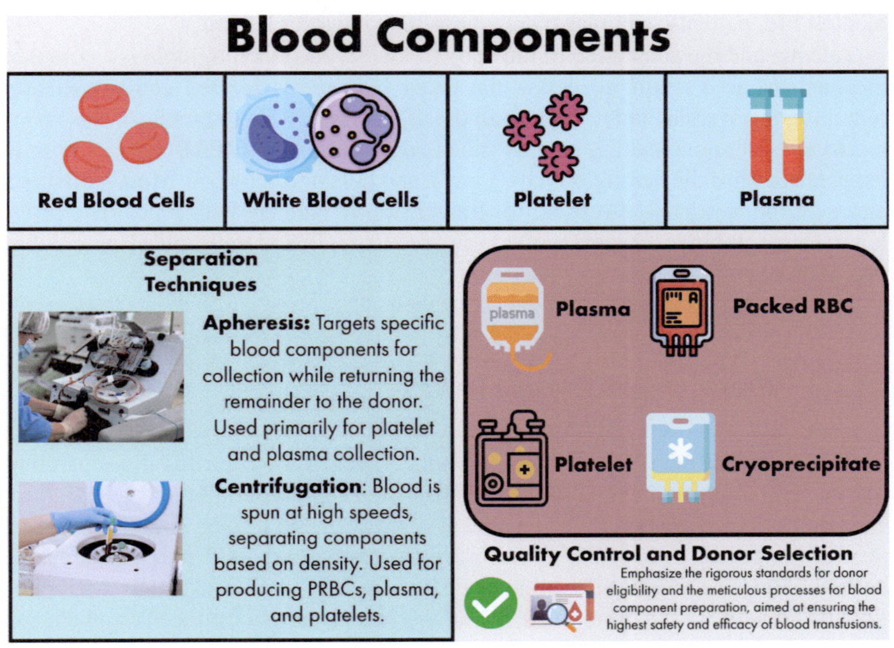

Fig. 13.1 Blood components

whole blood transfusion hence almost all collected whole blood gets processed into components.

We shall discuss the different components under the following headings: components, contents, storage, and indications.

13.2.1 Red Cell Transfusion

Commonly referred to as packed red cells. This is most commonly transfused to increase red cell mass. It is obtained by centrifugation of whole blood and removal of plasma. An average volume of PRBC is 250–300 ml. Depending upon the anticoagulant and additive solution used, PRBCs may be stored for 35–42 days at 2–4 degrees centigrade. Major crossmatch that entails crossmatching recipient plasma with donor red cells is performed. Crossmatched ABO compatible blood can be transfused.

Other types of PRBC include Leukoreduced PRBCs, in this, the red cell component is passed through a specialized filter either before storage or at the bedside. The advantages of leukoreduction include lesser febrile nonhemolytic reaction, alloimmunization, and CMV infection.

Washed RBCs: Washed RBCs have few indications, washing involves recentrifugation of the blood product with normal saline so as to remove residual plasma and additive solution, the process takes 1 h and results in loss of RBCs and shortening of shelf life, patients with plasma reactions may however benefit.

Anemia and the adaptation of the body to low levels of hemoglobin is a complex mechanism, as a result, to define the exact indications for red cell transfusion remains controversial and to discuss all the aspects is beyond the scope of this chapter. In a stable, nonbleeding average-sized adult, each unit of PRBC transfusion is expected to raise the hemoglobin by 1 gm% and hematocrit by 3%. Most guidelines agree on the restrictive threshold for transfusion in patients with no cardiac problems (Hemoglobin less than 8 g/dl) as opposed to the liberal threshold (Hemoglobin less than 10 g/dl).

13.2.2 Fresh Frozen Plasma (FFP)

Fresh Frozen Plasma (FFP) is a blood product obtained by centrifugally separating plasma from collected whole blood and then freezing it within 8 h of the donation. This quick-freeze process preserves the plasma, allowing it to be stored for up to a year at temperatures of −20° C or below. Typically, each FFP unit encompasses around 250 mL of plasma. Thawing of FFP, essential before transfusion, was traditionally done in a 37° C water bath, but advancements have introduced rapid plasma thawers that employ dry heat for this purpose.

FFP is rich in coagulation factors, maintaining a concentration of about 1 unit per mL. Although crossmatching is not a prerequisite for FFP transfusion, compatibility with the recipient's ABO blood group is crucial to avoid adverse reactions. The recommended dosage of FFP ranges from 10 to 15 mL per kilogram of the recipient's body weight and should be transfused within 20–30 min to ensure efficacy and safety.

The clinical applications of FFP are diverse, primarily addressing conditions associated with a deficiency in multiple coagulation factors. Such conditions include liver disease, which can impair the liver's ability to produce clotting factors, disseminated intravascular coagulation (DIC), where widespread clotting depletes these factors, and dilutional coagulopathy, often a result of massive fluid replacement or transfusion. FFP is also the treatment of choice in cases of congenital coagulation factor deficiencies when specific concentrates are unavailable, as well as for the urgent reversal of anticoagulation effects from Warfarin therapy.

Despite its valuable role in managing coagulopathies, FFP is not recommended for purposes like volume expansion, wound healing enhancement, or as a protein supplement in nutritional deficiencies. Its use is specifically geared toward correcting deficiencies in coagulation factors to prevent or control bleeding episodes.

13.2.3 Platelets

Platelet concentrates are a vital component in the management of thrombocytopenia and functional platelet disorders, offering a critical therapeutic option for patients with bleeding complications. The process of obtaining platelet concentrates involves two primary methods: centrifugation of donated whole blood, which yields random donor platelets (RDP), and apheresis, a more selective process that collects platelets directly from the donor's circulating blood.

Each unit of RDP contains a minimum of 55 × 10^10 platelets, suspended within approximately 50 mL of plasma. This contrasts with apheresis-derived platelet units, which are equivalent to 6–10 RDP units and are suspended in about 300 mL of plasma. The use of ABO-compatible platelets is preferred to minimize the risk of adverse reactions, though it is not absolutely required, allowing for greater flexibility in emergency situations or when compatible units are not readily available.

The expectation with a platelet transfusion is to achieve a significant rise in the platelet count of the recipient, typically by 10 × 10^9/L. This expected increase is a crucial benchmark in evaluating the effectiveness of the transfusion and in assessing the patient's response. The corrected platelet count increment (CCI) is calculated an hour after the transfusion to determine if the patient exhibits refractoriness to the platelet transfusion, a condition where the expected increase in platelet count is not observed, indicating a potential immune response or other complicating factors that might necessitate further medical intervention.

The formula for calculating the CCI is a critical tool in this assessment, factoring in the observed rise in platelet count, the patient's body surface area, and the number of platelets transfused. A satisfactory response to a platelet transfusion, seen as a rise in platelet count by 10 × 10^9/L, is an important indicator of the transfusion's success and the patient's capacity to benefit from this treatment.

Indications for platelet transfusion extend beyond simple thrombocytopenia to include cases with functional platelet defects. These transfusions are a cornerstone in the treatment of patients at risk of bleeding due to low platelet counts or dysfunctional platelets, providing a means to stabilize their condition and prevent potentially life-threatening hemorrhages. The strategic use of platelet transfusions, guided by a thorough understanding of the patient's condition and the specific indications for this therapy, is fundamental in optimizing patient outcomes and managing bleeding risks in vulnerable populations.

The following may be considered as a rough guideline for platelet transfusion:

Platelet count (10^9/L)	When should you transfuse
5 or less	Indication for transfusion as the risk of spontaneous bleed high
6–10	Consider transfusion in case of minor bleed, fever, or rapidly declining counts
11–20	If the patient is on heparin or some procedure is planned
21–50	Major bleeding or if surgery is planned
More than 50	Thrombocytopenia unlikely to be the cause of bleeding so unless there is evidence of platelet function defect or neurosurgical or ophthalmological surgery, transfusion is not indicated

Platelet transfusion is not recommended in thrombocytopenia due to: Immune destruction of platelets like ITP (Immune thrombocytopenic purpura).

13.2.3.1 Thrombotic Thrombocytopenic Purpura

Cryoprecipitate Cryoprecipitate, derived from fresh frozen plasma (FFP), is produced by a process that involves thawing the FFP at temperatures below 6 °C, followed by centrifugation. This process leads to the formation of a precipitate, which is then resuspended in 15–20 mL of plasma. This concentrated product serves as a rich source of several crucial blood coagulation factors. It contains 80–120 units of factor VIII, approximately 50% of the original plasma content of von Willebrand factor (vWF), 250 mg of fibrinogen, 30% of the original plasma content of factor XIII, and fibronectin.

The therapeutic applications of cryoprecipitate are specifically targeted toward conditions associated with deficiencies or dysfunctions of these factors. It is commonly indicated for the treatment of Hemophilia A, a genetic disorder characterized by the deficiency of factor VIII, and von Willebrand disease, which involves a deficiency or dysfunction of the von Willebrand factor. Additionally, cryoprecipitate is used in cases of factor XIII deficiency when specific factor concentrates are not available.

Another significant use of cryoprecipitate is for fibrinogen replacement therapy. This is particularly relevant in situations where fibrinogen levels are depleted, either due to inherited disorders or consumptive conditions, such as disseminated intravascular coagulation (DIC), where fibrinogen is used up in the widespread activation of the coagulation system.

Moreover, cryoprecipitate has shown efficacy in improving platelet function in patients with uremia, a condition often associated with a functional platelet defect, thereby aiding in the management of bleeding tendencies in these patients.

The dosing of cryoprecipitate typically begins with an initial 10 bags or units, followed by maintenance doses of 6–10 bags or units every 8 h, or as required to maintain fibrinogen levels above 100 mg/dL. This dosing strategy is crucial for ensuring the effectiveness of cryoprecipitate in managing the aforementioned conditions and requires careful monitoring to optimize treatment outcomes.

References

Burnouf T (2012) Plasma fractionation. ISBT Sci Ser 7(1):62–67

Cohn EJ, Oncley JL, Strong LE, Hughes WL, Armstrong SH (1944) Chemical, clinical, and immunological studies on the products of human plasma fractionation. I. The characterization of the protein fractions of human plasma. J Clin Invest 23(4):417–432

Hartley S, Foy R, Walwyn RE, Cicero R, Farrin AJ, Francis JJ et al (2017) The evaluation of enhanced feedback interventions to reduce unnecessary blood transfusions (AFFINITIE): protocol for two linked cluster randomised factorial controlled trials. Implement Sci 12:1–11

Kipkulei JC, Buziba NG, Mining SK (2019) Documentation of the clinical blood transfusion practice at a teaching and referral Hospital in Western Kenya. Am J Health Res 7(1):8–11

Marshall JC (2004) Transfusion trigger: when to transfuse? Crit Care 8:1–3

Murphy EL (2013) Health outcomes in recipients of blood transfusion–observational studies versus randomized clinical trials. ISBT Sci Ser 8(1):172–176

Murphy MF, Edbury C, Wickenden C (2003) Survey of the implementation of the recommendations in the Health Services Circular 1998/224 'Better Blood Transfusion'. Transfus Med 13(3):121–126

Murphy MF, Howell C, National Blood Transfusion Committee in England (2005) Survey of the implementation of the recommendations in the Health Service Circular 2002/009 'Better Blood Transfusion'. Transfus Med 15(6):453–460

Pine AB, Lee EJ, Sekeres M, Steensma DP, Zelterman D, Prebet T et al (2017) Wide variations in blood product transfusion practices among providers who care for patients with acute leukemia in the United States. Transfusion 57(2):289–295

Radosevich M, Burnouf T (2010) Intravenous immunoglobulin G: trends in production methods, quality control and quality assurance. Vox Sang 98(1):12–28

Secher EL, Stensballe J, Afshari A (2013) Transfusion in critically ill children: an ongoing dilemma. Acta Anaesthesiol Scand 57(6):684–691

Soliman HM, Elhapashy HM (2021) Nurses' competence in safety blood transfusion: the impact of a training module. Int J Nurs Educ 13(3):25

Chapter 14
Point-of-Care-Guided Transfusion of Blood Products in ICU

Pragya Kafley and Soonam John

Learning Points

1. Understand the limitations of traditional coagulation tests and the advantages of using POC diagnostics in ICU settings.
2. Learn the operational principles and interpretation of key POC techniques: TEG and ROTEM.
3. Explore the clinical applications and benefits of viscoelastic hemostatic assays in reducing transfusion needs and improving patient outcomes.
4. Assess the challenges and limitations of implementing POC techniques in the management of hemorrhage in critically ill patients.

14.1 Introduction

This chapter examines the shift in managing acute hemorrhage within the Intensive Care Unit (ICU) from traditional methods to innovative Point-of-Care (POC) technologies. Managing bleeding in critically ill patients involves navigating high risks of morbidity and mortality, complicated by factors such as surgical interventions, trauma, coagulopathies, and anticoagulant therapies. Traditionally, this management relied heavily on coagulopathy monitoring and blood product administration guided by tests like Prothrombin Time (PT) and Activated Partial Thromboplastin Time (aPTT). However, these conventional methods often delay necessary interventions due to their slow processing times and limited diagnostic scope.

The advent of POC technologies, specifically Thromboelastography (TEG) and Rotational Thromboelastometry (ROTEM), has revolutionized ICU hemorrhage management. These technologies offer rapid, detailed evaluations of a patient's coagulation status, allowing for more precise and effective treatment strategies. This chapter delves into how these technologies overcome the limitations of traditional

P. Kafley
Medical Genetics, SGPGI, Lucknow, Uttar Pradesh, India

S. John (✉)
Transfusion Medicine, Government Medical College, Parippally, Kollam, Kerala, India

S. B. Mishra (ed.), *Critical Care Hematology*,
https://doi.org/10.1007/978-981-97-5565-3_14

approaches and discusses their potential limitations and considerations in clinical practice.

14.2 Overview of Traditional Versus POC Approaches to Hemorrhage Management

14.2.1 Traditional Approaches

Traditionally, the management of acute hemorrhage in the Intensive Care Unit (ICU) has relied heavily on conventional diagnostic tests such as Prothrombin Time (PT) and Activated Partial Thromboplastin Time (aPTT). These tests assess the extrinsic and intrinsic pathways of the coagulation cascade, respectively. Management strategies have generally involved the surveillance for signs of coagulopathies, followed by the administration of blood products and coagulation-supporting medications based on these test results. This approach, while standardized, often leads to delays in intervention. The tests require blood samples to be sent to and processed in a laboratory, resulting in a time gap between sampling and obtaining results, which may not reflect the patient's current coagulation status due to the dynamic nature of hemorrhage and resuscitation.

14.2.2 Point-of-Care (POC) Approaches

In contrast, Point-of-Care (POC) testing technologies like Thromboelastography (TEG) and Rotational Thromboelastometry (ROTEM) offer real-time, bedside assessments of a patient's coagulation status. These technologies analyze the viscoelastic properties of blood, providing a dynamic picture of clot formation and stability. This includes not only the initiation and development of a clot but also its resistance to fibrinolysis, offering a comprehensive overview that traditional tests cannot match.

14.2.3 Advantages of POC Testing

The primary advantage of POC testing lies in its immediacy and relevance. Results from POC devices are available within minutes, allowing clinicians to make rapid, informed decisions about interventions such as the administration of Fresh Frozen Plasma, platelets, or coagulation factors. This timeliness is crucial in a critical care setting where conditions can deteriorate rapidly. Moreover, POC tests provide actionable insights into specific aspects of the coagulation process, such as clot firmness and fibrinolysis, which are pivotal in tailoring individualized treatment plans.

POC technologies also integrate well into algorithm-based approaches for managing hemorrhages, allowing for protocol-driven, systematic interventions that are consistent and easy to teach across multidisciplinary teams. For example, ROTEM-guided algorithms have been used successfully in settings ranging from cardiac surgery to trauma and liver transplantation, demonstrating a reduction in unnecessary transfusions and improvements in patient outcomes (Sahli et al. 2020).

14.2.4 Point-of-Care Diagnostic Techniques

This section elaborates on viscoelastic testing modalities and whole blood platelet function assays that are integral in the ICU for rapid diagnostics:

14.2.5 Viscoelastic Tests

Thromboelastography (TEG): Assesses the viscoelastic properties of blood clot formation.

Rotational Thromboelastometry (ROTEM): Similar to TEG, provides a comprehensive analysis of clot dynamics.

Whole Blood Platelet Function Tests: Evaluate platelet function and aggregation dynamics, crucial for assessing bleeding risks and guiding transfusion strategies.

Impedance Aggregometry: Measures platelet aggregation in response to specific agonists using changes in electrical impedance.

Turbidimetric Aggregometry: Assesses platelet aggregation by measuring changes in light transmission through the sample.

14.2.6 Thromboelastography (TEG)

Thromboelastography (TEG) is a noninvasive method that evaluates clot formation in whole blood. The device operates on the principle of viscoelastometry, where a pin is suspended in a blood-filled cup maintained at body temperature (37 °C). This pin is attached to a torsion wire that connects to a mechanical-electrical transducer. As the clot forms and evolves, its changing viscoelastic properties alter the pin's motion. These changes are converted into electrical signals, which are then processed to produce both graphical and numerical outputs. This continuous, real-time analysis provides insights into all phases of clot development and resolution, making it invaluable in clinical decision-making (Wirtz et al. 2017; Whiting et al. 2015).

TEG parameters that represent the three phases of hemostasis: initiation, amplification, and propagation are.

(A) R-value = reaction time (s) time of latency from the start of the test to initial fibrin formation (amplitude of 2 mm) initiation phase. It is dependent on clotting factors.
(B) K = kinetics (s)—time taken to achieve a certain level of clot strength (amplitude of 20 mm) amplification phase dependent on fibrinogen.
(C) alpha = angle (slope of line between R and K) measures the speed at which fibrin buildup and cross-linking take place, hence assesses the rate of clot formation "thrombin burst"/propagation phase dependent on fibrinogen,
(D) TMA = time to maximum amplitude(s).
(E) MA = maximum amplitude (mm)—represents the ultimate strength of the fibrin clot; i.e., the overall stability of the clot dependent on platelets (80%) and fibrin (20%) interacting via GPIIb/IIIa.
(F) A30 or LY30 = amplitude at 30 minutes-percentage decrease in amplitude at 30 min post-MA fibrinolysis phase.
(G) CLT = clot lysis time (s). Approximate normal values (kaolin-activated TEG, values differ if native blood is used, and between types of the assay).

R: 4–8 min
K: 1–4 min
α-Angle: 47–74°
MA: 55–73 mm
LY 30%: 0–8%

Guiding Treatment with Thromboelastography (TEG)
TEG provides actionable insights for specific therapeutic interventions:

Increased R time: Suggests a need for Fresh Frozen Plasma (FFP) to address coagulation factor deficiencies.
Decreased alpha angle: Indicates a potential deficiency in fibrinogen, typically managed with cryoprecipitate.
Decreased MA (Maximum Amplitude): Reflects a deficiency in platelet function or count, commonly addressed with platelet transfusion and potentially with desmopressin (DDAVP).
Presence of Fibrinolysis: Managed with antifibrinolytics such as tranexamic acid, aprotinin, or aminocaproic acid.

14.2.7 ROTEM

The ROTEM system is an advanced point-of-care analyzer crucial for detecting, managing, and monitoring hemostasis, particularly in surgical settings with significant blood loss. It utilizes thromboelastometry to evaluate the coagulation dynamics of a whole blood sample, applying five specific assays—INTEM, EXTEM, FIBTEM, APTEM, and HEPTEM—to comprehensively profile coagulation.

INTEM and EXTEM: Assess the presence of clotting factor deficiencies.
FIBTEM: Targets fibrinogen levels, indicating fibrinogen deficiencies.
APTEM: Detects hyperfibrinolysis.
HEPTEM: Evaluates the impact of heparin on coagulation, useful in identifying residual heparin-induced coagulopathies.

This multifaceted approach provides a detailed view of a patient's hemostatic status, facilitating tailored interventions based on real-time data (Benes et al. 2015; Dias et al. 2019) (Fig. 14.1).

Correlation of Variables Between ROTEM and TEG
Understanding the equivalent variables between ROTEM and TEG provides a comprehensive approach to interpreting coagulation data:

Clotting Time (CT): Corresponds to the R-value in TEG, indicating the reaction time or the time until clot initiation.
α Angle and Clot Formation Time (CFT): Equivalent to the K-value and α angle in TEG, these parameters assess the kinetics of clot formation and the rate of fibrin buildup and stabilization.
Maximum Clot Firmness (MCF): Matches the maximum amplitude (MA) in TEG, reflecting the ultimate strength and stability of the formed clot.
Clot Lysis (CL): Correlates with LY30 in TEG, measuring the degree of clot breakdown or fibrinolysis after its peak formation.

Clinical Interpretation of Hemostatic Data
Interpreting the data from hemostatic tests involves recognizing patterns that guide specific treatments:

Prolonged R Time: Indicates deficiencies in coagulation factors, typically managed with Fresh Frozen Plasma (FFP), prothrombin complex concentrates, or anticoagulant reversal agents.
Extended K Time or Decreased α Angle: Suggests a fibrinogen deficiency, addressable with cryoprecipitate or lyophilized fibrinogen concentrates.

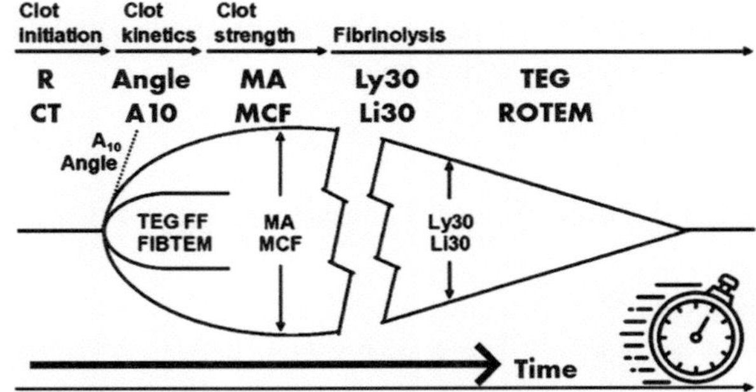

Fig. 14.1 Illustration of a thromboelastography (TEG) and Rotational thromboelastometry (ROTEM) tracing

Reduced Maximum Amplitude (MA): Points to either quantitative or functional platelet deficiencies, correctable with platelet concentrates or desmopressin.
Increased LY30 Value: Denotes active fibrinolysis, treatable with inhibitors such as aminocaproic acid or tranexamic acid.
Contrary Changes in TEG Parameters: May indicate a prothrombotic state, necessitating a careful reassessment of anticoagulant needs (Table 14.1).

14.2.8 Platelet Function Analyzer (PFA)

The Platelet Function Analyzer (PFA) is a valuable tool used in clinical settings to assess platelet function and coagulation processes. It measures various aspects of hemostasis, including coagulation, fibrin gel formation, clot retraction (platelet function), and fibrinolysis by evaluating platelet aggregation in response to different agonists like adenosine-diphosphate (ADP), arachidonic acid (AA), collagen, and epinephrine (EPI) (Mulliez et al. 2015).

Studies have shown that the PFA is effective in detecting bleeding disorders, monitoring platelet inhibition by antiplatelet drugs, and screening for conditions like von Willebrand disease (VWD) (Favaloro et al. 2022). It has also been utilized in assessing platelet function during pregnancy (Vincelot et al. 2001), in patients with thalassemia (Theodoridou et al. 2014), and in individuals with von Willebrand factor deficiency (Ardillon et al. 2015). Moreover, the PFA has been instrumental in establishing reference intervals for platelet function in conditions like anemia and thrombocytopenia (Kuiper et al. 2017).

The PFA has been compared to traditional bleeding time tests and is highly accurate in discriminating normal from abnormal platelet function, making it a valuable tool in diagnosing platelet disorders (Blaicher et al. 2004). Additionally, the PFA has been used in various clinical scenarios such as evaluating primary hemostasis in patients with menorrhagia (Philipp et al. 2005), neurofibromatosis type 1 (Favaloro et al. 2004), and hip fracture surgery (Thaler et al. 2010).

Furthermore, the PFA has been employed in research settings to study the effects of different drugs on platelet function, such as antirheumatic agents (Nielsen et al. 2020), and to investigate prothrombotic changes due to factors like an increase in thyroid hormone levels (Horacek et al. 2015). Overall, the PFA serves as a versatile instrument in assessing platelet function and coagulation processes in a wide range of clinical and research applications.

14.2.9 Benefits of Viscoelastic Hemostatic Assays

Viscoelastic hemostatic assays, such as TEG and ROTEM, offer several benefits in clinical practice. These assays have shown superiority in predicting the need for transfusion of blood products like FFP, RBCs, and platelets compared to traditional

Table 14.1 Differences between TEG (thromboelastography) and ROTEM (rotational thromboelastometry)

Feature	TEG (thromboelastography)	ROTEM (rotational thromboelastometry)
Principle of operation	Measures the elasticity of clot formation as a pin rotates in a blood sample	Measures the elasticity of clot formation using a rotation pin in a stationary blood sample
Assays used	Uses whole blood. Can be modified with reagents like kaolin, heparinase, or reptilase	Utilizes specific assays like INTEM, EXTEM, FIBTEM, APTEM, and HEPTEM for detailed analysis
Clotting time (CT)	R-value: indicates the reaction time or time clot initiation	Clotting time (CT): equivalent to TEG's R-value, indicating the time to clot initiation
Kinetics of clotting	K-value: time taken to achieve a certain level of clot strength. Alpha angle: rate of clot formation	Clot formation time (CFT): similar to TEG's K value. A angle: reflects the kinetics of clot formation
Clot firmness	Maximum amplitude (MA): represents the ultimate strength and stability of the clot	Maximum clot firmness (MCF): corresponds to MA in TEG, indicating the clot's strength
Fibrinolysis	LY30: percentage decrease in amplitude at 30 min post-MA	Clot lysis (CL): measures the degree of clot breakdown after peak formation, similar to LY30
Diagnostic focus	Broadly assesses coagulation status including clot initiation, formation, and lysis	Offers a more detailed diagnostic focus due to different assays that can pinpoint specific issues
Usage	Widely used in trauma, surgery, and obstetrics for overall coagulation assessment	Extensively used in surgery, especially cardiac and liver transplantation for detailed analysis
Data presentation	Provides a graphical representation of the clot's life cycle	Produces a graphical and numerical output that is highly detailed
Clinical implementation	Often used to guide transfusion requirements and manage coagulopathies	Used to guide specific therapeutic interventions and optimize patient blood management

coagulation tests like PT, aPTT, INR, platelet count, and fibrinogen (Peng et al. 2018). Additionally, these assays provide rapid results, with many outcomes available within 5–10 min of initiating the test, enabling quick clinical decision-making (Peng et al. 2018).

14.2.10 Disadvantages of Viscoelastic Hemostatic Assays

Despite their advantages, viscoelastic hemostatic assays also come with certain limitations. These assays exhibit marked interoperator variability and poor precision, which can affect result consistency (Da Luz et al. 2014). Moreover, the sensitivity and specificity of these assays may vary significantly across different patient populations, potentially impacting their reliability in certain clinical scenarios (Da Luz et al. 2014).

14.2.11 Massive Hemorrhage

Management of Massive Hemorrhage

In cases of massive hemorrhage among critically ill patients, rapid depletion of coagulation factors, beginning with fibrinogen, is a common complication (Peng et al. 2018). The preference for blood component therapy over whole blood transfusion is recommended to more specifically address these deficits (Peng et al. 2018). Viscoelastic tests such as Thromboelastography (TEG) and Rotational Thromboelastometry (ROTEM) have proven more effective than traditional coagulation tests (e.g., PT, PTT) in predicting the need for transfusions and in assessing the severity of bleeding (Da Luz et al. 2014). For example, TEG's α-angle has shown a higher predictive value for plasma transfusions than fibrinogen levels, and its maximum amplitude (MA) provides better guidance for platelet transfusions than does a simple platelet count (Da Luz et al. 2014).

Research indicates that TEG and ROTEM are critical in diagnosing fibrinogen deficiencies, assessing bleeding risks, and guiding transfusions across various clinical settings, including trauma, cardiac surgery, liver transplantation, and postpartum care (Nogami 2016). Integrating these tests with standard coagulation assays can improve our understanding of hemostasis, helping to predict bleeding tendencies and tailor long-term management strategies for patients with bleeding disorders (Nogami 2016).

Moreover, the application of TEG and ROTEM in perioperative settings has informed guidelines that minimize the use of transfusions without compromising safety. Notably, ROTEM has been instrumental in predicting outcomes and managing risks in liver transplantation procedures, thereby underscoring its utility in critical care and surgical contexts (Reinhöfer et al. 2008; Hartmann et al. 2022).

14.2.12 Cardiovascular Surgery

Point-of-care (POC) technologies such as Thromboelastography (TEG) and Rotational Thromboelastometry (ROTEM) have proven to be invaluable in managing postoperative blood loss in cardiovascular surgeries, significantly reducing the use of transfused blood products (Weber et al. 2015). These technologies are especially crucial in ICU settings for patients on mechanical circulatory support, where they help mitigate the risks of bleeding and thromboembolic complications (Wright et al. 2020). Evidence from various studies supports the efficacy of TEG/ROTEM-guided interventions in decreasing blood product use in bleeding patients during cardiac surgeries (Dias et al. 2019; Wahlen et al. 2018). Moreover, their implementation in trauma centers has demonstrated effective management of coagulation in severely injured patients, enhancing overall treatment outcomes (Fahrendorff et al. 2017). Systematic reviews and meta-analyses have further validated the role of viscoelastic hemostatic assays in optimizing blood product use, thereby improving patient safety without compromising survival rates or other important clinical outcomes (Li et al. 2021). The use of thromboelastography with platelet mapping has also been integrated into the management of patients undergoing intracranial aneurysm procedures, effectively preventing bleeding complications.

14.2.13 Sepsis and Coagulopathy Monitoring

In severe sepsis, hemostatic changes are often marked by increased levels of biomarkers such as procalcitonin and interleukin-6. However, Rotational Thromboelastometry (ROTEM) has emerged as a superior indicator of sepsis severity, providing a more reliable measure than traditional biomarkers like procalcitonin, interleukin-6, and C-reactive protein (Adamzik et al. 2010). ROTEM's ability to detect hyperfibrinolysis has proven particularly valuable, with studies linking it to increased mortality rates in trauma patients and suggesting its potential as a critical prognostic tool (Veigas et al. 2016). Additionally, ROTEM's assessments of fibrinolysis have been correlated with outcomes related to organ failure in septic patients, further establishing its importance in clinical diagnostics and management (Prakash et al. 2015).

The utility of thromboelastometry, particularly ROTEM, in diagnosing coagulopathy and predicting mortality in trauma patients has been well-documented (Veigas et al. 2016). Additionally, the application of viscoelastic coagulation monitoring in neonatal intensive care units has shown promise in predicting bleeding risk and assessing coagulopathy in critically ill neonates (Sokou et al. 2023). The use of thromboelastometry in diagnosing neonatal sepsis-associated coagulopathy has also been explored, indicating the versatility of this technique across different patient populations (Sokou et al. 2017).

14.3 Conclusion

The aggregometric and viscoelastic methods are recommended in an ICU setting. The POC coagulation testing is faster and more comprehensive than conventional laboratory tests of blood coagulation. POC techniques should be an integral part of a patient blood management program.

References

Adamzik M, Eggmann M, Frey UH, Görlinger K, Bröcker-Preuß M, Marggraf G et al (2010) Comparison of thromboelastometry with procalcitonin, interleukin 6, and C-reactive protein as diagnostic tests for severe sepsis in critically ill adults. Crit Care 14:1–7

Ardillon L, Ternisien C, Fouassier M, Sigaud M, Lefrançois A, Pacault M et al (2015) Platelet function analyser (PFA-100) results and von Willebrand factor deficiency: a 16-year 'real-world' experience. Haemophilia 21(5):646–652

Benes J, Zatloukal J, Kletecka J (2015) Viscoelastic methods of blood clotting assessment–a multidisciplinary review. Front Med 2:62

Blaicher AM, Landsteiner HT, Zwerina J, Leitgeb U, Volf I, Hoerauf K (2004) Effect of non-selective, non-steroidal anti-inflammatory drugs and cyclo-oxygenase-2 selective inhibitors on the PFA-100 closure time. Anaesthesia 59(11):1100–1103

Da Luz LT, Nascimento B, Shankarakutty AK, Rizoli S, Adhikari NK (2014) Effect of thromboelastography (TEG®) and rotational thromboelastometry (ROTEM®) on diagnosis of coagulopathy, transfusion guidance and mortality in trauma: descriptive systematic review. Crit Care 18:1–26

Dias JD, Sauaia A, Achneck HE, Hartmann J, Moore EE (2019) Thromboelastography-guided therapy improves patient blood management and certain clinical outcomes in elective cardiac and liver surgery and emergency resuscitation: a systematic review and analysis. J Thromb Haemost 17(6):984–994

Fahrendorff M, Oliveri RS, Johansson PI (2017) The use of viscoelastic haemostatic assays in goal-directing treatment with allogeneic blood products–A systematic review and meta-analysis. Scand J Trauma Resusc Emerg Med 25:1–12

Favaloro EJ, Zafer M, Nair SC, Hertzberg M, North K (2004) Evaluation of primary haemostasis in people with neurofibromatosis type 1. Clin Lab Haematol 26(5):341–345

Favaloro EJ, Mohammed S, Vong R, Chapman K, Kershaw G, Just S et al (2022) Harmonizing platelet function analyzer testing and reporting in a large laboratory network. Int J Lab Hematol 44(5):934–944

Hartmann M, Lorenz B, Brenner T, Saner FH (2022) Elevated pre-and postoperative ROTEM™ clot lysis indices indicate reduced clot retraction and increased mortality in patients undergoing liver transplantation. Biomedicines 10(8):1975

Horacek J, Maly J, Svilias I, Smolej L, Cepkova J, Vizda J et al (2015) Prothrombotic changes due to an increase in thyroid hormone levels. Eur J Endocrinol 172(5):537–542

Kuiper GJ, Houben R, Wetzels RJ, Verhezen PW, Oerle RV, Ten Cate H et al (2017) The use of regression analysis in determining reference intervals for low hematocrit and thrombocyte count in multiple electrode aggregometry and platelet function analyzer 100 testing of platelet function. Platelets 28(7):668–675

Li Y, Zhang X, Guo Z, Zhu J, Xu R, He Z, Sun X (2021) Standard vs. modified antiplatelet therapy based on thromboelastography with platelet mapping for preventing bleeding events in patients undergoing stent-assisted coil for a ruptured intracranial aneurysm. Front Neurol 11:615829

Mulliez S, Hallaert G, Van Roost D, Vantilborgh A, Devreese K (2015) Influence of platelet clumps on platelet function analyser (PFA)-200® testing. Int J Lab Hematol 37(5):E103–E105

Nielsen CB, Nielsen C, Nybo M, Just SA, Vinholt PJ (2020) The in vitro effect of antirheumatic drugs on platelet function. Platelets 31(2):248–257

Nogami K (2016) The utility of thromboelastography in inherited and acquired bleeding disorders. Br J Haematol 174(4):503–514

Peng HT, Nascimento B, Beckett A (2018) Thromboelastography and thromboelastometry in assessment of fibrinogen deficiency and prediction for transfusion requirement: a descriptive review. BioMed Res Int 2018:7020539

Philipp CS, Miller CH, Faiz A, Dilley A, Michaels LA, Ayers C et al (2005) Screening women with menorrhagia for underlying bleeding disorders: the utility of the platelet function analyser and bleeding time. Haemophilia 11(5):497–503

Prakash S, Verghese S, Roxby D, Dixon D, Bihari S, Bersten A (2015) Changes in fibrinolysis and severity of organ failure in sepsis: a prospective observational study using point-of-care test—ROTEM. J Crit Care 30(2):264–270

Reinhöfer M, Brauer M, Franke U, Barz D, Marx G, Lösche W (2008) The value of rotation thromboelastometry to monitor disturbed perioperative haemostasis and bleeding risk in patients with cardiopulmonary bypass. Blood Coagul Fibrinolysis 19(3):212–219

Sahli SD, Rössler J, Tscholl DW, Studt JD, Spahn DR, Kaserer A (2020) Point-of-care diagnostics in coagulation management. Sensors 20(15):4254

Sokou R, Georgiadou P, Tsantes AG, Parastatidou S, Konstantinidi A, Ioakeimidis G et al (2023) The utility of NATEM assay in predicting bleeding risk in critically ill neonates. In: Seminars in thrombosis and hemostasis, vol 49, No. 02. Thieme Medical Publishers, Inc, pp 182–191

Thaler HW, Frisee F, Korninger C (2010) Platelet aggregation inhibitors, platelet function testing, and blood loss in hip fracture surgery. J Trauma Acute Care Surg 69(5):1217–1221

Theodoridou S, Economou M, Vyzantiadis TA, Teli A, Vlachaki E, Neokleous N et al (2014) Laboratory investigation of platelet function in patients with thalassaemia. Acta Haematol 132(1):45–48

Veigas PV, Callum J, Rizoli S, Nascimento B, da Luz LT (2016) A systematic review on the rotational thrombelastometry (ROTEM®) values for the diagnosis of coagulopathy, prediction and guidance of blood transfusion and prediction of mortality in trauma patients. Scand J Trauma Resusc Emerg Med 24:1–14

Vincelot A, Nathan N, Collet D, Mehaddi Y, Grandchamp P, Julia A (2001) Platelet function during pregnancy: an evaluation using the PFA-100 analyser. Br J Anaesth 87(6):890–893

Wahlen BM, El-Menyar A, Peralta R, Al-Thani H (2018) World academic Council of Emergency Medicine experience document: implementation of point-of-care thromboelastography at an academic emergency and trauma center. J Emerg Trauma Shock 11(4):265–270

Weber C, Deppe AC, Kuhn EW, Scherner M, Slottosch I, Liakopoulos OJ et al (2015) Point-of-care TEG/ROTEM based coagulation Management in Cardiac Surgery: a meta-analysis of 8,321 patients. Thorac Cardiovasc Surg 63(S 01):OP27

Whiting P, Al M, Westwood M, Ramos IC, Ryder S, Armstrong N et al (2015) Viscoelastic point-of-care testing to assist with the diagnosis, management and monitoring of haemostasis: a systematic review and cost-effectiveness analysis. Health Technol Assess. https://doi.org/10.3310/hta19580

Wirtz MR, Baumann HM, Klinkspoor JH, Goslings JC, Juffermans NP (2017) Viscoelastic testing in trauma. In: Seminars in thrombosis and hemostasis, vol 43, No. 04. Thieme Medical Publishers, pp 375–385

Wright FL, Vogler TO, Moore EE, Moore HB, Wohlauer MV, Urban S et al (2020) Fibrinolysis shutdown correlation with thromboembolic events in severe COVID-19 infection. J Am Coll Surg 231(2):193–203

Chapter 15
Transfusion Reactions in ICU

Pragya Kafley and Soonam John

Learning Points

1. Identification and Management of Transfusion Reactions: Understanding the signs and appropriate management responses for different types of transfusion reactions can significantly enhance patient outcomes.
2. Prevention Strategies: The review highlights the importance of prevention strategies such as proper donor selection, use of leukoreduced blood products, and meticulous monitoring of transfusion practices to minimize the risk of adverse transfusion reactions.
3. Role of ICU Staff in Managing Transfusion Reactions: ICU staff play a crucial role in the detection and management of transfusion reactions. Their ability to respond quickly and effectively is critical in preventing severe outcomes, including death.
4. Improving Patient Safety with Updated Protocols: Updated protocols and continuous education for ICU healthcare providers are essential for improving transfusion safety.

15.1 Introduction

Transfusion reactions are important, as these are representative of a highly problematic issue at the intensive care unit, given that they represent the set of very different adverse events that may happen during or after blood transfusion. Reaction severity

P. Kafley
Medical Genetics, SGPGI, Lucknow, Uttar Pradesh, India

S. John (✉)
Transfusion Medicine, Government Medical College, Parippally, Kollam, Kerala, India

S. B. Mishra (ed.), *Critical Care Hematology*,
https://doi.org/10.1007/978-981-97-5565-3_15

might differ from a mere allergic response to acute hemolytic reactions or transfusion-related acute lung injury (TRALI) (Goel et al. 2019). From another perspective, this review helps to appreciate the pathophysiology, clinical presentation, management, and prevention strategies of the various types of transfusion reactions. It also becomes easily appreciated that this is an important aspect of patient safety by the bedside ICU practitioner (Goel et al. 2019).

Some studies have underscored the importance of both the need to manage non-infectious transfusion-associated adverse events and highlight the roles played by donors, products, and patients in lowering these events (Goel et al. 2019). Consider: (1) there may be transfusion-related acute lung injury (TRALI) following administration of plasma transfusions, and (2) Febrile-hemolytic transfusion reactions (FNHTRs) and transfusion-associated circulatory overload may occur. It is possible to identify and analyze the reported reactions in transfusions among different hospitals, which would help a lot toward their reduction of incidence and, therefore, an increase in security in the transfusion process (Kumar et al. 2013).

Research has been done to compare the rate, types, and associated products of transfusion reactions in pediatric and adult patients, bringing out differences and offering essential clinical practice insights. Global audits showed differences in the practice of transfusion and outcome effects in critically ill patients.

As a result of efforts to monitor and analyze hospital transfusion practices, errors in these processes have been put to light. Stopping adverse events associated with blood transfusions calls for proper documentation and vigilance (Reis et al. 2016). Additionally, several transfusion reactions, specifically the hemolytic and febrile nonhemolytic reactions, have been some of the greatest subjects of pathophysiologic studies to explain the mechanisms involved in such cases (Davenport 2005; Heddle 1999).

15.2 Classification of Transfusion Reactions

The reactions are further classified according to the time the reactions occur in the transfusion procedure. This allows, of course, an improvement in the diagnostic and management possibilities in case complications occur (Sakhalkar et al. 2005; Garratty 2004).

Acute transfusion reactions are those reactions that occur within 24 h after the blood is transfused. It may range from various responses to blood transfusion, such as mild allergic to severe life-threatening, including acute febrile nonhemolytic transfusion reactions, acute hemolytic reactions, or transfusion-related acute lung injury (TRALI).

Delayed Transfusion Reactions This may range from days to weeks after the transfusion. From various clinical diseases like delayed hemolytic transfusion reaction, transfusion-associated graft-versus-host disease, and transfusion-transmitted infections. It is important to monitor for and recognize the delayed responses so as to institute long-term care of the patient who is receiving transfusions appropriately.

15.3 Types of Transfusion Reactions

Transfusion reactions represent a spectrum of unfavorable adverse effects that could be implicated after the administration of the blood products. There are several principal types of transfusion reactions, which are divided according to the mechanisms and clinical implications:

Febrile Nonhemolytic Transfusion Reactions (FNHTRs): One of the most common of all reactions, FNHTRs are fever and chills without any evidence of hemolysis. Generally, the cause is an immune response to white cells, platelets, or donor plasma proteins by the recipient.

Acute Hemolytic Reimmunologic Reaction: This is a reaction taking place against rapidly destroyed transfused red blood cells from aggressive activity of the host immune system. Quite often, this kind of reaction follows ABO incompatibility; hence, it is a life-threatening reaction because it shows up with symptoms such as fever, back pain, dark urine, and renal failure.

Allergic Reactions: The reactions may be mild or severe, according to the immune response against plasma proteins in transfused blood. They include itching, rash, hives, or anaphylaxis in severe cases.

Transfusion-Associated Circulatory Overload (TACO): TACO occurs as a result of transfusing a large volume of blood or blood component, which exceeds the blood receiving capacity of the heart, leading to fluid overload, increased blood pressure, and respiratory distress, including signs of heart failure.

Transfusion-Related Acute Lung Injury (TRALI): An extremely serious reaction, including acute, serious, and respiratory distress following the transfusion, characterized by a very sudden beginning of hypoxia, bilateral pulmonary edema, and fever. It is produced through the action of antibodies in the donor against the white cells of the host or other immune factors.

Bacterial Contamination and Endotoxemia: Blood products are liable to be contaminated with bacteria at the time of collection or during storage, and at times, it causes a severe reaction—hallmark fever, chills, hypotension, and at its worst, septic shock.

Such data are useful for prompt identification and management of adverse events and would thus be very valuable in improving the outcome of patient safety in transfusion practices.

15.4 Febrile Nonhemolytic Transfusion Reactions (FNHTRs)

Febrile nonhemolytic transfusion reactions (FNHTRs) are the most common type of posttransfusion complication, with fever, chills, and rigors occurring within a few hours of transfusion (Cohen et al. 2017). Majorly, these reactions are triggered by the accumulation of cytokines during storage of cellular components, specifically in platelet units, and result in an inflammatory response of the recipient (Hei et al. 1999). FNHTRs are one of the most common transfusion reactions, rated from 0.5% to 6.8% of transfusions (King et al. 2004).

Signs of FNHTRs, among which fever (≥38 °C/100.4 °F) or chills prevail, should alert health workers to consider this set of reactions in addition to other possible problems related to blood transfusion (Geiger and Howard 2007). Management entails stopping the transfusion promptly, as it will help in ruling out other severe reactions, such as hemolytic transfusion reactions. After cessation, a full transfusion reaction workup shall be done as per hospital protocols. Symptomatic relief with antipyretics, especially acetaminophen, is recommended, considering its high-safety profile, while aspirin should be avoided in some patient populations (Geiger and Howard 2007).

The transfusion can then cautiously be restarted at a lower rate in case other causative factors have been appropriately ruled out, with close monitoring that would take place to optimize patient safety and symptom relief (Geiger and Howard 2007). Studies have demonstrated that decreasing the number of white blood cells in blood products leads to a reduction in the rate of FNHTR. However, in nonleukoreduced blood products, febrile reactions were estimated to occur in 0.5–6.8% of the red cell units transfused (King et al. 2004). It also studied the possibility of prophylactic pretreatment with acetaminophen and diphenhydramine against the occurrence of FNHTRs. It was found to be promising for reducing the likelihood of such reactions, especially during the administration of leukoreduced blood products (Kennedy et al. 2008). Observational studies have also indicated a decrease in the incidence of allergic and fejsoon anemolytic reactions among the recipients of platelet additive solution C platelets (Weisberg et al. 2018).

15.5 Suspecting Acute Hemolytic Transfusion Reactions

Acute hemolytic transfusion reactions are severe, life-threatening events that must be addressed immediately. These are characterized by pyrexia, loin pain, and dark urine; however, not all may necessarily occur at the same time (Talano et al. 2003). The major cause for hemolytic transfusion reactions is the immune response against an incompatible blood group, mainly referring to the ABO blood group system, although others critically implicated are Duffy and Kell (Chou et al. 2020). These reactions may also be caused by nonimmune factors, such as thermal, osmotic, or mechanical stress on the red blood cells (Chou et al. 2020).

Its different categories include: intravascular, where red cells contained wholly within the blood system are destroyed, unbound, or a free release of hemoglobin into the plasma; and extravascular hemolysis, where destruction by the reticuloendothelial system, principally the spleen, occurs because of bound antibody (Scheunemann and Ataga 2010). In a delayed hemolytic transfusion reaction, antigens are often of a minor blood group nature and, again, are likely to reflect an anamnestic response due to sensitization from a previous transfusion or, in females, from pregnancy (Scheunemann and Ataga 2010).

Management of hemolytic transfusion reactions should include immediate cessation of the infusion to prevent any further exposure to incompatible blood and initiate diagnostic and supportive measures. Diagnostics will involve contacting Hospital Transfusion Services; meanwhile, ensure intravenous access of the patient (Linder and Chou 2021). Protection of the renal by aggressive hydration with normal saline is mandatory to forestall the occurrence of renal failure, with close monitoring of its complications, such as disseminated intravascular coagulation (DIC) (Linder and Chou 2021).

The critical considerations include maintenance of airway patency and being ready for major difficulties in airway management, as well as line intravenous access. Toxins and cytokines have to be removed, and it should be done by continuous renal replacement therapy if needed. Accesses to dialysis therapies were also underscored in light of the potential future need for long-term renal replacement therapy.

15.6 Suspecting Allergic Transfusion Reactions

Allergic transfusion reactions present in various spectra of response, from mild hypersensitivity reactions such as urticaria to severe, life-threatening anaphylaxis. The reactions may present as localized mucocutaneous reactions, mild angioedema, or manifest severe symptoms such as those resembling respiratory compromise and hypotension (Hirayama 2013). The transfusion reactions are mostly allergic reactions due to an individual's hypersensitivity to foreign proteins carried by the blood donated from the donor. In particular, people who do not have any immunoglobulin A (IgA) are more susceptible to an anaphylactic reaction brought about by the immune response to this new protein (Hirayama 2013).

This involves termination of transfusion immediately to prevent continued exposure to the allergen, then administration of antihistamines to relieve the allergic symptoms. The combined use of H1 and H2 receptor antagonists has shown efficacy in managing these reactions (Hirayama 2013). Symptoms may progress, and the patient should be kept under close observation. In such a situation, anaphylaxis should be treated with the administration of epinephrine as early as possible because this is the mainstay of treatment for severe allergic reactions (Hirayama 2013).

Some of the specific considerations for an intubated and mechanically ventilated patient in the ICU setup include monitoring changes in peak inspiratory pressure, end-tidal CO_2, heart rate, and blood pressure, since they are among the signals of an anaphylactic reaction. Thus, advanced hemodynamic monitoring tools will help provide valuable information regarding reductions in the Global End-Diastolic Volume Index (GEDVI) and Systemic Vascular Resistance Index (SVRI), both of which will point toward systemic vasodilation, or increases in the Extravascular

Lung Water Index (EVLWI) and Pulmonary Vascular Resistance Index (PVRI), both of which help to represent pulmonary edema due to the complications of anaphylaxis.

15.7 Transfusion-Associated Circulatory Overload (TACO) in ICU Settings

15.7.1 Definition and Clinical Importance

Transfusion-associated circulatory overload (TACO) is recognized as a significant transfusion-related adverse event, particularly prevalent in intensive care units (ICU) where patients are often critically ill and have complex medical histories. TACO is defined by the acute onset of pulmonary edema following the administration of blood products, typically manifesting within 6 h of transfusion. It is characterized by hydrostatic pulmonary edema indicating a cardiogenic origin and is a leading cause of transfusion-related morbidity and mortality.

15.7.2 Epidemiology

The incidence of TACO varies widely, reported as high as 8% in certain high-risk patient groups, such as the elderly and those with preexisting cardiac or renal conditions. The condition is also frequently underdiagnosed or misreported due to overlapping symptoms with other transfusion-related and cardiac complications.

15.7.3 Pathophysiology

The pathophysiology of TACO involves volume overload and cardiac stress, which are not adequately compensated by the patient's physiological mechanisms due to underlying health conditions or the acute volume challenge of transfusion. This overload results in increased hydrostatic pressure in the pulmonary capillaries, leading to fluid transudation into the alveolar spaces, manifesting as pulmonary edema.

15.7.4 Risk Factors

Several factors increase the risk of TACO, including:

- Advanced age, which often correlates with decreased cardiac reserve.
- Existing cardiovascular disease, especially heart failure.

- Chronic renal insufficiency, which impairs fluid excretion.
- Acute or chronic pulmonary conditions.
- Volume and rate of blood product transfusion, with rapid transfusions being particularly risky.
- Concomitant administration of other fluids during transfusion.

15.7.5 Clinical Presentation

The clinical presentation of TACO typically includes:

- Sudden respiratory distress and dyspnea.
- Observations of increased central venous pressure.
- Signs of fluid overload such as peripheral edema.
- Radiographic evidence of pulmonary edema.
- Elevated brain natriuretic peptide (BNP) levels, often more than 1.5 times the baseline, which help differentiate it from other causes of respiratory distress.

15.7.6 Diagnostic Criteria

Diagnosis of TACO relies on a combination of clinical presentation and temporal association with blood transfusion. The major criteria for diagnosis include:

- Acute respiratory distress.
- Evidence of positive fluid balance.
- Radiographic signs of pulmonary edema.
- Elevated BNP levels.
- No alternative plausible explanation for the symptoms.

15.7.7 Management

Management strategies focus on preventing the development of TACO and mitigating its effects once it has occurred:

- Meticulous fluid management and monitoring during transfusion, especially in high-risk patients.
- Use of diuretics to manage fluid overload.
- Oxygen therapy and ventilatory support for severe cases.
- Slow and controlled transfusion rates.
- Pretransfusion assessment of cardiac function in vulnerable patients may help tailor transfusion protocols to minimize risk.

15.7.8 *Prevention*

Preventive measures include:

- Rigorous assessment of the patient's volume status and cardiac function before transfusion.
- Adjusting the transfusion volume and rate according to the patient's capacity to handle the fluid.
- Consideration of premedication with diuretics in patients at high risk for fluid overload.
- Close monitoring of vital signs and oxygen saturation throughout the transfusion process.

15.7.9 *Transfusion-Related Acute Lung Injury (TRALI) in ICU Settings*

15.7.9.1 Definition and Clinical Significance

Transfusion-related acute lung injury (TRALI) is a severe pulmonary complication associated with blood transfusion and represents one of the leading causes of transfusion-related deaths. TRALI is characterized by noncardiogenic pulmonary edema that occurs within 6 h of receiving blood products. Unlike TACO, TRALI involves increased pulmonary capillary permeability, leading to fluid leakage into the alveoli that is not related to left atrial hypertension or volume overload.

15.7.9.2 Epidemiology

TRALI is relatively rare but extremely serious, with an incidence that can vary significantly depending on the patient population and the types of blood products administered. It is particularly prevalent in patients with existing risk factors such as current smoking, recent surgery, or underlying sepsis.

15.7.9.3 Pathophysiology

The pathophysiology of TRALI is complex and thought to involve a "two-hit" model:

- First Hit: The patient's existing condition, such as inflammation or endothelial activation due to surgery, infection, or severe illness, primes the pulmonary vasculature.

- Second Hit: Bioactive substances within the transfused blood product, including antibodies against leukocyte antigens or other biologic response modifiers, trigger a robust immune response in the recipient's lungs. This response includes the activation of neutrophils, which adhere to the pulmonary endothelium and release mediators that increase capillary permeability, leading to pulmonary edema.

15.7.10 Risk Factors

15.7.10.1 Factors That Increase the Risk of Developing TRALI Include

- Intensive care unit (ICU) stays, particularly with mechanical ventilation.
- Recent major surgery or trauma.
- Active infection or sepsis.
- History of alcohol abuse or smoking.
- Transfusion of plasma-rich blood products from multiparous female donors or donors with specific leukocyte antibodies.

15.7.10.2 Clinical Presentation

Symptoms of TRALI are acute and include:

- Sudden onset of respiratory distress.
- Hypoxemia, which is severe and refractory to supplemental oxygen.
- Bilateral pulmonary infiltrates on chest X-rays without elevated pulmonary capillary wedge pressure, distinguishing it from cardiogenic pulmonary edema.

15.7.10.3 Diagnosis

Diagnosis of TRALI is primarily clinical, based on the temporal relationship to transfusion and the exclusion of other potential causes of acute lung injury. Diagnostic criteria include:

- Development of acute lung injury during or within 6 h after transfusion.
- No preexisting acute lung injury prior to transfusion.
- Hypoxemia and bilateral infiltrates on chest radiographs.
- Lack of left heart failure or fluid overload, confirmed via invasive hemodynamic monitoring if necessary.

15.7.10.4 Management

Management of TRALI is supportive and includes:

- Immediate cessation of the transfusion.
- Supportive care with oxygen therapy and mechanical ventilation if necessary.
- Monitoring in an ICU setting for severe cases.
- Use of conservative fluid management strategies to avoid exacerbating pulmonary edema.
- Corticosteroids and diuretics have been used anecdotally but lack evidence-based support for their effectiveness in TRALI.

15.7.10.5 Prevention

Preventive strategies are critical given the severity of TRALI and include:

- Screening and exclusion of blood donors with known HLA and HNA antibodies.
- Preferential use of male donor plasma or plasma from females without a history of pregnancy.
- Reduction in the use of high-plasma volume blood products when possible, especially in at-risk patients.

15.8 Bacterial Contamination and Endotoxemia

Transfusion-transmitted bacterial infections are a significant concern in healthcare settings, particularly during or after blood transfusions. Symptoms such as high fever, chills, rigors, and circulatory collapse should raise suspicion of such infections (Ahmad et al. 2021). Bacterial contamination of blood products can occur through various sources, including donor skin, unrecognized bacteremia in donors, and environmental contaminants during blood component preparation and storage (Brecher and Hay 2005). Platelets, stored at room temperature, are especially vulnerable to bacterial growth, with Staphylococcus aureus commonly found in platelets and Yersinia enterocolitica in red cell transfusions (Levy et al. 2018).

Immediate cessation of transfusion is crucial when a bacterial infection is suspected, followed by diagnostic procedures like gram staining and culture to identify the offending organism (Kuehnert et al. 2001). It is essential to isolate the same bacteria from both the patient and the blood product to confirm the source of infection (Jutzi et al. 2018). Medical management involves initiating broad-spectrum antibiotics and providing cardiorespiratory support as needed to stabilize the patient and manage sepsis symptoms (Bihl et al. 2007).

Preventative measures include rigorous screening of blood donors, sterile techniques during blood collection, and controlled environments during component preparation to minimize contamination risks (Hillyer et al. 2003). Bacterial contamination of platelets poses a significant infectious risk, with platelet transfusions associated with a higher risk of sepsis and death compared to other blood products (Levy et al. 2018). Implementing pathogen inactivation for platelet concentrates has been suggested to reduce the risk of septic transfusion reactions (Levy et al. 2018).

15.9 Transfusion-Associated Graft-Versus-Host Disease

Transfusion-associated graft-versus-host disease (TA-GVHD) is a rare but severe complication of blood transfusion, primarily affecting immunocompromised individuals. This condition arises when donor lymphocytes in transfused blood recognize the recipient's tissues as foreign and mount an immune response against them, leading to widespread tissue damage and potentially fatal outcomes (Kopolovic et al. 2015).

Immunocompromised patients, including those with congenital immunodeficiency or undergoing treatments that suppress the immune system like chemotherapy, are at heightened risk for TA-GVHD (Kopolovic et al. 2015). Individuals with hematological malignancies, such as leukemia or lymphoma, are also more susceptible due to their underlying conditions and the immunosuppressive effects of cancer therapies (Kopolovic et al. 2015).

Prevention of TA-GVHD primarily involves irradiating cellular blood components before transfusion. This process deactivates the lymphocytes present in the blood product, preventing them from attacking the recipient's tissues (Cid 2017). Irradiated blood products are crucial for high-risk patients, especially those who are immunocompromised or undergoing treatments that compromise their immune function (Cid 2017).

Given the high-mortality rate and limited treatment options for TA-GVHD, prevention is paramount. Close monitoring of high-risk patients for any signs of the disease is essential even after using irradiated products. Management of TA-GVHD focuses on supportive and symptomatic care, aiming to control the immune response and provide organ system support. However, outcomes remain poor once TA-GVHD develops (Kopolovic et al. 2015) (Fig. 15.1).

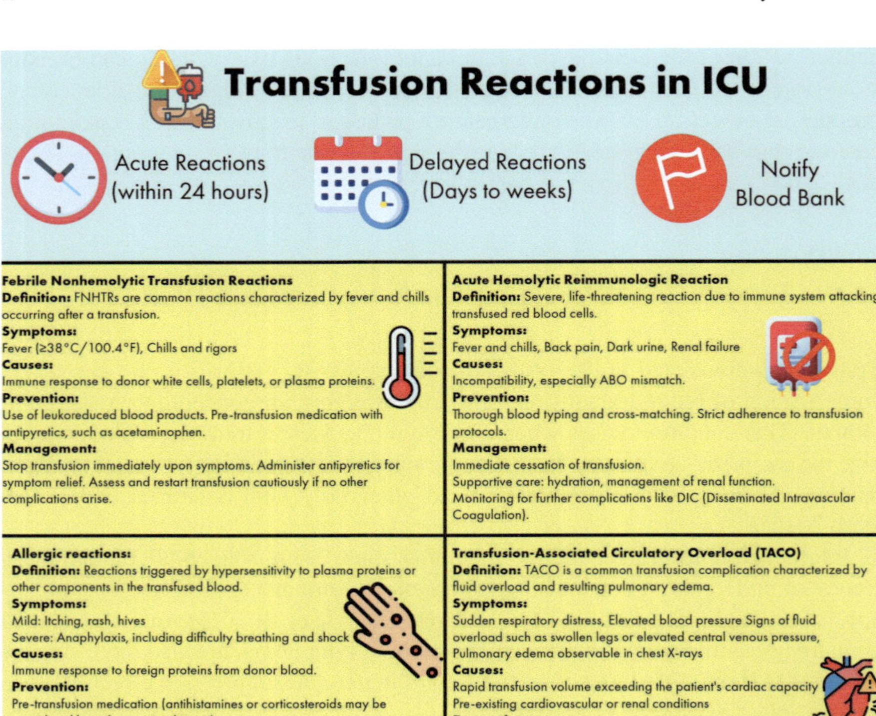

Fig. 15.1 Transfusion reactions in ICU

<a href="https://www.flaticon.com/free-icons/calendar" title="calendar icons">Calendar icons created by Freepik - Flaticon</a>
<a href="https://www.flaticon.com/free-icons/temperature" title="temperature icons">Temperature icons created by Freepik - Flaticon</a>
<a href="https://www.flaticon.com/free-icons/cancel" title="cancel icons">Cancel icons created by Freepik - Flaticon</a>
<a href="https://www.flaticon.com/free-icons/blood-bag" title="blood bag icons">Blood bag icons created by Freepik - Flaticon</a>
<a href="https://www.flaticon.com/free-icons/skin" title="skin icons">Skin icons created by Freepik - Flaticon</a>
<a href="https://www.flaticon.com/free-icons/lungs" title="lungs icons">Lungs icons created by Vitaly Gorbachev - Flaticon</a>
<a href="https://www.flaticon.com/free-icons/immune-system" title="immune system icons">Immune system icons created by Backwoods - Flaticon</a>
<a href="https://www.flaticon.com/free-icons/notify" title="notify icons">Notify icons created by hqrloveq - Flaticon</a>

References

Ahmad Y, Heroes AS, Hume HA, Farouk M, Owusu-Ofori A, Gehrie EA et al (2021) Bacterial contamination of blood products in Africa. Transfusion 61(3):767–780

Bihl F, Castelli D, Marincola F, Dodd RY, Brander C (2007) Transfusion-transmitted infections. J Transl Med 5:1–11

Brecher ME, Hay SN (2005) Bacterial contamination of blood components. Clin Microbiol Rev 18(1):195–204

Chou ST, Alsawas M, Fasano RM, Field JJ, Hendrickson JE, Howard J et al (2020) American Society of Hematology 2020 guidelines for sickle cell disease: transfusion support. Blood Adv 4(2):327–355

Cid J (2017) Prevention of transfusion-associated graft-versus-host disease with pathogen-reduced platelets with amotosalen and ultraviolet A light: a review. Vox Sang 112(7):607–613

Cohen R, Escorcia A, Tasmin F, Lima A, Lin Y, Lieberman L et al (2017) Feeling the burn: the significant burden of febrile nonhemolytic transfusion reactions. Transfusion 57(7):1674–1683

Davenport RD (2005, July) Pathophysiology of hemolytic transfusion reactions. In: Seminars in hematology, vol 42, No. 3. WB Saunders, pp 165–168

Garratty G (2004) Autoantibodies induced by blood transfusion. Transfusion 44(1):5–9

Geiger TL, Howard SC (2007) Acetaminophen and diphenhydramine premedication for allergic and febrile nonhemolytic transfusion reactions: good prophylaxis or bad practice? Transfus Med Rev 21(1):1–12

Goel R, Tobian AA, Shaz BH (2019) Noninfectious transfusion-associated adverse events and their mitigation strategies. Blood J Am Soc Hematol 133(17):1831–1839

Heddle NM (1999) Pathophysiology of febrile nonhemolytic transfusion reactions. Curr Opin Hematol 6(6):420

Hei DJ, Grass JA, Lin L, Corash L, Cimino GD (1999) Elimination of cytokine production in stored platelet concentrate aliquots by photochemical treatment with psoralen plus ultraviolet A light. Transfusion 39(3):239–248

Hillyer CD, Josephson CD, Blajchman MA, Vostal JG, Epstein JS, Goodman JL (2003) Bacterial contamination of blood components: risks, strategies, and regulation: joint ASH and AABB educational session in transfusion medicine. ASH Educ Program Book 2003(1):575–589

Hirayama F (2013) Current understanding of allergic transfusion reactions: incidence, pathogenesis, laboratory tests, prevention and treatment. Br J Haematol 160(4):434–444

Jutzi M, Mansouri Taleghani B, Rueesch M, Amsler L, Buser A (2018) Nationwide implementation of pathogen inactivation for all platelet concentrates in Switzerland. Transfus Med Hemother 45(3):151–156

Kennedy LD, Case LD, Hurd DD, Cruz JM, Pomper GJ (2008) A prospective, randomized, double-blind controlled trial of acetaminophen and diphenhydramine pretransfusion medication versus placebo for the prevention of transfusion reactions. Transfusion 48(11):2285–2291

King KE, Shirey RS, Thoman SK, Bensen-Kennedy D, Tanz WS, Ness PM (2004) Universal leukoreduction decreases the incidence of febrile nonhemolytic transfusion reactions to RBCs. Transfusion 44(1):25–29

Kopolovic I, Ostro J, Tsubota H, Lin Y, Cserti-Gazdewich CM, Messner HA et al (2015) A systematic review of transfusion-associated graft-versus-host disease. Blood J Am Soc Hematol 126(3):406–414

Kuehnert MJ, Roth VR, Haley NR, Gregory KR, Elder KV, Schreiber GB et al (2001) Transfusion-transmitted bacterial infectionin the United States, 1998 through 2000. Transfusion 41(12):1493–1499

Kumar P, Thapliyal R, Coshic P, Chatterjee K (2013) Retrospective evaluation of adverse transfusion reactions following blood product transfusion from a tertiary care hospital: a preliminary step towards hemovigilance. Asian J Transfus Sci 7(2):109–115

Levy JH, Neal MD, Herman JH (2018) Bacterial contamination of platelets for transfusion: strategies for prevention. Crit Care 22(1):271

Linder GE, Chou ST (2021) Red cell transfusion and alloimmunization in sickle cell disease. Haematologica 106(7):1805

Reis VND, Paixão IB, Perrone ACADSJ, Monteiro MI, Santos KBD (2016) Transfusion monitoring: care practice analysis in a public teaching hospital. Einstein (São Paulo) 14:41–46

Sakhalkar VS, Roberts K, Hawthorne LM, McCaskill DM, Veillon DM, Caldito GC, Cotelingam JD (2005) Allosensitization in patients receiving multiple blood transfusions. Ann N Y Acad Sci 1054(1):495–499

Scheunemann LP, Ataga KI (2010) Delayed hemolytic transfusion reaction in sickle cell disease. Am J Med Sci 339(3):266–269

Talano JAM, Hillery CA, Gottschall JL, Baylerian DM, Scott JP (2003) Delayed hemolytic transfusion reaction/hyperhemolysis syndrome in children with sickle cell disease. Pediatrics 111(6):e661–e665

Weisberg SP, Shaz BH, Tumer G, Silliman CC, Kelher MR, Cohn CS (2018) PAS-C platelets contain less plasma protein, lower anti-A and anti-B titers, and decreased HLA antibody specificities compared to plasma platelets. Transfusion 58(4):891–895

Chapter 16
Management of Patients with Massive Transfusion

Srivalli and Soonam John

Learning Points

1. Definition and Criteria of Massive Transfusion: Understand the various definitions and clinical criteria used to identify massive transfusion needs, including the replacement of blood volumes and the specific conditions that trigger the initiation of massive transfusion protocols.
2. Components and Implementation of Massive Transfusion Protocol (MTP): Learn about the elements that make up the MTP, including the coordination among multidisciplinary teams, the use of tranexamic acid, and the importance of maintaining a balance in blood component therapy to manage and mitigate complications effectively.
3. Adjunct Therapies and Complications: Learn about adjunct therapies, such as the use of prothrombin complex concentrates and fibrinogen, and potential complications arising from massive transfusions, including immunological and metabolic issues.
4. Recent Advances in Massive Transfusion Management: Explore the latest updates and studies related to massive transfusion, including outcomes from different transfusion ratios and the effectiveness of new protocols in improving patient survival and recovery.

Srivalli (✉)
Transfusion Medicine, Velammal Medical College Hospital & Research Institute, Madurai, India

S. John
Transfusion Medicine, Government Medical College, Parippally, Kollam, India

S. B. Mishra (ed.), *Critical Care Hematology*,
https://doi.org/10.1007/978-981-97-5565-3_16

16.1 Introduction

Massive blood loss remains to be the important cause of mortality that can be prevented. Management of such massive life-threatening hemorrhage with prompt blood component therapy and hemorrhage control are key steps in resuscitation.

Massive blood loss occurs in various settings of medicine such as obstetric hemorrhage, polytrauma, ruptured aortic aneurysm, surgical bleeding, gastrointestinal bleeds, and bleeding in patients on anticoagulants.

16.2 Massive Transfusion—Definition

Massive transfusion is traditionally defined as transfusion of 10 units of packed red blood cells (PRBCs) within a 24-hour period which would not be practical for clinical decision-making.

In adults, replacement of more than one blood volume in 24 hours or more than 50% of blood volume in 4 hours is defined as massive transfusion (adult blood volume is 70 mL/kg approximately) (Patil and Shetmahajan 2014). In children, transfusion of more than 40 mL/kg is defined as massive transfusion (blood volume in children over 1 month old is approximately 80 mL/kg). Massive hemorrhage can also be clinically defined as bleeding which causes a drop in systolic blood pressure less than 90 mm Hg or a heart rate of more than 110 beats per minute. Prevention of critical hypoperfusion and complications while surgical hemostasis can be achieved is major goal of massive transfusion.

16.3 Pathophysiology

Massive haemorrhage occurs in settings such as severe bleeding due to trauma, ruptured aortic aneurysm, surgery, and obstetric complications (Fig. 16.1).

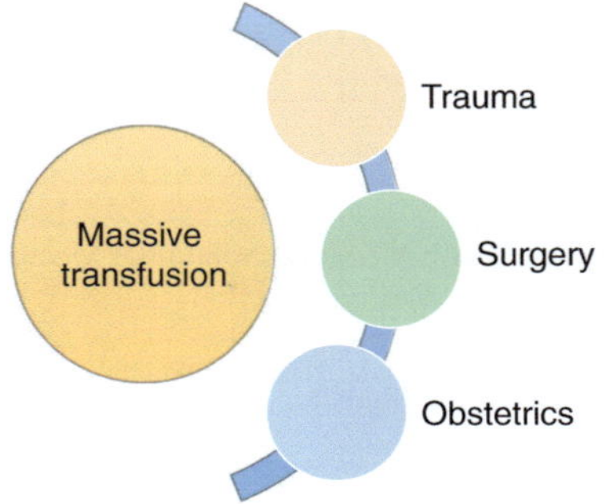

Fig. 16.1 Causes of massive haemorrhage

16.3.1 Trauma

In the setting of severe traumatic bleeding, aggressive replacement of fluids and rapid mechanical/surgical control of bleeding can often mitigate the extent of tissue hypoperfusion, injury, and inflammation. However, failure or inadequacy in control of massive bleeding can cause systemic consumptive coagulopathy with hemodilution and endothelial damage (Hsu et al. 2016).

The physiology of massive injury leads to both rapid degradation of the body's already limited coagulation capacity and the release of inflammatory mediators further enhancing the coagulopathy. Dilution, acidosis, hypothermia, consumption, and fibrinolysis add to the inability to utilize the limited coagulation capacity available in the body (Simon et al. 2022).

16.3.2 Obstetrics

Postpartum hemorrhage (PPH) is defined as estimated blood loss of more than 500 mL after a vaginal birth or 1000 mL after cesarean section, or any blood loss sufficient to cause hemodynamic instability. Postpartum hemorrhage due to abruption, amniotic fluid embolus, and severe bleeding with pre-eclampsia is commonly associated with severe early consumptive coagulopathy. Atonic or traumatic postpartum hemorrhage is unlikely to be associated with hemostatic impairment unless there is gross delay in diagnosis (Klein et al. 2016).

16.3.3 Surgery

Massive blood loss occurs in various surgical settings resulting from extensive surgical trauma or inadequate surgical hemostasis or inadequate reversal of anticoagulants. Cardiopulmonary bypass, oncological surgeries, neurosurgeries, surgical procedures on patients taking anticoagulants, management of gastrointestinal bleeds, and aneurysm repair are common surgical procedures causing massive blood loss. The major cause of bleeding during cardiopulmonary bypass is due to platelet dysfunction caused by heparin given before cardiopulmonary bypass and hypothermia. Extensive surgical trauma, prolonged contact of blood with the bypass circuit, hypothermia, and high doses of heparin lead to dysfunction of the coagulation, and inflammation further worsens the postoperative coagulopathy (Patil and Shetmahajan 2014).

The clinical hallmark of severe hemorrhagic shock is the lethal triad of acidosis, hypothermia, and coagulopathy as shown in Fig. 16.2.

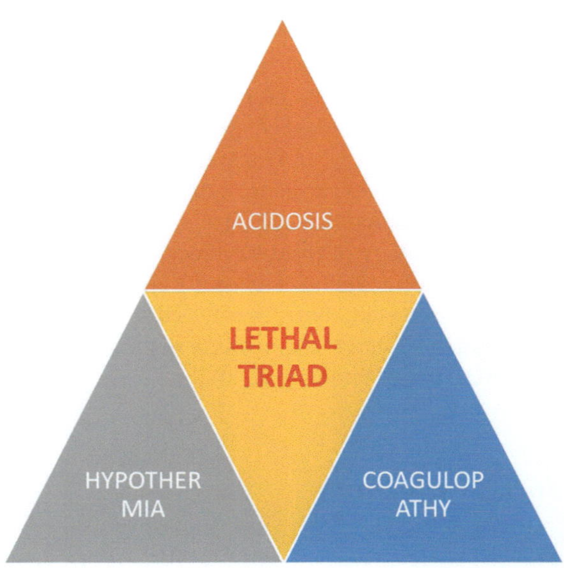

Fig. 16.2 Lethal triad of haemorrhagic shock

16.4 Goals in Management of Massive Transfusion

The major goals of management of massive transfusion are

- Early identification of blood loss
- Maintaining tissue perfusion and oxygenation by restoring blood volume and hemoglobin (Hb)
- Arrest bleeding by using early surgical or radiological interventions in combination, and
- Judicious use of blood and blood component therapy to correct coagulopathy.

16.4.1 Management of Massive Transfusion

The management of massive transfusion protocol involves prevention of hypothermia, acidosis, and coagulopathy. Damage control resuscitation (DCR) includes set of principles for resuscitation with the goal of arresting bleeding or limiting coagulopathy and the physiologic complications associated with resuscitation. The major steps in damage control resuscitation are,

1. Early Control of Hemorrhage

   Control of ongoing hemorrhage with direct pressure, topical or truncal hemostatic dressings, and/or tourniquets or intrauterine balloon devices, manual compression, and oxytocic agents for PPH preventing the development of shock (Spinella et al. 2021).

2. Minimal Volume Resuscitation and Permissible Hypotension

   Permissive hypotension and minimal volume resuscitation are strategies in which systolic blood pressures of 80–100 mm Hg are tolerated while bleeding is controlled. Aggressive volume resuscitation might worsen anemia, coagulopathy, bleeding due to clot disruption, compartment syndrome, and lung injury. Thus, minimal volume resuscitation is preferable. However, permissive hypotensive strategy is contraindicated in brain injury.
3. Massive Transfusion Protocol with the Right Ratio of Components

   The advent of massive hemorrhage protocols has aided in rapid damage control resuscitation of massive bleeding and provides organized utilization of blood and blood components in a systematic manner.

   The components of MHP are represented comprehensively in terms of 7 Ts:

- *T*rigger,
- *T*eam,
- *T*ranexamic acid,
- *T*esting,
- *T*ransfusion,
- *T*emperature, and
- *T*ermination

16.4.1.1 Trigger

Early recognition and identification of the patient who will require a massive transfusion is critical to successful resuscitation.

The transfusion triggers included an:

1. INR >1·5
2. SBP <90 mmHg
3. Base deficit ≥6
4. Positive hemoperitoneum by FAST
5. Heart rate ≥120 beats per minute and
6. A penetrating trauma mechanism.
7. pH—7.25 (Schreiber et al. 2007)

Certain comprehensive validated tools are available which includes individual clinical, laboratory, and ultrasound triggers in combination. Such tools appear to be effective in quick decision-making. The four widely used and practical tools are listed in Fig. 16.3.

Other critical considerations to decide the initiation of massive transfusion protocol are,

- Persistent hemodynamic instability.
- Active bleeding requiring operation or angioembolization.
- Resuscitation with blood transfusion in the trauma bay.

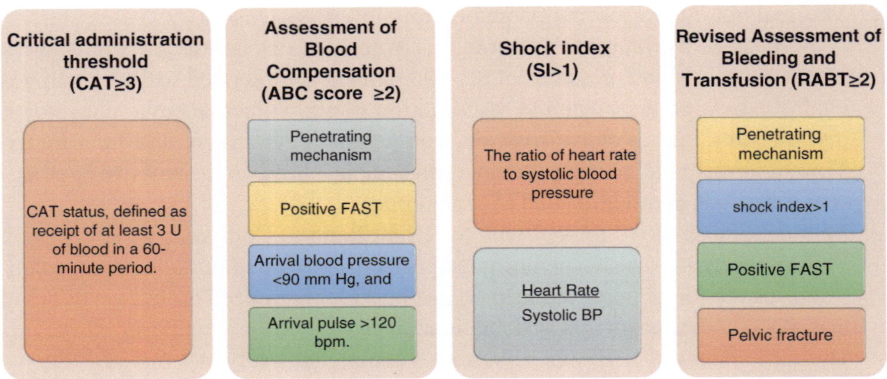

Fig. 16.3 Predictors of massive transfusion

16.4.1.2 Team

The development of massive transfusion protocol and the implementation should involve members from multidisciplinary team such as:

- Blood bank/transfusion services
- Anesthesia
- Emergency department
- Surgical departments
- Trauma service

Effective communication between the team members at the time of activation, execution, and deactivation of massive transfusion protocol is critical for it to be successful.

16.4.1.3 Tranexamic Acid

- Tranexamic acid is a synthetic derivative of lysine which acts by inhibiting fibrinolysis by blocking binding sites of lysine on plasminogen. This prevents the formation of plasmin and subsequent fibrin degradation.
- TXA has been shown to reduce the rate of bleeding and improve survival rates in acute hemorrhage (in cases of trauma and postpartum hemorrhage) (Godbey and Schwartz 2018).
- TXA does not reduce death from gastrointestinal (GI) bleeding and should not be used to treat upper or lower GI bleeding (Roberts et al. 2020).
- Every 15-minute delay in time to administration of TXA decreases survival benefit by 10%.
- The dosage and infusion rate should be determined by the local institution.

- Dosing options include:
  - 1-g bolus followed by a second 1-g bolus 1 hour later
  - 1-g bolus followed by 1 g infusion over subsequent 8 hours
  - 2-g bolus upfront (can be used in resource-challenged locations where second dose is frequently missed)

16.4.1.4 Testing

- Once MHP is initiated, patient's blood testing (CBC, PT, aPTT, fibrinogen, Ca, and arterial blood gas as shown in Fig. 16.4) must be performed to have baseline and then must be repeated at least every hour thereafter until stabilized.
- These laboratory tests help to identify patients receiving oral anticoagulant therapy and in need of reversal of same, assess quality of resuscitation required, and guide blood component administration.

16.4.1.5 Transfusion with Targets

- Balanced resuscitation is a key factor for successful massive hemorrhage protocol.
- For ongoing bleeding with hemorrhagic shock, administration of excessive crystalloids may dilute out coagulation factors and hemoglobin concentration. Ultimately, blood products must be transfused in the right proportions. Figure 16.5 shows the composition of each blood component and storage conditions.

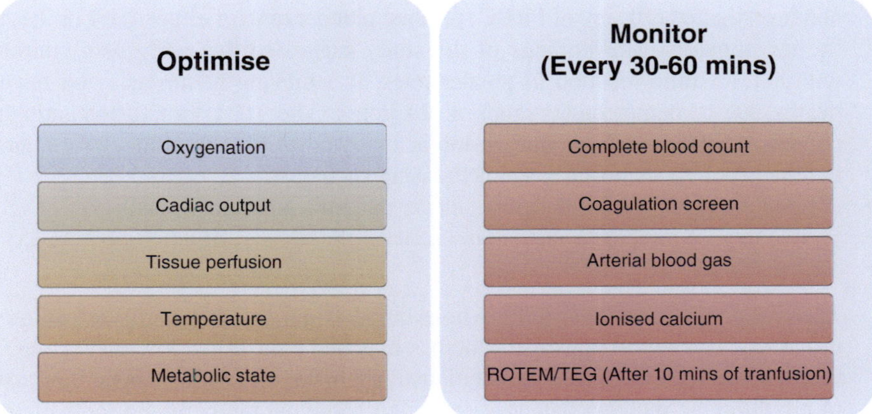

Fig. 16.4 Monitoring MTP

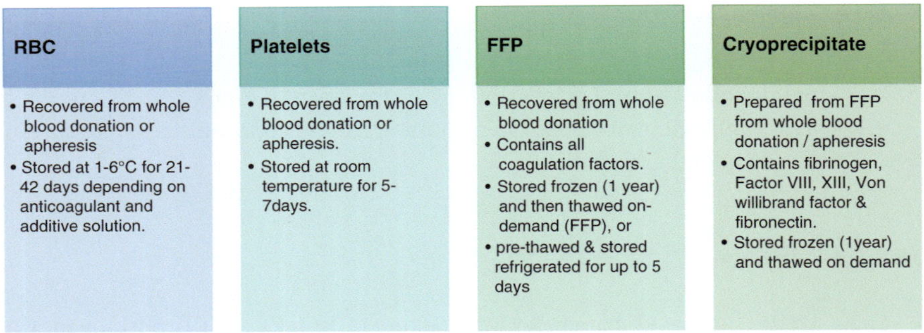

RBC	Platelets	FFP	Cryoprecipitate
• Recovered from whole blood donation or apheresis • Stored at 1-6°C for 21-42 days depending on anticoagulant and additive solution.	• Recovered from whole blood donation or apheresis. • Stored at room temperature for 5-7days.	• Recovered from whole blood donation • Contains all coagulation factors. • Stored frozen (1 year) and then thawed on-demand (FFP), or • pre-thawed & stored refrigerated for up to 5 days	• Prepared from FFP from whole blood donation / apheresis • Contains fibrinogen, Factor VIII, XIII, Von willibrand factor & fibronectin. • Stored frozen (1year) and thawed on demand

Fig. 16.5 Blood components

- In the early phases of resuscitation, when bleeding is rapid, transfusion should be guided by the institution's MHP, with replacement of blood components (red blood cell, plasma, and platelets) in a predetermined ratio, with early consideration for the addition of fibrinogen replacement (fibrinogen concentrate or cryoprecipitate). As time permits, transfusion can then be guided by either standard laboratory tests and/or viscoelastic tests of whole blood clotting (ROTEM® or TEG®) (Brill et al. 2021).
- The PROMMTT study revealed improved survival at 6 hours, for patients that received higher ratios of plasma to RBC or platelets to RBC. 1:1:1 (plasma: platelets: RBC) vs 1:1:2 transfusion strategies in 680 severely injured patients (median injury severity score (ISS) 26.5). There was a 3.7% reduction in 30-day mortality in patients who received higher ratio of plasma (22.4% vs 26.1%, respectively). In addition, patients in the 1:1:1 group achieved earlier hemostasis and had fewer deaths because of exsanguination at 24 hours (Holcomb et al. 2013).
- The Pragmatic Randomized Optimal Platelet and Plasma Ratios (PROPPR) study:
- The PROPPR study was a randomized control trial involving multiple centers and investigated efficacy of PRBC: plasma: platelet ratio of either 1:1:1 or 2:1:1. the investigators. The findings of the study suggested that early resuscitation with a 1:1:1 ratio resulted in greater rates of achieving hemostasis and fewer deaths due to hemorrhagic shock at 24 hours. The 1:1:1 transfusion ratio in patients receiving massive transfusion is a very cost-effective strategy for maintaining adequate hemostasis and decreasing such deaths.
- Administer fibrinogen replacement as per patient's laboratory results.
- Switch to goal-directed transfusion whenever the clinical situation permits.
- Whole blood:

  The use of fresh group-specific whole blood is gaining popularity in military usage as it is ready to transfuse. Uncross-matched cold-stored low-titer group O whole blood (LTOWB) has been demonstrated to be safe, with the benefit of ease of providing an inherent balanced resuscitation, allowing increased shelf-life of a platelet-containing product, and decreasing exposure to multiple donors.

16.4.1.6 Temperature

Hypoperfusion causes decreased heat production leading to hypothermia. Hypothermia dramatically leads to worsening of platelet and coagulation function, decreases citrate metabolism, increases hemoglobin-oxygen affinity leading to hypoxia of tissue, and decreases myocardial function. Aggressive management of temperature is imperative to success of massive transfusion.

- Temperature should be measured within 15 minutes of massive hemorrhage protocol initiation or hospital arrival and should be monitored every 30 minutes from then on till stabilization.
- Every 1 °C decrease in body temperature leads to increase in blood loss by 20% due to impaired coagulation, which eventually causes increased mortality.
- Application of warm blankets, radiant warmers, warm IV fluid infusion, and removal of wet clothes are few interventions to maintain temperature.

16.4.1.7 Termination

Termination of massive transfusion protocol at the right time is critical to ensure that resources are used in appropriate manner. This requires clear criteria for termination of massive transfusion protocol. All team members should be aware about criteria and should be communicated at the time of termination. Criteria for stopping the MTP should include both anatomic (control of bleeding) and physiologic criteria (normalizing hemodynamic, hematologic, and metabolic status).

- Frequent communication between the members of the resuscitation and surgical teams cannot be overemphasized to guide the resuscitation, plan for continued need for blood products and adjuncts, and determine when to move toward data-based resuscitation and when to end active resuscitation.
- Transfer care to the most appropriate department and return any blood components to blood bank.

16.5 Clinical Criteria for Termination

The surgeon/anesthesiologists declare,

- Achievement of hemostasis based on the absence of bleeding, requiring intervention in the surgical field or resolution of blush after angioembolization.
- Adequate resuscitation shown by stabilized blood pressure/heart rate/urine output/decreasing requirement for vasopressors to maintain a stable blood pressure.

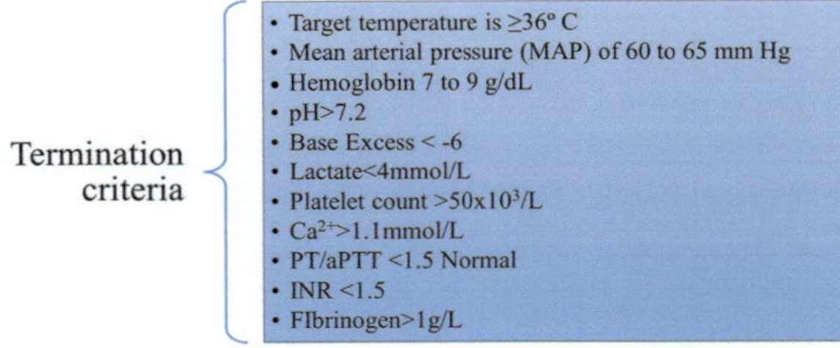

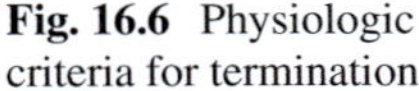
Fig. 16.6 Physiologic criteria for termination

16.5.1 Physiological and Laboratory Criteria for Termination

Physiological and laboratory criteria for termination of massive transfusion protocol are listed in Fig. 16.6.

16.5.2 Adjunctive Therapy

- *Calcium*:
- Transfusion of large volume of blood and components is associated with severe hypocalcemia due to citrate toxicity. In addition to several factors, hypocalcemia contributes to mortality and coagulopathy in patients receiving massive transfusion.
- Recommendation of calcium dosage from "The Joint Trauma System Clinical Practice Guideline" for damage control resuscitation:
  - Administration of 1 g of calcium chloride or 3 g of calcium gluconate to patients in hemorrhagic shock during or immediately after the first unit of blood product transfusion
  - During ongoing resuscitation, Ca dose after every 4 units of blood products, with monitoring of iCa and repletion if <1.2 mmol/L (Spinella et al. 2021).
- *Prothrombin Complex Concentrate (PCC)*:
- PCC is a pathogen-reduced and lyophilized concentrate that contains vitamin K-dependent coagulation factors (factor II, VII, IX, and X) in therapeutic levels. The use of PCC has been proposed as potential adjunct therapy in trauma-induced coagulopathy. Currently, only approved indication for the use of PCC is correction of warfarin-induced coagulopathy in the setting of major bleeding (Ash 2023).
- *Fibrinogen Concentrate*:
- Fibrinogen concentrate can be utilized for fibrinogen replacement therapy, and the concentrate has the advantage of being pathogen-reduced and available in a freeze-dried, powdered form, which makes it easier to reconstitute and administer than cryoprecipitate, which must remain frozen until use.

- *Recombinant VIIa*:
- Recombinant VIIa is generally not recommended for the management of refractory hemorrhage in trauma.

16.6 Complications of Massive Transfusion Protocol

Massive transfusion is associated with numerous infectious, immunological, and metabolic complications. Risks and complications associated with large-volume resuscitation with blood components and products are listed in Fig. 16.7.

METABOLIC
- Hypothermia
- Hypocalcemia
- Hypomagnesemia
- Hypokalemia
- Hyperkalemia
- Acidosis
- Metabolic alkalosis

TRANSFUSION REACTION
- Allergic reaction
- Anaphylactic reaction
- Febrile non hemolytc reaction
- Tranfusion associated circulatory overload
- Transfusion associate sepsis

IMMUNOLOGICAL
- Hemolytic transfusion reaction
- Alloimmunisation
- TRALI
- TRIM
- TA-GVHD
- Post transfusion purpura

OTHERS
- Impaired hemostasis
- Air embolism
- Renal injury

Fig. 16.7 Complications of massive transfusion. TRALI—transfusion-related acute lung injury, TRIM—transfusion-related immunomodulation, TA-GVHD—transfusion-associated graft-vs-host disease

Flowchart

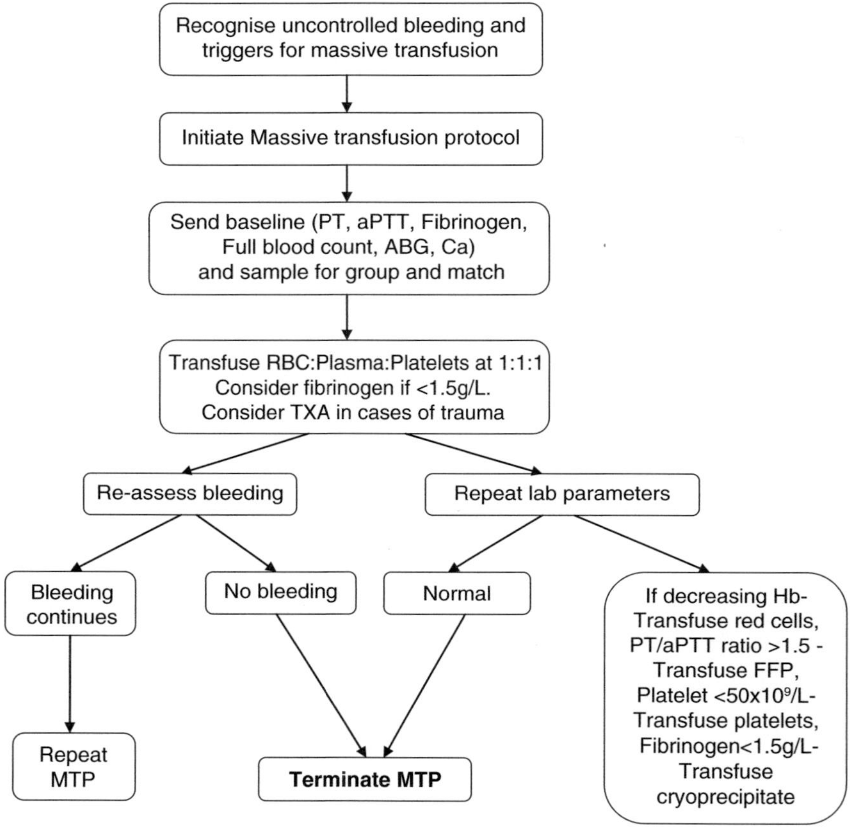

References

Ash T (2023) Massive transfusion protocol. Arch Hematol Case Rep Rev 8(1):004–007

Brill JB, Brenner M, Duchesne J, Roberts D, Ferrada P, Horer T et al (2021) The role of TEG and ROTEM in damage control resuscitation. Shock 56(1S):52–61

Godbey EA, Schwartz J (2018) Massive transfusion protocols and the use of tranexamic acid. Curr Opin Hematol 25(6):482–485

Holcomb JB, Del Junco DJ, Fox EE, Wade CE, Cohen MJ, Schreiber MA et al (2013) The prospective, observational, multicenter, major trauma transfusion (PROMMTT) study: comparative effectiveness of a time-varying treatment with competing risks. JAMA Surg 148(2):127–136

Hsu YMS, Haas T, Cushing MM (2016) Massive transfusion protocols: current best practice. Int J Clin Transfus Med 4:15–27

Klein AA, Arnold P, Bingham RM, Brohi K, Clark R, Collis R et al (2016) AAGBI guidelines: the use of blood components and their alternatives 2016. Anaesthesia 71(7):829–842

Patil V, Shetmahajan M (2014) Massive transfusion and massive transfusion protocol. Indian J Anaesth 58(5):590–595

Roberts I, Shakur-Still H, Afolabi A, Akere A, Arribas M, Brenner A et al (2020) Effects of a high-dose 24-h infusion of tranexamic acid on death and thromboembolic events in patients with acute gastrointestinal bleeding (HALT-IT): an international randomised, double-blind, placebo-controlled trial. Lancet 395(10241):1927–1936

Schreiber MA, Perkins J, Kiraly L, Underwood S, Wade C, Holcomb JB (2007) Early predictors of massive transfusion in combat casualties. J Am Coll Surg 205(4):541–545

Simon TL, McCullough J, Snyder EL, Solheim BG, Strauss RG (eds) (2022) Rossi's principles of transfusion medicine. John Wiley & Sons, Incorporated

Spinella PC, Strandenes CG, Forces NS (2021) Damage control resuscitation (CPG ID: 18)

Part IV
Oncological Emergencies and Critical Care

Chapter 17
Hyperviscosity in Plasma Cell Dyscrasias

Faheema Hasan

Learning Points

1. *Understanding Hyperviscosity*: Recognize hyperviscosity syndrome as a pathologic condition characterized by increased blood viscosity, primarily due to excessive paraprotein secretion in plasma cell dyscrasias, and appreciate its significant impact on patient morbidity and mortality.
2. *Clinical Presentation and Diagnosis*: Identify the classic triad of HVS symptoms, including visual changes, neurological disturbances, and mucosal bleeding, and understand the importance of ophthalmoscopic examination and serum viscosity measurement in the diagnostic process.
3. *Therapeutic Plasma Exchange (TPE)*: Grasp the critical role of TPE in the acute management of HVS, including its mechanisms, efficacy, and the need for subsequent chemotherapy to address the underlying malignancy causing the syndrome.
4. *Chemotherapy and Management Strategies*: Learn about the strategic use of chemotherapy, including the timing and selection of agents, in conjunction with TPE to treat the root cause of HVS and improve long-term patient outcomes, with a particular focus on addressing WM and MM.

17.1 Introduction

Viscosity is essentially the measure of a fluid's resistance to flowing, often likened to its "thickness." Hyperviscosity syndromes (HVS) refer to pathological conditions where blood viscosity increases (Gertz 2018). This can occur due to an increase in (1) cellular elements like erythrocytes and leukocytes, as seen in conditions such as

F. Hasan (✉)
Hematology, UIMS, Allahabad, India

S. B. Mishra (ed.), *Critical Care Hematology*,
https://doi.org/10.1007/978-981-97-5565-3_17

polycythemia, acute leukemia, and sickle cell anemia, or (2) acellular factors like proteins, typical in plasma cell dyscrasias, type 1 or 2 cryoglobulinemia, Sjogren's syndrome associated with polyclonal hyperglobulinemia, and uncontrolled HIV infection with polyclonal hyperglobulinemia. HVS predominantly affects individuals with hematologic cancers known for high paraprotein secretion. It is notably prevalent in Waldenstrom macroglobulinemia (WM), impacting 10–30% of patients, and is also observed in about 2% of multiple myeloma (MM) cases. Recognized as an urgent oncological condition, HVS demands swift clinical identification and appropriate intervention (Khan et al. 2017) (Table 17.1).

17.2 Basic Physics of Viscosity

Newtonian Fluids These fluids exhibit a constant viscosity regardless of the applied shear stress. Their viscosity remains unchanged under the influence of force. Common examples include water and alcohol.

Non-Newtonian Fluids In contrast, non-Newtonian fluids display varying viscosity levels in response to shear stress. Examples include everyday substances like ketchup and shampoo, as well as whole blood. Whole blood comprises cellular elements (red blood cells, white blood cells, and platelets) and a non-cellular component, plasma.

Measurement of Viscosity Viscosity can be quantified in two ways: as an absolute value, measured in centipoises (cP). For instance, water's viscosity is 0.894 cP, while healthy serum has a viscosity of less than or equal to 1.5 cP. Relative to water, where water's viscosity is set as 1.0 (unitless). In this scale, the relative viscosity of serum is about 1.7. Whole blood viscosity, not typically measured in clinical labs, is often deduced from hematocrit levels or absolute white blood cell counts (Dintenfass 1966).

Table 17.1 Cellular and acellular causes of hyperviscosity

Serum/plasma hyperviscosity		Whole blood/cellular hyperviscosity	
Monoclonal/malignant causes	Polyclonal/reactive causes	RBC's	WBC's
Waldenstrom macroglobulinemia (WM)	High-titer rheumatoid factor	Polycythemia vera	CLL
Multiple myeloma (Ig M,G3,A)	Sjögren's syndrome	HbSS	CML
Type 1/II cryoglobulinemia	IgG4 disease	Cyanotic heart disease	Acute leukemia
	HIV infection		

Factors Influencing Blood Viscosity The viscosity of whole blood is influenced by factors such as temperature, pressure, shear forces, and the radius of blood vessels. Under normal conditions, red blood cells majorly contribute to blood viscosity. For example, an increase in hematocrit to 70% doubles blood viscosity. Similarly, a decrease in body temperature leads to an increase in blood viscosity. The relationship between vessel size and viscosity is complex; while smaller vessels like capillaries would theoretically exhibit higher viscosity, the central streaming of deformable red blood cells alters this dynamic. The highest viscosity is typically observed in the postvenule system, a phenomenon described by Fahraeus in 1929.

Serum and Plasma Viscosity Unlike whole blood, the viscosity of serum and plasma is predominantly determined by proteins. Spherical proteins have a minimal effect on viscosity, whereas large linear proteins like fibrinogen and immunoglobulins significantly influence it. The impact of immunoglobulins on viscosity varies with their type and concentration. For instance, IgM, being pentameric and large (970 kDA), can notably increase serum viscosity at levels as low as 3 g/dL. IgA, smaller in size (320 kDA), affects viscosity at levels of 6 g/dL or higher. IgG, comparatively smaller (180 kDA), influences viscosity at levels above 10 g/dL. However, the IgG3 subtype, with its elongated hinge region, can impact viscosity at lower levels. Generally, HVS is rare unless serum viscosity exceeds 4 cP, but it should always be considered in patients with paraprotein-secreting malignancies exhibiting clinical symptoms (Weaver et al. 2020).

17.3 Clinical Features of HVS

The hallmark presentation of hyperviscosity syndrome typically encompasses a triad of symptoms: alterations in vision, neurological irregularities, and bleeding from mucosal surfaces. The most frequent clinical signs of this condition are bleeding from the nasal and oral regions (oronasal bleeding) and disturbances in vision, making ophthalmoscopic examination a critical step in evaluating suspected cases. A particularly severe complication associated with this syndrome is the bilateral blockage of central retinal veins. During an eye examination, one might observe dilated retinal veins with a distinctive, irregular "sausage-like" or segmented appearance, alongside signs of bleeding within the eye (flame hemorrhages), swelling of the optic disc (papilledema), fluid leakage (exudates), and small vascular bulges (microaneurysms) (Kwaan 2013) (Fig. 17.1).

This increased viscosity is most pronounced in smaller blood vessels, such as venules, where the thickened blood can damage the vessel walls in less supported tissues, including the retina, nasal cavity, gastrointestinal tract, brain surface, and gums. Consequently, a thorough examination of the retina is advised even for patients who exhibit bleeding from the nose (epistaxis) or mouth, but do not have visual symptoms.

Symptoms like headache, a general sense of unsteadiness or light-headedness, and loss of hearing have also been associated with hyperviscosity. However, these symptoms are less specific and do not possess the same diagnostic clarity as nosebleeds, bleeding from the gums, and hemorrhaging in the retina.

Currently, hyperviscosity syndrome (HVS) is less frequently observed in patients with Waldenstrom macroglobulinemia (WM) due to advancements in early diagnosis and effective treatment strategies. Symptomatic HVS is uncommon in patients where the concentration of immunoglobulin M (IgM) is below 4000 mg/dl. Consequently, there is no necessity for viscosity measurement in patients with IgM levels under this threshold. The symptoms associated with HVS are largely attributable to the shear forces disrupting the fragile venous channels. Common presentations include nosebleeds (epistaxis), bleeding of the gums (gingival bleeding), and changes in vision due to bleeding in the retina (retinal hemorrhage). Central nervous system symptoms like dizziness, light-headedness, and a pervasive sense of fatigue are rather vague and require confirmation through serum viscosity tests. The onset of HVS symptoms can occur at serum viscosity levels as low as 3 centipoise (cp), but they typically become evident when serum viscosity surpasses the 4–5 cp range (Castillo et al. 2016).

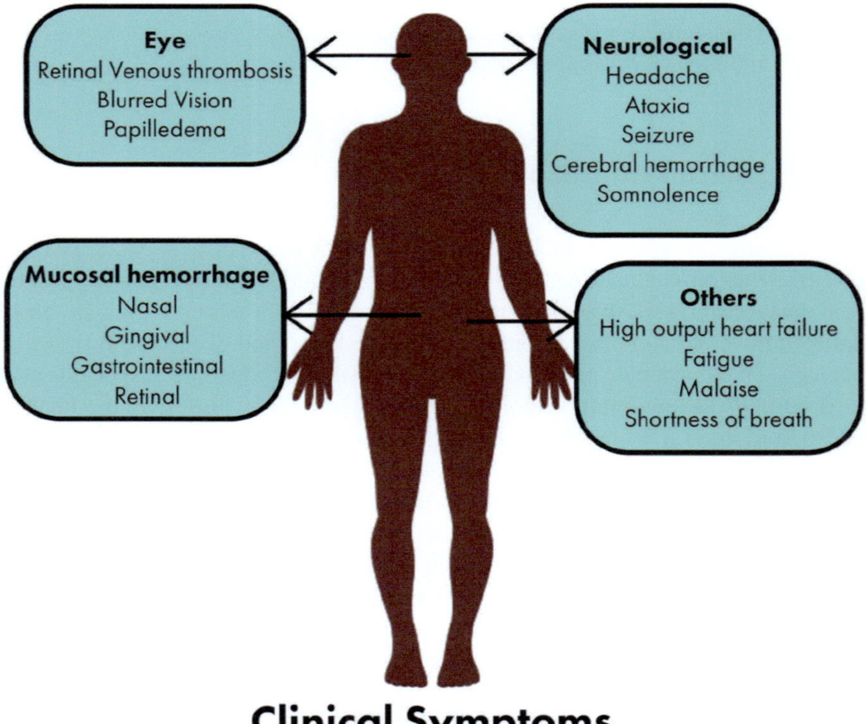

Fig. 17.1 Spectrum of symptomatology in hyperviscosity syndrome (HVS)

Treatment of hyperviscosity syndrome (HVS) is a critical and urgent medical intervention, as HVS is a hematological emergency. Timely and accurate diagnosis followed by the appropriate therapy is essential to prevent life-threatening complications such as cerebral or gastrointestinal hemorrhage and cardiac failure.

17.3.1 Understanding HVS and Indications for Treatment

HVS typically manifests in the setting of elevated immunoglobulin M (IgM) levels. However, a direct linear correlation between IgM levels and serum viscosity is not always evident. It is rare to observe HVS in patients with paraprotein levels less than 3 g/dL. Therefore, the presence of symptoms indicative of HVS or IgM levels exceeding 4 g/dL necessitates immediate clinical attention. These include comprehensive serum viscosity measurements and ophthalmologic evaluations, as visual disturbances are common in HVS.

17.3.2 Therapeutic Plasma Exchange (TPE) as a Primary Treatment Modality

TPE stands at the forefront of HVS management, particularly in acute settings, and has been a standard practice since the 1950s. The procedure aims to remove large molecular weight proteins, predominantly immunoglobulins, from the patient's plasma. This is achieved while reinfusing the cellular components back into the patient. The two prevalent methods of TPE are as follows:

- *Centrifugation Method*: In this method, whole blood is separated into cellular components and plasma using centrifugal force. The plasma is then discarded, and replacement fluid, typically 5% serum albumin or sometimes fresh frozen plasma, is infused back into the patient.
- *Double-Membrane Filtration*: This technique also involves filtering the plasma, but with a secondary membrane designed to remove high-molecular-weight molecules. The process allows smaller molecules, like albumin, to be reinfused into the patient.

Both centrifugation and double-membrane filtration have proven to be equally effective in reducing blood viscosity. A single session of TPE can lower viscosity by approximately 30%, helping to prevent further mucosal hemorrhages. TPE is generally considered safe with an adverse event rate of about 1%, as reported in a European registry study. The most common adverse events include hypotension and allergic reactions to the replacement fluids. Notably, while fibrinogen levels may decrease due to its filtration, significant bleeding complications have not been widely reported in major centers performing TPE.

Despite its efficacy in reducing serum viscosity, TPE does not address the underlying disease pathology. Serum IgM levels often return to baseline within 3–5 weeks post-TPE. Therefore, systemic chemotherapy aimed at treating the underlying malignant B-cell clones should be initiated immediately following TPE.

17.4 Concurrent Chemotherapy Treatment

Given that TPE does not impact the underlying disease process, the initiation of chemotherapy is often concurrent with TPE. This approach is especially pertinent in cases where plasma cell dyscrasias, like Waldenstrom macroglobulinemia (WM), are the underlying cause of HVS. In such scenarios, rapid-acting systemic chemotherapy can significantly reduce serum viscosity, potentially negating the need for plasma exchange.

It is important to consider the potential effects of certain chemotherapeutic agents, such as rituximab, which can lead to an IgM flare. This necessitates deferring rituximab in patients with high M protein levels (more than 4 g/dL) until after a TPE session if symptoms of HVS are present. The IgM flare following rituximab administration is sometimes immediate and may be related to IL-6 release triggered by the immune response. Consequently, rituximab is not typically used as monotherapy in patients at risk of HVS, particularly those with a high paraprotein burden.

Bruton tyrosine kinase inhibitors, like ibrutinib, have shown efficacy in rapidly reducing IgM levels in WM. Bortezomib-based therapies, commonly used in myeloma and in some cases of WM, can prompt quick responses in a majority of patients.

In most instances, an IgM reduction of as little as 25% can completely alleviate symptoms of hyperviscosity. This response rate underscores the effectiveness of these treatments in managing the condition. Research indicates that bortezomib-based triplet regimens result in the fastest decline in protein levels and are therefore considered crucial when hyperviscosity is observed in multiple myeloma cases.

In the rare instances of polyclonal hyperglobulinemia causing hyperviscosity, no pharmacologic technique has proven to be reliably and rapidly effective in reducing immunoglobulin levels. Therefore, in such cases, TPE remains the recommended treatment option.

17.4.1 Newly Diagnosed Waldenström Macroglobulinemia Treatment Algorithm

For patients diagnosed with IgM monoclonal gammopathy of undetermined significance (MGUS) showing less than 10% clonal infiltrate, or those with smoldering (asymptomatic) WM, observation is recommended, irrespective of IgM levels.

In the presence of IgM-related neuropathy, WM-associated hemolytic anemia, symptomatic cryoglobulinemia, bulky ($\geq$5 cm maximum diameter) or symptomatic lymphadenopathy, clinically significant cytopenias (hemoglobin $\leq$10 g/dL, platelets $<100 \times 10^9$/L), symptoms of hyperviscosity, constitutional symptoms, or concurrent AL amyloidosis, more proactive treatment approaches are indicated:

If the patient exhibits symptoms of hyperviscosity, single-agent rituximab for one cycle may be initiated. If there is a development of symptomatic hyperviscosity in the context of IgM flare, plasmapheresis should be initiated.

For more aggressive symptoms or clinical findings, treatment options include bendamustine plus rituximab (BR) for 4–6 cycles, or the use of the Bruton's tyrosine kinase inhibitor, zanubrutinib. It is noted that maintenance therapy with rituximab is not recommended following these treatments.

17.5 Monitoring and Follow-Up

Post-treatment, patients require careful monitoring for any recurrence of symptoms or complications arising from therapy. Regular follow-up appointments are essential, focusing on serum viscosity and IgM levels, to ensure the continued efficacy of the treatment and to adjust the therapeutic approach as necessary.

The management of HVS is a delicate balance between addressing the immediate symptoms through TPE and targeting the underlying disease with chemotherapy. This multifaceted approach ensures not only the rapid amelioration of symptoms but also a sustained response to treatment, thereby improving patient outcomes in this potentially life-threatening condition.

Flowchart

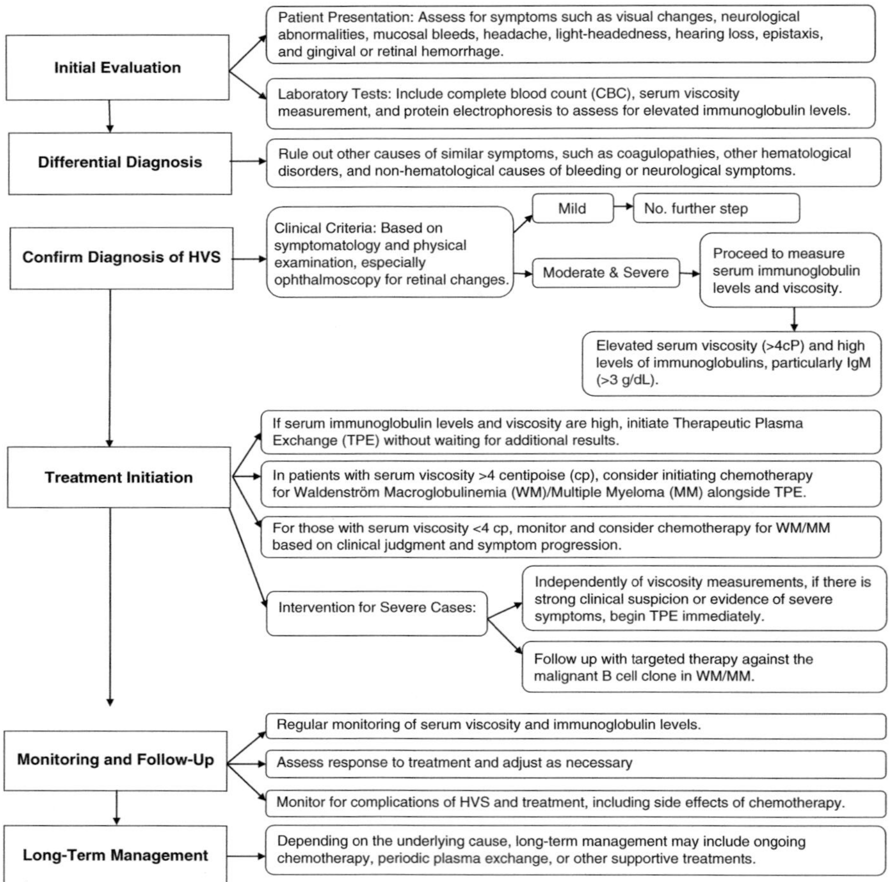

References

Castillo JJ, Garcia-Sanz R, Hatjiharissi E, Kyle RA, Leleu X, McMaster M et al (2016) Recommendations for the diagnosis and initial evaluation of patients with Waldenström Macroglobulinaemia: a Task Force from the 8th International Workshop on Waldenström Macroglobulinaemia. Br J Haematol 175(1):77–86

Dintenfass L (1966) A preliminary outline of the blood high viscosity syndromes. Arch Intern Med 118(5):427–435

Gertz MA (2018) Acute hyperviscosity: syndromes and management. Blood, J Am Soc Hematol 132(13):1379–1385

Gertz MA (2023) Waldenström macroglobulinemia: 2023 update on diagnosis, risk stratification, and management. Am J Hematol 98(2):348–358

Khan UA, Shanholtz CB, McCurdy MT (2017) Oncologic mechanical emergencies. Hematol Oncol Clinics 31(6):927–940

Kwaan HC (2013) Hyperviscosity in plasma cell dyscrasias. Clin Hemorheol Microcirc 55(1):75–83

Weaver A, Rubinstein S, Cornell RF (2020) Hyperviscosity syndrome in paraprotein secreting conditions including Waldenstrom macroglobulinemia. Front Oncol 10:815

Chapter 18
Disseminated Intravascular Coagulation (DIC)

Biswajit Nayak and Sushree Smita Behura

Learning Points

1. DIC Pathophysiology and Triggers: Understanding the systemic activation of coagulation and the role of various triggers such as sepsis, trauma, and malignancies in initiating DIC is crucial for early recognition and management of the condition.
2. Diagnostic Strategies: Familiarity with the International Society on Thrombosis and Haemostasis (ISTH) DIC score and other diagnostic criteria is essential for the accurate diagnosis of DIC, considering its multifactorial nature and the diverse clinical presentations.
3. Differential Diagnosis: The ability to differentiate DIC from other coagulopathies like heparin-induced thrombocytopenia (HIT), thrombotic thrombocytopenic purpura (TTP), and hemophagocytic lymphohistiocytosis (HLH) is critical for the appropriate management of patients.
4. Management Principles: A comprehensive understanding of the management strategies, including addressing the underlying cause of DIC, providing supportive care, and navigating the complexities of blood product replacement and anticoagulation therapy, is key to improving patient outcomes.

18.1 Introduction

Disseminated intravascular coagulation (DIC) is a critical health condition marked by widespread activation of the blood coagulation system within the vascular network, which results in significant fibrin accumulation and the development of microvascular clots across the body (Franchini et al. 2006). The International Society on Thrombosis and Haemostasis (ISTH) categorizes DIC as a syndrome acquired from various etiologies that prompts coagulation activation and disrupts its normal localization (Wada et al. 2020). This syndrome leads to the depletion of

B. Nayak (✉)
Critical Care Medicine, IMS & SUM Hospital, Bhubaneswar, India

S. S. Behura
Paediatric, KIMS, Bhubaneswar, India

S. B. Mishra (ed.), *Critical Care Hematology*,
https://doi.org/10.1007/978-981-97-5565-3_18

platelets and clotting factors, elevating the likelihood of hemorrhagic manifestations and thromboembolic complications, and may advance toward organ failure across multiple systems (Adelborg et al. 2021).

The onset of DIC is linked to a range of precipitating factors and conditions, underscoring the necessity for its swift identification and management to foster better patient prognoses (Adelborg et al. 2021). The syndrome manifests through a cascade of events that sequentially activate both the coagulation and fibrinolytic pathways, characterized by a widespread and rapid activation of the coagulation system. This results in clot formation within vessels and widespread bleeding due to the consumption of platelets and coagulation proteins (Papageorgiou et al. 2018).

DIC poses a significant risk in various clinical scenarios, often linked with systemic inflammation (Levi 2014). The hallmark of DIC is the extensive coagulation activation, culminating in fibrin deposit within blood vessels, dysfunction of organs, depletion of coagulation factors and platelets, and severe bleeding episodes (Hook and Abrams 2012). Particularly in patients with sepsis, DIC substantially escalates both morbidity and mortality rates (Hook and Abrams 2012). Effective management and vigilant monitoring of DIC are paramount due to its capacity to cause dire health outcomes. A comprehensive understanding of its pathophysiology and initiating factors is vital to ensure prompt and effective interventions, ultimately enhancing patient survival and recovery prospects.

18.2 Etiopathogenesis

The etiology of DIC is diverse and typically arises as a secondary response to an underlying disease or insult that initiates a cascade of events leading to defective coagulation. Some common underlying conditions are enumerated in Table 18.1.

One of the most common triggers for DIC is sepsis, a severe systemic infection with any gram-negative or gram-positive microbes as well as viral or fungal pathogens. There occurs activation of the endothelium in response to severe infection along with release of pro-inflammatory substances, including cytokines and tissue factors, thereby initiating platelet aggregation and coagulation cascade. Severe acute pancreatitis—a sterile systemic inflammation—also results in coagulation dysfunction from endothelial cell activation caused by release of cytokines.

Acute injuries, significant tissue damage, and traumatic events are known to incite a systemic inflammatory response, which can heighten fibrinolytic activity and activate the coagulation system. This cascade of events may culminate in disseminated intravascular coagulation (DIC), as documented by Poskitt et al. (1973). DIC represents a critical medical emergency, marked by the widespread formation of blood clots within the microvasculature, disrupting normal organ function and potentially leading to organ failure. The underlying mechanisms of DIC encompass a sophisticated interaction among factors that promote and inhibit coagulation, fostering an environment conducive to both excessive clot formation and bleeding tendencies.

Table 18.1 Etiology of DIC

1. Sepsis (most common)
2. Trauma (physical trauma/accidents/major surgeries)
3. Solid tumors/hematologic malignancies
4. Obstetrical complications (placental abruption, HELLP, amniotic fluid embolism, severe eclampsia, septic abortion, retained placental tissue, postpartum hemorrhage)
5. Acute pancreatitis
6. Severe transfusion reactions
7. Snake envenomation or exposure to certain toxins
8. Hyperthermia/heat stroke

Aggressive cancers can release tissue factor and cancer-related procoagulants, activating platelets and the coagulation pathway, contributing to thrombosis and DIC (Agrawal et al. 2019). Cancer-associated thrombosis is a common complication in cancer patients and is a major cause of morbidity and mortality. The risk of thrombosis is highest in patients with advanced stage cancer, those undergoing cancer treatment, and those with certain types of cancer, such as pancreatic and lung cancer.

Complications during pregnancy and childbirth, such as abruptio placentae, amniotic fluid embolism, pre-eclampsia, and HELLP syndrome, can lead to DIC through various complex mechanisms involving endothelial damage, platelet consumption, and clotting factor depletion (Bick 1992). These conditions are associated with a high risk of maternal and fetal morbidity and mortality. Early recognition and management of DIC in these patients are essential to prevent adverse outcomes.

Furthermore, exposure to toxins like bacterial, snake venom, or chemicals can induce a strong immune response, triggering inflammation and coagulation activation, potentially leading to DIC (Figtree et al. 2009). These toxins can directly activate platelets and endothelial cells, leading to the release of procoagulant factors and the activation of the coagulation pathway.

Conditions like heat stroke can also induce DIC through mechanisms such as dehydration, systemic inflammation, endothelial damage, and organ dysfunction (Vadasz and Toubi 2018). Heat stroke is a medical emergency that occurs when the body's core temperature rises to a dangerous level, leading to multiple organ dysfunctions. DIC is a rare but serious complication of heat stroke and is associated with a poor prognosis.

Although rare, severe reactions to blood transfusions can trigger disseminated intravascular coagulation (DIC), as highlighted by Pilli (2018). Such transfusion-associated DIC arises when the immune system of the transfusion recipient reacts to the introduced blood products, initiating a sequence that releases procoagulant factors and activates the blood coagulation cascade. This sequence can cause the formation of clots in the microcirculation, potentially leading to significant organ damage or failure. Given its severe implications, DIC represents a critical,

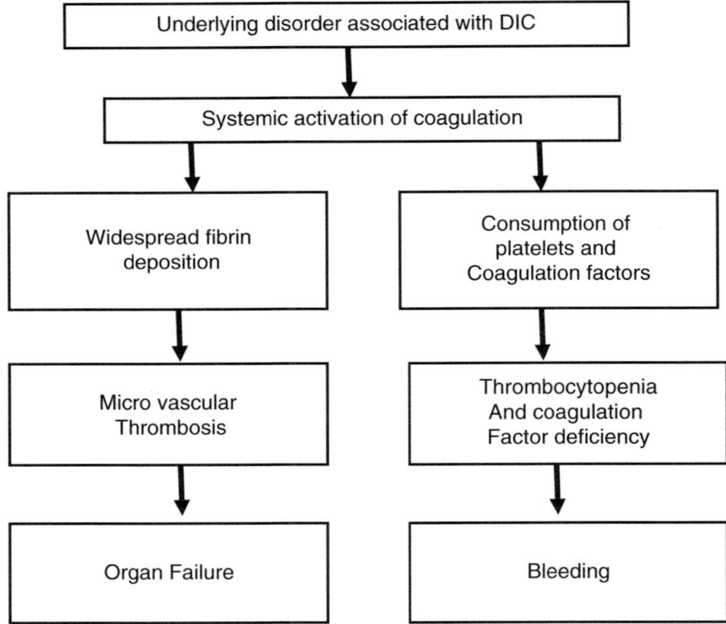

Fig. 18.1 Flowchart depicting pathogenesis of DIC

potentially fatal condition that can emerge across various medical scenarios. Prompt identification and intervention are crucial in mitigating the risk of negative outcomes associated with DIC (Fig. 18.1).

18.3 Diagnosis

The diagnosis of disseminated intravascular coagulation (DIC) is a complex process that requires a comprehensive approach that integrates clinical suspicion with a battery of laboratory tests. DIC is a multifactorial coagulation disorder that can present with diverse clinical features, making it challenging to diagnose accurately. Common clinical features of DIC include bleeding from various sites such as petechiae, ecchymosis, mucosal bleeding, and gastrointestinal bleeding. Patients may also exhibit altered mental status, respiratory distress, or renal impairment due to organ dysfunction resulting from microvascular thrombosis (Erez et al. 2014). Laboratory tests play a crucial role in assessing the coagulation status in DIC. These tests typically include a combination of coagulation assays, platelet counts, and markers of fibrinolysis. Thrombocytopenia, along with decreased hematocrit, is a common finding in DIC due to platelet consumption in microvascular thrombosis. The presence of schistocytes in the peripheral blood smear indicates intravascular hemolysis, a common feature of DIC. Additionally, an increase in activated partial thromboplastin time (aPTT) and prothrombin time (PT), along with decreased fibrinogen levels, is indicative of ongoing clotting cascade activation. Elevated levels of D-dimer and fibrin split products (FSPs) serve as markers of fibrinolysis and further support the diagnosis of DIC (Suzuki et al. 2018). Given the impact of underlying clinical conditions on laboratory tests, the International Society on Thrombosis and Haemostasis (ISTH) recommends a combination of tests to diagnose DIC with a reasonable degree of certainty, especially in patients with known associated disorders (Squizzato et al. 2020). The diagnosis of DIC requires a high level of clinical suspicion supported by relevant laboratory tests to accurately identify and manage this complex coagulation disorder.

18.4 Scoring System

To facilitate the assessment of disseminated intravascular coagulation (DIC), various scoring systems integrating both clinical and laboratory data have been developed, assisting healthcare professionals in navigating this intricate disorder. Among these, the International Society on Thrombosis and Haemostasis (ISTH) DIC scoring system is frequently applied, where a score equal to or greater than 5 signals overt DIC, according to Muddana et al. (2022). In addition to the ISTH system, the Japanese Association for Acute Medicine (JAAM) score and the sepsis-induced coagulopathy (SIC) score serve as specialized tools for determining DIC's presence and intensity, especially in septic conditions, as outlined by Soundar et al. (2013). These scoring systems are pivotal for clinicians in diagnosing and gauging the severity of DIC, providing a standardized approach to manage and monitor the condition effectively.

The choice of which scoring system to use often depends on the clinical relevance and familiarity with the parameters employed in each system. These scoring systems play a crucial role in aiding clinicians in diagnosing and managing DIC effectively, especially in challenging clinical scenarios such as sepsis-induced coagulopathy (Soundar et al. 2013) (Tables 18.2 and 18.3).

Table 18.2 International Society on Thrombosis and Haemostasis (ISTH) DIC score

International Society on Thrombosis and Haemostasis (ISTH) DIC score				
Test	0 points	1 point	2 points	3 points
INR, or, PT prolongation	INR ≤ 1.3 <3 seconds	INR 1.3–1.7 seconds 3–6 seconds	INR > 1.7 >6 seconds	
Fibrinogen	>100 mg/dL	<100 mg/dL		
D-dimer	<400 ng/dL		400–4000 ng/ml	>4000 ng/ml
Platelets	>100,000uL	50,000–100,000uL	<50,000/uL	

Interpretation of total score:

- ≥5 points: positive for DIC
- <5 points: negative, but patients could still have "non-overt DIC" which could evaluate into frank DIC. If there is ongoing concern for DIC, coagulation labs may be repeated in 12–24 hours.

Table 18.3 Sepsis-induced coagulopathy (SIC) score

Sepsis-induced coagulopathy (SIC) score			
Test	0 points	1 point	2 points
INR	INR ≤ 1.2	INR 1.2–1.4	INR > 1.4
Platelets	>150,000/μL	100,000—150,000/μL	<100,000/μL
SOFA score[a]	0	1	≥2

Interpretation of total score:
- ≥4 points: positive for SIC
- <4 points: negative for SIC

[a]Sequential Organ Failure Assessment score

18.5 Differential Diagnosis

Disseminated intravascular coagulation (DIC) involves the systemic activation of the coagulation cascade, leading to the formation and deposition of fibrin. This process results in the development of microvascular clots within various organs, potentially culminating in multiple organ dysfunction syndrome (MODS). Given the complexity of DIC and its clinical presentation, which often resembles other coagulation disorders, precise differential diagnosis is essential.

18.5.1 Heparin-Induced Thrombocytopenia (HIT)

One such condition that needs differentiation from DIC is heparin-induced thrombocytopenia (HIT). HIT is a condition where the immune system reacts negatively to heparin, leading to a substantial decrease in platelet count after exposure to the drug. Unlike DIC, HIT is characterized by the absence of widespread coagulation activation. The diagnosis of HIT is primarily based on the observation of a decrease in platelet count following heparin exposure, with confirmation coming from the detection of heparin-platelet factor 4 antibodies, as detailed by Minakata et al. (2019).

18.5.2 Thrombotic Thrombocytopenic Purpura (TTP)

TTP presents with a pentad of symptoms: severe thrombocytopenia, microangiopathic hemolytic anemia, neurological symptoms, renal dysfunction, and fever. The absence of significant coagulopathy differentiates it from DIC. ADAMTS13 activity assay, showing severely reduced levels, is crucial for diagnosis (Shimizu et al. 2018).

18.5.3 Mechanical Circulatory Support Devices

The use of mechanical circulatory support devices, such as ventricular assist devices, can induce platelet activation and consumption, mimicking thrombocytopenia seen in DIC. However, the presence of the device itself and the absence of widespread coagulation activation are key differentiating factors (Asakura et al. 2016).

18.5.4 Hemophagocytic Lymphohistiocytosis (HLH)

HLH is characterized by fever, hepatosplenomegaly, and hyperferritinemia, often triggered by infections, malignancies, or genetic predispositions. It involves hyperactivation of the immune system, leading to significant cytokine release and tissue damage. The diagnostic criteria include elevated ferritin, triglycerides, and soluble CD25 levels, along with hemophagocytosis in bone marrow or other tissues (Yoshinobu et al. 2021).

18.5.5 Hematological Malignancies

Hematological malignancies can present with coagulopathy and cytopenias similar to DIC. However, the presence of abnormal cells in peripheral blood or bone marrow biopsy, indicating malignancy, helps in differentiating from DIC (Duran and Tannock 2006).

18.5.6 Drug- and Alcohol-Induced Microangiopathy

Both drug-induced and alcohol-induced microangiopathy present with microangiopathic hemolytic anemia and thrombocytopenia. Detailed medication history and alcohol use history are essential for diagnosis, distinguishing them from DIC, which involves a broader spectrum of coagulation activation (Yildiz et al. 2022; Gando 2010).

18.5.7 Idiopathic Thrombocytopenic Purpura (ITP)

ITP is an autoimmune disorder characterized by isolated thrombocytopenia without the global coagulopathy seen in DIC. Diagnosis is primarily clinical, supported by exclusion of other causes of thrombocytopenia (Ling et al. 2021).

18.5.8 Post-Transfusion Purpura

Post-transfusion purpura is a rare disorder characterized by severe thrombocytopenia occurring 5–10 days after a blood transfusion. The temporal relationship with transfusion and the presence of specific platelet antibodies differentiate it from DIC (Franchini et al. 2013).

18.5.9 Hypersplenism

Hypersplenism involves an enlarged spleen leading to cytopenias, including thrombocytopenia. The absence of global coagulopathy and evidence of splenomegaly on imaging help differentiate it from DIC (Valade et al. 2015).

18.6 Management

Effective management of DIC necessitates a twofold approach: addressing the underlying condition that triggered the DIC and providing supportive care tailored to the patient's clinical manifestations (Fig. 18.2).

1. *Addressing Underlying Conditions*

   The management of underlying conditions is pivotal in the treatment of DIC. This includes the administration of antibiotics for sepsis, chemotherapy for cancer-related DIC, and specific interventions such as timely childbirth in obstetric complications and the use of all-trans retinoic acid (ATRA) for patients with acute promyelocytic leukemia (APML), as highlighted by Dixit et al. (2007).
2. *Supportive Care and Monitoring*

   Supportive care, including the use of the International Society on Thrombosis and Haemostasis (ISTH) DIC score, is crucial for diagnostic accuracy and guiding treatment strategies. The ISTH DIC score, as discussed by Squizzato et al. (2016), provides a quantitative measure of DIC severity, aiding in the monitoring of disease progression and the effectiveness of treatment interventions.
3. *Blood Product Replacement*

   Blood product replacement is a key component of DIC management, especially for patients with bleeding manifestations or those at a high risk of bleeding. Platelet transfusion guidelines suggest thresholds for transfusion, and the use of fresh frozen plasma and cryoprecipitate is recommended based on specific clinical parameters such as prothrombin time and fibrinogen levels. Le Trinh et al. (2020) provide a comprehensive overview of platelet transfusion practices in this context.

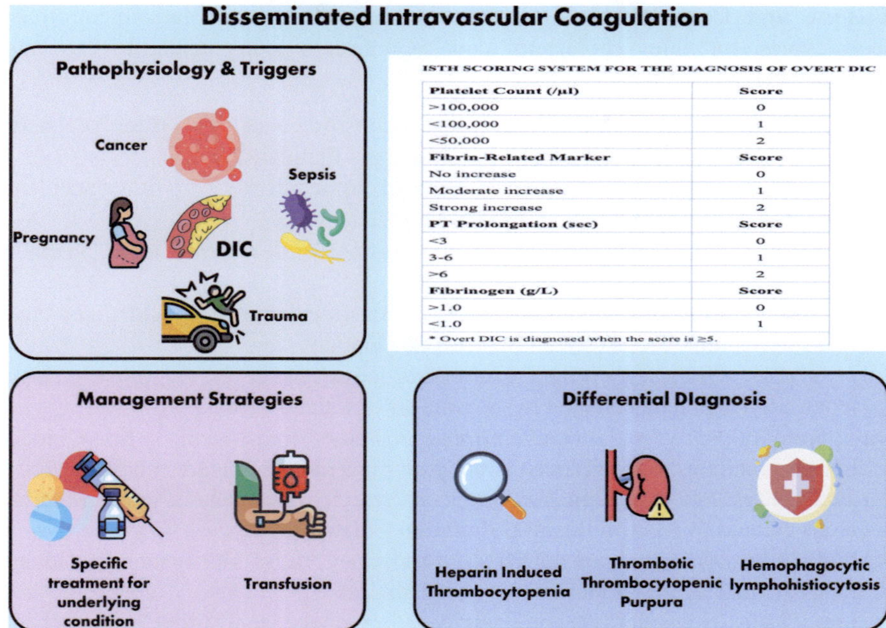

ISTH SCORING SYSTEM FOR THE DIAGNOSIS OF OVERT DIC

Platelet Count (/µl)	Score
>100,000	0
<100,000	1
<50,000	2
Fibrin-Related Marker	**Score**
No increase	0
Moderate increase	1
Strong increase	2
PT Prolongation (sec)	**Score**
<3	0
3-6	1
>6	2
Fibrinogen (g/L)	**Score**
>1.0	0
<1.0	1

* Overt DIC is diagnosed when the score is ≥5.

Fig. 18.2 Approach to management of disseminated intravascular coagulation

4. *Prophylactic and Therapeutic Anticoagulation*

   The role of prophylactic and therapeutic anticoagulation in DIC management involves a delicate balance between mitigating thrombotic risk and minimizing the potential for bleeding complications. Unfractionated heparin (UFH) and low-molecular-weight heparin (LMWH) are commonly employed, with their use tailored to the patient's clinical condition and bleeding risk.
5. *Antifibrinolytic Agents*

   The use of antifibrinolytic agents, such as tranexamic acid, in DIC is generally limited to specific hyperfibrinolytic states. Rosen et al. (2018) discuss the nuanced application of these agents, particularly in the context of acute promyelocytic leukemia (APML) and primary hyperfibrinolytic states within DIC.
6. *Anticoagulant Factor Concentrates*

   The chapter will also delve into the use of anticoagulant factor concentrates, including the therapeutic use of recombinant human-activated protein C and antithrombin concentrates. The literature, including studies by Saito et al. (2007) and Sletnes et al. (1995), provides insights into the effectiveness and risks associated with these treatments.

The management of disseminated intravascular coagulation (DIC) is multifaceted, requiring a comprehensive approach that addresses the underlying cause, provides supportive care, and navigates the complexities of anticoagulation and blood product replacement. Future research will continue to refine these strategies, improving outcomes for patients with this challenging condition.

Flowchart

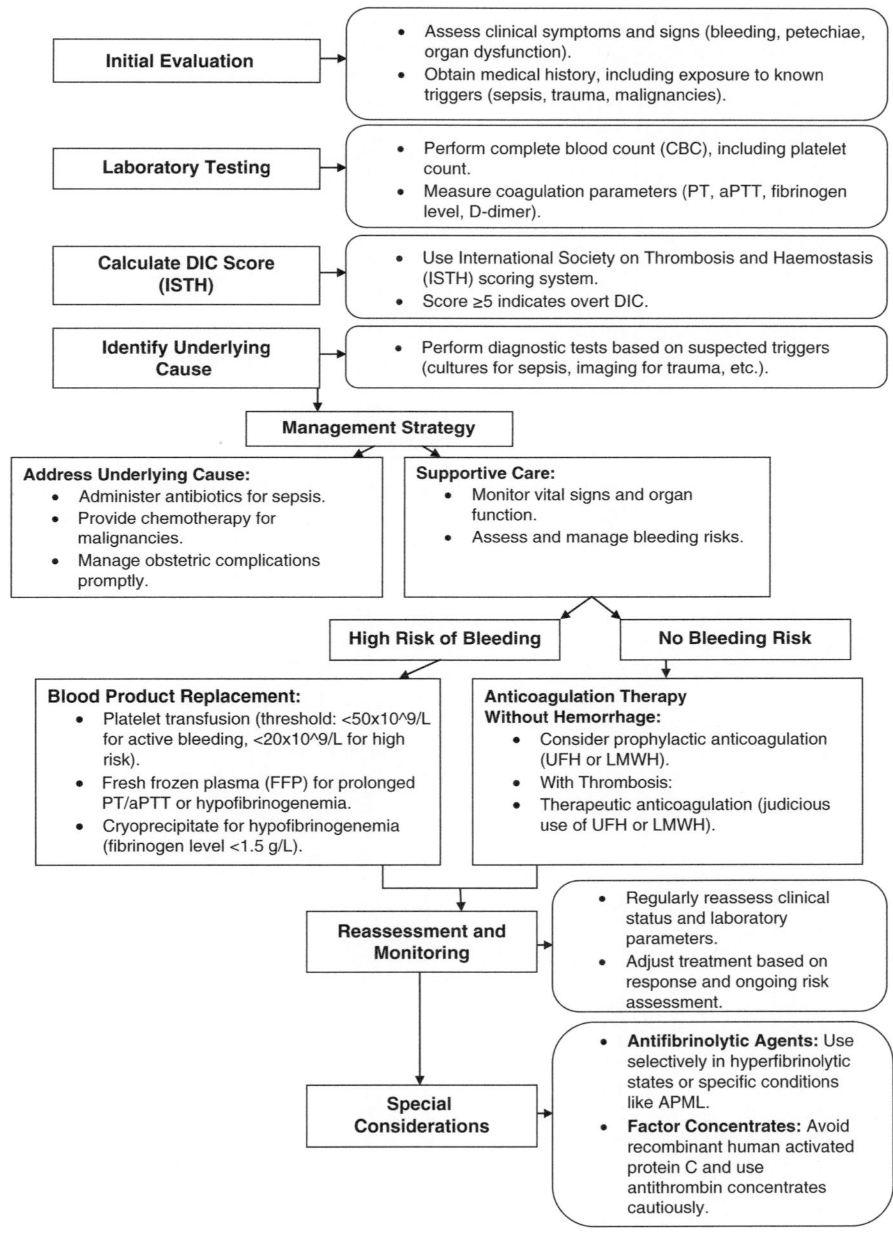
Initial Evaluation
• Assess clinical symptoms and signs (bleeding, petechiae, organ dysfunction).
• Obtain medical history, including exposure to known triggers (sepsis, trauma, malignancies).
Laboratory Testing
• Perform complete blood count (CBC), including platelet count.
• Measure coagulation parameters (PT, aPTT, fibrinogen level, D-dimer).
Calculate DIC Score (ISTH)
• Use International Society on Thrombosis and Haemostasis (ISTH) scoring system.
• Score ≥5 indicates overt DIC.
Identify Underlying Cause
• Perform diagnostic tests based on suspected triggers (cultures for sepsis, imaging for trauma, etc.).
Management Strategy
Address Underlying Cause:
• Administer antibiotics for sepsis.
• Provide chemotherapy for malignancies.
• Manage obstetric complications promptly.
Supportive Care:
• Monitor vital signs and organ function.
• Assess and manage bleeding risks.
High Risk of Bleeding
No Bleeding Risk
Blood Product Replacement:
• Platelet transfusion (threshold: <50x10^9/L for active bleeding, <20x10^9/L for high risk).
• Fresh frozen plasma (FFP) for prolonged PT/aPTT or hypofibrinogenemia.
• Cryoprecipitate for hypofibrinogenemia (fibrinogen level <1.5 g/L).
Anticoagulation Therapy Without Hemorrhage:
• Consider prophylactic anticoagulation (UFH or LMWH).
• With Thrombosis:
• Therapeutic anticoagulation (judicious use of UFH or LMWH).
Reassessment and Monitoring
• Regularly reassess clinical status and laboratory parameters.
• Adjust treatment based on response and ongoing risk assessment.
Special Considerations
• Antifibrinolytic Agents: Use selectively in hyperfibrinolytic states or specific conditions like APML.
• Factor Concentrates: Avoid recombinant human activated protein C and use antithrombin concentrates cautiously.

References

Adelborg K, Larsen JB, Hvas AM (2021) Disseminated intravascular coagulation: epidemiology, biomarkers, and management. Br J Haematol 192(5):803–818

Agrawal K, Agrawal N, Miles L (2019) Disseminated intravascular coagulation as an initial manifestation of metastatic prostate cancer emergently treated with docetaxel-based chemotherapy. Case Rep Oncol Med 2019:6092156

Asakura H, Takahashi H, Uchiyama T, Eguchi Y, Okamoto K, Kawasugi K et al (2016) Proposal for new diagnostic criteria for DIC from the Japanese Society on Thrombosis and Hemostasis. Thromb J 14:1–13

Bick RL (1992) Coagulation abnormalities in malignancy: a review. Semin Thromb Hemost 18(04):353–372. Copyright© 1992 by Thieme Medical Publishers, Inc

Dixit A, Chatterjee T, Mishra P, Kannan M, Choudhry DR, Mahapatra M et al (2007) Disseminated intravascular coagulation in acute leukemia at presentation and during induction therapy. Clin Appl Thromb Hemost 13(3):292–298

Duran I, Tannock IF (2006) Disseminated intravascular coagulation as the presenting sign of metastatic prostate cancer. J Gen Intern Med 21(11):C6–C8

Erez O, Novack L, Beer-Weisel R, Dukler D, Press F, Zlotnik A et al (2014) DIC score in pregnant women–a population based modification of the International Society on Thrombosis and Hemostasis score. PLoS One 9(4):e93240

Figtree MC, Miyakis S, Tanaka K, Martin L, Konecny P, Krilis S (2009) Unexpected outcome (positive or negative) including adverse drug reactions: Dapsone hypersensitivity syndrome causing disseminated intravascular coagulation. BMJ Case Rep 2009. https://doi.org/10.1136/bcr.11.2008.1257

Franchini M, Lippi G, Manzato F (2006) Recent acquisitions in the pathophysiology, diagnosis and treatment of disseminated intravascular coagulation. Thromb J 4:1–9

Franchini M, Frattini F, Crestani S, Bonfanti C (2013) Bleeding complications in patients with hematologic malignancies. Semin Thromb Hemost 39(1):94–100.

Gando S (2010) Microvascular thrombosis and multiple organ dysfunction syndrome. Crit Care Med 38:S35–S42

Hook KM, Abrams CS (2012) The loss of homeostasis in hemostasis: new approaches in treating and understanding acute disseminated intravascular coagulation in critically ill patients. Clin Transl Sci 5(1):85–92

Le Trinh H, Nguyen VT, Mai NK, Tran BT, Pham QN (2020) Successful chemotherapy management of disseminated intravascular coagulation presenting with metastatic clear cell renal carcinoma: a case report and review of the literature. J Med Case Rep 14:1–6

Levi M (2014) Diagnosis and treatment of disseminated intravascular coagulation. Int J Lab Hematol 36(3):228–236

Ling L, Huang X, Liu C, Liao J, Zhou J (2021) Monitoring coagulation-fibrinolysis activation prompted timely diagnosis of hemophagocytic lymphohistiocytosis-related disseminated intravascular coagulation. Thromb J 19:1–5

Minakata D, Fujiwara SI, Ikeda T, Kawaguchi SI, Toda Y, Ito S et al (2019) Comparison of gabexate mesilate and nafamostat mesilate for disseminated intravascular coagulation associated with hematological malignancies. Int J Hematol 109:141–146

Muddana PS, Kar SS, Kar R (2022) Evaluation of the International Society on Thrombosis & Haemostasis scoring system & its modifications in diagnosis of disseminated intravascular coagulation: a pilot study from southern India. Indian J Med Res 155(2):306–310

Papageorgiou C, Jourdi G, Adjambri E, Walborn A, Patel P, Fareed J et al (2018) Disseminated intravascular coagulation: an update on pathogenesis, diagnosis, and therapeutic strategies. Clin Appl Thromb Hemost 24(9_suppl):8S–28S

Pilli VS (2018) Understanding the clotting cascade, regulators, and clinical modulators of coagulation. In: Hematology-latest research and clinical advances. IntechOpen

Poskitt TR, Fortwengler HP Jr, Lunskis BJ (1973) Activation of the alternate complement pathway by autologous red cell stroma. J Exp Med 138(3):715–722

Rosen EA, Vallurupalli M, Choy E, Lennerz JK, Kuter DJ (2018) Management of disseminated intravascular coagulation in a patient with hepatic angiosarcoma: a case report. Medicine 97(47):e13321

Saito H, Maruyama I, Shimazaki S, Yamamoto Y, Aikawa N, Ohno R et al (2007) Efficacy and safety of recombinant human soluble thrombomodulin (ART-123) in disseminated intravascular coagulation: results of a phase III, randomized, double-blind clinical trial. J Thromb Haemost 5(1):31–41

Shimizu M, Konishi A, Nomura S (2018) Examination of biomarker expressions in sepsis-related DIC patients. Int J Gen Med 11:353–361

Sletnes KE, Godal HC, Wisløff F (1995) Disseminated intravascular coagulation (DIC) in adult patients with acute leukaemia. Eur J Haematol 54(1):34–38

Soundar EP, Jariwala P, Nguyen TC, Eldin KW, Teruya J (2013) Evaluation of the International Society on Thrombosis and Haemostasis and institutional diagnostic criteria of disseminated intravascular coagulation in pediatric patients. Am J Clin Pathol 139(6):812–816

Squizzato A, Hunt BJ, Kinasewitz GT, Wada H, Ten Cate H, Thachil J et al (2016) Supportive management strategies for disseminated intravascular coagulation. Thromb Haemost 116(05):896–904

Squizzato A, Gallo A, Levi M, Iba T, Levy JH, Erez O et al (2020) Underlying disorders of disseminated intravascular coagulation: communication from the ISTH SSC Subcommittees on Disseminated Intravascular Coagulation and Perioperative and Critical Care Thrombosis and Hemostasis. J Thromb Haemost 18(9):2400–2407

Suzuki K, Wada H, Imai H, Iba T, Thachil J, Toh CH (2018) A re-evaluation of the D-dimer cut-off value for making a diagnosis according to the ISTH overt-DIC diagnostic criteria: communication from the SSC of the ISTH. J Thromb Haemost 16(7):1442–1444

Vadasz Z, Toubi E (2018) Hemostasis in allergy. Semin Thromb Hemost 44(07):669–675. Thieme Medical Publishers

Valade S, Azoulay E, Galicier L, Boutboul D, Zafrani L, Stepanian A et al (2015) Coagulation disorders and bleedings in critically ill patients with hemophagocytic lymphohistiocytosis. Medicine 94(40):e1692

Wada H, Shiraki K, Shimaoka M (2020) The prothrombin time ratio is not a more effective marker for evaluating sepsis-induced coagulopathy than fibrin-related markers. J Thromb Haemost 18(6):1506–1507

Yildiz H, Castanares-Zapatero D, d'Abadie P, Bailly S, Yombi JC (2022) Hemophagocytic lymphohistiocytosis in adults: a retrospective study in a Belgian teaching hospital. Int J Gen Med 15:8111

Yoshinobu S, Honda G, Kawano N, Uchiyama T, Kawasugi K, Madoiwa S et al (2021) Clinical features of disseminated intravascular coagulation according to the French-American-British Classification in patients with acute leukemia and thrombomodulin alfa treatment—a cohort study using a postmarketing surveillance database. Clin Appl Thromb Hemost 27:10760296211054094

Chapter 19
Diagnosis and Management of Thrombotic Microangiopathies

Rohit Kumar Patnaik and Nupur Karan

Learning Points

1. *Complex Nature and Diagnosis of TMAs*: Thrombotic microangiopathies (TMAs) encompass a group of disorders characterized by microangiopathic hemolytic anemia, thrombocytopenia, and organ dysfunction due to microvascular thrombosis.
2. *Treatment Strategies and Challenges*: Effective management of TTP hinges on therapeutic plasma exchange (TPE) and immunosuppression, with the manuscript detailing the frontline role of TPE in treating TTP by replacing the deficient ADAMTS13 enzyme.
3. *Interdisciplinary Approach to Care*: The manuscript emphasizes the critical role of an interdisciplinary approach to the care of patients with TMAs, involving intensive care management, hematologists, nephrologists, and other specialists.
4. *Need for Personalized Medicine*: Acknowledging the varied clinical presentations and responses to treatment among TMA patients, the manuscript calls for further research and the development of personalized treatment strategies.

19.1 Introduction

The term thrombotic microangiopathies (TMAs) refers to a cluster of diseases that usually share common characteristics such as microvascular or macrovascular intraluminal thrombosis, microangiopathic hemolytic anemia (MAHA), and thrombocytopenia. The most common TMAs are thrombotic thrombocytopenic purpura (TTP) and atypical hemolytic uremic syndrome (aHUS).

R. K. Patnaik (✉)
Critical Care Medicine, IMS & SUM Hospital, Bhubaneswar, India

N. Karan
Anaesthesiology, Kalinga Institute of Medical Sciences (KIMS), Bhubaneswar, India

S. B. Mishra (ed.), *Critical Care Hematology*,
https://doi.org/10.1007/978-981-97-5565-3_19

19.1.1 Thrombotic Thrombocytopenic Purpura (TTP)

Thrombotic thrombocytopenic purpura (TTP) is an emergency condition in critical care. It is a life-threatening thrombotic microangiopathy characterized by microangiopathic hemolytic anemia (MAHA), severe consumption thrombocytopenia, and organ ischemia linked to disseminated microvascular platelet-rich thrombi. Limited evidence exists regarding the management of TTP in critically ill patients. Azoulay et al. have published an expert statement on the ICU management of patients with TTP (Azoulay et al. 2019).

19.1.2 Epidemiology

Annual incidence of one new case per million people. Twofold more common in women. Presents in adulthood and has relapsing tendency. (Joly et al. 2017) A rare non-immune inherited form of TTP is called as Upshaw-Schulman syndrome (USS). Mortality rate of 10–20% in spite of appropriate therapeutic management. Admission to ICU can be either due to severe end-organ dysfunction or due to requirement of therapeutic plasma exchange (TPE) under close monitoring.

19.1.3 Pathophysiology

TTP is caused by deficiency in the von Willebrand factor (vWF)-cleaving specific serine metalloprotease ADAMTS13 (a disintegrin and metalloprotease with a thrombospondin type 1 motif, member 13). ADAMTS13 deficiency causes the blood accumulation of platelet-hyperadhesive ultra-large VWF multimers, leading to the formation of platelet-rich microthrombi within small arterioles (Fig. 19.1).

19.2 Diagnosis

19.2.1 Clinical Features

Amorosi and Ultman proposed the class pentad for diagnosis of TTP which consists of fever, MAHA with schistocytes, peripheral thrombocytopenia, renal dysfunction (hematuria and/or proteinuria or elevated blood urea nitrogen), and neurological abnormalities. Classic pentad seen in less than 10% cases (Fodil and Zafrani 2022).

Approximately 60% patients have neurologic symptoms at presentation, with a broad range from headache and confusion to stroke, coma, seizures, and

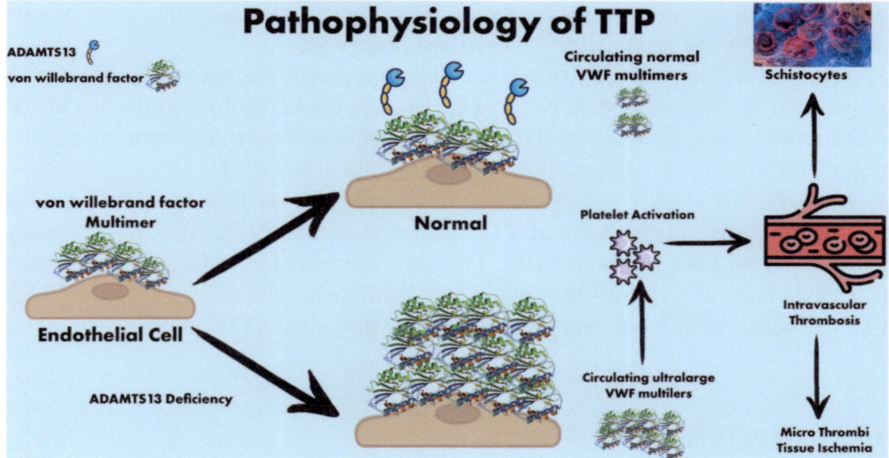

Fig. 19.1 Pathophysiology of TTP

hemiparesis. Neurological symptoms fluctuate over time due to formation and dissolution of cerebral microthrombi.

Approximately 25% patients have ischemic cardiovascular episode and approximately 35% patients have mesenteric ischemia. Cardiac manifestations include acute coronary syndrome, arrythmias, heart failure, cardiogenic shock, and cardiac arrest. Cardiac and cerebral events are more likely in patients with troponin level above 0.25 μg/L. Need for coronary angiography is done on a case-to-case basis.

Renal involvement is not obvious in most cases of TTP. Renal manifestations consist mainly of an isolated proteinuria/hematuria; acute renal failure is unusual in TTP, with typically a serum creatinine level below 2 mg/dL at presentation. Severe TTP (with confirmed ADAMTS13 activity <10%) has reported 10–27% acute kidney injury. Causes of renal dysfunction in TTP include TTP itself, hemolysis, BP variations, or drug toxicity. Approximately 40% of patients developing AKI after TTP can progress to chronic kidney disease after 6 months.

The PLASMIC score has been developed to predict severe ADAMTS13 deficiency and diagnosis of TTP (Bendapudi et al. 2017). Other similar scoring systems include the French score and Bentley score.

19.2.2 Laboratory Investigations

Microangiopathic hemolytic anemia with consumption thrombocytopenia with classic parameters of hemolysis includes elevated LDH, high reticulocyte count, high indirect hyperbilirubinemia, and an undetectable serum haptoglobin concentration. Proteinuria, hematuria, and sometimes increased BUN and creatinine are seen. 60% patients have elevated troponin I. Except in some associated autoimmune contexts (SLE), the erythrocyte Coombs test is negative.

Schistocytes are small, irregular triangular, or crescent-shaped cells, with pointed projections and lack of central pallor (Fig. 19.2). A confident threshold value of 1% is the morphologic hallmark of the disease. Schistocytes may be absent initially on peripheral smear, which may lead to diagnostic dilemma of TTP.

ADAMTS13 assay showing activity less than 10% of that in normal pooled plasma confirms the diagnosis of TTP. Although sampling for ADAMTS13 assay should be done prior to starting TPE, TPE should not be delayed waiting for results of ADAMTS13 assay. Anti-ADAMTS13 autoantibodies can also be assayed. Shiga toxin PCR on rectal swab may be done to rule out typical STEC-HUS.

19.3 Treatment

The initial management should rule out other causes of TMA such as Shiga toxin-related hemolytic and uremic syndrome (STEC-HUS), complement-mediated HUS, and secondary TMA syndromes. Despite severe thrombocytopenia seen in TTP, it should be noted that ischemia is a bigger concern in TTP than bleeding. Thus, platelet transfusions should be avoided as it is associated with worsening of TTP and increased relapse rates. TPE along with corticosteroid therapy is the mainstay of treatment of TTP. Therapy specific for TTP includes:

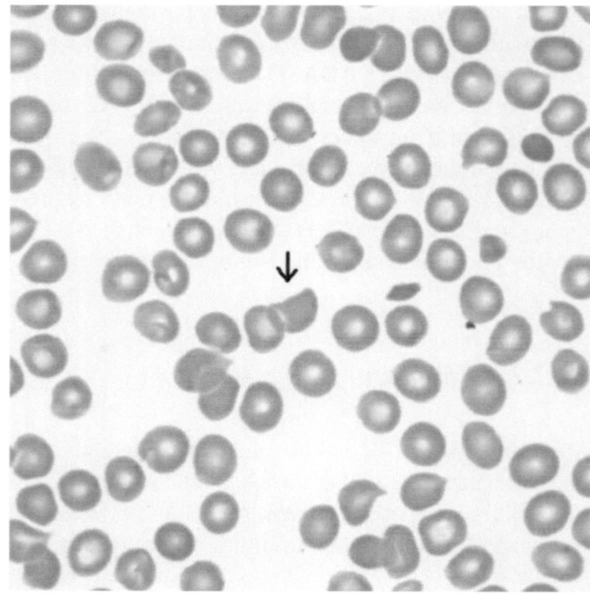

Fig. 19.2 Peripheral smear showing schistocyte (black arrow)

1. *Frontline therapy is therapeutic plasma exchange (TPE)*: TPE with fresh frozen plasma (FFP) works by supplying functional ADAMTS13. TPE is started as soon as the diagnosis of TTP is suspected (within 4–6 hours) and no obvious evidence of an alternative diagnosis. It is usually done at 1.5 times the plasma volume (60 ml/kg) exchange for the first procedures followed by 1.0 time plasma volume thereafter. TPE is performed daily until features related to organ involvement (cerebral manifestations, renal failure, increased troponin level, abdominal pain resulting from enteritis or pancreatitis) have resolved, the platelet count has stably recovered to more than 150×10^9/L for at least 48 hours, and hemolysis has ceased. Close monitoring is essential during initial sessions of TPE as sudden cardiac death can occur from cardiac microvasculature occlusion, arrythmias, or cardiogenic shock (Bendapudi et al. 2017). FFP infusion alone can be used if time to initiation of TPE is being delayed due to logistical reasons. Medications for patients receiving TPE should be given after a TPE session is completed.
2. *Steroids*: Corticosteroid therapy is recommended as first-line therapy for TTP in combination with TPE (Scully et al. 2012; Coppo et al. 2017). High-dose methylprednisolone (10 mg/kg/day for 3 days and then 2.5 mg/kg/day) may be more efficacious than standard dose (1 mg/kg/day) as an adjunctive treatment (Balduini et al. 2010). Steroids also help by reducing the side effects seen with TPE. Level of proof concerning steroid efficacy in the treatment of TTP remains quite low.
3. *Rituximab*: 375 mg/m^2 in 4 weekly doses after suboptimal response to standard treatment. Rituximab remarkably reduces the incidence of TTP relapse by diminishing the production of anti-ADAMTS13 antibodies and restoring ADAMTS13 activity, which parallels peripheral B-cell depletion. Due to its slow onset of action (10 days), it chiefly helps to prevent relapses.
4. *New drugs*: N-acetylcysteine, bortezomib, recombinant ADAMTS13 (BAX930), caplacizumab. Caplacizumab is an anti-vWF humanized immunoglobulin which inhibits the interaction between the vWF-A1 domain and platelet GPIb. Both the TITAN and the HERCULES trial which compared caplacizumab with placebo showed faster time to platelet count normalization and required fewer TPE sessions. However, bleeding was more common with caplacizumab compared to placebo in trials performed so far (Scully et al. 2019; Peyvandi et al. 2016). Based on available evidence, the expert panel on ICU management of TTP recommends caplacizumab as first-line therapy along with TPE, corticosteroids, and rituximab.
5. *Other immunomodulators*: Vincristine, Cyclosporine A
6. *Supportive management of ICU patients*: Folate supplementation for first 2 weeks, peptic ulcer prophylaxis, DVT prophylaxis, care of catheter used for TPE, ICU monitoring, and organ support (Table 19.1).

19.4 Treatment of More Severe Forms

No consensus on the best management strategy. Caplacizumab and rituximab in combination should be used if it has not been used as first-line therapy. Treatment options which have been tried beyond these two include performing twice-daily TPE (1.5 volume plasma per session), pulses of cyclophosphamide, bortezomib, or splenectomy. Splenectomy is a therapy of last resort once all first- and second-line therapies have failed. Newer methods such as immunoadsorption are being tried for severe forms of TTP. Refractory TTP has been defined as persistent thrombocytopenia and hemolysis after 7 days of first-line treatment (Scully et al. 2017; Mariotte et al. 2013). TTP relapse has been defined as recurrent TTP more than 30 days after TPE discontinuation (Scully et al. 2017).

19.5 Prognosis and Follow-Up

With prompt management, average survival rate from a first episode of TTP is 80–90%. Factors associated with worse outcomes include older age, very high lactate dehydrogenase, increased cardiac troponin level on diagnosis (troponin level > 0.25 ng/ml), seizures, coma, platelet transfusions, unresponsiveness to plasma exchange, and steroids. A substantial proportion of TTP survivors reported

Table 19.1 Advantages and disadvantages of treatments used for TTP

Treatment	Advantage	Disadvantage
Therapeutic plasma exchange (TPE)	1. First-line treatment 2. Most efficacious	1. Needs close monitoring 2. Risks of bleeding and infection with catheter insertion 3. Requirement of fresh frozen plasma
Corticosteroids	1. First-line treatment 2. Ease of administration	1. Risks of infection 2. Long-term administration needs prophylaxis against HSV and PCP
Rituximab	1. Second-line treatment 2. Ease of administration 3. Best for prevention of relapse	1. Slow onset of action 2. Risk of infection 3. Infusion-related reactions can occur
Caplacizumab	1. Second-line treatment 2. Ease of administration 3. New monoclonal antibody	1. Risk of bleeding, especially mucocutaneous sites

HSV Herpes simplex virus, *PCP* Pneumocystis carinii pneumonia incomplete recovery, with deficits in health-related quality of life. 40% cases of autoimmune TTP experience one or multiple relapses.

19.6 Hemolytic Uremic Syndrome (HUS)

Hemolytic uremic syndrome (HUS) can occur in critically ill patients as a complication of various underlying conditions. The development of HUS in critically ill individuals may have different characteristics compared to typical HUS seen in children or those associated with specific infections.

In critically ill patients, HUS can be classified into two categories: primary HUS and secondary HUS.

- *Primary HUS*: In some cases, HUS can occur without an identifiable underlying cause or trigger. This form of HUS is referred to as primary or de novo HUS. It is believed to involve a dysregulated complement system and endothelial dysfunction, which can lead to microangiopathic hemolytic anemia, thrombocytopenia, and kidney injury. Primary HUS in critically ill patients may have a multifactorial etiology and could be associated with systemic inflammatory response syndrome, sepsis, disseminated intravascular coagulation (DIC), or drug-induced complications.
- *Secondary HUS*: Secondary HUS in critically ill patients is often associated with an underlying condition or trigger. It can occur as a complication of severe infections (such as E. coli or other bacterial infections), certain medications, autoimmune disorders, malignancies, or organ transplantation. In critically ill patients, secondary HUS may present with a combination of factors, such as inflammation, infection, endothelial dysfunction, and other systemic complications, which contribute to the development of HUS.

The management of HUS in critically ill patients involves addressing the underlying cause or trigger, supportive care, and specific interventions as needed. Treatment may include fluid and electrolyte balance, blood transfusions, dialysis for kidney failure, and targeted therapies depending on the underlying condition or the presence of specific abnormalities in the complement system. It is important to note that the specific approach to managing HUS in critically ill patients may vary based on the individual's clinical condition, the underlying cause, and the expertise of the critical care team involved.

19.7 TMA Beyond TTP and HUS in the Critically Ill

(a) *TMA in pregnancy*

Approximately 5% of TTP cases occur during pregnancy. Recessively inherited ADAMTS13 deficiency (Upshaw-Shulman syndrome) is more common in pregnancy. Management of TTP during pregnancy is similar to non-pregnant patients. aHUS is more common in the post-partum period. A declining renal function despite blood pressure control and delivery of the fetus should raise suspicion of aHUS.

(b) *Drug-induced thrombotic microangiopathy (DI-TMA)*

Two mechanisms have been described for DI-TMA. These include immune mediated and toxin mediated. Immune mediated occurs via formation of antibodies against various cell types. Toxin mediated occurs via direct toxic effect. Thorough history remains the key to identifying the culprit drug. Stopping the offending drug remains the cornerstone of treatment. However, TPE has no role. Eculizumab has been used with mixed results.

(c) *TMA in patients with cancer*

TMA may be manifestation of metastatic disease and bone marrow involvement or because of a medication used in cancer treatment, most commonly seen in gastric and breast cancer, specifically mucin-producing adenocarcinomas. The mechanism triggering TMA includes upregulation of cytokines. Treatment of TMA in patients with cancer is treatment of the primary malignancy or removal of the offending drug. TPE has no role.

(d) *Hematopoietic stem cell transplant-associated TMA (TA-TMA)*

Syndrome of multifactorial endothelial injury commonly affects the kidneys and results in transfusion-dependent anemia and thrombocytopenia. Multisystem manifestations include pulmonary hypertension, intestinal TMA, posterior reversible encephalopathy syndrome (PRES) secondary to uncontrolled hypertension and polyserositis. Treatment is supportive and limited role of TPE. Role of eculizumab is questionable.

19.8 Conclusion

Multidisciplinary care with availability of ICU and long-term management is crucial to management of TMAs including TTP. Further multicenter studies with large registries are needed for a personalized approach to management of TMAs.

Flowchart

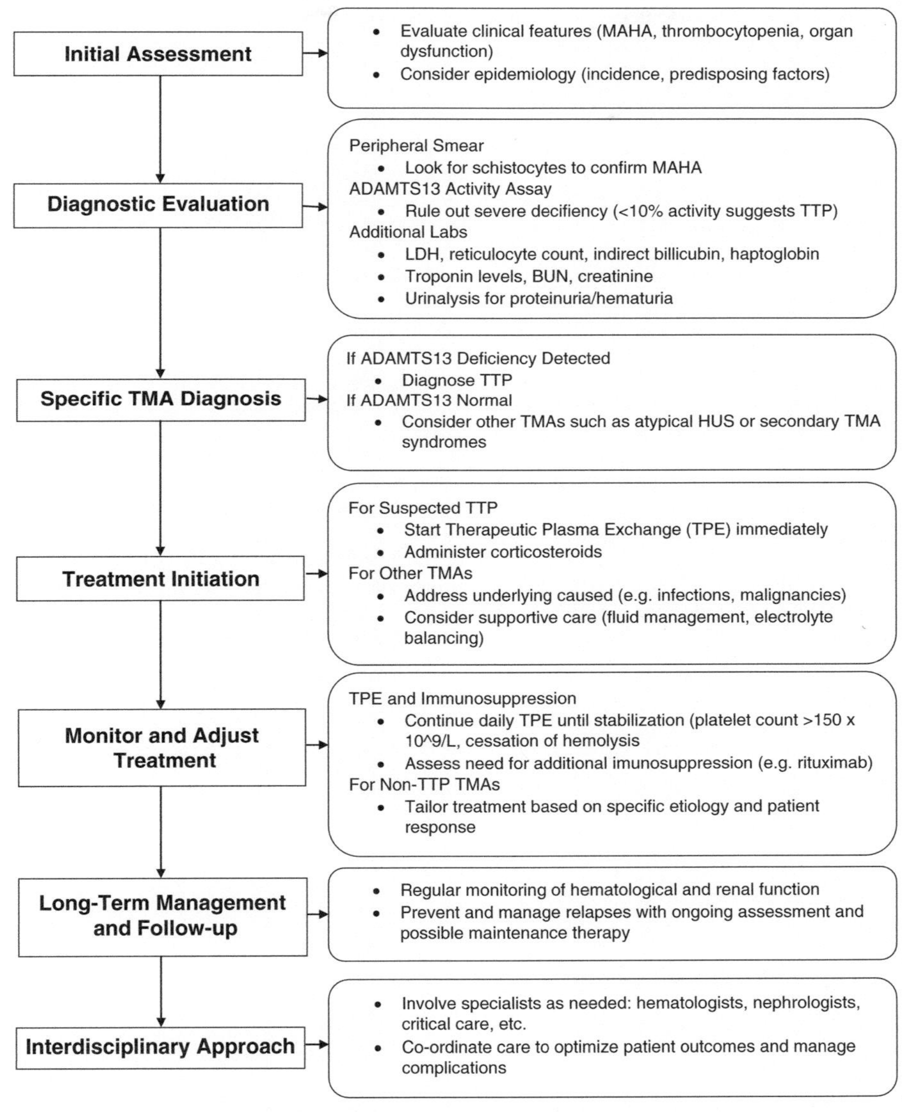

Diagnosis and Management of Thrombotic Microangiopathies Flowchart

References

Azoulay E, Bauer PR, Mariotte E, Russell L, Knoebl P, Martin-Loeches I et al (2019) Expert statement on the ICU management of patients with thrombotic thrombocytopenic purpura. Intensive Care Med 45:1518–1539

Balduini CL, Gugliotta L, Luppi M, Laurenti L, Klersy C, Pieresca C et al (2010) High versus standard dose methylprednisolone in the acute phase of idiopathic thrombotic thrombocytopenic purpura: a randomized study. Ann Hematol 89:591–596

Bendapudi PK, Hurwitz S, Fry A, Marques MB, Waldo SW, Li A et al (2017) Derivation and external validation of the PLASMIC score for rapid assessment of adults with thrombotic microangiopathies: a cohort study. Lancet Haematol 4(4):e157–e164

Coppo P, French Reference Center for Thrombotic Microangiopathies (2017) Management of thrombotic thrombocytopenic purpura. Transfus Clin Biol 24(3):148–153

Fodil S, Zafrani L (2022) Severe thrombotic thrombocytopenic Purpura (TTP) with organ failure in critically ill patients. J Clin Med 11(4):1103

Joly BS, Coppo P, Veyradier A (2017) Thrombotic thrombocytopenic purpura. Blood, J Am Soc Hematol 129(21):2836–2846

Mariotte E, Blet A, Galicier L, Darmon M, Parquet N, Lengline E et al (2013) Unresponsive thrombotic thrombocytopenic purpura in critically ill adults. Intensive Care Med 39:1272–1281

Peyvandi F, Scully M, Kremer Hovinga JA, Cataland S, Knöbl P, Wu H et al (2016) Caplacizumab for acquired thrombotic thrombocytopenic purpura. N Engl J Med 374(6):511–522

Scully M, Hunt BJ, Benjamin S, Liesner R, Rose P, Peyvandi F et al (2012) Guidelines on the diagnosis and management of thrombotic thrombocytopenic purpura and other thrombotic microangiopathies. Br J Haematol 158(3):323–335

Scully M, Cataland S, Coppo P, De La Rubia J, Friedman KD, Hovinga JK et al (2017) Consensus on the standardization of terminology in thrombotic thrombocytopenic purpura and related thrombotic microangiopathies. J Thromb Haemost 15(2):312–322

Scully M, Cataland SR, Peyvandi F, Coppo P, Knöbl P, Kremer Hovinga JA et al (2019) Caplacizumab treatment for acquired thrombotic thrombocytopenic purpura. N Engl J Med 380(4):335–346

Chapter 20
Leukostasis: A Comprehensive Overview

Swathi Kondala and Samir Samal

Learning Points

1. Scope of the Chapter: The chapter covers the pathophysiology of leukostasis, its clinical presentation in AML and CML patients, diagnostic methodologies, and the latest treatment strategies.
2. Significance in Clinical Practice: Leukostasis has significant implications for patient outcomes. It can lead to severe complications, including respiratory distress, neurological impairment, and multi-organ failure.
3. Prevalence and Impact: The prevalence of leukostasis in AML and CML and its impact on patient morbidity and mortality rates are discussed.
4. Importance of Early Diagnosis and Treatment: The chapter underscores the critical nature of the disease and how early diagnosis and timely treatment helps in improving patient outcomes.

20.1 Introduction

Leukostasis, a critical and potentially fatal condition, is most commonly observed in patients with high leukocyte counts, particularly those with acute myeloid leukemia (AML) and chronic myeloid leukemia (CML). Incidence of hyperleukocytosis as per randomized trials is about 8 – 12%, whereas it is 9 – 18% according to retrospective studies (Bewersdorf and Zeidan 2020). This chapter aims to provide a comprehensive understanding of leukostasis, highlighting its clinical importance in the management of AML and CML.

S. Kondala
Department of Critical Care Medicine, IMS & SUM Hospital, Bhubaneswar, Odisha, India

S. Samal (✉)
Critical Care Medicine, IMS & SUM Hospital, Bhubaneswar, India

S. B. Mishra (ed.), *Critical Care Hematology*,
https://doi.org/10.1007/978-981-97-5565-3_20

20.2 Pathophysiology

Leukostasis is generally caused due to rapidly rising very high counts of blast cells (immature leukocytes) in AML or CML. Leukostasis is mostly seen in M4 or M5 (myelomonocytic or monocytic) subtype of AML.

Abnormalities in MLL gene on 11q23 and FLT3-ITD mutations are the commonest risk factors for developing leukostasis (Thiede et al. 2002).

Leukostasis is generally seen in AML or CML patients with Total Leukocyte Count (TLC) > 100,000/μL. However, it may also be seen in patients with TLC > 50,000/μL. The higher cell counts lead to increase in blood viscosity and reduced deformability of myeloid blast cells.

This overt crisis leads to end-organ damage due to blocking/occlusion of microcirculation in the organs. The high numbers of TLCs stack up leading to mechanical obstruction and occluding the microvasculature or the small caliber vessels, cutting off blood flow/circulation to the organs leading to organ damage.

The high number of leukocytes and blast cells adhere to the vascular endothelium which sets up a vicious cascade leading to recruitment of more leukocytes to the site of adhesion. L, P, and E-selectin are present on the endothelial cells and leukocytes. These selectins interact with the integrin proteins and adhesion molecules on the leukocytes. CD43, CD44, P-selectin glycoprotein ligand 1 (PSGL-1) are the adhesion molecules on leukocytes that play a role in this interaction (Nourshargh and Alon 2014).

Secretion of TNF-α and IL-1ß activates the endothelial cells and the leukocytes leading to increased expression of selectins and integrin ligands. This results in upregulation of adhesion molecules (ICAM, VCAM, and E-selectin) culminating in endothelial adhesion and extravasation (Stucki et al. 2001). These interactions further lead to connective tissue damage by matrix metalloproteinases (MMPs) resulting in leukocyte stacking (leukostasis) (Reikvam et al. 2010).

20.3 Signs and Symptoms

Multisystem involvement in patients of AML and CML with hyperleukocytosis generally should create a suspicion of leukocytosis. The symptoms however may not be specific to leukostasis. Pulmonary involvement leading to dyspnea and respiratory distress is the most common presentation in the patients. The distress can range from being mild to life threatening needing mechanical ventilator support. Imaging (chest X-ray and HRCT chest) shows alveolar or interstitial infiltrates which can be of varying severity. Pseudohypoxemia is also seen in such patients on blood gas analysis due to oxygen consumption by the high number of leukocytes present in the drawn sample and is called as *leukocyte larceny*.

Symptoms of leukostasis are not very specific and depend on the organ affected because of the occlusion of microcirculation (Fig. 20.1). It is a clinical diagnosis

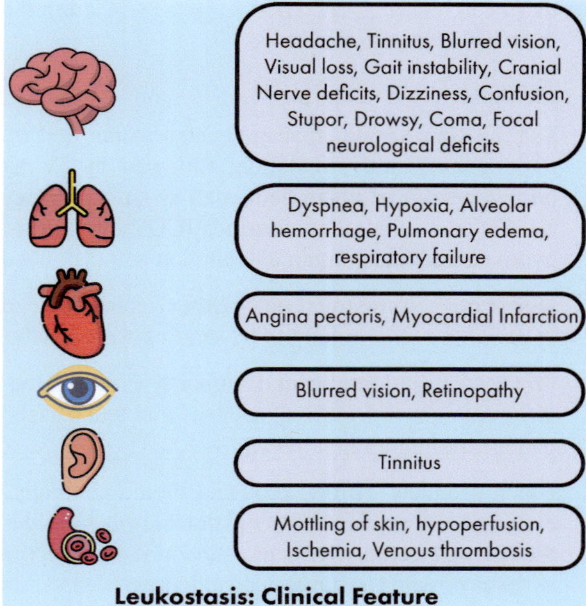

Fig. 20.1 Organ wise signs and symptoms of Leukostasis

needing high level of suspicion in patients of AML and CML with signs and symptoms can often be confused with sepsis, heart failure, acute coronary syndrome, or ischemic vasculitis and deep vein thrombosis.

20.4 Management

- *Diagnostic*

  Complete blood count with peripheral smear comment—Complete blood picture with peripheral smear comment clinches diagnosis most of the times. The TLC counts are generally found to be in excess of 50,000/μL and most of the times above 100,000/μL. Peripheral smear study shows presence of large number of immature blast cells. Concomitant anemia is also a common finding which is generally a compensatory mechanism adapted by the body to reduce the blood viscosity and also may be due to marrow proliferation by blast cells (Fig. 20.1).

  Arterial blood gas (ABG) analysis—ABG analysis may show falsely low oxygen saturation levels due to activity of high number of TLCs (*leukocyte larceny*) unless sent over ice packs to minimize the metabolic activity of the cells. Hyperkalemia can also be seen due to release of intracellular potassium into the serum by the high number of blast cells. Further investigations may be advised like ECG, chest X-ray, HRCT chest, NCCT brain depending on the symptoms indicating the organ involved.

- *Therapeutic*

  Stabilization—initial management remains that of airway, breathing (oxygen requirement), and circulation, followed by IV hydration. This suspected or proven condition has to be treated as an emergency. Patients may be shifted to tertiary care center. Patient needs ICU care in view of impending organ failure, hypoxia, and multi-organ dysfunction and may need ventilator support.

  Differentials to be ruled out—Other hemorrhagic and thromboembolic complications have to be ruled out by sending various laboratory tests as per the need.

  Prophylaxis and treatment of tumor lysis syndrome (TLS) should be initiated as any treatment of hyperleukocytosis and leukostasis has very high chance of the patient landing up in it (TLS).

  Blood products—Blood products should generally be avoided unless and until extremely emergency. Target platelet levels should be above 20,000/μL to reduce the risk of bleeding. RBC transfusion is avoided (inspite of presence of anemia) as far as possible as it may lead to increased viscosity of the blood and worsening of symptoms.

  Leukoreduction–Leukoreduced blood product are to be transfused if at all the need arises.

  Allopurinol and/or rasburicase and hydroxyurea (50–100 mg/kg/day) in divided doses should be administered to reduce the leukocyte counts. Hydroxyurea helps in cyto-reduction and this effect may take up to 24–48 hours to show. These measures are taken prior to the start of definitive chemotherapy. Chemotherapy cannot be started unless the patient is stable (Table 20.1).

Leukapheresis Mechanical separation or leukapheresis is also a modality of treatment that reduces CNS symptoms along with pulmonary system and metabolic abnormalities. Leukaphersis can reduce counts by upto 20–50, 000 (30–60%) leading to relief from symptoms. This should immediately be followed by definitive chemotherapy. Leukapheresis patients have the risk of developing thrombocytopenia due to their removal during the procedure. There is no direct correlation with reduced long-term mortality in patients who undergo leukapheresis (Nan et al. 2017). However, placement of lines, interdepartmental co-ordination, aphaeresis machine availability, and blood products availability can delay the procedure. The availability of this facility is also a concern in most centers.

Definitive therapy The patient should be planned for definitive chemotherapy (underlying primary malignancy/leukemia) after cytoreduction.

Other medications—Injection dexamethasone 10 mg bolus followed by 16 mg/day in singular or divided doses is to be given to patients with cerebral edema having neurological symptoms.

Table 20.1 Drugs and Modalities in Leukostasis

Drug/ Modality name	Mechanism of action	Dose	Disadvantages
Allopurinol	Inhibits xanthine oxidase and inhibits the conversion of xanthine and hypoxanthine to uric acid	Oral—200–600 mg/m^2/day in 3 divided doses Intravenous—200–400 mg/m^2/day single dose or 2 or 3 divided doses	Maculo-papular rash, gastrointestinal adverse effects, transaminitis, leukopenia, thrombocytopenia
Rasburicase	Recombinant urate oxidase that converts uric acid to more soluble allantoin	Intravenous—0.05–0.2 mg/kg over 30 min Reduce uric acid within 4–6 h of administration	Rash, hypersensitivity, and contraindicated in patients with glucose-6-phosphate dehydrogenase
Hydroxyurea	Inhibits deoxyribonucleic acid synthesis by inhibiting ribonucleotide diphosphatase reductase and blocking the conversion of ribonucleotides to deoxyribonucleotides	20–30 mg/kg/day Takes up to 24–48 h for cytoreduction	Sores in mouth and lips, black tarry stool, gastrointestinal discomfort, cough, sore throat, fever, marrow suppression, secondary leukemias, macrocytosis, transaminitis, infertility, interstitial pneumonitis, headache, dizziness, confusion
Leukapheresis	Mechanical separation of leukocytes from circulating blood	1–2 blood volume Reduces leukocytes by 30–60%	Risk of thrombocytopenia, placement of lines, interdepartmental coordination, apheresis machine availability, and blood products availability

20.5 Conclusion

Leukostasis is a condition that warrants immediate attention and treatment. Failure to detect and attend to this condition can have life-threatening complications, eventually leading to mortality. Since the tumor load is very high, there are risks of TLS (discussed in another chapter). Patients have very high rate of mortality if timely treatment is not initiated. Sepsis should be considered as an important differential in such cases and should be thoroughly investigated by sending bacteriological cultures from blood, endotracheal aspirate, and urine and starting appropriate antibiotics.

Flowchart

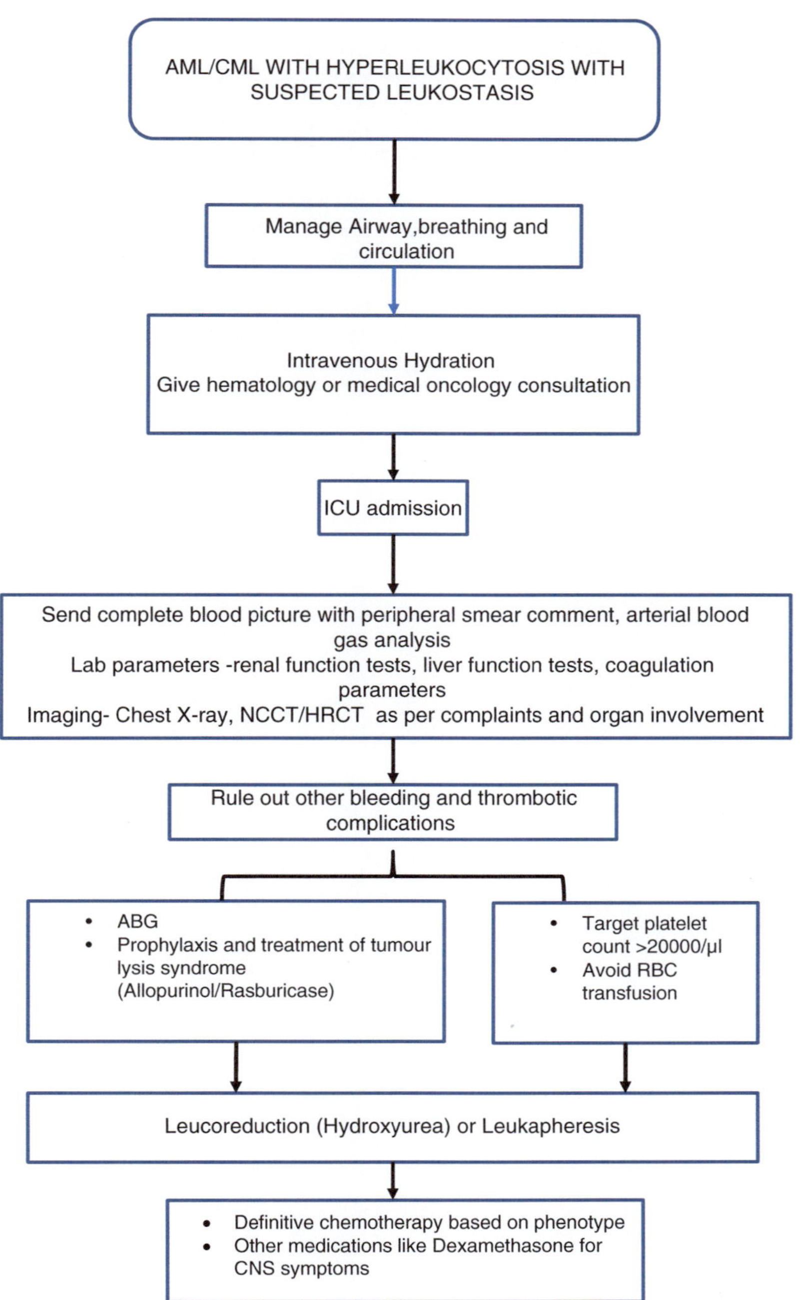
FLOW CHART- 1: STEP BY STEP MANAGEMENT OF LEUKOSTASIS
AML/CML WITH HYPERLEUKOCYTOSIS WITH SUSPECTED LEUKOSTASIS
Manage Airway,breathing and circulation
Intravenous Hydration
Give hematology or medical oncology consultation
ICU admission
Send complete blood picture with peripheral smear comment, arterial blood gas analysis
Lab parameters -renal function tests, liver function tests, coagulation parameters
Imaging- Chest X-ray, NCCT/HRCT as per complaints and organ involvement
Rule out other bleeding and thrombotic complications
• ABG
• Prophylaxis and treatment of tumour lysis syndrome (Allopurinol/Rasburicase)
• Target platelet count >20000/μl
• Avoid RBC transfusion
Leucoreduction (Hydroxyurea) or Leukapheresis
• Definitive chemotherapy based on phenotype
• Other medications like Dexamethasone for CNS symptoms

References

Bewersdorf JP, Zeidan AM (2020) Hyperleukocytosis and leukostasis in acute myeloid leukemia: can a better understanding of the underlying molecular pathophysiology lead to novel treatments? Cells 9(10):2310

Nan X, Qin Q, Gentille C, Ensor J, Leveque C, Pingali SR et al (2017) Leukapheresis reduces 4-week mortality in acute myeloid leukemia patients with hyperleukocytosis–a retrospective study from a tertiary center. Leuk Lymphoma 58(9):2110–2117

Nourshargh S, Alon R (2014) Leukocyte migration into inflamed tissues. Immunity 41(5):694–707

Reikvam H, Hatfield KJ, Øyan AM, Kalland KH, Kittang AO, Bruserud Ø (2010) Primary human acute myelogenous leukemia cells release matrix metalloproteases and their inhibitors: release profile and pharmacological modulation. Eur J Haematol 84(3):239–251

Stucki A, Rivier AS, Gikic M, Monai N, Schapira M, Spertini O (2001) Endothelial cell activation by myeloblasts: molecular mechanisms of leukostasis and leukemic cell dissemination. Blood, J Am Soc Hematol 97(7):2121–2129

Thiede C, Steudel C, Mohr B, Schaich M, Schäkel U, Platzbecker U et al (2002) Analysis of FLT3-activating mutations in 979 patients with acute myelogenous leukemia: association with FAB subtypes and identification of subgroups with poor prognosis: presented in part at the 42nd Annual Meeting of the American Society of Hematology, December 1–5, 2000, San Francisco, CA (abstract 2334). Blood, J Am Soc Hematol 99(12):4326–4335

Chapter 21
Tumor Lysis Syndrome

Tatikonda Chandra Mouli and Samir Samal

Learning Points

1. Pathophysiology of TLS: Understanding the biochemical cascade triggered by the rapid lysis of tumor cells is crucial.
2. Risk factors identification: The chapter details specific risk factors associated with TLS, including high tumor cell proliferation rates, the chemosensitivity of the malignancy, and pre-existing patient conditions like nephropathy or hyperuricemia.
3. Preventative measures: Emphasis is placed on proactive measures such as adequate hydration, dietary adjustments, and the use of medications like allopurinol and rasburicase to manage uric acid levels.
4. Management Strategies: Effective management of TLS includes not only emergency interventions to correct metabolic abnormalities but also careful monitoring and adjustment of ongoing cancer treatments.

21.1 Introduction

Tumor lysis syndrome (TLS) is one of the oncometabolite emergencies which usually result from cell lysis and warrants a physician's acute intervention. The cause for TLS is not readily intuitive, but the most common is secondary to initiation of chemotherapy to chemosensitive hematologic malignancies. Few case reports suggest that TLS can be noted spontaneously or secondary to steroid therapy (Wesemüller and Taverna 2021; Shafie et al. 2022). The common malignancies associated with

T. Chandra Mouli
RACC ICU Universal Hospital Danavai peta, Rajahmundry, India

S. Samal (✉)
Critical Care Medicine, IMS & SUM Hospital, Bhubaneswar, India

S. B. Mishra (ed.), *Critical Care Hematology*,
https://doi.org/10.1007/978-981-97-5565-3_21

TLS are Burkitt lymphoma and acute lymphoblastic leukemia (ALL). With ever improving diagnostic and treatment modalities of malignancies; coming across an oncomeatbolic emergency may become a common occurence rather than a rarity. This mandates intensivists to have a protocolized approach toward oncological emergencies. This chapter provides an overview on the pathophysiology of TLS, various risk factors, and detailed management of TLS in critical care settings

21.2 Pathophysiology of Tumor Lysis Syndrome

The initiation of cancer treatment, such as chemotherapy or radiation therapy, causes tumor cell death. The lysis of cancer cells releases intracellular contents which include electrolytes, inflammatory mediators like various cytokines, and deoxyribonucleic acid (DNA). Electrolytes such as potassium and phosphate released bind with extracellular calcium causing hypocalcemia. DNA further breaks down to purines by the action of DNAse enzyme and eventually accumulates as uric acid. Chemotherapy aims to destroy malignant cells, but when large number of tumor cells are destroyed simultaneously, it can overwhelm the body's ability to eliminate the cellular debris. These can directly impact the renal function and can lead to acute renal failure. The mechanism of cell destruction depends on the mechanism of the chemotherapy agent used. Sometimes it could also be due to spontaneous lysis of tumor cells leading to TLS. This cell destruction results in various metabolic abnormalities like hyperuricemia, hyperkalemia, hyperphosphatemia, and hypocalcemia (Fig. 21.1).

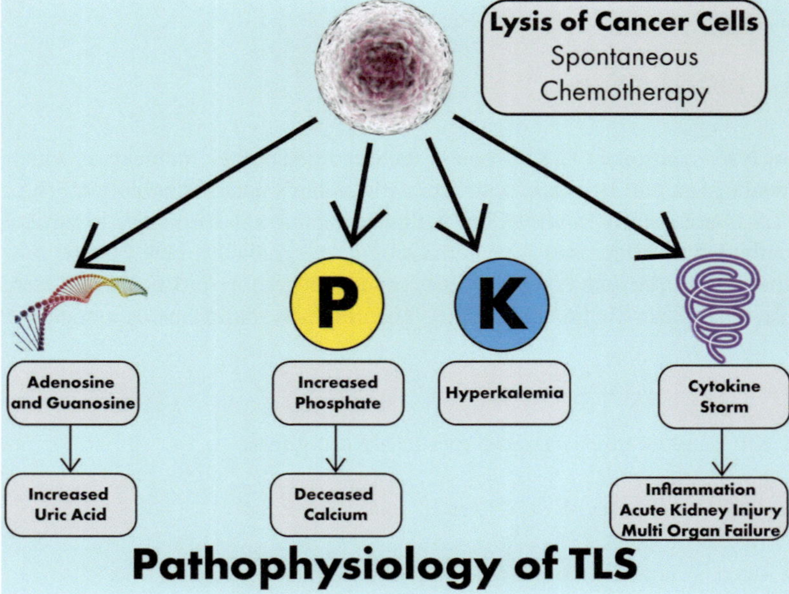

Fig. 21.1 Pathophysiology of TLS

As mentioned earlier, tumor lysis syndrome is associated with highly proliferative and chemosensitive hematological malignancies and few other solid tumors.

21.3 Hematologic Malignancies Associated with TLS

- Chronic lymphocytic leukemia
- Burkitt lymphoma
- Diffuse large B-cell lymphoma
- Acute lymphoblastic leukemia
- Rarely seen in retroperitoneal sarcomas (Zakharia et al. 2014)
- It can also be seen in patients with highly treatment-sensitive small cell carcinoma of the lungs.

Apart from the above-mentioned malignancies, *Bortezomib*, a proteasome inhibitor used in the treatment of multiple myeloma, has been reported to induce tumor lysis in patients with multiple myeloma (Singh et al. 2017).

21.3.1 Classification of TLS

TLS has been classified based on clinical parameters and laboratory values. Cairo-bishop definition proposed in 2004 provided specific laboratory criteria in the diagnosis of TLS both at presentation and within 7 days of treatment (Fig. 21.2) (Cairo and Bishop 2004).

Cairo-Bishop classification of TLS

Clinical	Laboratory
1. Serum creatinine increased more than 1.5 times the baseline value. 2. Seizures 3. Sudden death 4. Cardiac arrhythmia	1. Serum uric acid ≥ 8 mg/dl or 25% increase from baseline. 2. Serum potassium levels of ≥ 6mEq/L or 25% increase from baseline. 3. Serum phosphate ≥ 4.5 mg/dl or 25% increase from baseline. 4. Serum calcium < 7 mg/dl or 25% decrease from baseline.

Fig. 21.2 Cairo-Bishop Classification of TLS (Cairo and Bishop 2004)

TLS can be diagnosed when two or more of the above-mentioned laboratory criteria in the same 24 hour period are met in 3 days before to within 7 days of initiation of chemotherapy.

Clinical TLS - Laboratory TLS plus one or more of the clinical parameters (p.s. other causes of AKI must be excluded)

21.3.2 Risk Factors of TLS

The risk factors for TLS were highest in patients with hematologic malignancies.

- *Intrinsic tumor-related factors*
  - High tumor cell proliferation rate
  - Chemosensitivity to malignancy
  - Large tumor burden manifested by

    Bulky disease >10 cm in diameter
    WBC count >50,000/μL
    Pre-treatment serum LDH >2 times upper limit of normal
    Bone marrow involvement

- *Patient-related factors that predispose to TLS*
  - Pre-treatment hyperuricemia (serum uric acid >7.5 mg/dl)
  - Pre-treatment hyperphosphatemia
  - A pre-existing nephropathy or exposure to nephrotoxins
  - Inadequate hydration during the treatment
  - Intensity of chemotherapy, radiation therapy, and targeted therapies
  - Some degree of renal insufficiency prior to initiation of chemotherapy

21.3.3 Signs and Symptoms of TLS

Though not specific to TLS, patients may present with

- Generalized asthenia and fatigue
- Nausea, emesis, and diarrhea
- Dyspnea, Non-cardiogenic pulmonary edema (especially in children) (Flood et al. 2021)
- Altered mental status, stupor, seizures
- Myasthenia, tetany
- Tachycardia, arrhythmias, ECG changes (tall T waves, wide QRS, ventricular arrhythmias)
- Sudden cardiac arrest
- Signs and symptoms are due to the cellular metabolites released into the circulation

- Tumor cell lysis leads to hyperphosphatemia and hyperuricemia can lead to anorexia, lethargy, nausea, and vomiting and may lead to renal failure.
- Secondary hypocalcemia may cause arrhythmias, tetany, or seizures.
- Hyperkalemia can also cause muscular fatigue, arrhythmias, and sudden cardiac arrest.
- TLS is also known for its atypical presentation like intestinal perforation (Kunimoto et al. 2022).
- In a retrospective study of 161 patients with hematological malignancies undergoing chemotherapy, univariate analysis revealed that TLS is a significant risk factor for Posterior Reversible Encephalopathy Syndrome (PRES) (Suzuki et. al. 2014).

Key Signs and Symptoms
- Arrhythmias
- Muscle weakness
- Gastrointestinal symptoms such as nausea and emesis
- Tetany
- Seizures

21.3.4 Prevention of TLS

Prevention of TLS is the best possible practice, and identifying high-risk group of patients and applying preventive strategies is better in terms of effectivity and affordability. In a retrospective study, TLS is associated with increased economic burdens as compared to non-TLS cohort of patients among chronic lymphoid leukemia patients (Rogers et al. 2022). Apart from ear marking the high-risk patient groups, clinician should also eye on dietary intake of potassium and phosphate.

Hydration The main stay of prevention of TLS is adequate hydration, more than 3 L/m^2 of total body surface area per day. Patients should receive intravenous fluids of at least 3–4 mL/kg with a target urine output of more than 1 mL/kg/hour (Coiffier et al. 2008).

Urine Alkalinization Uric acid is highly soluble in alkaline pH, and this theoretically allows rapid elimination of uric acid by alkalinization. On flip side, the alkaline pH (achieved by infusing soda bicarbonate) precipitates purine metabolites like xanthine and hypoxanthine before formation of uric acid. This negates the potential advantage of uric acid elimination by urinary alkalization. Currently, there is no evidence in favor of urinary alkalization in prevention of TLS (Coiffier et al. 2008; Jones et al. 2015).

21.3.5 Prophylaxis with Uricosuric Drugs

Allopurinol belongs to a class of medications known as xanthine oxidase inhibitors. It works by reducing the production of uric acid in the body. Specifically, allopurinol decreases the conversion rate of hypoxanthine to xanthine and xanthine to uric acid (Fig. 21.1). By doing so, it helps to prevent the formation of uric acid crystals, particularly in the distal tubules of the renal system. This is important because the acidic environment in the distal tubules promotes the precipitation of uric acid as insoluble urate salts. It is important to note that allopurinol does not increase the breakdown of any existing uric acid that has already been formed. Therefore, its therapeutic effects are not immediate and may take 24–72 hours to become noticeable.

Rasburicase is a synthetic version of the enzyme urate oxidase (UO), which is naturally found in most mammals but not in humans due to a genetic mutation. Its primary function is to convert urate into allantoin which is considerably more soluble than uric acid, with a solubility of five to ten times higher (Fig. 21.1). Unlike allopurinol, rasburicase has an immediate effect and can act on already formed urate. It rapidly reduces plasma uric acid levels within 4 hours of intravenous administration, allowing for earlier initiation of chemotherapy compared to allopurinol, which is slower in its therapeutic response. Hence, in the treatment or prevention of tumor lysis syndrome (TLS), combining Rasburicase with Allopurinol is unnecessary and may compromise the efficacy of Rasburicase. The differences of these drugs are tabulated (Table 21.1).

The usage of the uricosuric drugs as prophylaxis to prevent TLS is based on risk stratification (Cairo et al. 2010; Ñamendys-Silva et al. 2015) (Table 21.2). In a retrospective propensity, matched analysis found that Rasburicase has high chances of prevention of TLS and significantly shorter ICU stay and economic burden (Cairo et al. 2017).

Table 21.1 Differences between allopurinol and Rasburicase

S. no	Allopurinol	Rasburicase
1.	Dose 300 mg/m^2/day	Dose 0.2 mg/kg
2.	Oral and easy to use	IV administration
3.	*Slow onset of action*: No effect on pre-existing uric acid levels	*Rapid onset of action:* lowers the pre-existing uric acid levels without accumulation of precursors and allows the start of chemotherapy agents without delay
4.	Ineffective sometimes	Lowers the uric acid in all patients
5.	1% incidence of allergic reactions	4–5% incidence of immune reactions
6.	No added risk for G6PD deficiency	Can lead to hemolysis in G6PD deficiency
7.	Inexpensive	Very expensive
8.	Interferes with metabolism of 6 mercaptopurine	No effect on drug metabolism

Table 21.2 Risk Stratification of Various Tumors for TLS (Jones et al. 2015)

Low-risk group	Intermediate-risk group	High-risk group
Low-risk patients can be managed with careful attention to the monitoring and measurement of fluid status and laboratory results with a low threshold for recourse to intravenous fluids and consideration of allopurinol if needed	Intermediate-risk patients should be offered up to 7 days of allopurinol prophylaxis along with increased hydration post-initiation of treatment or until risk of TLS has resolved.	High-risk patients should be offered prophylaxis with rasburicase along with increased hydration

Febuxostat is a xanthine oxidase inhibitor; it has been tried as an alternative to allopurinol. In a meta-analysis of studies involving a total of six studies with 658 patients, febuxostat demonstrated reduction in the incidence of tumor lysis syndrome with an odds ratio of 1.39, 95% CI: [0.55, 3.51]. It effectively lowered uric acid levels and improved clinical outcomes (Bellos et al. 2019).

21.3.6 Management of TLS

The best modality of management of TLS is risk stratifying the malignancies for TLS and incorporating preventive strategies or anticipating TLS and intervening before manifestation of complications.

- Airway, breathing, and circulation are to be evaluated and managed depending on the severity of symptoms and presentation. Patient may need mechanical ventilation if severe hemodynamic compromise or severe metabolic acidosis is present.
- Hydration—IV fluids—3–3.5 L/m^2/day
- Target urine output—100 mL/hour. Add diuretics if output falls or fluid overload.
- Serial lab monitoring (6–12 hourly, depending on the risk and severity) of serum uric acid, potassium, calcium, phosphorus, and lactic acids
- Chemotherapy deferral by 24–48 hours if patient not adequately hydrated or presence of deranged laboratory parameters
- Low-intensity treatment such as single-drug therapy/mono-regimen can be restarted based on the reversal of symptomatology and normalization of laboratory parameters.
- Treat hyperkalemia, hypocalcemia, hyperuricemia, hyperphosphatemia (Table 21.3)
- *Hyperuricemia:* Start allopurinol 1–2 days prior to chemo (300 mg/m^2/day, maxm 600 mg) and continue up to 7 days. Rasburicase (0.2 mg/kg in 50 ml NS over 30 minutes) can be given for up to 7 days if very high levels of uric acid are present. It should be avoided in G6PD deficiency patients. Hemodialysis should be initiated if uremic symptoms are present (Bose and Qubaiah 2011).
- *Hyperkalemia:* Should have low threshold for dialysis/renal replacement therapy. Continuous cardiac monitoring is required. Management includes calcium gluconate, insulin and dextrose, and loop diuretics.

Table 21.3 Management of Various Complications of TLS

Complications	Etiology	Manifestation	Management
Hyperkalemia	Intracellular potassium release rate exceeds the renal clearance capacity	Muscle cramps, weakness, and paresthesia Arrythmias Diarrhea	Aggressive hydration Intravenous calcium gluconate Intravenous 25% dextrose with insulin Loop diuretics. Renal replacement therapy.
Hyperphosphatemia	Intracellular phosphate release rate exceeds the renal clearance capacity	Acute renal failure Secondary hypocalcemia	Aggressive hydration 25% dextrose with insulin Oral phosphate binders (non-calcium based) based). Renal replacement therapy.
Hypocalcemia	Secondary to hyperphosphatemia and tissue precipitation of calcium phosphate	Muscle twitches, cramps, tetany, carpopedal spasm Mental status changes, confusion, and delirium Seizures rarely	Manage hyperphosphatemia because correcting hypocalcemia before hyperphosphatemia leads precipitation of calcium oxalate crystals
Hyperuricemia	Purine derivatives and nucleic acids released by cell lysis get converted to uric acid by a sequential process. Intracellular uric acid release rate exceeds the renal clearance capacity	Acute renal failure	Aggressive hydration Allopurinol Urate oxidase/rasburicase Hemodialysis

- *Hyperphosphatemia and Hypocalcemia:* Cardiac monitoring is to be done. Hypocalcemia is to be treated if there are symptoms e.g. tetany. Phosphate binders such as aluminum hydroxide (50–100 mg/kg/day orally for 1–2 days) or sevelamer (2.4–4.8 g/day) can be considered. Severe hyperphosphatemia mandates hemodialysis. Hemodialysis with large pore size filters helps in faster phosphate clearance.

Flowchart

Key signs and symptoms

- Arrhythmias
- Muscle weakness
- Gastrointestinal symptoms such as nausea and emesis
- Tetany
- Seizures

References

Bellos I, Kontzoglou K, Psyrri A, Pergialiotis V (2019) Febuxostat administration for the prevention of tumour lysis syndrome: a meta-analysis. J Clin Pharm Ther 44(4):525–533

Bose P, Qubaiah O (2011) A review of tumour lysis syndrome with targeted therapies and the role of rasburicase. J Clin Pharm Ther 36(3):299–326

Cairo MS, Bishop M (2004) Tumour lysis syndrome: new therapeutic strategies and classification. Br J Haematol 127(1):3–11

Cairo MS, Coiffier B, Reiter A, Younes A, TLS Expert Panel (2010) Recommendations for the evaluation of risk and prophylaxis of tumour lysis syndrome (TLS) in adults and children with malignant diseases: an expert TLS panel consensus. Br J Haematol 149(4):578–586

Cairo MS, Thompson S, Tangirala K, Eaddy MT (2017) A clinical and economic comparison of rasburicase and allopurinol in the treatment of patients with clinical or laboratory tumor lysis syndrome. Clin Lymphoma Myeloma Leuk 17(3):173–178

Coiffier B, Altman A, Pui CH, Younes A, Cairo MS (2008) Guidelines for the management of pediatric and adult tumor lysis syndrome: an evidence-based review. J Clin Oncol 26(16):2767–2778

Flood K, Rozmus J, Skippen P, Matsell DG, Mammen C (2021) Fluid overload and acute kidney injury in children with tumor lysis syndrome. Pediatr Blood Cancer 68(12):e29255

Jones GL, Will A, Jackson GH, Webb NJ, Rule S (2015) Guidelines for the management of tumour lysis syndrome in adults and children with haematological malignancies on behalf of the British Committee for Standards in Haematology. Br J Haematol 169(5):661

Kunimoto S, Tashima L, Ito K, Hori K (2022) Advanced ovarian cancer that resulted in death from intestinal perforation following tumor lysis syndrome: a case report. Int J Surg Case Rep 98:107518

Ñamendys-Silva SA, Arredondo-Armenta JM, Plata-Menchaca EP, Guevara-García H, García-Guillén FJ, Rivero-Sigarroa E, Herrera-Gómez A (2015) Tumor lysis syndrome in the emergency department: challenges and solutions. Open Access Emerg Med 7:39–44

Rogers KA, Lu X, Emond B, Côté-Sergent A, Kinkead F, Lafeuille MH et al (2022) Clinical and economic burden of tumor lysis syndrome among patients with chronic lymphocytic leukemia/small lymphocytic lymphoma: a real-world US retrospective study. J Manag Care Spec Pharm 28(9):1033–1045

Shafie M, Teymouri A, Parsa S, Sadeghian A, Zarei Jalalabadi N (2022) Spontaneous tumor lysis syndrome in adrenal adenocarcinoma: a case report and review of the literature. J Med Case Rep 16(1):52

Singh A, Gupta S, Yim B, Thekkekara R (2017) Tumor lysis syndrome in multiple myeloma: an increasingly recognized risk—a report of seven cases. Indian J Hematol Blood Transfus 33:41–44

Suzuki D, Kobayashi R, Iguchi A, Sano H, Kishimoto K, Yasuda K, Kobayashi K (2014) Tumor lysis syndrome as a risk factor for posterior reversible encephalopathy syndrome in children with hematological malignancies. Int J Hematol 100:485–489

Wesemüller W, Taverna C (2021) Spontaneous tumor lysis syndrome. Case Rep Oncol 13(3):1116–1124

Zakharia Y, Mansour J, Vasireddi S, Zakharia K, Fatakhov E, Koch C, Hrinczenko B (2014) Tumor lysis syndrome in a retroperitoneal sarcoma. J Investig Med High Impact Case Rep 2(3):2324709614542340

Chapter 22
Hypercalcemia of Malignancy

Monalisa Mishra and Samir Samal

Learning Points

1. *Etiology of Hypercalcemia in Malignancy*: Understanding the primary mechanisms—Parathyroid Hormone (PTH)-related Protein (PTHrP) secretion, osteolysis induced by metastases, and calcitriol production by cancer cells—provides insight into the diverse etiological landscape of hypercalcemia in cancer patients.
2. *Clinical Manifestations*: Recognizing the spectrum of symptoms associated with hypercalcemia, including neuropsychiatric effects, renal involvement, gastrointestinal symptoms, and cardiovascular manifestations, is crucial for early detection and management.
3. *Diagnostic Approach*: A structured diagnostic workflow, starting with the confirmation of hypercalcemia and proceeding through the measurement of PTH, PTHrP, and calcitriol levels, is vital for identifying the underlying cause of hypercalcemia in malignancy.
4. *Management Strategies*: Familiarity with the therapeutic options, including fluid resuscitation, calcitonin, bisphosphonates, Denosumab, corticosteroids, and dialysis, allows for a comprehensive and effective approach to managing hypercalcemia of malignancy.

22.1 Introduction

Hypercalcemia of malignancy refers to serum calcium levels exceeding the upper reference limit set by the testing laboratory. This condition is primarily caused by two major factors: primary hyperparathyroidism and malignancy-associated

M. Mishra
Apollo Multi-speciality Hospitals, Kolkata, India

S. Samal (✉)
Critical Care Medicine, IMS & SUM Hospital, Bhubaneswar, India

S. B. Mishra (ed.), *Critical Care Hematology*,
https://doi.org/10.1007/978-981-97-5565-3_22

hypercalcemia. Notably, hypercalcemia related to cancer is linked with significant morbidity and mortality, affecting 2–30% of all individuals diagnosed with cancer.

Normal calcium levels range from 8.5 to 10.2 mg/dL (2.13–2.55 millimol/L). Hypercalcemia is categorized based on the serum calcium (SCa) levels: mild hypercalcemia is indicated by SCa levels of 10.5 to <12 mg/dL, moderate hypercalcemia is defined by serum calcium levels from 12 to 14 mg/dL, and serum calcium levels exceeding 14 mg/dL are considered severe. The main symptoms reported by patients with mild to moderate hypercalcemia, regardless of its origin, include fatigue, constipation, increased urination (polyuria), and excessive thirst (polydipsia). In cases of severe hypercalcemia or a rapid increase in serum calcium levels, patients may experience cognitive dysfunction, kidney failure, and arrhythmias (Dickens et al. 2023).

22.2 Etiology

22.2.1 Etiology of Hypercalcemia of Malignancy

Hypercalcemia associated with malignancy can arise through three primary mechanisms.

Secretion of Parathyroid Hormone (PTH)-related Protein (PTHrP) by tumors This is a common mechanism wherein tumor cells produce PTHrP, which mimics the action of PTH, leading to increased calcium release from bones, enhanced calcium reabsorption in the kidneys, and increased intestinal calcium absorption. PTHrP-mediated hypercalcemia is often associated with solid tumors, such as breast and lung cancers.

Osteolysis Induced by Metastases This involves the direct destruction of bone tissue by metastatic cancer cells. The process is facilitated by cytokines and osteoclast activating factors released by the tumor cells, which stimulate osteoclasts to resorb bone, thereby releasing calcium into the bloodstream. This mechanism is frequently observed in cancers that metastasize to bone, such as breast, prostate, and lung cancers.

Production of 1,25-Dihydroxy Vitamin D (Calcitriol) by Cancer Cells Some lymphomas and other tumors possess the enzyme 1-α-hydroxylase, enabling them to convert 25-hydroxyvitamin D into its active form, calcitriol. Elevated levels of calcitriol lead to increased intestinal absorption of calcium, contributing to hypercalcemia. This mechanism is relatively less common compared to the first two but can significantly impact calcium metabolism.

22.2.2 PTH-Related Protein

The predominant mechanism, responsible for approximately 80% of hypercalcemia in cancer patients, involves the increased production of PTHrP by tumor cells, also referred to as humoral hypercalcemia of malignancy. PTHrP, secreted by cancerous cells, stimulates osteoblasts to produce RANK Ligand (RANKL), which in turn activates osteoclasts, leading to increased bone resorption and the subsequent release of calcium into the bloodstream. In addition, PTHrP promotes the reabsorption of calcium in the renal tubules, further elevating serum calcium levels. This mechanism is notably prevalent in squamous cell cancers, cancers of the urinary tract (including renal and bladder cancers), breast cancer, non-Hodgkin's lymphoma (NHL), and ovarian cancer. Typically associated with advanced disease stages, hypercalcemia via this route often signifies a poor prognosis.

22.2.3 Osteolytic Metastases

Approximately 20% of hypercalcemia cases in malignancy are due to osteolytic metastases, especially observed in breast carcinoma and multiple myeloma. Here, the elevated calcium levels result not directly from tumor cell activity but from osteoclast activation mediated by inflammatory cytokines released in the bone microenvironment. This process leads to bone destruction and the release of calcium into circulation, contributing to hypercalcemia.

22.2.4 1, 25-Dihydroxy Vitamin D

In the context of hematological malignancies, such as nearly all cases of Hodgkin's lymphoma (HL) and about one-third of NHL, there is an associated increase in the production of 1,25-dihydroxyvitamin D (calcitriol). The elevated calcitriol levels enhance calcium absorption from the gastrointestinal tract, significantly impacting the development of hypercalcemia in these diseases. Furthermore, it is hypothesized that the increased calcitriol may also promote bone resorption, further contributing to the hypercalcemic state observed in HL and NHL.

22.2.5 Ectopic PTH Secretion

Various malignancies, including ovarian carcinoma, small cell lung carcinoma, squamous cell lung carcinoma, primitive neuroectodermal tumors, thyroid papillary carcinoma, metastatic rhabdomyosarcoma, pancreatic malignancy, and gastric carcinoma, have been identified to produce PTH through ectopic PTH secretion, leading to hypercalcemia.

Therefore, hypercalcemia in the context of malignancy can arise from several key mechanisms. These include the overproduction of PTHrP by tumors, osteolysis triggered by metastatic lesions, the ectopic activity of 1-alpha-hydroxylase leading to increased calcitriol production, the overproduction of PTH by parathyroid carcinoma as well as ectopic PTH secretion by other malignancies, and hypercalcemia resulting from the binding of paraproteins. These diverse etiologies underscore the complexity of hypercalcemia associated with malignancy.

22.3 Clinical Features of Hypercalcemia

The clinical manifestations of hypercalcemia are influenced by the serum calcium concentration and the rate of increase in these levels. Patients with hypercalcemia due to malignancy often present with higher serum calcium levels and a rapid increase in these levels over a short duration compared to those with nonmalignant causes of hypercalcemia. This acute and significant elevation in calcium levels in cancer patients is the primary reason for their more pronounced symptoms compared to individuals with hypercalcemia of other origins (Fig. 22.1).

- *Major Affected Systems and Symptoms*
- *Neuropsychiatric Effects*
  The mnemonic "stones, bones, abdominal moans, and psychic groans" aptly summarize the spectrum of hypercalcemia symptoms. Neuropsychiatric manifestations can include cognitive dysfunction, mood changes, anxiety, and, in severe cases, profound confusion or coma. The latter is more commonly observed in malignancy-associated hypercalcemia, potentially leading to life-threatening conditions, such as posterior reversible leukoencephalopathy syndrome, characterized by headache, seizures, and specific findings on MRI imaging.
- *Renal Involvement*
  Renal symptoms are prevalent and include increased urination (polyuria), excessive thirst (polydipsia), and nephrogenic diabetes insipidus. Advanced cases can lead to nephrolithiasis, resulting in distal renal tubular acidosis. Immediate intervention is crucial to avert long-term renal damage, which could manifest as tubular atrophy, interstitial fibrosis, and calcification.
- *Gastrointestinal Symptoms*
  Gastrointestinal complaints can range from mild, such as constipation and anorexia, to more severe forms, such as pancreatitis and peptic ulcer disease. These symptoms arise due to decreased gastrointestinal smooth muscle tone and increased gastrin secretion, driven by elevated calcium levels. Specifically, hypercalcemia is recognized as a risk factor for pancreatitis through calcium deposition in the pancreatic ducts and activation of pancreatic enzymes.
- *Cardiovascular Manifestations*
  Cardiovascular signs include a shortened QT interval on the electrocardiogram. While mild to moderate hypercalcemia may not elicit cardiovascular symptoms, severe hypercalcemia can disrupt the heart's conduction system, leading to arrhythmias. In addition, severe hypercalcemia can precipitate a myocardial infarction and contribute to cardiovascular morbidity through calcific deposits in heart valves and coronary arteries.
  The acute and pronounced symptoms in malignancy-related hypercalcemia underscore the need for prompt diagnosis and management to mitigate the risk of severe complications across multiple organ systems (Fig. 22.1).

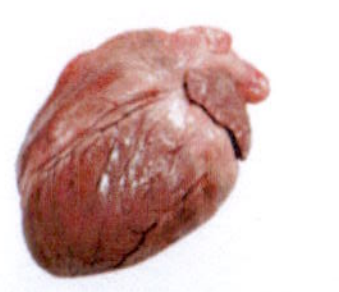

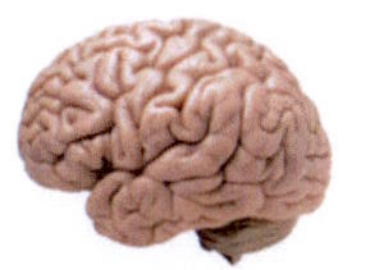

Neurological System:
- Anxiety and mood changes as a result of calcium affecting neurotransmitter levels.
- Cognitive decline due to disrupted calcium homeostasis in neuronal function.
- Potential for coma in severe hypercalcemia.
- Symptoms of PRES such as headaches and seizures, possibly related to vascular effects of calcium

Cardiovascular System:
- Shortened QT interval on electrocardiogram, indicating potential cardiac electrical abnormalities.
- Risk of arrhythmias from disturbed cardiac conduction.
- Calcium deposition in the heart valves and coronary arteries can lead to stenosis and ischemic heart disease.

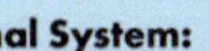

Hypercalcemia Clinical Features

Gastrointestinal System:
- Constipation due to decreased bowel motility.
- Anorexia and nausea influenced by altered digestive processes.
- Increased gastrin levels can promote peptic ulcer disease.
- Pancreatitis linked to calcium-mediated enzyme activation.

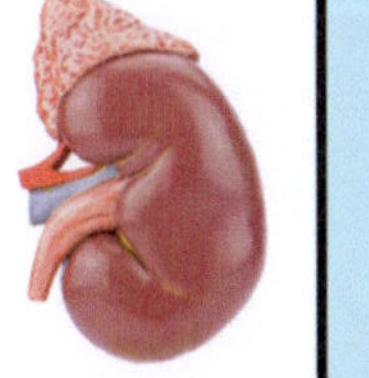

Renal System:
- Polyuria and polydipsia resulting from impaired kidney function and altered water reabsorption.
- Nephrogenic diabetes insipidus due to damaged renal tubules.
- Distal renal tubular acidosis from nephrolithiasis.
- Long-term complications like tubular atrophy, interstitial fibrosis, and nephrocalcinosis from sustained high calcium levels.

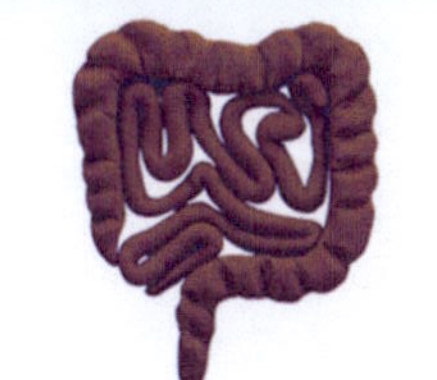

Fig. 22.1 Signs and symptoms of Hypercalcemia (system wise)

22.4 Diagnostic Approach to Hypercalcemia of Malignancy

After receiving a high serum calcium level from the lab, the first thing that should be done is to confirm with the lab by repeating a sample. The total levels should also be corrected for albumin [measured total Ca (mg/dl) + 0.8 (4 – serum albumin (g/dl))]. It should be confirmed if there is a true rise in serum levels of calcium. It is important to try to get a previous serum calcium level of the patient if available. This can help with the severity, duration, and acuteness of the current high serum calcium levels.

Once hypercalcemia is confirmed, the cause of the hypercalcemia needs to be established. Based on the etiologies discussed above, we need to send PTH and PTHrP levels to ascertain if these are the cause of the rise in serum calcium levels. Elevated PTH levels suggest a primary pathology with the parathyroid gland.

The rise in PTHrP levels with a low to normal PTH level suggests that malignancy can be the cause, as discussed in the etiology section. A rise in serum calcium levels with low PTH and no significant levels of PTHrP usually point toward osteoclastic/lytic activity due to bone invasion/metastases as the culprit.

We need to measure serum 1, 25-dihydroxyvitamin D levels if we get low PTHrP levels. Vit D-induced hypercalcemia is generally seen in lymphomas. Low levels of PTH, PTHrP, and 1, 25-dihydroxy vitamin D must raise the suspicion of hypercalcemia due to osteolysis. Osteolysis can be seen in patients with bony metastases or multiple myeloma (Mirrakhimov 2015). If, in such cases, we do not find any evidence of bony metastasis, then we should suspect myeloma and/or monoclonal gammopathy. This mandates looking for serum protein and urine electrophoresis and immunofixation. We should also look for serum-free light chain levels and may order a skeletal survey to look out for bony lesions due to myeloma.

It needs to be kept in mind, however, that more than one mechanism can contribute to the hypercalcemia of malignancy.

22.5 Treatment of Hypercalcemia

Lowering the serum calcium levels to achieve relief from the symptoms should be the primary goal, along with treating the cause of hypercalcemia. The various methods to reduce calcium levels can be increased urinary excretion, reduced absorption from the gut, and inhibited bone resorption. Hemodialysis can also be taken as a modality for acute reduction in serum calcium levels and relief of symptoms. Coming to a conclusive etiology can take several days, and the hypercalcemia can worsen patient outcomes in the meantime. Thus, it is prudent to keep the serum calcium levels in check before initiating the definitive treatment of the underlying cause. Hypercalcemia of malignancy is to be treated as an oncological emergency. This requires immediate attention and an aggressive approach to lowering serum calcium levels to increase the chances of survival in such patients.

Treatment consists of volume expansion and calcitonin along with bisphosphonates for the management of hypercalcemia of malignancy. Initial treatment remains aggressive resuscitation with intravenous fluids (IV fluids—crystalloids). The IV fluids help lower calcium levels by dilution and diuresis and can lower the calcium levels by approximately 2 mg/dL (0.5 mmol/L). The rate and volume of fluids depend on the patient's volume status, age, and underlying comorbidities, especially cardiac and renal disease. The addition of loop diuretics is needed in patients with oliguric renal failure and congestive heart failure to prevent the unwanted effects of volume expansion in this subset of patients (Dickens et al. 2023).

We can start with a bolus of around 1–2 L of crystalloids and then follow it with 100–150 mL every hour. We should be targeting a urine output of 100 ml/h, which leads to effective removal and thus lowering of calcium levels. We can target a total fluid intake of around 4–6 L on day 1 in patients with severe hypercalcemia if the condition permits. It should be kept in mind that the goal of this resuscitation with IV fluids is to make them euvolemic. Hypervolemic fluid resuscitation must be avoided at all costs to prevent the deleterious effects of organ congestion. It also must be kept in mind that fluid resuscitation lowers the calcium levels by 2 mg/dL only and does not normalize the serum calcium levels. This will not help in patients with moderate-to-severe hypercalcemia. Thus, we need adjuvant therapies to normalize serum calcium levels, such as bisphosphonates and calcitonin.

- *Calcitonin*
  Derived from the thyroid gland, calcitonin helps regulate calcium levels in the body by inhibiting osteoclast activity, thereby reducing bone resorption and calcium release. However, calcitonin administration provides a rapid but short-term solution by directly suppressing bone resorption, which effectively lowers serum calcium levels (Vakiti et al. 2024). It takes about 4 h for calcitonin to show maximal effect, and like IV fluids, it can also cause a maximal drop of 2 mg/dL (Vaughn and Vaitkevicius 1974; Dumon et al. 1992; Wisneski 1990).
  Calcitonin is administered at a dosage of 4–8 International Units (IU) per kilogram per day, through either subcutaneous or intramuscular injections. An alternative method involves a continuous intravenous infusion at the same rate of 4–8 IU/kg/day. Typically, the duration of treatment with calcitonin is restricted to 2–3 days due to the onset of tachyphylaxis, which diminishes the drug's efficacy over time. The administration intervals for calcitonin are generally every 6–12 h, with adjustments made based on the individual's response to the treatment in terms of lowering calcium levels. The adaptability in both dosage and frequency of administration is crucial to achieving the desired hypocalcemic effect. However, its efficacy may vary among individuals and tumor types. In addition, calcitonin's effects are transient, often necessitating concurrent therapy with bisphosphonates for sustained control of hypercalcemia.
  Intranasal spray calcitonin can also be utilized in the management of hypercalcemia of malignancy. Typically, a dose of 200 IU is administered every 12 h. This route offers convenience and ease of administration, especially in patients where intravenous access may be challenging. However, its efficacy may be less pronounced compared to injectable forms.
- *Bisphosphonates*
  Bisphosphonates are the treatment of choice for severe hypercalcemia, particularly when serum calcium levels exceed 14 mg/dl, and for the sustained manage-

ment of hypercalcemia. These compounds are effective against hypercalcemia that results from excessive bone resorption, as they inhibit the activity of osteoclasts in a dose-dependent manner and contribute to bone matrix stabilization by adhering to extracellular calcium and phosphorus. Pamidronate and zoledronic acids are primarily employed in the treatment of hypercalcemia. Among bisphosphonates, zoledronic acid is noted for its superior potency, with a recommended dosage of 4 mg administered intravenously over a period of 15–30 min. While pamidronate and ibandronate are considered less potent than zoledronic acid, they offer comparable efficacy, with pamidronate being administered in doses ranging from 60 mg to 90 mg intravenously over 2–24 h. Although intravenous bisphosphonates are generally well-received, potential side effects include fever, arthralgias, myalgias, fatigue, bone pain, ocular inflammation (such as uveitis), hypocalcemia, hypophosphatemia, and renal function impairment, which may manifest as proteinuria. Prolonged bisphosphonate therapy carries risks of osteonecrosis of the jaw and atypical fractures of the femur (Xu et al. 2013).

- *Denosumab*
  Denosumab, a human monoclonal antibody, specifically targets the receptor activator of nuclear factor-kappa B ligand (RANKL), effectively diminishing osteoclast activity. This reduction in bone resorption leads to decreased release of calcium into the bloodstream, making Denosumab an essential treatment for hypercalcemia, especially when it arises from malignancy and is not sufficiently managed by bisphosphonates (Hu et al. 2013). Its metabolism predominantly occurs through proteolytic degradation into amino acids and smaller peptides, with renal excretion playing a negligible role in its elimination. Consequently, Denosumab not only offers a therapeutic option for hypercalcemia but has also been observed to enhance renal function in patients with multiple myeloma and associated hypercalcemia. For individuals with bone metastases stemming from solid tumors, the suggested regimen is a subcutaneous injection of 120 mg every 4 weeks.
  Adjustments in dosage may be necessary, taking into account factors like renal functionality, with a 60 mg dose being considered for patients experiencing renal failure. The hypocalcemic effects of Denosumab typically manifest within 2–4 days (Russell et al. 2007; Hanley et al. 2012).
- *Corticosteroids*
  In instances of hypercalcemia attributed to elevated concentrations of 1, 25-dihydroxyvitamin D (calcitriol), the application of corticosteroid therapy is advisable. Corticosteroids act by obstructing the conversion of 25-hydroxyvitamin D (calcidiol) to 1, 25-dihydroxyvitamin D (calcitriol) by inhibiting 1-α-hydroxylase. This inhibition results in decreased calcitriol levels, leading to diminished intestinal absorption and consequently reduced serum calcium levels. The regimen for treating hypercalcemia related to calcitriol involves administering 200–400 mg/day of intravenous hydrocortisone for 3–5 days, succeeded by 10–20 mg/day of oral prednisone for a subsequent 7 days. Notable adverse effects associated with corticosteroid use include hyperglycemia, hypertension, psychiatric disorders, muscle weakness, and peptic ulcer disease, among others.

- *Dialysis*
  Patients who are highly symptomatic with impending multi-organ failure or patients who do not respond to the pharmacological methods of calcium-lowering agents are ideal candidates for hemodialysis. Congestive cardiac failure and patients with renal injury who cannot be adequately resuscitated with IV fluids should also undergo dialysis. Although hemodialysis is usually the last resort, it should not be delayed if there are no significant early improvements by pharmacological therapies or if there is multi-organ involvement. It should be kept in mind to use dialysate fluids with no or minimal calcium present in them.
  To summarize, the management of symptomatic hypercalcemia should commence with prompt fluid resuscitation for individuals not affected by severe renal or cardiac conditions. The employment of calcitonin is advisable due to its rapid onset and minimal adverse effects. The administration of bisphosphonates is recommended alongside, as their effect on lowering calcium levels begins within 2–4 days. In cases where there is excessive production of 1,25-dihydroxycholecalciferol, corticosteroids are to be considered. For hypercalcemia that remains unresponsive, treatment with Denosumab should be contemplated, followed by hemodialysis if necessary (Fig. 22.2).

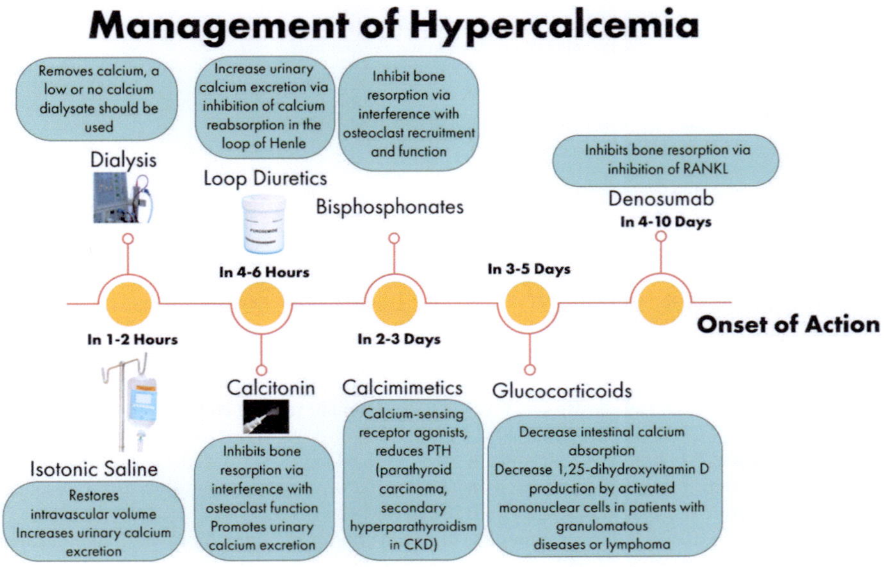

Fig. 22.2 Management of hypercalcemia

Flowchart

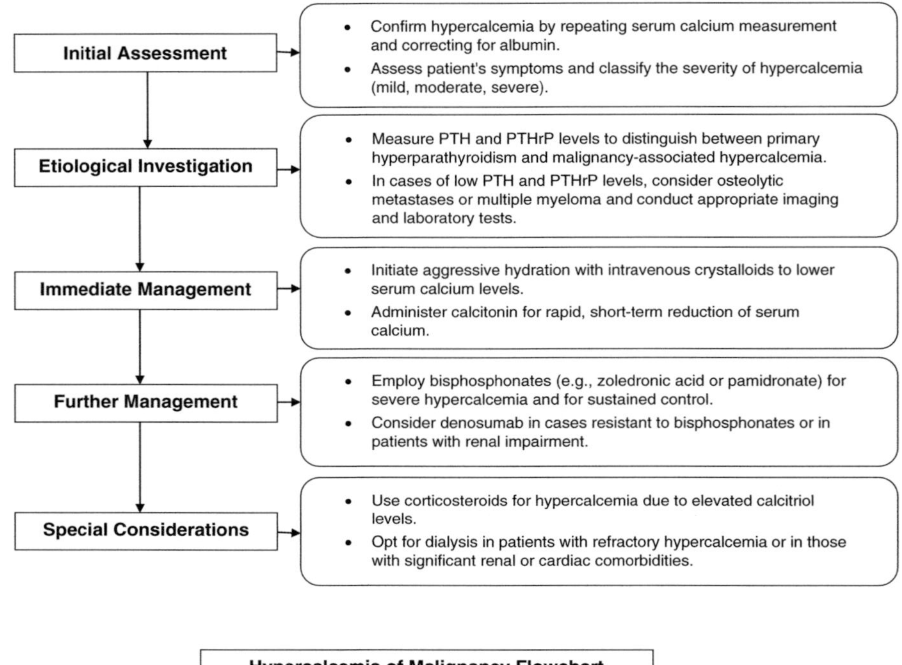

Flowchart 22.1 Stepwise assessment and management of Hypercalcemia

References

Dickens LT, Derman B, Alexander JT (2023) Endocrine Society hypercalcemia of malignancy guidelines. JAMA Oncol 9(3):430–431

Dumon JC, Magritte A, Body JJ (1992) Nasal human calcitonin for tumor-induced hypercalcemia. Calcif Tissue Int 51:18–19

Hanley DA, Adachi JD, Bell A, Brown V (2012) Denosumab: mechanism of action and clinical outcomes. Int J Clin Pract 66(12):1139–1146

Hu MI, Glezerman I, Leboulleux S, Insogna K, Gucalp R, Misiorowski W et al (2013) Denosumab for patients with persistent or relapsed hypercalcemia of malignancy despite recent bisphosphonate treatment. J Natl Cancer Inst 105(18):1417–1420

Mirrakhimov AE (2015) Hypercalcemia of malignancy: an update on pathogenesis and management. N Am J Med Sci 7(11):483

Russell RGG, Xia Z, Dunford JE, Oppermann UDO, Kwaasi A, Hulley PA et al (2007) Bisphosphonates: an update on mechanisms of action and how these relate to clinical efficacy. Ann N Y Acad Sci 1117(1):209–257

Vakiti A, Anastasopoulou C, Mewawalla P (2024) Malignancy-Related Hypercalcemia. [Updated 2023 Apr 16]. In: StatPearls [Internet]. Treasure Island (FL): StatPearls Publishing. Available from: https://www.ncbi.nlm.nih.gov/books/NBK482423/

Vaughn CB, Vaitkevicius VK (1974) The effects of calcitonin in hypercalcemia in patients with malignancy. Cancer 34(4):1268–1271

Wisneski LA (1990) Salmon calcitonin in the acute management of hypercalcemia. Calcif Tissue Int 46:S26–S30

Xu XL, Gou WL, Wang AY, Wang Y, Guo QY, Lu Q et al (2013) Basic research and clinical applications of bisphosphonates in bone disease: what have we learned over the last 40 years? J Transl Med 11:1–8

Chapter 23
Advancements in Chemotherapeutic Drugs for Intensive Care Management of Hematological Malignancies

Shakti Bedanta Mishra

Learning Points

1. Precision of Targeted Therapies: Targeted therapies, categorized into small molecule and macromolecule drugs, offer a precise approach to treating hematological malignancies by focusing on specific genetic markers and pathways.
2. Role of Protein Kinase Inhibitors: Protein kinase inhibitors, including tyrosine kinase inhibitors and multi-kinase inhibitors, play a pivotal role in blocking key signaling pathways, halting cancer cell proliferation and survival.
3. Advancements in Macromolecule Anticancer Drugs: Monoclonal antibodies, bispecific antibodies, antibody–drug conjugates, and recombinant immunotoxins represent significant advancements, targeting cancer cells while sparing healthy tissue.
4. Combating Drug Resistance: The chapter underscores the importance of developing second- and third-generation inhibitors and combination therapies to overcome resistance to treatment, enhancing efficacy and patient outcomes.

23.1 Introduction

Hematological malignancies encompass a diverse group of cancers affecting the blood, bone marrow, and lymph nodes, characterized by the clonal proliferation of blood-forming cells derived from myeloid and lymphoid lineages. Significant advancements in their treatment have been achieved over the last decade, notably with the FDA approval and development of targeted therapies, which are categorized into small molecule and macromolecule agents, offering more precise and effective treatment options (Sochacka-Ćwikła et al. 2021). These malignancies are

S. B. Mishra (✉)
Department of Critical Care Medicine, IMS and SUM Hospital, Bhubaneswar, Odisha, India

S. B. Mishra (ed.), *Critical Care Hematology*,
https://doi.org/10.1007/978-981-97-5565-3_23

highly heterogeneous, with specific genetic lesions associated with each disease type, underlining the necessity for tailored treatment approaches (Pang et al. 2018; Przybylski 2020). The prevalence of these diseases, with non-Hodgkin's lymphomas being the most common among male patients, followed by Hodgkin's lymphoma and acute myeloid leukemia (AML), underscores their significant impact on human health (Hamid 2012). Recent research has focused on the development of novel agents and regimens, including selective inhibitors of nuclear export and proteasome inhibitors, aiming to enhance treatment efficacy and patient outcomes (Hou et al. 2021; Das et al. 2015; Whittle and Desai 2015) (Table 23.1).

A. *Small Molecule Anticancer Drugs*

   I. Protein kinase inhibitors
   II. PI3K inhibitors
   III. Enzyme inhibitors
   IV. Receptor antagonists
   V. Proteasome inhibitors
   VI. Tubulin inhibitor

B. *Macromolecule Anticancer Drugs*

   I. Monoclonal antibodies
   II. Bispecific antibody
   III. Antibody–drug conjugates
   IV. Recombinant immunotoxins

23.2 Small Molecule Anticancer Drugs

These include a variety of protein kinase inhibitors [e.g., tyrosine kinase inhibitors (TKIs) and multi-kinase inhibitors], Phosphatidylinositol 3-Kinase (PI3K) inhibitors, enzyme inhibitors [e.g., histone deacetylase (HDAC) inhibitors and isocitrate dehydrogenase (IDH) inhibitors], receptor antagonists, and inhibitors targeting specific proteins, such as BCL-2, exportin-1, proteasome, and tubulin. These drugs work by blocking essential pathways in cancer cells, leading to cell death or halting proliferation.

23.2.1 Protein Kinase Inhibitors

Protein kinase inhibitors have revolutionized the treatment landscape for various cancers, including hematological malignancies, by offering targeted therapies that specifically inhibit the activity of protein kinases—enzymes crucial for the regulation of cell functions such as division, growth, and apoptosis. By targeting these

Table 23.1 Chemotherapeutic drugs for hematological malignancies

Class	Drug	Mechanism of action (inhibits tumor growth)	Resistance	Indication
Tyresine Kinase Inhibitors (TKIs)	Imatinib (Greevec)	Binds to BCR–ABL tyrosine kinase, blocking proliferative signaling pathways	Mutations in kinase domain, activation of alternative pathways	Chronic myeloid leukemia (CML)
	Erlotinib (Tarceva)	Targets EGFR tyrosine kinase, blocking signaling pathways driving cell proliferation and survival	Mutations in EGFR, activation of alternative pathways	Non-small cell lung cancer (NSCLC) with EGFR mutations
Multi Kinase Inhibitors	Sorafenib (Nexavar)	Inhibits multiple tyrosine protein kinases and Raf kinases, blocking tumor cell proliferation and angiogenesis	Mutations in kinase domain, activation of alternative pathways	Advanced renal cell carcinoma, hepatocellular carcinoma
	Sunitinib (Sutent)	Blocks activity of multiple receptor tyrosine kinases involved in angiogenesis and tumor cell proliferation	Mutations in kinase domain, activation of alternative pathways	Gastrointestinal stromal tumors (GISTs), advanced renal cell carcinoma
PI3K Inhibitors	Idelalisib	Blocks PI3K delta (δ) inhibiting PI3K/AKT/mTOR signaling pathway, reducing cell growth and survival	Activation of alternative signaling pathways	Relapsed chronic lymphocytic leukemia (CLL), follicular lymphoma, small lymphocytic lymphoma
	Copanlisib	Inhibits PI3K-alpha (α) and delta (δ), targeting a broad range of signaling pathways, leading to tumor suppression	Activation of alternative signaling pathways	Relapsed follicular lymphoma

(continued)

Table 23.1 (continued)

Class	Drug	Mechanism of action (inhibits tumor growth)	Resistance	Indication
Histone Deacetylase (HDAC) Inhibitors	Vorinostat (Zolinza)	Increases acetylation of histones, promoting transcription of genes that induce apoptosis and cell cycle arrest	Changes in histone acetylation patterns	Cutaneous T-cell lymphoma (CTCL)
	Romidepsin	Selectively inhibits Class I HDACs, altered gene expression, and induction of cancer cell death	Changes in histone acetylation patterns	CTCL, peripheral T-cell lymphoma (PTCL)
Isocitrate Dehydrogenase (IDH) Inhibitors	Ivosidenib (Tibsovo)	Inhibits mutant IDH1 enzyme, reducing oncometabolite levels and promoting differentiation of leukemic cells.	Unknown	Acute myeloid leukemia (AML) with IDH1 mutation
	Enasidenib (Idhifa)	Targets mutant IDH2 enzyme, decreases 2-HG production and inducing apoptosis and differentiation of cancer cells	Unknown	AML with IDH2 mutation
SMO Receptor Antagonist	Glasdegib (Daurismo)	Binds to SMO receptor, blocking Hedgehog signaling and disrupting cancer cell survival and proliferation	Unknown	Newly diagnosed AML in older adults or those with comorbidities
Proteasome Inhibitors	Bortezomib (Velcade)	Directly inhibits the proteasome, leading to accumulation of proteins that induce apoptosis and block proliferation	Development of proteasome mutation or alternative survival pathways	Multiple myeloma mantle cell lymphoma
Tubulin Inhibitors	Vincristine (Oncovin)	Inhibits tubulin polymerization, preventing mitosis and triggering apoptosis in tumor cells	Alterations in tubulin or efflux mechanisms	Leukemia, lymphoma, certain solid tumors

(continued)

Table 23.1 (continued)

Class	Drug	Mechanism of action (inhibits tumor growth)	Resistance	Indication
Monoclonal Antibodies (mAbs)	Rituximab (Rituxan)	Targets CD20 on B cells, directly inducing apoptosis and activating immune response against B cells	Loss or mutation of CD20, immune escape mechanisms	Non-Hodgkin lymphoma, chronic lymphocytic leukemia
	Trastuzumab (Herceptin)	Bind to HER2, blocking cell proliferation and activating immune-mediated mechanisms against tumor cells	HER2 mutation or loss, activation of bypass pathways	HER2-positive breast cancer
Bispecific Antibodies	Blinatumomab (Blincyto)	Connect CD19-positive B-cell leukemia/lymphoma cells with CD3-positive T-cells.	Loss or mutation of CD19, immune escape mechanisms	Acute lymphoblastic leukemia (ALL) refractory or relapsed
Antibody-Drug Conjugates (ADCs)	Brentuximab Vedotin (Adcetris)	Targets CD30, delivers cytotoxic agent MMAE	CD30 down regulation or mutation, drug resistance	

enzymes, these inhibitors can block key signaling pathways, ultimately leading to the cessation of cancer cell proliferation and survival.

1. *Tyrosine Kinase Inhibitors (TKIs)*

   Tyrosine kinases are a subset of protein kinases that phosphorylate tyrosine residues on certain proteins, which can activate a cascade of signaling pathways leading to cell proliferation, differentiation, migration, and survival. The aberrant activation of tyrosine kinases is a common feature in many cancers, making them prime targets for cancer therapy:

   - *Imatinib (Gleevec)*: A breakthrough in the treatment of chronic myeloid leukemia (CML), Imatinib specifically targets the BCR–ABL tyrosine kinase, a fusion protein resultant from the Philadelphia chromosome mutation characteristic of CML. Imatinib binds to the ATP-binding site of BCR–ABL, inhibiting its activity and thus the proliferative signaling, leading to significant improvements in patient outcomes.
   - *Erlotinib (Tarceva)*: Targets the epidermal growth factor receptor (EGFR), a receptor tyrosine kinase involved in the signaling pathways that drive cell proliferation and survival. Erlotinib is particularly effective in non-small cell lung cancer patients who harbor mutations in the EGFR gene, offering a personalized treatment approach that has been shown to improve survival rates.

2. *Multi Kinase Inhibitors*

   Unlike TKIs that target a single tyrosine kinase, multi-kinase inhibitors block the activity of multiple kinases simultaneously. This broad-spectrum activity can be beneficial in treating cancers where multiple signaling pathways are aberrantly activated:

   - *Sorafenib (Nexavar)*: This inhibitor targets several tyrosine protein kinases, such as those associated with the VEGF receptors (VEGFRs) and the platelet-derived growth factor receptor (PDGFR), as well as the Raf kinases. By inhibiting these kinases, Sorafenib blocks tumor cell proliferation and angiogenesis (the formation of new blood vessels that supply the tumor with nutrients), making it effective in treating advanced renal cell carcinoma and hepatocellular carcinoma (Westerdijk et al. 2020).
   - *Sunitinib (Sutent)*: Similar to Sorafenib, Sunitinib inhibits multiple receptor tyrosine kinases, including those involved in angiogenesis (VEGFRs and PDGFRs) and tumor cell proliferation (KIT, FLT3). Its ability to target these various pathways makes Sunitinib an effective treatment for gastrointestinal stromal tumors and advanced renal cell carcinoma (Westerdijk et al. 2020).

Mechanism of Action and Resistance

The primary mechanism of action of protein kinase inhibitors involves the competitive inhibition of the ATP-binding site of the kinase, preventing ATP from binding and thus halting the kinase's ability to phosphorylate its substrates. This inhibition disrupts the downstream signaling pathways that promote cancer cell growth and survival.

However, resistance to kinase inhibitors can develop, often through mutations in the kinase domain that prevent drug binding or through the activation of alternative signaling pathways that can bypass the blockade. To combat resistance, second- and third-generation inhibitors have been developed, and combination therapies are increasingly used to target multiple pathways simultaneously.

23.2.2 PI3K Inhibitors

PI3Ks play a pivotal role in various cellular processes, including growth, proliferation, differentiation, and survival, by activating the AKT/mTOR signaling pathway. The dysregulation of this pathway is a hallmark of many cancers, making PI3Ks attractive targets for anticancer therapy. PI3K inhibitors, by blocking this pathway, offer a targeted approach to cancer treatment, particularly for tumors with upregulated PI3K/AKT/mTOR signaling (Niu et al. 2019).

Understanding PI3K/AKT/mTOR Pathway

The PI3K/AKT/mTOR pathway is an intracellular signaling pathway important in regulating the cell cycle. It is directly related to cellular quiescence, proliferation, cancer, and longevity. PI3K activation phosphorylates and activates AKT, localizing it in the plasma membrane. AKT can then phosphorylate and inactivate components of the apoptotic machinery, leading to enhanced survival and growth of the cell. mTOR is a downstream target of AKT and serves as a central regulator of cell growth and survival, integrating signals from PI3K and AKT to mediate cell responses to growth factors, nutrient availability, and energy status (Niu et al. 2019):

1. *Idelalisib*:

   - *Target*: Specifically inhibits PI3K delta (δ), a class I PI3K enzyme isoform that is predominantly expressed in hematopoietic cells. This selective inhibition is crucial because it minimizes the impact on other PI3K isoforms that are essential for the normal functions of non-hematologic tissues, potentially reducing side effects.
   - *Clinical Use*: Approved for the treatment of several types of non-Hodgkin lymphoma, including relapsed chronic lymphocytic leukemia (CLL), follicular lymphoma, and small lymphocytic lymphoma, especially in patients who have received at least two prior systemic therapies.

2. *Copanlisib*:

   - *Target*: Acts as a pan-PI3K inhibitor with potent activity against PI3K-alpha (α) and delta (δ) isoforms. The ability to inhibit multiple isoforms of PI3K allows Copanlisib to target a broader range of signaling pathways within cancer cells, potentially leading to more effective tumor suppression.
   - *Clinical Use*: Approved for the treatment of adult patients with relapsed follicular lymphoma who have received at least two prior systemic therapies. Its efficacy in inhibiting both α and δ isoforms makes it valuable in treating follicular lymphoma, where these pathways contribute to the survival and proliferation of lymphoma cells.

Mechanism of Action

PI3K inhibitors bind to the PI3K enzymes, preventing their ability to phosphorylate the 3′ position of the inositol ring of phosphatidylinositol. This inhibition blocks the PI3K/AKT/mTOR pathway downstream signaling, resulting in reduced cell growth, proliferation, and survival. By curtailing this pathway, PI3K inhibitors can induce apoptosis in cancer cells and potentially reduce tumor growth and spread.

23.2.3 Enzyme Inhibitors

Enzyme inhibitors in cancer therapy target enzymes critical for the survival, proliferation, and metastasis of cancer cells. By inhibiting these enzymes, these drugs can interfere with the metabolic and regulatory processes essential for cancer cell growth. Among the enzyme inhibitors, HDAC inhibitors and IDH inhibitors stand out for their unique mechanisms of action and clinical applications (Teppo et al. 2017).

1. *Histone Deacetylase (HDAC) Inhibitors*

HDAC inhibitors represent a class of compounds that play a pivotal role in modulating gene expression through epigenetic mechanisms. By inhibiting HDAC enzymes, these drugs increase the acetylation of histone proteins, leading to a more open chromatin structure and promoting the transcription of genes involved in cell cycle arrest, apoptosis, and differentiation (Ku et al. 2022).

- *Vorinostat (Zolinza)*: Approved for the treatment of cutaneous T-cell lymphoma (CTCL), Vorinostat targets various HDAC enzymes, inducing apoptosis and cell cycle arrest in cancer cells. Its broad-spectrum HDAC inhibitory activity modulates gene expression and disrupts cellular processes vital for tumor growth and survival.
- *Romidepsin (Istodax)*: Like Vorinostat, Romidepsin is used for CTCL and peripheral T-cell lymphoma. It selectively inhibits Class I HDACs, leading to increased histone acetylation, altered gene expression, and induction of cancer cell death.

Mechanism of Action
HDAC inhibitors increase the acetylation of histones, resulting in a less compact and more transcriptionally active chromatin structure. This change in chromatin architecture leads to the upregulation of tumor suppressor genes and downregulation of oncogenes, inducing apoptosis, cell cycle arrest, and differentiation in cancer cells (Montoya et al. 2021).

2. *Isocitrate Dehydrogenase (IDH) Inhibitors*

IDH inhibitors target mutations in the IDH1 and IDH2 enzymes, which are frequently found in certain leukemias and other cancers. These mutations lead to the production of an oncometabolite, 2-hydroxyglutarate (2-HG), which contributes to the oncogenic process through epigenetic dysregulation.

Types and Examples
- *Ivosidenib (Tibsovo)*: A targeted inhibitor of the mutant IDH1 enzyme, Ivosidenib, is used for treating AML with an IDH1 mutation. By inhibiting mutant IDH1, Ivosidenib reduces the levels of the oncometabolite 2-HG, leading to the differentiation of leukemic cells.
- *Enasidenib (Idhifa)*: Targets the mutant IDH2 enzyme and is approved for AML patients with an IDH2 mutation. Similar to Ivosidenib, Enasidenib's inhibition of mutant IDH2 decreases 2-HG production, promoting the differentiation and apoptosis of cancer cells.

Mechanism of Action
IDH inhibitors target the abnormal enzymatic activity of mutant IDH enzymes, preventing the production of the oncometabolite 2-HG. The reduction in 2-HG levels reverses the epigenetic changes associated with the IDH mutation, leading to the differentiation of leukemic cells into normal cells and the restoration of normal hematopoiesis (Ikram et al. 2019; Friday and Adjei 2008).

23.2.4 Receptor Antagonists

Receptor antagonists play a crucial role in the arsenal against cancer by specifically targeting and inhibiting the activity of receptors involved in the signaling pathways that promote tumor growth and progression. Among these, the Smoothened (SMO) receptor antagonists have gained attention for their role in inhibiting the Hedgehog (Hh) signaling pathway, which is pivotal in various cancers, including AML (Savona et al. 2018).

Smoothened (SMO) Receptor and the Hedgehog Signaling Pathway
The Hedgehog signaling pathway is essential for embryonic development and tissue regeneration. However, its aberrant activation is implicated in the growth and spread of various cancers. The pathway is initiated by the binding of Hedgehog ligands to the Patched (PTCH) receptor, relieving PTCH-mediated suppression of the SMO receptor. Activated SMO then propagates intracellular signals that lead to the transcription of genes, promoting cell proliferation, survival, and differentiation.

Glasdegib: A Novel SMO Receptor Antagonist
Glasdegib (Daurismo) stands out as a potent inhibitor of the SMO receptor, designed to block the aberrant activation of the Hedgehog signaling pathway seen in certain cancers, notably AML (Wu et al. 2020).

Clinical Application
- *Acute Myeloid Leukemia (AML)*: Glasdegib has been approved for use in combination with low-dose cytarabine for the treatment of newly diagnosed AML in adult patients who are aged 75 years or older or who have comorbidities that preclude the use of intensive chemotherapy. This approval was based on the clinical benefit observed in trials, demonstrating an improvement in overall survival among patients treated with the glasdegib combination compared to those treated with low-dose cytarabine alone.

Mechanism of Action
- Glasdegib binds to and inhibits the SMO receptor, effectively blocking the Hedgehog signaling pathway. By doing so, it interrupts the downstream signaling that would otherwise promote the survival and proliferation of cancer cells. The inhibition of this pathway is particularly crucial in cancers like AML, where it plays a role in the maintenance of leukemic stem cells that contribute to the disease's progression and relapse (Cortes et al. 2018).

Benefits and Considerations
- *Targeted Therapy*: Glasdegib offers a targeted approach to treating AML, providing an option for patients unable to tolerate more aggressive chemotherapy regimens (Fersing and Mathias 2022).
- *Combination Therapy*: When used in combination with low-dose cytarabine, glasdegib has been shown to improve treatment outcomes, underlining the potential benefits of combining targeted therapies with traditional treatments (Lin et al. 2020).

23.2.5 *Proteasome Inhibitors*

Proteasome inhibitors represent a critical class of anticancer drugs that target the ubiquitin–proteasome system, a pivotal pathway responsible for degrading unneeded or damaged proteins within the cell. By inhibiting the proteasome, these drugs disrupt the delicate balance of protein homeostasis (proteostasis) in cancer cells, leading to an accumulation of proteins that induces cellular stress, cell cycle arrest, and apoptosis. This mechanism has proven particularly effective against multiple myeloma and mantle cell lymphoma, where proteasome inhibitors have become a cornerstone of treatment (Nawrocki et al. 2008).

23.2.5.1 Bortezomib: The First Proteasome Inhibitor

Mechanism of Action

- *Bortezomib (Velcade)* directly inhibits the 26S proteasome's catalytic core, preventing the targeted degradation of proteins involved in cell cycle regulation and apoptosis. This inhibition leads to an accumulation of polyubiquitinated proteins, disrupting various cell signaling pathways, inducing apoptosis, and blocking proliferation in cancer cells (Łuczkowska et al. 2020).

Clinical Applications

- Primarily used in the treatment of *multiple myeloma* and *mantle cell lymphoma*, Bortezomib has dramatically improved outcomes for patients. It can be administered as a single agent or in combination with other therapies, including corticosteroids and immunomodulatory drugs, enhancing its efficacy (Nawrocki et al. 2008).

Considerations

- Bortezomib is known for its neuropathic side effects, which can be a limiting factor in its use. The route of administration (intravenous or subcutaneous) and dosing schedule can impact its tolerability and effectiveness (Jayaweera et al. 2021).

23.2.5.2 Carfilzomib: A Second-Generation Proteasome Inhibitor

Mechanism of Action

- *Carfilzomib (Kyprolis)* works by irreversibly binding to the N-terminal threonine-containing active sites of the 20S proteasome, leading to more sustained inhibition compared to bortezomib. This irreversible binding enhances the drug's ability to induce apoptosis in myeloma cells (Taylor-Harding et al. 2012).

Clinical Applications

- Carfilzomib is approved for the treatment of patients with *multiple myeloma* who have received one or more prior therapies. It is often used in combination with dexamethasone or with both dexamethasone and immunomodulatory agents, offering a potent treatment option that has been shown to improve survival rates in relapsed or refractory cases (Taylor-Harding et al. 2012).

Considerations

- Carfilzomib is generally well-tolerated, with a lower incidence of peripheral neuropathy than bortezomib, making it a suitable option for patients who cannot tolerate bortezomib's neuropathic side effects. However, it is associated with an increased risk of cardiovascular events, which necessitates careful monitoring of patients (Nawrocki et al. 2008).

23.2.6 Tubulin Inhibitor

Tubulin inhibitors target microtubules, which are pivotal for cell division and intracellular transport. By disrupting microtubule dynamics, these drugs inhibit mitosis, leading to cell cycle arrest and apoptosis in rapidly dividing tumor cells (Xiong et al. 2021).

Vincristine (Oncovin) A classic example of a tubulin inhibitor, Vincristine, binds to tubulin dimers, inhibiting their polymerization into microtubules and thus preventing spindle formation during mitosis. It is widely used in various chemotherapy regimens for the treatment of leukemia, lymphoma, and certain solid tumors. Due to its mechanism of action, Vincristine is particularly effective against rapidly dividing cancer cells, but it also affects rapidly dividing normal cells, which accounts for its side effect profile (Lazzarino et al. 2005).

Mechanism of Action

Vincristine's anti-cancer effects are primarily achieved through the disruption of microtubule formation. By binding to the tubulin protein, Vincristine prevents its polymerization, which is essential for microtubule assembly. As a result, the mitotic spindle cannot form, halting cell division at the metaphase–anaphase boundary. This disruption triggers apoptosis, eliminating cancer cells. However, the impact on normal cells, especially those with high proliferative rates, such as hair follicles and gastrointestinal tract cells, leads to side effects, such as alopecia and gastrointestinal disturbances (Hernández-Téllez et al. 2021) (VanderPorten et al. 2009).

23.3 Macromolecule Anticancer Drugs

Macromolecule anticancer drugs represent a significant advancement in the treatment of cancer, offering targeted therapies that leverage the specificity of antibodies and the potency of cytotoxic agents. These drugs have transformed the therapeutic landscape for numerous cancers, providing options that can selectively target cancer cells while sparing healthy tissue to a greater extent than traditional chemotherapies.

23.3.1 Monoclonal Antibodies (mAbs)

Monoclonal antibodies (mAbs) represent a cornerstone of modern cancer therapy, offering targeted treatment options that leverage the immune system's precision to combat malignancies. These laboratory-engineered proteins are designed to bind selectively to specific antigens found on the surface of cancer cells. This binding can achieve several therapeutic effects: direct inhibition of cancer cell growth, recruitment of immune cells to destroy the cancer cells, or the delivery of cytotoxic agents directly to the cancer cells, minimizing damage to healthy tissues (Tassone et al. 2004).

- *Rituximab (Rituxan)*: Rituximab is a pioneering monoclonal antibody that targets the CD20 protein found on the surface of B cells. It is primarily used in the treatment of non-Hodgkin lymphoma and CLL (Morales 2017). Rituximab works through several mechanisms, including the direct induction of apoptosis in B cells and the activation of the body's immune response to attack and destroy the B cells. It may also sensitize cancer cells to the effects of chemotherapy and radiation therapy.
- *Trastuzumab (Herceptin)*: Trastuzumab specifically targets the human EGFR 2 (HER2), which is overexpressed in about 20% of breast cancers. By binding to the HER2 protein, Trastuzumab inhibits the proliferation of tumor cells that overexpress HER2 (Kosaka et al. 2010; Goldstein and Cagan 1982). It also activates immune-mediated mechanisms to further target and destroy the cancer cells. Trastuzumab has significantly improved outcomes for patients with HER2-positive breast cancer, both as a standalone treatment and in combination with chemotherapy.

Enhanced Efficacy and Precision

The development of monoclonal antibodies has revolutionized cancer treatment by offering therapies that are both effective and precise. Unlike traditional chemotherapy, which can indiscriminately affect rapidly dividing cells, monoclonal antibodies selectively target cancer cells, resulting in fewer side effects and improved quality of life for patients. Furthermore, the ability of mAbs to engage the immune system adds a layer of biological complexity to cancer treatment, enabling a more robust and durable response against cancer (Mahmood and Green 2007).

23.3.2 Bispecific Antibody

Bispecific antibodies represent a novel class of therapeutic agents in oncology, designed through advanced genetic and protein engineering techniques to possess two distinct antigen-binding sites. This dual specificity allows these antibodies to simultaneously engage with two different antigens, a feature that can be harnessed to bridge cancer cells with immune effector cells, thereby enhancing the immune system's ability to detect and eliminate cancer cells (Ren et al. 2023).

Example and Mechanism

- *Blinatumomab (Blincyto)*: Blinatumomab is one of the most well-known bispecific T-cell engagers, designed to connect CD19-positive B-cell leukemia and lymphoma cells with CD3-positive cytotoxic T cells. The CD19 antigen is a common marker on the surface of B cells, making it an ideal target for B-cell malignancies. On the other side, CD3 is part of the T-cell receptor complex involved in activating T cells. By binding to both CD19 and CD3, Blinatumomab brings the T cells into close proximity with the cancer cells, facilitating a more efficient and directed immune response against the cancer cells. The engagement of T cells leads to their activation and the subsequent release of cytotoxic enzymes and signaling molecules that induce apoptosis in the targeted B cells (Yi et al. 2012; Yang et al. 2019).

Therapeutic Impact

Blinatumomab's ability to recruit and activate T cells directly at the site of cancer cells provides a potent mechanism for inducing cancer cell death, even in cases where traditional therapies may have failed. This has led to significant therapeutic success, particularly in acute lymphoblastic leukemia patients who are refractory or have relapsed after standard treatments.

Advantages of bispecific antibodies:

- *Enhanced Specificity*: By simultaneously targeting two antigens, bispecific antibodies can more precisely identify and bind to cancer cells, reducing off-target effects and improving therapeutic outcomes (Jana et al. 2016).
- *Immune System Engagement*: The ability to directly engage and activate components of the immune system represents a significant advantage, providing a robust and potentially long-lasting anti-cancer response.
- *Versatility*: The concept of bispecific antibodies can be applied to various combinations of targets, offering a platform for developing treatments for a wide range of cancers.

23.3.3 Antibody–Drug Conjugates (ADCs)

Antibody–drug conjugates (ADCs) represent a sophisticated amalgamation of targeted therapy and chemotherapy, designed to combine the specificity of monoclonal antibodies with the potent cytotoxicity of chemotherapy agents. By targeting specific antigens present in cancer cells, ADCs deliver their cytotoxic payload directly to the tumor site, thereby maximizing tumor cell destruction while minimizing the impact on healthy tissues (Su et al. 2016).

Key Examples and Their Mechanisms

- *Brentuximab Vedotin (Adcetris)*: This ADC targets CD30, a surface antigen expressed on Hodgkin lymphoma and anaplastic large-cell lymphoma cells. The monoclonal antibody component of Brentuximab Vedotin binds specifically to CD30, facilitating the internalization of the ADC into the cancer cell (King et al. 2023). Once inside, the linker connecting the antibody to the cytotoxic payload, a microtubule-disrupting agent (monomethyl auristatin E, MMAE) is cleaved, releasing MMAE to inhibit microtubule assembly. This inhibition leads to cell cycle arrest and apoptosis of the cancer cell.
- *Trastuzumab Emtansine (Kadcyla)*: Designed for the treatment of HER2-positive breast cancer, Trastuzumab Emtansine combines the HER2-targeting capabilities of Trastuzumab with the cytotoxic activity of DM1 (a microtubule inhibitor). Similar to Brentuximab Vedotin, the binding of the antibody component to HER2 facilitates the internalization of the ADC, whereupon the cytotoxic DM1 is released to induce cell death (Filntisi et al. 2016).

Therapeutic Impact

ADCs such as Brentuximab Vedotin and Trastuzumab Emtansine have significantly impacted the treatment landscape for certain cancers, offering new hope to patients with previously limited treatment options. Their ability to deliver highly potent cytotoxic agents directly to cancer cells translates to improved efficacy and reduced systemic toxicity compared to conventional chemotherapy (Li et al. 2022).

Advantages of ADCs

- *Targeted Delivery*: The precision targeting of antigens specific to cancer cells minimizes the exposure of healthy cells to cytotoxic agents, reducing the side effects associated with traditional chemotherapy (Miret et al. 2020).
- *Potent Efficacy*: The use of highly potent cytotoxic drugs, which would be too toxic to administer systemically, becomes possible when their delivery is restricted to cancer cells (Kozak et al. 2013).
- *Versatility and Expansion*: The concept of ADCs can be applied to a wide array of targets and toxic payloads, providing a versatile platform for developing treatments for diverse types of cancer (Li et al. 2022).

23.3.4 Recombinant Immunotoxins

Recombinant immunotoxins represent an innovative class of cancer therapeutics that ingeniously combine the precise targeting capabilities of antibodies (or other ligand-binding domains) with the potent cytotoxicity of toxins derived from bacteria, plants, or animals. These engineered proteins exploit the specificity of antibody–antigen interactions to deliver lethal toxins directly into cancer cells, offering a targeted approach to cancer treatment with the potential for high efficacy and reduced side effects compared to conventional therapies (Chen et al. 2008).

Example and Mechanism

- *Moxetumomab Pasudotox (Lumoxiti)*: This recombinant immunotoxin targets CD22, a cell surface antigen expressed on B cells and widely present in the cells of certain leukemias and lymphomas. Moxetumomab Pasudotox consists of a monoclonal antibody fragment that binds specifically to CD22, fused to a truncated form of pseudomonas exotoxin A (PE38). Upon binding to CD22, the immunotoxin–receptor complex is internalized into the cancer cell, where the toxin portion is released into the cytoplasm. PE38 then catalytically inactivates elongation factor-2 (EF-2) by ADP-ribosylation, halting protein synthesis, and triggering apoptotic cell death (Ochiai et al. 2008).

Therapeutic Impact

Moxetumomab Pasudotox has shown significant efficacy in treating hairy cell leukemia, particularly in patients who have relapsed or are refractory to traditional treatments. Its approval marks a significant advancement in the treatment options available for this rare cancer, providing a new therapeutic avenue for patients with limited alternatives (Dieffenbach and Pastan 2020; Allahyari et al. 2017).

Advantages of Recombinant Immunotoxins

- *High Specificity and Potency*: By harnessing the targeting precision of antibodies and the potent cytotoxic activity of toxins, recombinant immunotoxins can effectively kill cancer cells while minimizing impact on healthy tissues.
- *Mechanism of Action*: The ability to inhibit protein synthesis offers a unique mechanism of action compared to other cancer therapies, potentially overcoming resistance to drugs that target different cellular pathways (Mazor et al. 2018).
- *Versatile Platform*: The recombinant immunotoxin platform allows for the development of new therapies by substituting different targeting ligands and toxins, broadening the potential applications across various types of cancer (Pak et al. 2014).

23.4 Conclusion

This chapter underscores the transformative impact of targeted therapies on the treatment landscape of hematological malignancies. By focusing on specific molecular targets, these therapies offer a more precise, effective, and personalized approach to treatment, significantly improving patient outcomes. Continued research and development in this field holds the promise of further advancements, including overcoming drug resistance and expanding the arsenal of targeted therapies available to clinicians.

References

Allahyari H, Heidari S, Ghamgosha M, Saffarian P, Amani J (2017) Immunotoxin: a new tool for cancer therapy. Tumour Biol 39(2):1010428317692226

Chen KC, Kim J, Li X, Lee B (2008) Modeling recombinant immunotoxin efficacies in solid tumors. Ann Biomed Eng 36:486–512

Cortes JE, Douglas Smith B, Wang ES, Merchant A, Oehler VG, Arellano M et al (2018) Glasdegib in combination with cytarabine and daunorubicin in patients with AML or high-risk MDS: phase 2 study results. Am J Hematol 93(11):1301–1310

Das A, Wei G, Parikh K, Liu D (2015) Selective inhibitors of nuclear export (SINE) in hematological malignancies. Exp Hematol Oncol 4:1–4

Dieffenbach M, Pastan I (2020) Mechanisms of resistance to immunotoxins containing pseudomonas exotoxin a in cancer therapy. Biomol Ther 10(7):979

Fersing C, Mathias F (2022) Update on glasdegib in acute myeloid leukemia–broadening horizons of Hedgehog pathway inhibitors. Acta Pharma 72(1):9–34

Filntisi A, Vlachakis D, Matsopoulos GK (2016) A bioinformatics method for the production of antibody-drug conjugates through site-specific cysteine conjugation. In: Bioinformatics-updated features and applications. IntechOpen

Friday BB, Adjei AA (2008) Advances in targeting the Ras/Raf/MEK/Erk mitogen-activated protein kinase cascade with MEK inhibitors for cancer therapy. Clin Cancer Res 14(2):342–346

Goldstein NI, Cagan RH (1982) Biochemical studies of taste sensation: monoclonal antibody against L-alanine binding activity of catfish taste epithelium. Proc Natl Acad Sci 79(23):7595–7597

Hamid GA (2012) The pattern of hematological malignancies at Al-Gamhouria teaching hospital, Aden, Yemen, from 2008 to 2010. Turk J Hematol 29:342–347

Hernández-Téllez CN, Luque-Alcaraz AG, Plascencia-Jatomea M, Higuera-Valenzuela HJ, Burgos-Hernández M, García-Flores N et al (2021) Synthesis and characterization of a Fe3O4@ PNIPAM-chitosan nanocomposite and its potential application in vincristine delivery. Polymers 13(11):1704

Hou JZ, Ye JC, Pu JJ, Liu H, Ding W, Zheng H, Liu D (2021) Novel agents and regimens for hematological malignancies: recent updates from 2020 ASH annual meeting. J Hematol Oncol 14:1–25

Ikram N, Mirza MU, Vanmeert M, Froeyen M, Salo-Ahen OM, Tahir M et al (2019) Inhibition of oncogenic kinases: an in vitro validated computational approach identified potential multi-target anticancer compounds. Biomol Ther 9(4):124

Jana B, Mohapatra S, Mondal P, Barman S, Pradhan K, Saha A, Ghosh S (2016) α-Cyclodextrin interacts close to vinblastine site of tubulin and delivers curcumin preferentially to the tubulin surface of cancer cell. ACS Appl Mater Interfaces 8(22):13793–13803

Jayaweera SPE, Wanigasinghe Kanakanamge SP, Rajalingam D, Silva GN (2021) Carfilzomib: a promising proteasome inhibitor for the treatment of relapsed and refractory multiple myeloma. Front Oncol 11:740796

King TA, Walsh SJ, Kapun M, Wharton T, Krajcovicova S, Glossop MS, Spring DR (2023) Disulfide re-bridging reagents for single-payload antibody-drug conjugates. Chem Commun 59(65):9868–9871

Kosaka N, Ogawa M, Paik DS, Paik CH, Choyke PL, Kobayashi H (2010) Semiquantitative assessment of the microdistribution of fluorescence-labeled monoclonal antibody in small peritoneal disseminations of ovarian cancer. Cancer Sci 101(3):820–825

Kozak KR, Tsai SP, Fourie-O'Donohue A, dela Cruz Chuh J, Roth L, Cook R et al (2013) Total antibody quantification for MMAE-conjugated antibody–drug conjugates: impact of assay format and reagents. Bioconjug Chem 24(5):772–779

Ku GC, Chapdelaine AG, Ayrapetov MK, Sun G (2022) Identification of lethal inhibitors and inhibitor combinations for mono-driver versus multi-driver triple-negative breast cancer cells. Cancers 14(16):4027

Lazzarino M, Arcaini L, Orlandi E, Iacona I, Bernasconi P, Calatroni S et al (2005) Immunochemotherapy with rituximab, vincristine and 5-day cyclophosphamide for heavily pretreated follicular lymphoma. Oncology 68(2–3):146–153

Li L, Zhang D, Liu B, Lv D, Zhai J, Guan X et al (2022) Antibody-drug conjugates in HER2-positive breast cancer. Chin Med J 135(03):261–267

Lin S, Shaik N, Martinelli G, Wagner AJ, Cortes J, Ruiz-Garcia A (2020) Population pharmacokinetics of glasdegib in patients with advanced hematologic malignancies and solid tumors. J Clin Pharmacol 60(5):605–616

Łuczkowska K, Rogińska D, Ulańczyk Z, Paczkowska E, Schmidt CA, Machaliński B (2020) Molecular mechanisms of bortezomib action: novel evidence for the miRNA–mRNA interaction involvement. Int J Mol Sci 21(1):350

Mahmood I, Green MD (2007) Drug interaction studies of therapeutic proteins or monoclonal antibodies. J Clin Pharmacol 47(12):1540–1554

Mazor R, King EM, Onda M, Cuburu N, Addissie S, Crown D et al (2018) Tolerogenic nanoparticles restore the antitumor activity of recombinant immunotoxins by mitigating immunogenicity. Proc Natl Acad Sci 115(4):E733–E742

Miret J, Camps M, Farràs M, Román R, Erb S, Cianferani S et al (2020) Insight on the impact of the reduction step on the site-directed conjugation of an anti-HER2 cysteine-engineered antibody. ChemistrySelect 5(11):3187–3190

Montoya S, Soong D, Nguyen N, Affer M, Munamarty SP, Taylor J (2021) Targeted therapies in cancer: to be or not to be, selective. Biomedicines 9(11):1591

Morales JO (2017) Formulation and delivery of macromolecules. AAPS PharmSciTech 18(1):1–2

Nawrocki ST, Carew JS, Maclean KH, Courage JF, Huang P, Houghton JA et al (2008) Myc regulates aggresome formation, the induction of Noxa, and apoptosis in response to the combination of bortezomib and SAHA. Blood, J Am Soc Hematol 112(7):2917–2926

Niu J, Wang X, Liang C, Zhang YD, Liu FY, Li HY et al (2019) Suppression of epidermal growth factor receptor-mediated β-catenin nuclear accumulation enhances the anti-tumor activity of phosphoinositide 3-kinase inhibitor in breast cancer. Cell Biol Int 43(8):931–939

Ochiai H, Archer GE, Herndon JE, Kuan CT, Mitchell DA, Bigner DD et al (2008) EGFRvIII-targeted immunotoxin induces antitumor immunity that is inhibited in the absence of CD4+ and CD8+ T cells. Cancer Immunol Immunother 57:115–121

Pak Y, Pastan I, Kreitman RJ, Lee B (2014) Effect of antigen shedding on targeted delivery of immunotoxins in solid tumors from a mathematical model. PLoS One 9(10):e110716

Pang X, Li H, Guan F, Li X (2018) Multiple roles of glycans in hematological malignancies. Front Oncol 8:364

Przybylski GK (2020) Mouse models to study genes involved in hematological malignancies. Blood Sci 2(02):50–53

Ren Y, Wang Y, Liu J, Liu T, Yuan L, Wu C et al (2023) X-ray crystal structure-guided discovery of novel indole analogues as colchicine-binding site tubulin inhibitors with immune-potentiating and antitumor effects against melanoma. J Med Chem 66(10):6697–6714

Savona MR, Pollyea DA, Stock W, Oehler VG, Schroeder MA, Lancet J et al (2018) Phase Ib study of glasdegib, a hedgehog pathway inhibitor, in combination with standard chemotherapy in patients with AML or high-risk MDS. Clin Cancer Res 24(10):2294–2303

Sochacka-Ćwikła A, Mączyński M, Regiec A (2021) FDA-approved drugs for hematological malignancies—the last decade review. Cancers 14(1):87

Su D, Ng C, Khosraviani M, Yu SF, Cosino E, Kaur S, Xu K (2016) Custom-designed affinity capture LC-MS F (ab′) 2 assay for biotransformation assessment of site-specific antibody drug conjugates. Anal Chem 88(23):11340–11346

Tassone P, Goldmacher VS, Neri P, Gozzini A, Shammas MA, Whiteman KR et al (2004) Cytotoxic activity of the maytansinoid immunoconjugate B-B4–DM1 against CD138+ multiple myeloma cells. Blood 104(12):3688–3696

Taylor-Harding B, Agadjanian H, Nassanian H, Kwon S, Guo X, Miller C et al (2012) Indole-3-carbinol synergistically sensitises ovarian cancer cells to bortezomib treatment. Br J Cancer 106(2):333–343

Teppo HR, Soini Y, Karihtala P (2017) Reactive oxygen species-mediated mechanisms of action of targeted cancer therapy. Oxid Med Cell Longev 2017:1485283

VanderPorten EC, Taverna P, Hogan JN, Ballinger MD, Flanagan WM, Fucini RV (2009) The Aurora kinase inhibitor SNS-314 shows broad therapeutic potential with chemotherapeutics and synergy with microtubule-targeted agents in a colon carcinoma model. Mol Cancer Ther 8(4):930–939

Westerdijk K, Desar IM, Steeghs N, van der Graaf WT, van Erp NP, Dutch Pharmacology and Oncology Group (DPOG) (2020) Imatinib, sunitinib and pazopanib: from flat-fixed dosing towards a pharmacokinetically guided personalized dose. Br J Clin Pharmacol 86(2):258–273

Whittle JR, Desai J (2015) Histone deacetylase inhibitors in cancer: what have we learned? Cancer 121(8):1164–1167

Wu F, Zhang C, Zhao C, Wu H, Teng Z, Jiang T, Wang Y (2020) Prostaglandin E1 inhibits GLI2 amplification–associated activation of the Hedgehog pathway and drug refractory tumor growth. Cancer Res 80(13):2818–2832

Xiong C, Chua KC, Stage TB, Priotti J, Kim J, Altman-Merino A et al (2021) Human induced pluripotent stem cell derived sensory neurons are sensitive to the neurotoxic effects of paclitaxel. Clin Transl Sci 14(2):568–581

Yang J, Li Y, Yan W, Li W, Qiu Q, Ye H, Chen L (2019) Covalent modification of Cys-239 in β-tubulin by small molecules as a strategy to promote tubulin heterodimer degradation. J Biol Chem 294(20):8161–8170

Yi X, Zhong B, Smith KM, Geldenhuys WJ, Feng Y, Pink JJ et al (2012) Identification of a class of novel tubulin inhibitors. J Med Chem 55(7):3425–3435

Chapter 24
Comprehensive ICU Management of Chemotherapy for Hematological Malignancies

Shakti Bedanta Mishra

Learning Points

1. Multidisciplinary Collaboration: The delivery of chemotherapy in the ICU demands close coordination among oncologists, ICU specialists, pharmacists, and nursing staff to manage the disease and its critical complications effectively.
2. Indications for Urgent Chemotherapy: Identifying conditions requiring urgent chemotherapy, such as high-grade lymphomas and acute leukemias, is vital for timely interventions that can significantly influence patient outcomes.
3. Management of Chemotherapy-Related Complications: Proactive and reactive strategies to manage complications such as neutropenic sepsis and tumor lysis syndrome are critical to maintaining patient safety and improving survival rates.
4. Dosing Adjustments and Special Considerations: Adjustments based on organ function and consideration of the broader clinical context, including pharmacokinetic changes and the potential for drug interactions, are essential for the effective administration of chemotherapy in critically ill patients.

24.1 Introduction

Hematologic malignancies, including leukemias, lymphomas, and myelomas, pose significant challenges due to their ability to rapidly proliferate abnormal blood cells, thereby impairing the functionality of normal blood cells (Kanji et al. 2020). The cornerstone of treatment for these malignancies is chemotherapy, which is designed to eradicate cancer cells, achieve remission, and extend patient survival (Kanji et al. 2020). Nonetheless, the inherent aggressiveness of these conditions and their treatments frequently necessitates intensive care unit (ICU) admissions to manage both

S. B. Mishra (✉)
Department of Critical Care Medicine, IMS and SUM Hospital, Bhubaneswar, Odisha, India

S. B. Mishra (ed.), *Critical Care Hematology*,
https://doi.org/10.1007/978-981-97-5565-3_24

therapy-induced complications and disease-associated acute incidents (Vijenthira et al. 2020). The administration of chemotherapy within the ICU is vital for managing the malignancy and simultaneously addressing acute complications, such as significant infections, respiratory distress, and multi-organ failure (Hong et al. 2022).

The care of patients with hematologic malignancies in the ICU setting demands specialized attention due to an increased susceptibility to infections, potential for organ toxicity, and the intricacies of handling chemotherapy's adverse effects in critically ill patients (Rivera et al. 2020). The collaborative efforts of oncologists, intensive care specialists, and pharmacists are crucial to ensuring the safe and efficacious administration of chemotherapy, particularly in adjusting dosages for patients with renal or hepatic dysfunction (Pastores et al. 2018). Decisions regarding the initiation or continuation of chemotherapy in the ICU are laden with ethical considerations, balancing the advantages of treatment against potential risks and taking into account the patient's prognosis and quality of life (Barth et al. 2018).

Research has demonstrated that the outcomes of patients with hematologic malignancies undergoing chemotherapy in the ICU are distinct and vary according to the type of anticancer medication employed (Shaz et al. 2022). The ICU emerges as a pivotal center for comprehensive multidisciplinary care, harmonizing aggressive cancer therapy with supportive critical care measures to optimize patient results (Getz et al. 2015). Recognizing the intricacies involved in administering chemotherapy in such a critical setting is essential for effectively navigating the complexities of care, ensuring both effective cancer treatment and supportive patient care (Namendys-Silva et al. 2013).

24.2 ICU Management of Hematological Malignancies

The management of hematological malignancies within the ICU demands an integrated approach that adeptly combines rigorous cancer therapy with precise critical care, as delineated by Ileri et al. (2020). Critical factors influencing the decision to admit patients with hematological malignancies to the ICU include the severity of the patient's condition, the potential for treatment reversibility, complications arising from treatment, disease progression, and considerations of the patient's wishes and expected outcomes (Demandt et al. 2017). Notably, common complications that necessitate ICU intervention in these patients include neutropenic sepsis, respiratory failure, acute kidney injury, tumor lysis syndrome (TLS), gastrointestinal complications, as well as hemorrhagic and thrombotic events, and cardiac issues (Rawson et al. 2019).

The effective navigation of these challenges requires the concerted efforts of a multidisciplinary team, which should include oncologists, hematologists, intensivists, pharmacists, nursing personnel, and various support staff (Hung et al. 2013). Research has illuminated that the survival rates of patients with hematological malignancies admitted to the ICU are significantly impacted by their functional status and existing comorbidities (Horster et al. 2012). Ethical considerations, alongside patient preferences and prognostic insights, are pivotal in guiding decisions related to ICU admissions and the scope of interventions administered (Claustre et al. 2020).

The ICU acts as an essential hub for the specialized care of patients with hematological malignancies, emphasizing the importance of timely interventions, proactive management of adverse effects, and the prioritization of patient-centric care (Malak et al. 2014). A deep understanding of the factors predictive of ICU admission, patient outcomes, and mortality influencers is indispensable for enhancing the quality of care and patient survival rates (Mo et al. 2021). Moreover, the dynamic nature of therapeutic advancements, improvements in supportive care measures, and the rising prevalence of hematological malignancies highlight the critical need for ongoing research and collaborative endeavors within this domain (Fujiwara et al. 2016).

24.3 Chemotherapy in the ICU: Feasibility and Indications

Administering chemotherapy in the ICU for patients with hematologic malignancies represents a critical and nuanced approach, gaining acknowledgment for its viability and importance (Darmon et al. 2005). The feasibility of this approach is underpinned by the concerted efforts of a multidisciplinary healthcare team, adherence to protocols for the safe handling of chemotherapeutic agents, advanced patient monitoring systems, and rigorous selection of patients (Kanji et al. 2020). The exigency of chemotherapy in the context of hematologic malignancies is particularly pronounced for conditions such as high-grade lymphomas, acute leukemias, cases of leukostasis, imminent organ failure, TLS, neutropenic sepsis, and as interim therapy pending more definitive treatment strategies (Shaz et al. 2022). Critical to the decision-making process for chemotherapy administration in the ICU are considerations of the patient's prognosis, potential for recuperation, and personal treatment preferences (Rivera et al. 2020).

The effective execution of chemotherapy in the ICU setting demands a robust collaboration among oncologists, ICU specialists, pharmacists, and nursing staff, supported by appropriate infrastructure and monitoring facilities, alongside stringent criteria for patient eligibility (Darmon et al. 2005). This multidisciplinary team is pivotal in managing urgent chemotherapy for patients facing rapidly advancing diseases and life-threatening complications such as leukostasis and potential organ failure (Shaz et al. 2022). The ICU provides a critical environment for the safe administration of chemotherapy, offering vital support to critically ill patients battling hematologic malignancies, thereby underscoring the essential role of comprehensive care in these high-risk scenarios (Rivera et al. 2020).

Multidisciplinary Collaboration The successful delivery of chemotherapy in the ICU hinges on the close collaboration of a multidisciplinary team, including oncologists, hematologists, intensivists, pharmacists, and specially trained nursing staff.

This team approach ensures comprehensive care that addresses both malignancy and critical illness:

- *Infrastructure and Protocols*: Modern ICUs are equipped with the necessary infrastructure to safely administer chemotherapy, including facilities for the preparation and safe handling of cytotoxic drugs. Protocols are in place for the management of potential side effects and complications, ensuring patient safety.
- *Monitoring and Support*: The ICU setting offers advanced monitoring and support capabilities, such as continuous hemodynamic monitoring and access to rapid intervention for complications like TLS or sepsis, which are crucial for patients undergoing chemotherapy.
- *Patient Selection*: Feasibility also depends on careful patient selection, prioritizing individuals who are likely to benefit from ICU-level care and whose condition is potentially reversible with intensive support and chemotherapy.

Indications for Urgent Chemotherapy in Hematological Patients

- *High-Grade Lymphomas and Acute Leukemias*: Patients with rapidly progressing diseases such as high-grade lymphomas or acute leukemias may require urgent chemotherapy to control disease progression and mitigate life-threatening complications.

  1. *Hyperleukocytic Acute Myeloid Leukemia (AML)* is characterized by markedly elevated leukocyte counts, which can precipitate risks such as leukostasis, TLS, and disseminated intravascular coagulation (Bewersdorf et al. 2020). The therapeutic approach prioritizes immediate chemotherapy and supportive interventions, with initial cytoreductive strategies (for instance, hydroxyurea) being advocated to lessen TLS risks (Cortes et al. 2020). The utility of leukapheresis in rapidly reducing leukocyte counts is debated, particularly in terms of its effectiveness in improving patient survival.
  2. *Acute Promyelocytic Leukemia (APL)*, a distinct variant of AML, is notorious for its association with severe coagulopathy, elevating the risk of hemorrhage. Prompt initiation of therapy with all-transretinoic acid (ATRA) and anthracyclines is deemed critical, more so in instances of hyperleukocytosis. Moreover, preventative measures against bleeding through supportive care are paramount. APL differentiation syndrome, a grave complication arising from treatment with ATRA or arsenic trioxide, necessitates swift intervention with corticosteroids.
  3. *Hemophagocytic Lymphohistiocytosis (HLH)* is indicative of an overactive immune response, potentially culminating in life-threatening, sepsis-like organ dysfunction. The diagnosis hinges on specific markers, including persistent fever, splenomegaly, and cytopenias. Management strategies emphasize supportive care and addressing the root cause, frequently employing a regimen of etoposide and corticosteroids for immediate impact.
  4. *Acute Lung Injury in Acute Monocytic Leukemia* is particularly prevalent among patients diagnosed with specific leukemia subtypes (FAB classifica-

tions M4 or M5), often manifesting pulmonary complications attributable to leukostasis or infiltration. The therapeutic regimen may incorporate corticosteroids in conjunction with traditional cytoreduction and chemotherapy, aiming to diminish mortality rates.

- *Leukostasis and Hyperleukocytosis*: In conditions such as acute myeloid leukemia with leukostasis, immediate chemotherapy is necessary to reduce leukocyte counts and prevent or treat organ dysfunction.
- *Impending Organ Failure*: Urgent chemotherapy may be indicated for tumors causing imminent risk of organ failure, such as spinal cord compression or superior vena cava syndrome.
- *Tumor Lysis Syndrome (TLS)*: Although TLS is a complication of chemotherapy, in some instances, urgent chemotherapy is required to reduce tumor burden in a controlled manner alongside aggressive supportive measures to manage or prevent TLS.
- *Neutropenic Sepsis*: While not an indication for chemotherapy per se, patients with neutropenic sepsis may require continuation or initiation of chemotherapy once infections are under control, especially if the underlying malignancy contributes to the immune-compromised state.
- *Chemotherapy as Bridge to More Definitive Treatment*: For some patients, chemotherapy in the ICU may serve as a bridging therapy to stabilize them for more definitive treatments such as stem cell transplantation.
- The decision to administer chemotherapy in the ICU involves a complex interplay of factors, including the patient's overall prognosis, potential for recovery, and, critically, the patient and family's preferences and goals of care. The ICU setting, with its comprehensive support services, offers a unique environment where chemotherapy can be administered safely to critically ill patients, potentially improving outcomes for those with hematological malignancies (Fig. 24.1).

24.4 Specific Complications and Management

Chemotherapy, while a cornerstone in the treatment of hematological malignancies, is associated with a range of complications. The ICU setting demands not only a proactive approach to the prevention of these complications but also a swift and effective management strategy when they arise.

Chemotherapy-Related Complications and Management Strategies

- *Neutropenic Sepsis*

Management: Immediate empirical antibiotic therapy is crucial, following guidelines that cover a broad spectrum of potential pathogens. The choice of antibiotics may be adjusted based on culture results and patient-specific factors, including any known drug allergies and renal or hepatic function. Granulocyte colony-stimulating factor can be used to expedite neutrophil recovery (Catania et al. 2017).

Comprehensive ICU Management of Chemotherapy for Hematological Malignancies

Overview of ICU Chemotherapy Management

- Multidisciplinary teams, including **oncologists, ICU specialists, pharmacists, and nurses,** collaborate to deliver specialized chemotherapy within the ICU.
- This approach focuses on managing critical complications and adjusting chemotherapy doses according to patient organ function.

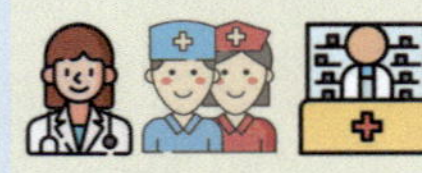

Key Indications for Chemotherapy in the ICU

- Chemotherapy in the ICU is crucial for conditions like **high-grade lymphomas and acute leukemias,** where immediate treatment can control disease progression and **manage severe complications such as tumor lysis syndrome and neutropenic sepsis.**

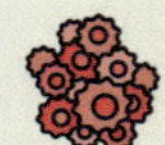

Patient Monitoring and Infrastructure

- ICUs are equipped with **advanced monitoring systems** and infrastructure to safely administer chemotherapy.
- This includes specialized facilities for the preparation and handling of cytotoxic drugs, ensuring **patient safety.**

Dosing Adjustments

- Chemotherapy dosing in the ICU is carefully adjusted based on **renal and hepatic** function to prevent toxicity.
- This includes considerations for patients with multi-organ dysfunction, ensuring effective and safe treatment.

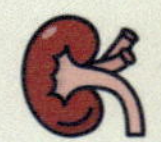
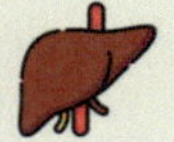

Ethical and Quality of Life Considerations

- ICU chemotherapy involves ethical decisions balancing treatment **benefits against risks.**
- Discussions focus on aligning care with **patient and family goals,** emphasizing quality of life and informed decision-making.

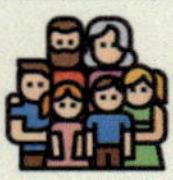

Fig. 24.1 Comprehensive ICU management of chemotherapy for hematological malignancies

- *Tumor Lysis Syndrome (TLS)*

Management: TLS requires aggressive hydration to maintain high urine output, allopurinol or rasburicase to reduce uric acid levels, and careful monitoring and correction of electrolyte imbalances. In severe cases, renal replacement therapy may be necessary (Tosi et al. 2008).

- *Acute Kidney Injury (AKI)*

Management: Management includes ensuring adequate hydration, adjusting doses of nephrotoxic agents or discontinuing them if possible, and monitoring renal function closely. In cases where AKI is severe, dialysis may be required (Krishnappa et al. 2016).

- *Gastrointestinal Toxicity*

Management: Prophylactic use of anti-emetics for nausea and vomiting, aggressive management of diarrhea with anti-motility agents, and monitoring for signs of typhlitis (neutropenic enterocolitis). Supportive care, including nutritional support and, in severe cases, parenteral nutrition, may be necessary (Catania et al. 2017).

- *Hemorrhagic Complications*

Management: Thrombocytopenia, common during chemotherapy, is managed with platelet transfusions to maintain platelet counts above a critical threshold, typically 10,000–20,000/μL or higher if there is active bleeding or a planned invasive procedure. The use of agents such as tranexamic acid may be considered to control bleeding (Rivera-Gamma and Davis 2023).

- *Hepatotoxicity*

Management: Monitoring liver function tests (LFTs) before and during chemotherapy, avoiding or adjusting the dose of hepatotoxic drugs, and using supportive treatments for liver dysfunction. In severe cases, management may involve discontinuing the offending agent and supportive care while the liver recovers.

- *Cardiotoxicity*

Management: Early recognition of cardiotoxicity involves monitoring cardiac function (e.g., echocardiograms) before and during treatment with cardiotoxic agents. Management includes using cardioprotective agents (e.g., dexrazoxane), adjusting doses, or discontinuing the offending agent. Treatment of congestive heart failure symptoms follows standard guidelines, including the use of ACE inhibitors, beta-blockers, and diuretics.

- *Pulmonary Toxicity*

Management: Early identification of chemotherapy-induced lung injury is critical using imaging and pulmonary function tests. Management involves discontinuing the offending agent and initiating corticosteroids for inflammatory lung injury. Supportive care includes supplemental oxygen and, in severe cases, mechanical ventilation.

- *Neurotoxicity*

Management: Monitoring for signs of neurotoxicity, such as peripheral neuropathy or central nervous system effects. Adjusting chemotherapy doses or discontinuing the offending agent may be necessary. Symptomatic treatment includes pain management for neuropathy and seizure prophylaxis if indicated.

For all these complications, a key aspect of management in the ICU is the close collaboration between oncologists, intensivists, pharmacists, and nursing staff, ensuring that complications are anticipated, promptly recognized, and effectively managed. This integrated approach maximizes the safety and efficacy of chemotherapy administration in critically ill patients with hematological malignancies.

24.5 Dosing Adjustments and Special Considerations

Administering chemotherapy to patients with hematological malignancies in the ICU requires meticulous attention to dosing adjustments, particularly in the context of organ failure. In addition, the ICU setting presents unique challenges that necessitate special considerations to ensure the safe and effective delivery of chemotherapy.

Adjusting Chemotherapy Doses in Organ Failure

- *Renal Impairment*:

  - Many chemotherapy agents are excreted via the kidneys, and renal impairment can lead to increased toxicity due to decreased drug clearance. Dose adjustments are often necessary based on the level of renal function, typically estimated using creatinine clearance or glomerular filtration rate.
  - Drugs such as methotrexate, platinum compounds (e.g., cisplatin), and certain alkylating agents may require significant dose reductions or avoidance in patients with reduced renal function (Pastores et al. 2018).

- *Hepatic Dysfunction*:

  - Hepatic impairment affects drug metabolism, necessitating dose adjustments for agents metabolized primarily in the liver. This includes drugs such as anthracyclines (doxorubicin), taxanes, and some monoclonal antibodies.
  - Monitoring LFTs is crucial, and doses may be adjusted based on specific parameters such as bilirubin levels and hepatic enzyme elevations (Pastores et al. 2018).

- *Combined Organ Dysfunction*:

  - Patients with multi-organ dysfunction present a particularly complex scenario for chemotherapy dosing. In such cases, a careful evaluation of the risks and benefits of chemotherapy is necessary, often requiring consultation with a pharmacist specializing in oncology for individualized dosing strategies (Pastores et al. 2018).

Special Considerations for Administering Chemotherapy in ICU Settings

- *Pharmacokinetic and Pharmacodynamic Variability*:

  - Critical illness can alter drug pharmacokinetics and pharmacodynamics, affecting drug absorption, distribution, metabolism, and excretion. Close monitoring of drug levels and effects, when possible, is advised to guide dosing adjustments (Lew et al. 2017).

- *Drug Interactions*:

  - The risk of drug–drug interactions is heightened in the ICU due to the complex medication regimens often required for critically ill patients. Potential interactions between chemotherapy agents and other medications (e.g., antibiotics, antifungals, and cardiovascular drugs) necessitate thorough review and management strategies to avoid adverse effects (Brunstein et al. 2019).

- *Nutritional and Fluid Status*:

  - Changes in fluid balance and nutritional status can impact chemotherapy dosing and toxicity. Fluid overload or depletion and alterations in albumin levels can affect drug distribution and efficacy, requiring adjustments in fluid management and nutritional support (Barth et al. 2018).

- *Infection Control and Neutropenic Precautions*:

  - Infection control is paramount in the ICU, particularly for patients receiving chemotherapy who are at increased risk for neutropenia. Strict adherence to neutropenic precautions and aggressive management of infections are critical (Yeary et al. 2020).

- *Patient and Family Communication*:
  - Discussing the goals of care, potential benefits, and risks of chemotherapy in the ICU setting is essential. Transparent communication with patients (when possible) and families about the expected outcomes and possible side effects of treatment is crucial for informed decision-making (de Man et al. 2019).

- *End-of-Life Care Considerations*:
  - For some patients, the focus may shift from aggressive treatment to palliative care. Decisions regarding the continuation or withholding of chemotherapy in the ICU should be made in the context of the patient's overall prognosis, quality of life considerations, and wishes (Garcia Borrega et al. 2023).

Administering chemotherapy in the ICU demands a highly individualized approach, with adjustments based on organ function, careful management of potential drug interactions, and consideration of the broader clinical context. A multidisciplinary team effort is essential to navigate these complexities and optimize patient outcomes (Song et al. 2011).

24.6 Long-Term Outcomes and Quality of Life

Long-term outcomes and quality of life are crucial considerations in the management of hematological malignancies in the ICU, especially with the use of chemotherapy. Short-term survival rates have seen improvements due to advancements in ICU care and chemotherapy, although mortality rates for this patient group remain significant (Vanhorebeek et al. 2020). Factors such as cancer type, stage, age, comorbidities, and critical illness leading to ICU admission influence survival rates. Long-term survival outcomes post-ICU care and chemotherapy vary, with some patients achieving remission while others face relapse or long-term complications (Orwelius et al. 2010). The integration of targeted therapies and personalized medicine shows promise in enhancing long-term survival rates but requires continuous monitoring for late-onset side effects.

24.7 Conclusion

The administration of chemotherapy for hematological malignancies within the ICU setting presents a unique intersection of oncologic precision and critical care. This approach, though complex, offers a vital lifeline to patients facing life-threatening complications of their disease or treatment. The key points outlined in this chapter underscore the necessity of a nuanced, multidisciplinary approach to patient care, emphasizing the need for dose adjustments in the presence of organ failure and addressing the myriad challenges and special considerations inherent to the ICU setting.

Summary of Key Points

- *Feasibility and Indications*: Administering chemotherapy in the ICU is feasible with the appropriate infrastructure and a multidisciplinary team. Indications for such an approach often include managing acute complications of hematological malignancies or the side effects of chemotherapy itself.
- *Complications and Management*: The array of potential complications, from neutropenic sepsis to TLS, requires vigilant monitoring, rapid intervention, and tailored management strategies to mitigate risk and optimize patient outcomes.
- *Dosing Adjustments*: Critical illness and organ dysfunction necessitate careful adjustment of chemotherapy doses, with special considerations given to the pharmacokinetic and pharmacodynamic changes that can affect drug efficacy and toxicity.
- *Quality of Life*: The impact of ICU care and chemotherapy on patients' quality of life and long-term survival rates is profound, emphasizing the importance of clear communication, shared decision-making, and, when appropriate, discussions about goals of care and end-of-life preferences.

Future Directions for Research and Clinical Practice

- *Personalized Medicine*: Advances in genomics and pharmacogenetics offer the promise of more personalized, targeted therapies that could reduce toxicity and improve outcomes for patients receiving chemotherapy in the ICU.
- *Integration of Palliative Care*: Early integration of palliative care principles into the management of critically ill patients with hematological malignancies could improve quality of life, aid in the navigation of complex treatment decisions, and ensure that care aligns with patients' values and preferences.
- *Technological Advances*: The development of novel drug delivery systems and monitoring technologies could enhance the safety and precision of chemotherapy administration in critically ill patients.
- *Interdisciplinary Training*: Enhancing the training of oncologists, intensivists, pharmacists, and nursing staff in the nuances of delivering chemotherapy in the ICU setting can improve patient care. This includes expanding knowledge on dose adjustments for organ dysfunction and managing the unique challenges of critical illness.

- *Patient-Centered Outcomes Research*: Further research focusing on patient-centered outcomes, including quality of life and functional status post-ICU discharge, is essential to inform future clinical guidelines and support shared decision-making processes.

Flowchart

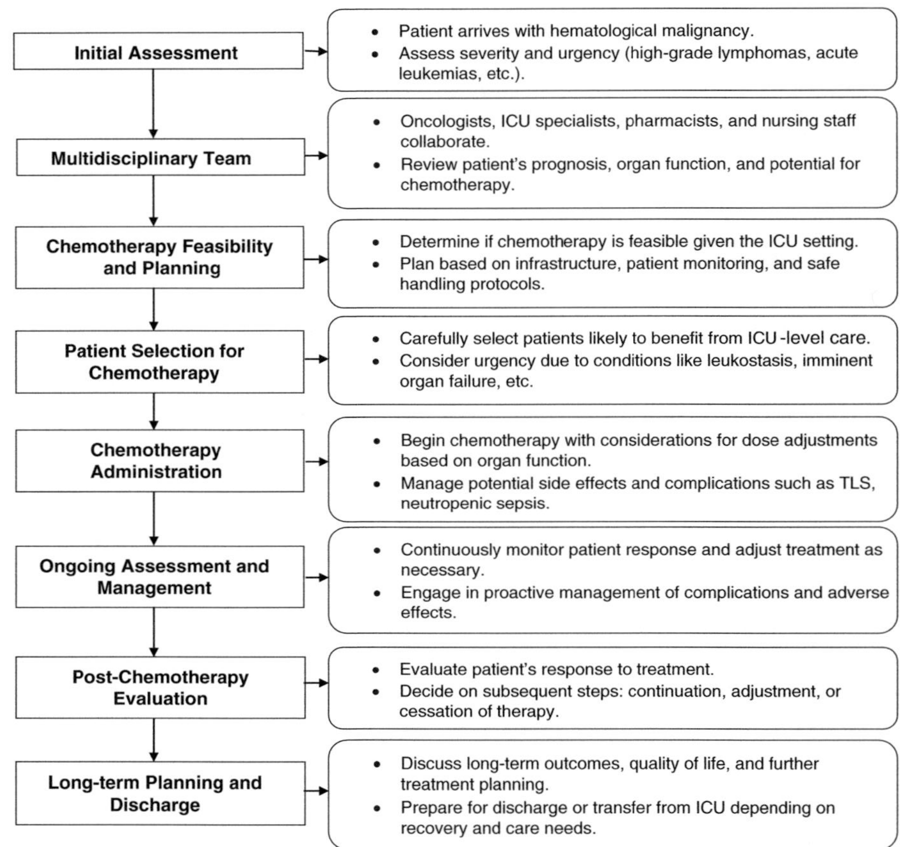

References

Barth C, Soares M, Toffart AC, Timsit JF, Burghi G, Irrazabal C et al (2018) Characteristics and outcome of patients with newly diagnosed advanced or metastatic lung cancer admitted to intensive care units (ICUs). Ann Intensive Care 8:1–9

Bewersdorf JP, Giri S, Tallman MS, Zeidan AM, Stahl M (2020) Leukapheresis for the management of hyperleukocytosis in acute myeloid leukemia—a systematic review and meta-analysis. Transfusion 60(10):2360–2369

Brunstein CG, Pasquini MC, Kim S, Fei M, Adekola K, Ahmed I et al (2019) Effect of conditioning regimen dose reduction in obese patients undergoing autologous hematopoietic cell transplantation. Biol Blood Marrow Transplant 25(3):480–487

Catania VE, Vecchio M, Malaguarnera M, Madeddu R, Malaguarnera G, Latteri S (2017) Tumor lysis syndrome in an extraskeletal osteosarcoma: a case report and review of the literature. J Med Case Rep 11:1–5

Claustre J, Larcher R, Jouve T, Truche AS, Nseir S, Cadiet J et al (2020) Mucormycosis in intensive care unit: surgery is a major prognostic factor in patients with hematological malignancy. Ann Intensive Care 10:1–12

Cortes JE, de Lima M, Dombret H, Estey EH, Giralt SA, Montesinos P et al (2020) Prevention, recognition, and management of adverse events associated with gemtuzumab ozogamicin use in acute myeloid leukemia. J Hematol Oncol 13:1–8

Darmon M, Thiery G, Ciroldi M, de Miranda S, Galicier L, Raffoux E et al (2005) Intensive care in patients with newly diagnosed malignancies and a need for cancer chemotherapy. Crit Care Med 33(11):2488–2493

de Man Y, Atsma F, Oosterveld-Vlug MG, Brom L, Onwuteaka-Philipsen BD, Westert GP, Groenewoud AS (2019) The intensity of hospital care utilization by Dutch patients with lung or colorectal cancer in their final months of life. Cancer Control 26(1):1073274819846574

Demandt AM, Geerse DA, Janssen BJ, Winkens B, Schouten HC, van Mook WN (2017) The prognostic value of a trend in modified SOFA score for patients with hematological malignancies in the intensive care unit. Eur J Haematol 99(4):315–322

Fujiwara Y, Yamaguchi H, Kobayashi K, Marumo A, Omori I, Yamanaka S et al (2016) The therapeutic outcomes of mechanical ventilation in hematological malignancy patients with respiratory failure. Intern Med 55(12):1537–1545

Garcia Borrega J, Böll B, Kochanek M, Naendrup JH, Simon F, Sieg N et al (2023) Characteristics and outcomes of patients undergoing high-dose chemotherapy and autologous stem cell transplantation admitted to the intensive care unit: a single-center retrospective analysis. Ann Hematol 102(1):191–197

Getz KD, Miller TP, Seif AE, Li Y, Huang YS, Bagatell R et al (2015) A comparison of resource utilization following chemotherapy for acute myeloid leukemia in children discharged versus children that remain hospitalized during neutropenia. Cancer Med 4(9):1356–1364

Hong Y, Hong JY, Park J (2022) Differences in ICU outcomes according to the type of anticancer drug in lung cancer patients. Front Med 9:824266

Horster S, Stemmler HJ, Mandel PC, Mück A, Tischer J, Hausmann A et al (2012) Mortality of patients with hematological malignancy after admission to the intensive care unit. Oncol Res Treat 35(10):556–561

Hung YS, Wu JH, Chang H, Wang PN, Kao CY, Wang HM et al (2013) Characteristics of patients with hematologic malignancies who received palliative care consultation services in a medical center. Am J Hosp Palliat Med 30(8):773–780

Ileri I, Coskun R, Temel S, Gundogan K, Sungur M (2020) Evaluation of national early warning system for mortality in hematological malignancy patients admitted to intensive care unit: prospective, single center, observational study. J Crit Intensive Care 11(2):NA–NA

Kanji S, MacLean E, Rashid FJ, Pittman M, Trinacty M, Allan D, Rosenberg E (2020) Chemotherapy in the intensive care unit: an evaluation of context and outcomes. Can J Hosp Pharm 73(4):279

Krishnappa V, Gupta M, Manu G, Kwatra S, Owusu OT, Raina R (2016) Acute kidney injury in hematopoietic stem cell transplantation: a review. Int J Nephrol 2016:5163789

Lew CCH, Wong GJY, Cheung KP, Chua AP, Chong MFF, Miller M (2017) Association between malnutrition and 28-day mortality and intensive care length-of-stay in the critically ill: a prospective cohort study. Nutrients 10(1):10

Malak S, Sotto JJ, Ceccaldi J, Colombat P, Casassus P, Jaulmes D et al (2014) Ethical and clinical aspects of intensive care unit admission in patients with hematological malignancies: guidelines of the ethics commission of the French society of hematology. Adv Hematol 2014:1

Mo L, Urbauer DL, Bruera E, Hui D (2021) Recommendations for palliative and hospice care in NCCN guidelines for treatment of cancer. Oncologist 26(1):77–83

Namendys-Silva S, Correa-García P, López-Basave H, García-Guillùn F, Texcocano-Becerra J, Herrera-Gómez A (2013) Organ dysfunction in critically ill cancer patients undergoing cytoreductive surgery with hyperthermic intraperitoneal chemotherapy. Chest 144(4):548A

Orwelius L, Nordlund A, Nordlund P, Simonsson E, Bäckman C, Samuelsson A, Sjöberg F (2010) Pre-existing disease: the most important factor for health related quality of life long-term after critical illness: a prospective, longitudinal, multicentre trial. Crit Care 14:1–10

Pastores SM, Goldman DA, Shaz DJ, Kostelecky N, Daley RJ, Peterson TJ et al (2018) Characteristics and outcomes of patients with hematologic malignancies receiving chemotherapy in the intensive care unit. Cancer 124(14):3025–3036

Rawson JL, Fagan FM, Burrough GC, Tang HM, Cuncannon MA, Ellem KL, Enjeti AK (2019) Intensive care unit outcomes in patients with hematological malignancy. Blood Sci 1(03):189–193

Rivera MJ, Do B, Bryan JC, Shigle TL, Patel R (2020) Complications and toxicities associated with cancer therapies in the intensive care unit. Oncol Crit Care:201–227

Rivera-Gamma S, Davis ME (2023) CE: Tumor lysis syndrome: an oncologic emergency. Am J Nurs 123(3):30–35

Shaz D, Pastores SM, Dayal L, Berkowitz J, Kostelecky N, Tan KS, Halpern N (2022) Analysis of intent and reason for oncologic therapy administration in cancer patients admitted to the intensive care unit. J Intensive Care Med 37(10):1305–1311

Song JU, Suh GY, Chung MP, Kim H, Kwon OJ, Jung CW et al (2011) Risk factors to predict outcome in critically ill cancer patients receiving chemotherapy in the intensive care unit. Support Care Cancer 19:491–495

Tosi P, Barosi G, Lazzaro C, Liso V, Marchetti M, Morra E et al (2008) Consensus conference on the management of tumor lysis syndrome. Haematologica 93:1877–1885

Vanhorebeek I, Latronico N, Van den Berghe G (2020) ICU-acquired weakness. Intensive Care Med 46(4):637–653

Vijenthira A, Chiu N, Jacobson D, Freedman Z, Cheung MC, Goddard S et al (2020) Predictors of intensive care unit admission in patients with hematologic malignancy. Sci Rep 10(1):21145

Yeary J, Greco A, McKnight R, Petros K, Schaefer G, Garavaglia J (2020) Adjusted vs total body weight–based dosing of sedation and analgesia used in the intensive care unit. Hosp Pharm 55(6):400–404

Chapter 25
Hematopoietic Stem Cell Transplantations (HSCT) and Implications in Critically Ill

Kishore Kumar

Learning Points

1. Understanding Hematopoietic Stem Cell Transplantation (HSCT) Types and Their Implications: Learning about the two primary types of HSCT-autologous (using the patient's own stem cells) and allogeneic (using donor stem cells) is crucial.
2. Management of HSCT Recipients in the Intensive Care Unit (ICU): The management of HSCT recipients in the ICU is complex due to their severe immunosuppression and susceptibility to opportunistic infections.
3. Complications Associated with HSCT: HSCT recipients are prone to a range of complications, including but not limited to severe graft-versus-host disease, sepsis, and atypical viral infections. Understanding these complications, their presentation, and management strategies is vital for ICU clinicians.
4. Role of Multidisciplinary Approach in HSCT Patient Care: The care of HSCT recipients, especially when they become critically ill, requires a multidisciplinary approach. This involves collaboration among hematologists, transplant specialists, intensivists, nurses, and pharmacists.

K. Kumar (✉)
Haemato-Oncology & BMT, MIOT International Hospital, Chennai, India

S. B. Mishra (ed.), *Critical Care Hematology*,
https://doi.org/10.1007/978-981-97-5565-3_25

25.1 Introduction

25.1.1 Basics of Bone Marrow Transplant: Agriculture in an HEPA-Filtered Room

Hematopoietic stem cells play a crucial role in the continuous division and replacement of cells in the peripheral blood. These master cells undergo division and differentiate into various blood cell types within the bone marrow. Defective stem cells pose a challenge in blood cancers such as leukemias or inherited diseases such as immunodeficiency, thalassemia, or sickle cell anemia. To treat these entities, healthy stem cells from a donor are required to replace the faulty ones. Conversely, conditions such as myeloma, lymphoma, and certain autoimmune disorders are characterized by normal stem cells but abnormalities in mature differentiated cells like lymphocytes. In such cases, a high dose of chemotherapy is administered to eliminate these mature cells, which, unfortunately, may also affect the stem cells as a side effect. Therefore, before treatment, the patient's stem cells are collected and reinfused after the chemotherapy to rescue the bone marrow. This process can be likened to agricultural practices where weeds are physically removed or eradicated with weed killer.

Similarly, cancer cells or genetically defective cells are targeted using intensive chemotherapy or immunotherapy over multiple cycles. Once the unwanted cells are eliminated, the bone marrow needs to be prepared for new stem cells, comparable to ploughing the land to make it receptive to new seeds. This is achieved through conditioning therapy, which involves intensified chemotherapy, and in some cases, similar to a mini nuclear explosion, total body irradiation is delivered to create a receptive environment in the marrow. The collected stem cells are then returned to the patient's bloodstream through the peripheral vein, eventually settling and growing in the bone marrow to produce new blood cells, similar to the growth of crops. However, this process takes several weeks, and patients undergoing this transition may require intensive care unit (ICU) care. Before the transplant, patients are started on various prophylactic medications to mitigate expected side effects, as the drugs used during the conditioning regimen can potentially cause significant organ failures. In allogeneic transplants, the cells perceive themselves as in a new body after the infusion of stem cells. They may initiate an immune response against the recipient's body, known as graft-versus-host disease (GVHD) (Scales et al. 2008).

Consequently, drugs are administered to prevent or treat GVHD in the allograft, although GVHD itself or drug-related side effects can still occur. During the neutropenic period, such as a culture medium, the patient becomes highly susceptible to atypical infections, uncommon in immunocompetent ICU patients. Therefore, having a thorough understanding of the phases involved in bone marrow transplantation procedures is crucial for providing optimal care to patients in the ICU.

25.1.2 Timepoints When Intensivists Encounter BMT Patients

There are four distinct timelines when a bone marrow transplant (BMT) patient may require transfer to the ICU (Fig. 25.1).

A. *The First Timeline Occurs During the Start of the Conditioning Regimen*:

   In these cases, the patient would have been recently cleared by various physicians, such as pulmonologists, nephrologists, cardiologists, dental surgeons, and psychiatrists, in preparation for the BMT procedure. Most conditioning regimens typically last for 5–6 days, except for myeloma, which is usually a 1-day regimen. During this period, patients transferred to the ICU are mainly affected by pharmacotoxicity or total-body irradiation-induced adverse effects, which may manifest as hyper-acute drug reactions such as seizures or acute radiation sickness. In some instances, individuals with conditions such as aplastic anemia may have a significantly low platelet count, leading to life-threatening hemorrhage. It is crucial to consider pharmacotoxicity and hemorrhagic complications as the primary differential diagnosis for such cases. In addition, it is important to remember that conditioning chemotherapy is myelotoxic, leading to prolonged cytopenia and presenting unique related issues. If stem cell reinfusion is scheduled, performing it in the ICU on day 0 is essential to restore counts.

B. *The Second Scenario Involves Patients Being Transferred to the ICU Within the First Week After Stem Cell Infusion but Before Engraftment*:

   During this phase, patients experience severe cytopenia and are susceptible to developing Gram-negative bacterial sepsis and bleeding manifestations. Due to the absence of neutrophils, their ability to respond to infections is compromised compared to healthy individuals. Therefore, training staff and junior doctors to promptly recognize the slightest changes in vital signs and administer antibiotics when necessary is crucial. These patients may experience sepsis-

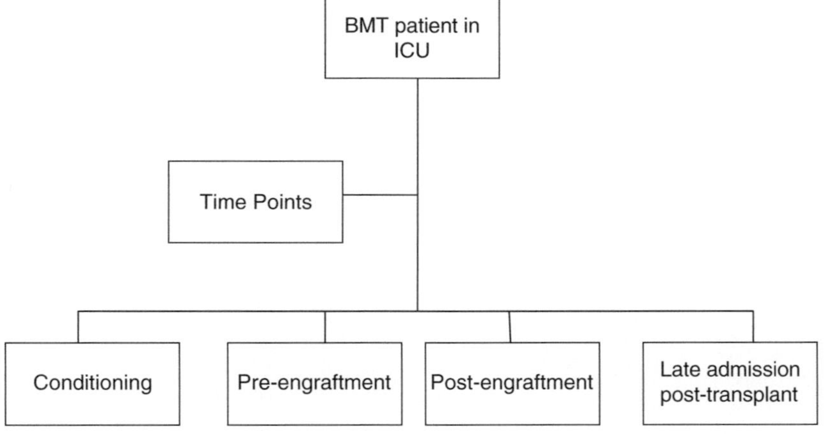

Fig. 25.1 Understanding phase of BMT patient in ICU

related mortality within a few hours. Extra caution should be taken to avoid puncture site hematomas and bleeding when dealing with procedures such as a central line or blood gas samples. Transfusion of sufficient irradiated hemocomponents before procedures is essential, considering potential differences in blood groups between donors and recipients, which may lead to mixed-field reactions. Preferred products for fresh frozen plasma and random donor platelets include O+ve irradiated leukodepleted packed red blood cells (PRBCs) and AB products. Management of febrile neutropenia is crucial during this phase.

C. *The Third Scenario Involves Patients Shifted to the ICU Post-engraftment*:

Mostly severe GVHD, sepsis, and atypical viral infections such as disseminated cytomegalovirus infection, adenoviral hemorrhagic cystitis, and thrombotic microangiopathy are due to immunosuppressants. Hemophagocytosis leading to delayed engraftment should also be considered. Therefore, it is essential to remain vigilant for cases that resemble multi-organ failure, which could indicate thrombotic microangiopathy, GVHD, or hemophagocytosis. When a patient is transferred to the ICU, obtaining a proper medical history and liaising with the primary transplant physician are crucial to understanding the phase of the transplant and managing patient expectations.

D. *The Fourth Scenario Is Late Admission Posttransplant*:

With either relapse, chronic GVHD, or sepsis, where they will be treated nearly like other transplant patients except for immunosuppressants and chronic GVHD-related side effects.

25.2 How to Prime Intensive Care Nurses While Caring for BMT Patients

To prepare ICU nurses for the care of BMT patients, it is crucial to provide specific instructions and reminders tailored to their unique challenges and requirements. Here are some critical points to prime ICU nurses for BMT patients (Fig. 25.2).

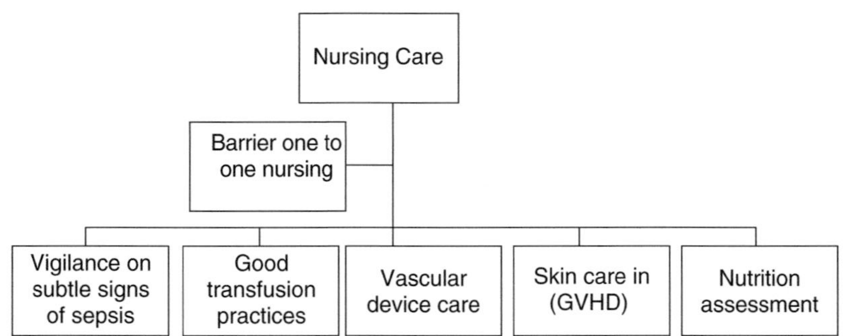

Fig. 25.2 Nursing care in critically ill BMT patients

Emphasize Hand Hygiene and Barrier Nursing Reinforce the importance of rigorous handwashing techniques and barrier nursing to prevent cross-infections, as most die from sepsis. Keeping these patients in an individual cubicle with dedicated one-to-one nursing is highly advisable.

Be Mindful of Long Lines Most BMT patients have peripherally inserted central catheter lines or Hickman catheters with lower maximum flow rates than central lines and vascath. Nurses need to be cautious while administering fluids and consider the limitations of these lines, especially the flow rate.

Follow Transfusion Protocols BMT patients often require frequent blood product transfusions. Ensure that nurses strictly adhere to standard transfusion protocols to prevent complications. The selection of blood products is separately discussed at the end of this chapter.

Be Alert to Subtle Signs of Infection Due to low neutrophil counts, BMT patients may not exhibit typical signs of sepsis-like fever and toxicity. Nurses should take mild tachycardia or hypotension seriously and promptly inform doctors of appropriate action.

Manage Nutrition Challenges BMT patients may experience mucositis and gut GVHD, leading to compromised nutrition. Nurses should be familiar with total parenteral nutrition and Ryles tube feeding practices for critically ill patients in liaison with dieticians.

Electrolyte Correction Most of these patients will be hypokalemic along with other electrolyte abnormalities. The correction cycles should be adequately monitored, and doctors should be informed of real-time lab results for modification.

Address Skin GVHD Skin peeling and dryness are expected due to skin GVHD. Nurses should prioritize skin and back care to prevent additional comorbidities and improve patient outcomes.

Be Knowledgeable About Medications BMT patients receive numerous immunosuppressants, antivirals, and antifungals that are not commonly used in most ICU patients. Pharmacists and nurses should be well-informed about drug preparation, infusion techniques, and potential drug interactions.

Reiterate the Importance of Training While some of these points are part of standard ICU nursing training, it is essential to reemphasize their significance when receiving BMT patients in the ICU.

By providing focused training and reminders, ICU nurses will be better equipped to handle the unique challenges presented by BMT patients, ultimately ensuring better patient outcomes and safety (Fig. 25.3).

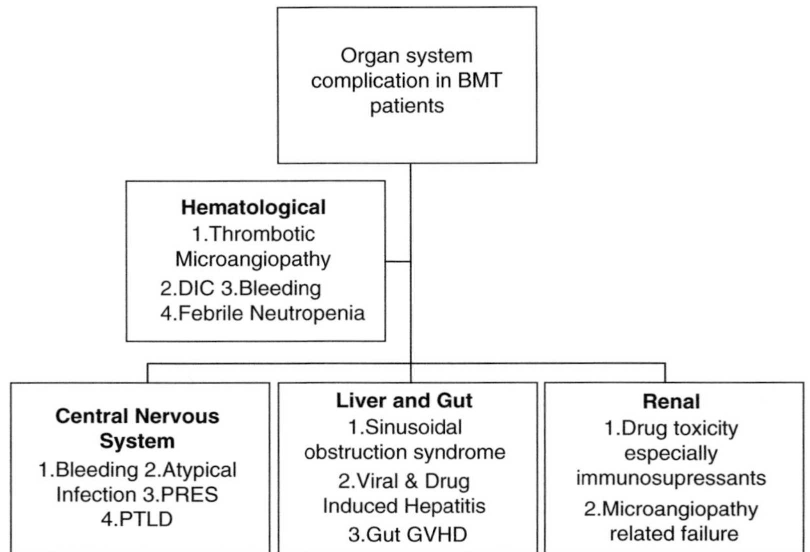

Fig. 25.3 Systemwise complications in BMT patients

25.3 Systemwise Points in Critically Ill Patients Bone Marrow Transplant (BMT): (Fig. 25.3)

25.3.1 Central Nervous System

Regarding the central nervous system (CNS), BMT is associated with various complications that can arise due to the underlying disease, prolonged myelosuppression, and the use of immunosuppressive drugs. These complications encompass hemorrhage, infections, vascular conditions, posterior reversible encephalopathy (PRES), drug-induced neurotoxicity, metabolic disturbances, and post-BMT carcinogenesis, including posttransplant lymphoproliferative disorder (PTLD). Some specific CNS complications include atypical infections such as fungal and viral encephalitis, drug-induced toxicity like PRES, and long-term complications like secondary malignancies such as PTLD. To ensure the best possible care for these critically ill BMT patients, it is crucial to conduct timely imaging and cerebrospinal fluid analysis when appropriate. In addition, transfusion should be administered as required, and anti-seizure measures should be implemented (Yoshida et al. 2008).

25.3.2 Renal Failure

Acute renal failure is a frequent and potentially life-threatening complication after bone marrow transplantation. Renal issues occur at different post-BMT times. Immediate failure includes tumor lysis syndrome and marrow-infusion toxicity within 5 days. Early renal failure, such as hepatorenal-like syndrome, can happen within 1 month. Late failure has BMT-associated nephropathy and cyclosporin nephrotoxicity after 4 weeks. Non-specific causes such as sepsis, hypotension, and nephrotoxic agents can occur anytime. Renal supportive intensive care treatment is vital, and renal replacement backup will be lifesaving in many of these cases (Pulla et al. 1998).

25.3.3 Gastrointestinal and Liver Disease

Pre-existing liver disease affects transplant choice and posttransplant hepatic complications (e.g., SOS and fulminant hepatitis B). Sinusoidal obstruction is a unique complication of BMT with a grave prognosis. Continuing prophylaxis is vital during immune suppression to prevent hepatic infections (HSV, VZV, HBV for at-risk patients, and fungi). Differential diagnosis depends on conditioning therapy, stem cell donor, and timing of liver issues. Elevated serum ALT (>1000 U/L) may be due to various factors, not just infection. Ursodiol prophylaxis reduces jaundice frequency and improves survival. In extreme failure cases, plasma exchange may be indicated. In the case of acute gut GVHD, voluminous diarrhea in liters is expected, and adequate hydration, antimotility medications, and investigations are to differentiate from infective causes like clostridium.

25.3.4 Cardiac Complications

Severe heart-related issues can arise during hematopoietic cell transplantation, including acute heart failure, arrhythmias, pericardial tamponade, or cardiac arrest. The increased cardiovascular risk in transplant is attributed to exposure to cardiotoxic chemotherapy, especially anthracyclines, radiation, and direct and indirect detrimental effects on cardiovascular function (Tuzovic et al. 2019).

25.3.5 Sorting the Transfusion Confusion

Due to the lack of blood group matching required in allogeneic bone marrow transplantations, transfusion services face unique serologic challenges. Many ICUs opt for transfusing group O erythrocytes (PRBCs) when non-ABO-matched transplantation is admitted. For ABO-identical transplantations, ABO-identical or ABO-compatible erythrocytes and plasma are suitable choices. The criteria for platelet transfusion follow those of plasma transfusions. The most commonly required plasma for ABO-mismatched HPC transplantation recipients is group AB (universal donor) plasma. In most cases, transfusion triggers are kept to a minimum of <8 gm% for hemoglobin and bleeding as a trigger for platelets and plasma products. Leukodepletion and irradiation are not to be forgotten at any cost in these patients. Be prepared for a blood group change in these patients when comparing them with the previously filed group (Gajewski et al. 2008).

Points to Remember Before the Next BMT ICU Rounds
The primary objective of this chapter is not to instruct intensivists in managing critically ill patients, as they are already proficient in this skill. Instead, the aim is to acquaint intensivists with unique situations when caring for critically ill patients undergoing BMTs, highlighting the differences from other scenarios.

The following points serve as a quick and convenient reminder

- Most BMT patients have experienced prolonged and multiple hospital admissions as part of their therapy, potentially harboring pre-existing infections and organ dysfunction. A comprehensive medical history can help narrow down the current diagnosis.
- Due to abnormal blood counts, these patients may not exhibit typical physical reactions to sepsis, necessitating a cautious approach when titrating anti-infective treatments.
- Several transplant medications must be continued during intensive care admission, requiring vigilant monitoring for potential drug interactions and complications.
- Unique complications, such as sinusoidal obstruction syndrome, drug-induced thrombotic microangiopathy, GVHD, and PRES, should be remembered when dealing with these patients.
- ABO compatibility is not mandatory for BMTs, leading to potential mixed-field reactions in blood grouping and cross-matching. As discussed in the text, properly informing and educating the staff about the appropriate transfusion guidelines is crucial.
- In most cases, the decision for a BMT is based on the patient's minimum fitness for the procedure. Consequently, the current intensive care admission likely results from an acute and reversible event in most patients, making them highly amenable to successful treatment.
- A multidisciplinary approach involving different specialties, especially the primary treating physician, is vital to ensure favorable outcomes for these patients. Collaboration and communication among the medical team are crucial in managing these cases effectively (Fig. 25.4).

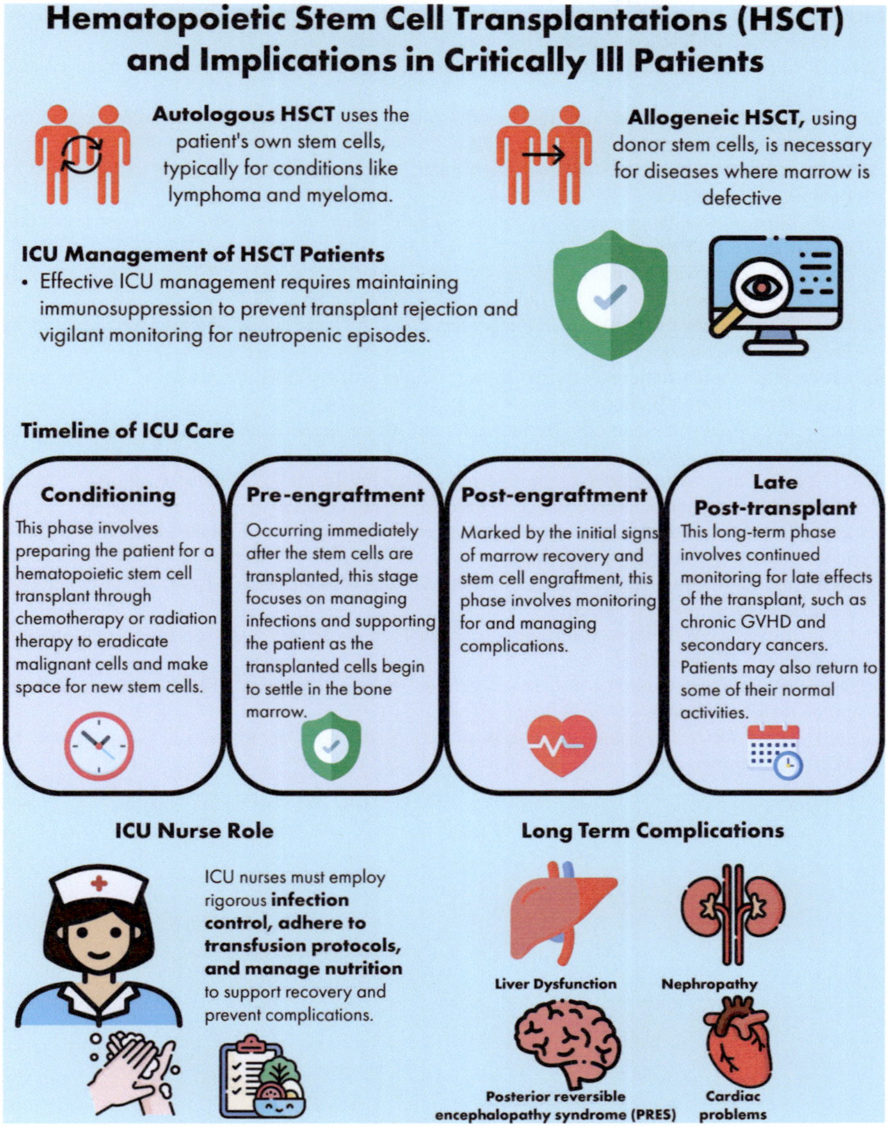

Hematopoietic Stem Cell Transplantations (HSCT) and Implications in Critically Ill Patients

Autologous HSCT uses the patient's own stem cells, typically for conditions like lymphoma and myeloma.

Allogeneic HSCT, using donor stem cells, is necessary for diseases where marrow is defective

ICU Management of HSCT Patients

- Effective ICU management requires maintaining immunosuppression to prevent transplant rejection and vigilant monitoring for neutropenic episodes.

Timeline of ICU Care

Conditioning
This phase involves preparing the patient for a hematopoietic stem cell transplant through chemotherapy or radiation therapy to eradicate malignant cells and make space for new stem cells.

Pre-engraftment
Occurring immediately after the stem cells are transplanted, this stage focuses on managing infections and supporting the patient as the transplanted cells begin to settle in the bone marrow.

Post-engraftment
Marked by the initial signs of marrow recovery and stem cell engraftment, this phase involves monitoring for and managing complications.

Late Post-transplant
This long-term phase involves continued monitoring for late effects of the transplant, such as chronic GVHD and secondary cancers. Patients may also return to some of their normal activities.

ICU Nurse Role

ICU nurses must employ rigorous **infection control, adhere to transfusion protocols, and manage nutrition** to support recovery and prevent complications.

Long Term Complications

Liver Dysfunction

Nephropathy

Posterior reversible encephalopathy syndrome (PRES)

Cardiac problems

Fig. 25.4 Hematopoietic stem cell transplantations (HSCT) and implications in critically ill

Flowchart

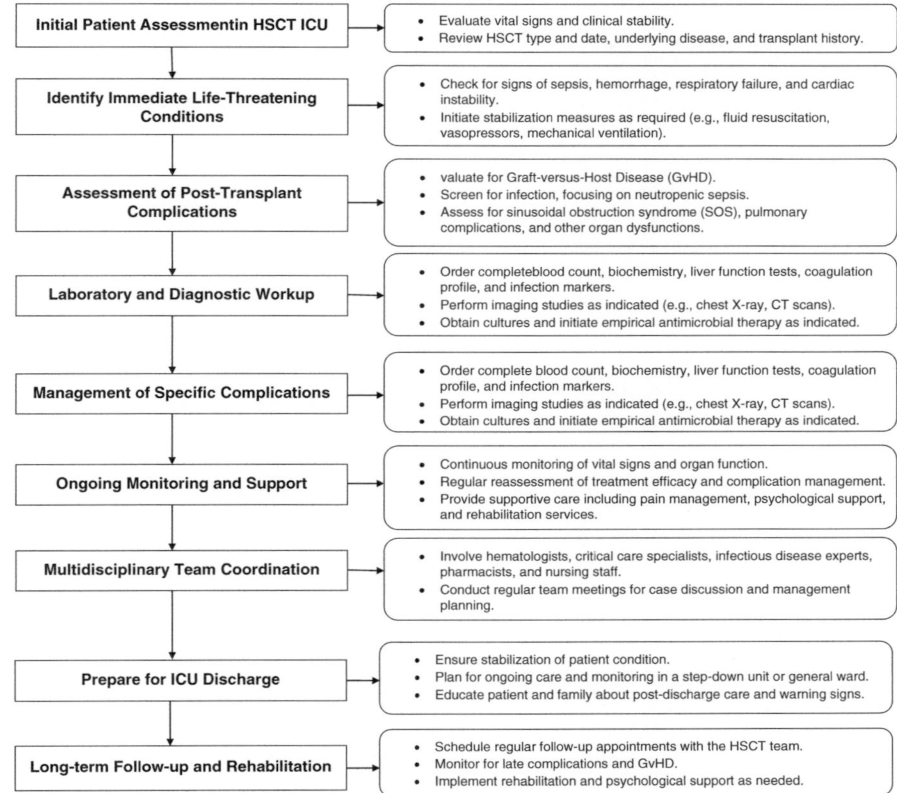

References

Gajewski JL, Johnson VV, Sandler SG, Sayegh A, Klumpp TR (2008) A review of transfusion practice before, during, and after hematopoietic progenitor cell transplantation. Blood, J Am Soc Hematol 112(8):3036–3047

Pulla B, Barri YM, Anaissie E (1998) Acute renal failure following bone marrow transplantation. Ren Fail 20(3):421–435

Scales DC, Thiruchelvam D, Kiss A, Sibbald WJ, Redelmeier DA (2008) Intensive care outcomes in bone marrow transplant recipients: a population-based cohort analysis. Crit Care 12:1–9

Tuzovic M, Mead M, Young PA, Schiller G, Yang EH (2019) Cardiac complications in the adult bone marrow transplant patient. Curr Oncol Rep 21:1–16

Yoshida S, Hayakawa K, Yamamoto A, Kuroda H, Imashuku S (2008) The central nervous system complications of bone marrow transplantation in children. Eur Radiol 18:2048–2059

Chapter 26
Patients on CAR T Cell Therapy

Priyanka Samal and Sasmita Das

Learning Points

1. Chimeric antigen receptor -T (CAR T)-Cell Mechanism: CAR T therapy modifies T cells to target tumor antigens, showing high efficacy in treating hematologic malignancies.
2. Managing Adverse Events: Key to CAR T therapy's success is managing adverse events such as cytokine release syndrome and immune effector cell-associated neurotoxicity syndrome to ensure patient safety and treatment effectiveness.
3. Generational Advances: CAR T therapy's evolution through generations has improved its efficacy, persistence, and safety, underscoring the therapy's growing potential.
4. Facing Challenges: Despite CAR T's progress, challenges such as treatment resistance, relapse, high costs, and accessibility persist, guiding future research directions.

26.1 Introduction

Cancer has long been a formidable adversary in the field of medicine, affecting millions of lives worldwide and presenting a complex challenge to healthcare professionals. Despite significant advancements in traditional cancer treatments such as chemotherapy and radiation therapy, these often result in severe adverse events and

P. Samal (✉)
Department of Clinical Hematology and BMT, IMS & SUM Hospital, Bhubaneswar, India
e-mail: priyankasamal@soa.ac.in

S. Das
Centre for Good Governance, GAA, Government of Odisha, Bhubaneswar, India

S. B. Mishra (ed.), *Critical Care Hematology*,
https://doi.org/10.1007/978-981-97-5565-3_26

have limited efficacy in certain cases. In recent years, novel approaches in adoptive T-cell therapies for cancer treatment have emerged, including T cells with modified T-cell receptors (TCR), tumor-infiltrating lymphocytes, and T cells with chimeric antigen receptors (CARs), also known as CAR T cell (CAR T) (Skorka et al. 2020; June et al. 2018; Rohaan et al. 2019). Among these, CAR T therapy stands as a beacon of hope for cancer patients (June et al. 2018; Sterner and Sterner 2021). This groundbreaking immunotherapy utilizes the body's immune system to combat cancer by genetically modifying a patient's T cells to identify and target cancer cells, resulting in impressive effectiveness against various hematological malignancies such as lymphoma and leukemia (Davila and Sadelain 2016; Mavi et al. 2023). Numerous clinical trials and real-world cases have shown remarkable response rates and long-term remissions in patients who had exhausted all available treatments (Havard and Stephens 2018). The approval of Kymriah, the first CAR T-cell therapy, by the US FDA in 2017 for pediatric and young adult patients with acute B lymphoblastic leukemia marked a historic milestone in cancer treatment, opening doors for further advancements in this field. Combining cutting-edge science with compassionate care, this therapy has emerged as a transformative force in the fight against cancer, offering hope for a future where cancer is no longer a terminal illness but a treatable condition (Mitra et al. 2023). However, relapse is a major drawback with CAR T therapy, as patients have very few options left after undergoing this treatment.

26.2 Hematological Malignancy

Hematological malignancies encompass a range of cancers and disorders affecting the blood, bone marrow, and lymphatic system, posing a significant health burden worldwide. In India, there has been a consistent rise in the occurrence of hematological malignancies over the years (Keykhaei et al. 2021; Zhang et al. 2023). Although obtaining accurate and up-to-date nationwide statistics may be challenging, regional studies and cancer registries offer valuable insights into the prevalence of these conditions. Leukemia, a cancer of the blood and bone marrow, stands among the most common hematological malignancies. The incidence of leukemia varies across different regions in India. According to data from the Indian Council of Medical Research's National Cancer Registry Program, leukemia accounts for approximately 6–8% of all cancers in the country. This highlights the substantial impact of leukemia on the population and emphasizes the need for effective treatment options. Lymphomas, which include Hodgkin lymphoma and non-Hodgkin lymphoma, affect the lymphatic system. The incidence of lymphomas is also increasing in India (Cai et al. 2021). The Indian Journal of Medical and Pediatric Oncology reports that non-Hodgkin lymphoma is the third most prevalent cancer in Indian adults, with a notable high occurrence in urban areas. Multiple myeloma, a cancer of plasma cells, is yet another prevalent hematological malignancy in India. The Indian Cancer Society estimates that multiple myeloma accounts for 1–2% of all cancers in India (Haslauer et al. 2021). As the elderly population continues to grow, the prevalence of multiple myeloma is also expected to increase. This highlights the need for better treatment strategies to cope with the rising burden of this disease.

26.3 What Is CAR T Cell?

CAR T-cell therapy involves modifying a patient's own T cells through genetic engineering to express CARs that specifically recognize antigens on tumor cell surface in a major histocompatibility complex-independent manner. This personalized technique has demonstrated remarkable efficacy in treating specific hematologic cancers, especially refractory or relapsed B-cell lymphomas and B-acute lymphoblastic leukemia (B-ALL) (Haslauer et al. 2021).

26.4 History of CAR T Therapy

The therapy has a fascinating history spanning several generations of advancements.

The first CAR T cells were developed against 2,4,6-trinitrophenyl more than two decades ago when (Teoh and Chng 2021) scientists discovered in 1960 that immune cells may eradicate cancer in mice. Immunologist Jacques Miller found out the thymus gland as the location of T cell development in 1961 (Maus 2022; Bourbon et al. 2021) (Fig. 26.1).

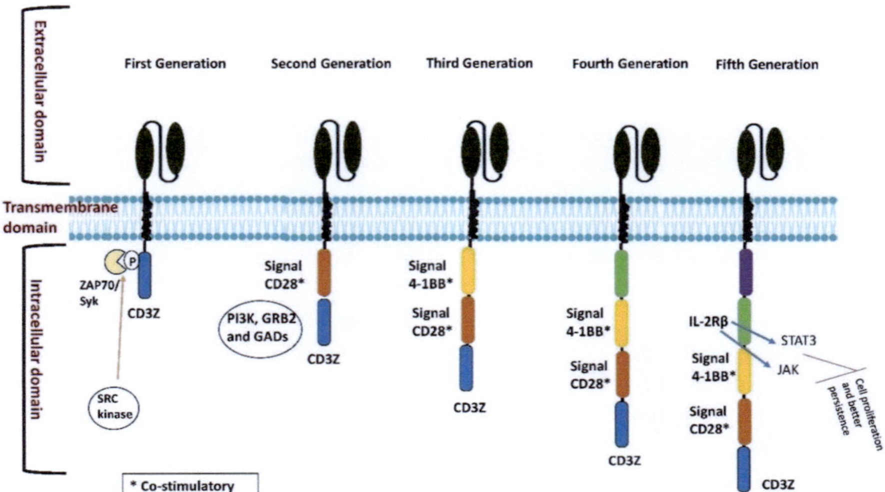

Fig. 26.1 Process of fifth generation CAR, each building upon the previous one

1. *First Generation CAR T Cells*:

   In the early 1990s, Immunologist Zelig Eshhar engineered the first chimeric molecule, combining a part of an antibody with a component of a T-cell receptor (Gross and Eshhar 1992; Goverman et al. 1990). These synthetic receptors were engineered to redirect T-cell specificity, function, and metabolism. The first generation CARs had an intracellular signaling domain that typically included the zeta chain of the CD3 complex to activate T cells upon antigen recognition and an extracellular part derived from immunoglobulins that provided specificity for the target tumor antigens without major histocompatibility restriction. However, these CAR T cells lacked sufficient interleukin-2 (IL-2) production and, hence, needed exogenous IL-2 or other cytokines to destroy tumor cells. However, their signaling capability was limited, resulting in transient T-cell responses (Maus 2022).
2. *Second Generation CAR T Cells*:

   In the early 2000s, researchers developed second generation CAR T cells to address the drawbacks of first generation CARs. The first successful cells, however, directed against a prostate cancer antigen, were created by the MSK team in 2002. This second generation demonstrated the viability of this treatment by surviving and multiplying, as well as killing prostate cancer cells in the laboratory. These CARs included additional chimeric costimulatory receptors, such as CD28 or CD 137 (or 4-1BB) and CD 134 (OX40), which, when activated by an antigen, gave T cells strong co-stimulatory signals. This enhancement led to improved T-cell proliferation, survival, and effect or functions. As a result, second generation CAR T cells demonstrated greater efficacy and persistence, setting the stage for more effective "living drugs" in cancer therapy. In 2010, these second generation cells successfully demonstrated the eradication of advanced chronic lymphocytic leukemia in a patient targeting the CD19 protein (Asmamaw Dejenie et al. 2022; Eshhar et al. 1993; Eshhar 2014; Mancikova and Smida 2021).
3. *Third Generation CAR T Cells*:

   In the years that followed, third generation CAR T cells developed, building on the success of second generation CARs. Combinations of multiple costimulatory domains, including CD28 and 4-1BB, were integrated into these enhanced CARs to augment potency with stronger cytokine production and tumor destruction along with prolonged persistence of the third generation CARs in the hostile tumor microenvironment. While these CARs showed promise in preclinical studies, their complex design raised concerns about potential toxicities and manufacturing challenges.
4. *Fourth Generation CAR T Cells (TRUCKs) Cytokine Expressing CAR T Cells*

   The success of these CAR T cells is not yet harnessed in the solid tumors. To use this concept of adoptive cell therapy to eradicate tumor cells, T cells redirected for antigen-unrestricted cytokine-initiated killing (TRUCKs) are being developed. These fourth generation cells are known as TRUCKS. The concept was to engage CAR to the targeted tumor antigen and direct the antitumor activity of CAR T with the immunomodulatory capacity of the delivered transgenic transcripted cytokines which are released close to the tumor antigen. This enabled more efficacious killing of tumor cells with local deposition of cytokines, causing acute inflammation in the stromal tumor and minimal systemic adverse events. The cytokines released also cause stimulation and remain in the body of the CAR T cells. The most common cytokines used in these models are IL-7, IL-1, IL-15, IL-18, IL-23, and also their combinations. These are in the early phase of clinical trials and need to be further validated before they are commercially available. The TRUCKs are being developed not only to address the solid tumors but also to treat autoimmune disorders, viral infections, and metabolic disorders (Asmamaw Dejenie et al. 2022; Eshhar et al. 1993; Mancikova and Smida 2021).

5. *Fifth Generation CAR T Cells*

   The fifth generation CAR T cells are similar to second generation, but have further integrated an extra intracellular domain of a cytokine receptor. The most common is the IL 2Rβ. This is incorporated in between CD25/4-1BB and CD 3ζ costimulatory molecules, activated JAK–STAT signaling, and causes cell proliferation (Davila and Sadelain 2016; Asmamaw Dejenie et al. 2022; Mancikova and Smida 2021; Lu and Jiang 2022).

6. *Breakthroughs and Expanding Indications*

   The tremendous progression of the therapy has led to significant clinical successes. Two CAR T-cell treatments received FDA approval in 2017: Yescarta for adult diffuse large B-cell lymphoma and Kymriah for pediatric B-ALL (Seimetz et al. 2019). These approvals marked a turning point in cancer treatment, providing hope for patients with previously untreatable or refractory diseases.

26.5 Evolution of CAR T-Cell Therapy

It can be attributed to several factors:

- Advances in Genetic Engineering: Over the years, transformations in gene transfer techniques, such as viral vectors, and gene-editing technologies such as CRISPR–Cas9, have enabled more efficient and precise modification of T cells (Li et al. 2020). These advancements have played a crucial role in the evolution of next generation CAR T-cell therapies.
- Identification of Novel Targets: Researchers have made significant findings regarding novel tumor-associated antigens expressed on cancer cells' surfaces. Utilizing CAR T cells designed to target these specific antigens allows for a personalized approach to therapy, broadening the potential applications of this treatment for various types of cancer (June et al. 2018).
- Improved CAR Designs: Significant progress has been made in optimizing CAR designs to enhance their efficacy. These enhancements involve integrating co-stimulatory domains such as CD28 or 4-1BB into the CAR structure. By doing so, modified T cells receive extra activation signals, resulting in improved persistence and increased anti-tumor activity (Gross and Eshhar 1992; Asmamaw Dejenie et al. 2022).

- Clinical Trial Results and Iterative Improvements: Clinical trials have played a vital role in refining the therapy. The insight gained from these clinical trials has helped in refining treatment protocols, addressing possible side effects, such as cytokine release syndrome (CRS), and enhancing overall patient results (Asmamaw Dejenie et al. 2022).
- Combination Therapies: To increase the efficacy of this therapy, it has also been combined with additional treatments such checkpoint inhibitors, targeted therapies, or traditional chemotherapy. These combination approaches aim to overcome tumor resistance mechanisms and improve response rates (Mitra et al. 2023; Asmamaw Dejenie et al. 2022).
- The evolution of therapy continues to progress rapidly, with ongoing research focusing on expanding its application to solid tumors, improving safety profiles, and developing off-the-shelf CAR T-cell products. The field holds great promise for revolutionizing cancer treatment and achieving long-term remissions for patients.

CAR T-Cell Therapy Consists of Several Essential Stages, which are depicted in Fig. 26.2

1. *Leukapheresis*: The patient's blood is collected through leukapheresis, a procedure that separates and collects white blood cells, including T cells, from the rest of the blood components (Fig. 26.3).
2. *T-Cell Genetic Modification*: The collected T cells are sent to the laboratory, where they are genetically modified to express CARs on their surface. CARs consist of an antigen-binding domain specific to a cancer cell surface antigen, a spacer domain, a transmembrane domain, and an intracellular signaling domain.
3. *T-Cell Expansion*: The modified T cells are cultured and expanded in the laboratory to generate a large population of CAR-expressing T cells. This process typically takes several days.
4. *Conditioning Regimen*: Prior to CAR T-cell infusion, the patient may undergo a conditioning regimen, which involves receiving chemotherapy or other treatments to create an optimal environment for CAR T-cell therapy.
5. *CAR T-Cell Infusion*: The expanded CAR T cells are infused back into the patient's bloodstream. These CAR T cells recognize and bind to cancer cells that express the targeted antigen.
6. *Targeting Cancer Cells*: Once infused, the CAR T cells target and bind to cancer cells expressing the specific antigen recognized by the CAR. This triggers the activation of the CAR T cells, leading to the destruction of the cancer cells.
7. *Proliferation and Persistence*: CAR T cells can multiply within the patient's body, leading to a sustained anti-cancer effect. They can persist for months or even years after infusion, providing long-term immune surveillance against cancer recurrence.

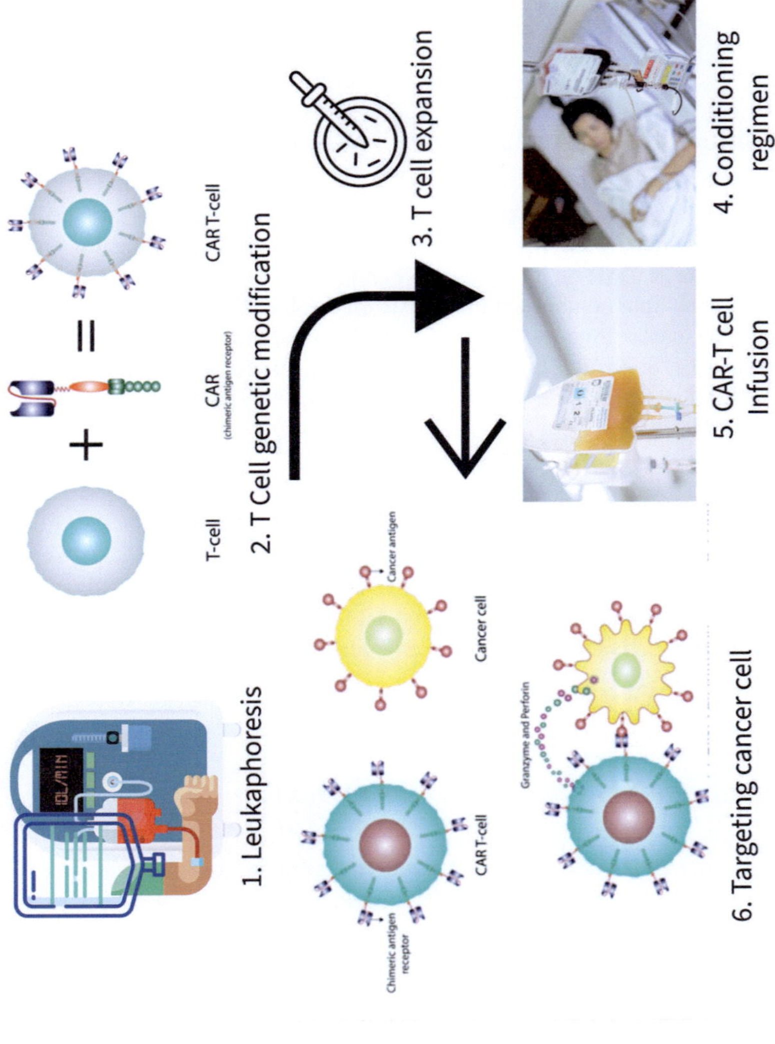

Fig. 26.2 Diagram depicting the steps involved in CAR T-cell therapy

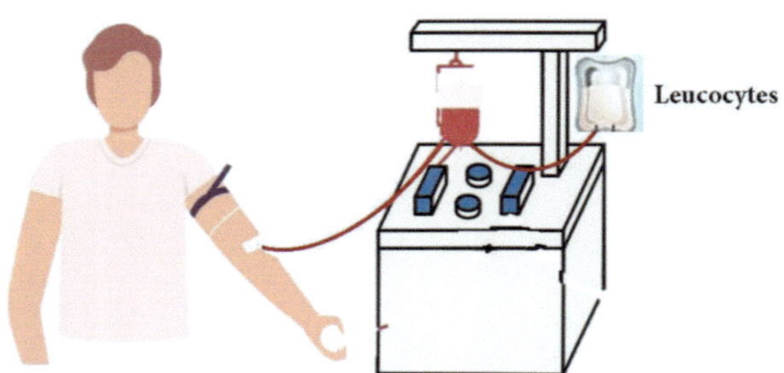

Fig. 26.3 Leukapheresis process

26.6 Inside the Cell Mechanism of CAR T-Cell Therapy

CAR T cells are engineered to express a synthetic receptor on their surface. The CAR T cell continuously circulates through blood vessels in looking for cancer cells, because it has a CAR on its surface. When the target antigen on the surface of a cancer cell comes into contact with the CAR on the T cell, it binds exclusively to that antigen. The extracellular domain of CARs, known as the single-chain variable fragment, which is often derived from an antibody, serves as crucial for antigen recognition (Lu and Jiang 2022; Whitlow et al. 1993).

26.6.1 CAR Signaling Activation

Intracellular signaling events start when the CAR binds to the target antigen. The CAR's intracellular domain, which contains elements, such as CD3-ζ, is responsible for transmitting activation signals to the T cell (Lu and Jiang 2022; Pulè et al. 2005; Song et al. 2012).

26.6.2 Activation of CAR Intracellular Domain

There is an intracellular domain in the CAR that contains crucial signaling elements, such as CD3-ζ and, on occasion, co-stimulatory domains, such as CD28 or 4-1BB. These intracellular regions become phosphorylated following effective antigen binding, triggering a series of subsequent signaling events (Lu and Jiang 2022; Pulè et al. 2005; Song et al. 2012).

26.6.3 T-Cell Receptor (TCR)-Like Signaling

The natural TCR signaling cascade is often triggered by the phosphorylation of CD3- and other intracellular domains in CAR T cells. This process results in the creation of immune receptor tyrosine-based activation motifs (ITAMs), which is accomplished by the activation of kinases, such as linkage for activation of T cells and ZAP-70 (Lu and Jiang 2022; Wurdeman et al. 2018).

26.6.4 Amplification of Signals

Activation of ITAMs amplifies the signaling cascade, resulting in heightened intracellular calcium levels and the activation of protein kinase pathways.

26.6.5 Activation of Transcription Factors

Numerous downstream signaling pathways, such as the PI3K and mitogen-activated protein kinase pathways, are triggered by the activated kinases which result in the expression of transcription factors, such as NF-B and nuclear factor of activated T cells (NFATs) translocate (Lu and Jiang 2022; Kilic-Erkek et al. 2023).

26.6.6 Gene Expression Changes

Gene expression profiles within the CAR T cell are modified by transcription factors, such as NF-β and NFAT. This leads to the release of several cytokines, such as interferon-gamma (IFN-γ), tumor necrosis factor-alpha (TNF-α), and interleukin-2 (IL-2), all of which have potent anti-cancer capabilities (Lu and Jiang 2022; Li et al. 2018).

26.6.7 Cytotoxic Activity

The activated CAR T cell also releases cytotoxic molecules, including perforin and granzyme, which are packaged in cytotoxic granules. Perforin creates pores within the target cancer cell's membrane, allowing granzyme to penetrate the cancer cell. Granzyme initiates a cascade of events within the target cell, leading to apoptosis or cell death (Lu and Jiang 2022; Grosser et al. 2019; Lee et al. 2014).

26.6.8 Memory Formation

Some CAR T cells have the capacity to mature into memory cells, which remain in the patient's body for years after completing the initial therapy. Memory CAR T cells offer continual monitoring and defense against probable cancer recurrence (Lu and Jiang 2022; Grosser et al. 2019; Lee et al. 2014).

26.6.9 Checkpoints and Regulation

Checkpoint receptors such as PD-1 and CTLA-4 may reduce the activity of CAR T cells to fine-tune immune responses. These inhibiting signals can be blocked by immunotherapy agents known as checkpoint inhibitors, which will increase the potency of CAR T cells (Lu and Jiang 2022; Grosser et al. 2019; Lee et al. 2014).

26.7 Antigen Escape Challenges and Solutions for CAR T-Cell Therapy

Antigen escape is one of the difficulties facing in this therapy despite the fact that it has demonstrated significant promise in treating several forms of cancer. Antigen escape is the process by which cancer cells change or adapt to avoid being recognized and eliminated by CAR T cells, which causes the disease to reappear. Antigen-negative or low antigen variations in tumors present an obstacle to CAR-based therapy. This happens as a result of immunological pressure from CAR T cells, which encourage cancer to advance by expressing their target antigens. Antigen escape and lineage switching are the two main pathways that can lead to antigen loss. Lineage switch causes a phenotypic shift in the tumor, such as the transition from lymphoid to myeloid lineage, whereas antigen escape includes the selection of tumor cells expressing alternate forms of the target antigen. Researchers are investigating methods, such as multispecific CARs capable of simultaneously targeting numerous antigens, to circumvent antigen loss. These strategies include coadministration of several CAR T-cell products, tandem CARs, and bicistronic CARs. Another approach is called epitope spreading, in which the immune system targets additional tumor antigens.

26.8 Need for CAR T-Cell Therapy

This therapy has become a hopeful treatment choice for hematological malignancies, particularly in situations where conventional therapies have demonstrated limited efficacy. The burden of hematological malignancies, along with the need for the therapy, can be summarized as follows:

26.8.1 Limited Treatment Options

While conventional treatments such as chemotherapy and radiation therapy have been effective in some cases, approximately 30–40% of hematological malignancies may be resistant to these treatments or relapse after the initial response. There is a need to address these relapsed and refractory diseases which require more aggressive therapy and, hence, are associated with greater adverse events. This therapy appears to have the potential to cure with manageable side effects in such subgroup of patients (Haslauer et al. 2021; Lu and Jiang 2022; Boyiadzis et al. 2018; Gill and Brudno 2021; Zhao et al. 2018; Abbasi et al. 2023; Huang et al. 2022; Zhang et al. 2022).

26.8.2 High Disease Burden

Hematological malignancies can significantly impact the quality of life and survival rates of affected individuals. The burden of these diseases on patients, their families, and the healthcare system is substantial. It offers hope for enhanced outcomes and higher QOL for individuals facing limited treatment alternatives (Haslauer et al. 2021; Lu and Jiang 2022; Boyiadzis et al. 2018; Gill and Brudno 2021; Zhao et al. 2018; Abbasi et al. 2023; Huang et al. 2022; Zhang et al. 2022).

26.8.3 Rising Demand for Innovative Therapies

As the incidence of hematological malignancies increases in India, the demand for advanced and effective therapies grows. The remarkable success of therapy in managing specific types of blood cancers on a global scale makes it a much-needed and vital solution for patients who have already explored other treatment options (Haslauer et al. 2021; Lu and Jiang 2022; Boyiadzis et al. 2018; Gill and Brudno 2021; Zhao et al. 2018; Abbasi et al. 2023; Huang et al. 2022; Zhang et al. 2022).

26.8.4 Access and Affordability

Making sure that access and affordability are fair is one of the difficulties in tackling the burden of this therapy in India. For many patients, the high cost of CAR T-cell therapy will remain a financial hurdle. Government initiatives, health insurance coverage, and collaborations with pharmaceutical companies as well as research institutions are needed to make CAR T-cell therapy more accessible and affordable to those in need (Haslauer et al. 2021; Lu and Jiang 2022; Boyiadzis et al. 2018; Gill and Brudno 2021; Zhao et al. 2018; Abbasi et al. 2023; Huang et al. 2022; Zhang et al. 2022).

26.9 Patient Selection and Preparation

Prerequisites for CART therapy

1. Tumor should express a CAR target (e.g., CD19, CD20, CD22, and BCMA) predominantly in cancer cells and not in healthy cells.
2. Patient or donor should have adequate number of T cells for collection.
3. Recipient of CAR T cells should have no active, uncontrolled infections, including hepatitis B, hepatitis C, or HIV.
4. Patient should have good organ function and ECOG performance status.
5. The absence of clinically significant comorbidities (e.g., immunological, neurological, or cardiovascular problems).
   Eastern Cooperative Oncology Group performance status (ECOG PS)

26.10

Currently, CAR T-cell therapy has been approved for the medical treatment of select hematologic malignancies, particularly B-cell leukemias and lymphomas. Before undergoing the therapy, patients are evaluated to determine their eligibility and assess the potential risks and benefits of the treatment. Other factors considered include the cancer type and stage and previous treatments received (Nasta et al. 2019).

After determining a patient's eligibility for therapy, they will undergo a procedure known as leukapheresis.

26.11 Treatment Process and Monitoring

After modifying the T cells genetically, they are cultivated and multiplied in the lab until an adequate quantity is achieved. The patient next undergoes a conditioning program to prepare their immune system for the injection of CAR T cells, which frequently entails chemotherapy. The patient receives the CAR T-cell infusion as a single, one-time treatment after the conditioning period is over. In addition, a patient stays in the hospital for 1–2 weeks on average (Obaisi et al. 2022; Nasta et al. 2019). The post-infusion response of the disease is evaluated by monitoring peripheral blood or bone-marrow aspirate B-cell levels by flow cytometry, bone-marrow biopsy, IHC, RT-PCR, and CT scan. CAR T-cell persistence is also tracked by flow cytometry.

26.12 Immediate Toxicity

1. *Cytokine Release Syndrome (CRS)*

   Following the infusion, patients are closely monitored for potential side effects and complications. CAR T cells can trigger a widespread inflammatory response called CRS due to their activation and rapid multiplication in the body. Specifically observed in patients who respond positively to the treatment. CRS commonly appears 2–14 days after the CAR T-cell infusion but may manifest within a month and is mediated primarily by IL-6 and IFN γ, as a result of T-cell activation.

   The symptoms of CRS are similar to those seen in severe flu-like syndrome or sepsis due to infection. These symptoms may include:

   - High fevers
   - Rapid heart rate (Tachycardia)
   - Low oxygen levels (Hypoxia)
   - Low blood pressure (Hypotension)
   - Decrease in liver or kidney function
   - Prolonged partial thromboplastin time and a risk of bleeding

Patients can experience varying degrees of CRS severity, and in extreme situations, hospitalization to the intensive care unit may be necessary (Table 26.1).

Table 26.1 CRS grading system (Lee et al. 2014; Boyiadzis et al. 2018; Brudno and Kochenderfer 2016; Maude et al. 2018; Maude et al. 2014) along with its management

Grades	Symptoms	Treatment
Grade-1	Mild reaction Fever (Temperature > 38 °C) Nausea, Fatigue, Headache, Malaise	Interruption of infusion not needed Supportive care Antipyretics Antiemetics
Grade-2	Moderate reaction Grade 3 LFTs and Grade 2 creatinine dysfunction Hypoxia with Oxygen requirement below 40%FiO_2 Hypotension not requiring Vasopressor.	Interruption of infusion NSAIDS, Antihistamines, narcotics IV Fluids for hypotension +/– Low dose Vasopressor +/– IL-6 receptors agonist Tocilizumab 8 mg/kg IV
Grade-3	More severe reaction Hypoxia requiring more than equal to 40% Oxygen Hypotension requiring high dose or multiple vasopressor Grade-3 creatinine and/or grade 4 LFT dysfunction	Treat symptoms as grade-2 Tocilizumab Low dose Corticosteroids High-flow nasal cannula (>6 L/min), face mask, non-rebreather mask, or venturi mask High dose vasopressor +/– vasopressin
Grade-4	Life threatening Hypoxia requiring positive airway pressure/ventilator. Hypotension requiring multiple vasopressor. Grade 4 organ toxicity, excluding transaminitis	Treat symptoms as grade-2 High dose corticosteroids CPAP, bilevel positive airway pressure, intubation, mechanical ventilation Multiple vasopressors

2. *Neurotoxicity*

Immune effector cell-associated neurotoxicity syndrome (ICANS): It is a known neurologic complication seen in patients undergoing CAR T-cell therapy. The severity of this syndrome is associated with young age of patient, high tumor burden, and those experiencing early onset and high-grade CRS. Other contributing factors may be the type of costimulatory molecule used in the CAR as well as the lymphodepleting conditioning regimen used prior to the CAR infusion. Similar to the CRS, ICANS is also mediated by the inflammatory cytokines released and occurs within days to 2–3 week post-CAR T-cell infusion. The following symptoms should be considered as manifestations of ICANS and may exhibit various symptoms, such as:

- Confusion
- Somnolence (drowsiness)
- Tremors
- Gait instability
- Seizures
- Impaired language comprehension and speech
- Occasionally hallucinations

It is important to emphasize that these neurologic toxicities can occur independently from CRS and their exact cause is not fully understood. As similar adverse effects have been documented with a bispecific anti-CD19, blinatumomab, and anti-CD3 monoclonal antibody, these toxic consequences are thought to be a class effect associated with medicines targeting CD19. Fortunately, these toxicities are usually temporary and tend to resolve within a few days or weeks. Prompt recognition and management of these neurologic side effects are crucial to ensure the safety of patients and to optimize treatment outcomes (Zhao and Cao 2019; Mikkilineni and Kochenderfer 2017; Brudno and Kochenderfer 2019; Su and Vale 2018; Ghilardi et al. 2022; Asmamaw Dejenie et al. 2022). IV corticosteroids, Anakirna, Tocilizumab, and Siltuximab are some drugs used to manage ICANS.

26.13 Long-Term Effects and Follow-Up

CAR T-cell therapy has shown impressive effectiveness, leading to numerous patients achieving complete remission. After receiving the treatment, patients are strictly advised to remain in close proximity to the hospital for a minimum of 30 days for follow-up care and continuous health assessments. The recovery process may extend for 2–3 months. However, the long-term effects of this treatment are still being studied. Though some of its toxicities are B-cell aplasia/cytopenias, hypogammaglobulinemia, infection, and HLH/MAS. It is important for patients to undergo regular follow-up visits to monitor their response to therapy, assess for disease recurrence, and manage any potential late effects (Zhao and Cao 2019, Mikkilineni and Kochenderfer 2017, Brudno and Kochenderfer 2019, Su and Vale 2018, Ghilardi et al. 2022, Asmamaw Dejenie et al. 2022). A significant concern associated with this therapy is the possibility of relapse. It has also been seen that after undergoing the therapy, cancer cells were either reduced or completely eliminated in 80% of patients. Though, in some cases, cancer cells can evolve to evade recognition by the modified T cells, leading to disease recurrence. Strategies to overcome this challenge, such as combination therapies and modifications to the CAR T-cell design are evolving (Lee et al. 2014; Boyiadzis et al. 2018; Brudno and Kochenderfer 2016; Maude et al. 2018; Maude et al. 2014).

26.14 Psychosocial Impact and Supportive Care

Undergoing CAR T-cell therapy can present both physical and emotional challenges for patients. The treatment process can be lengthy and intense, requiring prolonged hospitalization and isolation to minimize the risk of infections. Patients may experience anxiety, depression, and uncertainty about the expenses and outcome of their treatment.

However, psychosocial support is crucial for patients on CAR T-cell therapy. Multidisciplinary teams, including hemato-oncologists, nurses, psychologists, and social workers, collaborate to provide comprehensive care (Johnson et al. 2023; Mao et al. 2023; Borreani et al. 2020; Oerlemans et al. 2013).

26.15 Expected Cost of Therapy in India

The cost of CAR T-cell therapy varies widely in India depending on a number of variables. However, the expected cost ranges from approximately INR 1 crore (10 million) to INR 3 crores (30 million) or more. It is crucial to note that this range is only an estimate and may change based on the specific treatment protocol, the center chosen, and the patient's individual requirements. However, the expected cost of CAR T-cell therapy in India is influenced by variety of factors (Zhu et al. 2020; Choi et al. 2022).

26.15.1 Factor Influencing the Cost of CAR T-Cell Therapy

- Treatment Centre and Infrastructure:
- The cost of this therapy can be significantly influenced by the choice of treatment center. Specialized medical centers with state-of-the-art infrastructure and expertise often have higher treatment charges.
- Manufacturing and Processing of CAR T Cells:
- The production and processing of this cells involve complex laboratory procedures and specialized personnel. The cost associated with isolating, modifying, and expanding the patient's T cells can significantly impact the overall therapy cost. In addition, the need for advanced equipment, consumables, and quality control measures contributes to the expenses involved in manufacturing CAR T cells.
- Pre-treatment Evaluation and Diagnosis:
- Before receiving CAR T-cell therapy, patients undergo thorough evaluations and diagnostic tests to assess their eligibility and prepare for treatment. These pre-treatment assessments, including laboratory tests, imaging studies, and consultations with healthcare professionals, contribute to the overall cost.
- Treatment Administration and Follow-Up:
- CAR T-cell therapy requires meticulous monitoring, hospitalization, and post-treatment follow-up. The duration and intensity of these services can vary depending on the individual patient's response and requirements. Consequently, the cost of treatment administration and follow-up adds to the overall therapy expenses.

26.16 Conclusion

CAR T-cell therapy has revolutionized cancer treatment, particularly for certain hematologic malignancies. It utilizes the patient's immune system to target and eliminate cancer cells, presently offering hope for those with limited treatment options. Despite impressive response rates and long-term remissions, challenges such as CRS and neurologic toxicities require careful management. Understanding the treatment process, potential side effects, and long-term effects is crucial for healthcare. The high cost of therapy and the need for improved access remain concerns. Multidisciplinary care is vital to address the physical and emotional impacts on patients. With ongoing research and advancements, this therapy holds promise for transforming cancer treatment and improving patient outcomes.

Flowchart

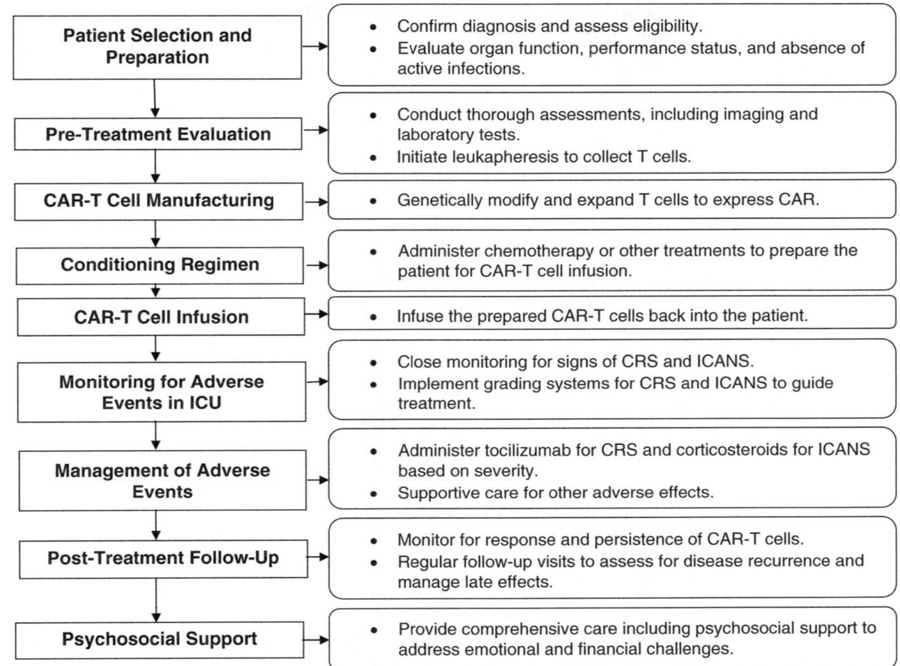

References

Abbasi S, Totmaj MA, Abbasi M, Hajazimian S, Goleij P, Behroozi J et al (2023) Chimeric antigen receptor T (CAR-T) cells: novel cell therapy for hematological malignancies. Cancer Med 12(7):7844–7858

Asmamaw Dejenie T, Tiruneh G, Medhin M, Dessie Terefe G, Tadele Admasu F, Wale Tesega W, Chekol Abebe E (2022) Current updates on generations, approvals, and clinical trials of CAR T-cell therapy. Hum Vaccin Immunother 18(6):2114254

Borreani C, Alfieri S, Farina L, Bianchi E, Corradini P (2020) Fear of cancer recurrence in haematological cancer patients: exploring socio-demographic, psychological, existential and disease-related factors. Support Care Cancer 28:5973–5982

Bourbon E, Ghesquières H, Bachy E (2021) CAR-T cells, from principle to clinical applications. Bull Cancer 108(10):S4–S17

Boyiadzis MM, Dhodapkar MV, Brentjens RJ, Kochenderfer JN, Neelapu SS, Maus MV et al (2018) Chimeric antigen receptor (CAR) T therapies for the treatment of hematologic malignancies: clinical perspective and significance. J Immunother Cancer 6:1–12

Brudno JN, Kochenderfer JN (2016) Toxicities of chimeric antigen receptor T cells: recognition and management. Blood, J Am Soc Hematol 127(26):3321–3330

Brudno JN, Kochenderfer JN (2019) Recent advances in CAR T-cell toxicity: mechanisms, manifestations and management. Blood Rev 34:45–55

Cai W, Zeng Q, Zhang X, Ruan W (2021) Trends analysis of non-hodgkin lymphoma at the national, regional, and global level, 1990–2019: results from the global burden of disease study 2019. Front Med 8:738693

Choi G, Shin G, Bae S (2022) Price and prejudice? The value of chimeric antigen receptor (CAR) T-cell therapy. Int J Environ Res Public Health 19(19):12366

Davila ML, Sadelain M (2016) Biology and clinical application of CAR T cells for B cell malignancies. Int J Hematol 104:6–17

Eshhar Z (2014) From the mouse cage to human therapy: a personal perspective of the emergence of T-bodies/chimeric antigen receptor T cells. Hum Gene Ther 25(9):773–778

Eshhar Z, Waks T, Gross G, Schindler DG (1993) Specific activation and targeting of cytotoxic lymphocytes through chimeric single chains consisting of antibody-binding domains and the gamma or zeta subunits of the immunoglobulin and T-cell receptors. Proc Natl Acad Sci 90(2):720–724

Ghilardi G, Chong EA, Svoboda J, Wohlfarth P, Nasta SD, Williamson S et al (2022) Bendamustine is safe and effective for lymphodepletion before tisagenlecleucel in patients with refractory or relapsed large B-cell lymphomas. Ann Oncol 33(9):916–928

Gill S, Brudno JN (2021) CAR T-cell therapy in hematologic malignancies: clinical role, toxicity, and unanswered questions. Am Soc Clin Oncol Educ Book 41:e246–e265

Goverman J, Gomez SM, Segesman KD, Hunkapiller T, Laug WE, Hood L (1990) Chimeric immunoglobulin-T cell receptor proteins form functional receptors: implications for T cell receptor complex formation and activation. Cell 60(6):929–939

Gross G, Eshhar Z (1992) Endowing T cells with antibody specificity using chimeric T cell receptors. FASEB J 6(15):3370–3378

Grosser R, Cherkassky L, Chintala N, Adusumilli PS (2019) Combination immunotherapy with CAR T cells and checkpoint blockade for the treatment of solid tumors. Cancer Cell 36(5):471–482. https://doi.org/10.1016/j.ccell.2019.09.006

Haslauer T, Greil R, Zaborsky N, Geisberger R (2021) CAR T-cell therapy in hematological malignancies. Int J Mol Sci 22(16):8996

Havard R, Stephens DM (2018) Anti-CD19 chimeric antigen receptor T cell therapies: harnessing the power of the immune system to fight diffuse large B cell lymphoma. Curr Hematol Malig Rep 13:534–542

Huang J, Huang X, Huang J (2022) CAR-T cell therapy for hematological malignancies: limitations and optimization strategies. Front Immunol 13:1019115

Johnson PC, Dhawale T, Newcomb RA, Amonoo HL, Lavoie MW, Vaughn D et al (2023) Longitudinal patient-reported outcomes in patients receiving chimeric antigen receptor T-cell therapy. Blood Adv 7(14):3541–3550

June CH, O'Connor RS, Kawalekar OU, Ghassemi S, Milone MC (2018) CAR T cell immunotherapy for human cancer. Science 359(6382):1361–1365

Keykhaei M, Masinaei M, Mohammadi E, Azadnajafabad S, Rezaei N, Saeedi Moghaddam S et al (2021) A global, regional, and national survey on burden and Quality of Care Index (QCI) of hematologic malignancies; global burden of disease systematic analysis 1990–2017. Exp Hematol Oncol 10:1–15

Kilic-Erkek O, Gundogdu G, Adiguzel E, Coguplugil A, Bor-Kucukatay M (2023) Influences of alternate-day fasting and time-restricted feeding alone and in combination with swimming exercise on hypothalamic lipid homeostasis. Available at SSRN 4563592

Lee DW, Gardner R, Porter DL, Louis CU, Ahmed N, Jensen M et al (2014) Current concepts in the diagnosis and management of cytokine release syndrome. Blood, J Am Soc Hematol 124(2):188–195

Li G, Boucher JC, Kotani H, Park K, Zhang Y, Shrestha B et al (2018) 4-1BB enhancement of CAR T function requires NF-κB and TRAFs. JCI Insight 3(18):e121322

Li H, Yang Y, Hong W, Huang M, Wu M, Zhao X (2020) Applications of genome editing technology in the targeted therapy of human diseases: mechanisms, advances and prospects. Signal Transduct Target Ther 5(1):1

Lu J, Jiang G (2022) The journey of CAR-T therapy in hematological malignancies. Mol Cancer 21(1):194

Mancikova V, Smida M (2021) Current state of CAR T-cell therapy in chronic lymphocytic leukemia. Int J Mol Sci 22(11):5536

Mao Y, Huang L, Ruan H, Guo Y, Ni S, Ling Y (2023) Patients' experience with chimeric antigen receptor T-cell therapy for DLBCL in China: a qualitative study. Support Care Cancer 31(5):303

Maude SL, Frey N, Shaw PA, Aplenc R, Barrett DM, Bunin NJ et al (2014) Chimeric antigen receptor T cells for sustained remissions in leukemia. N Engl J Med 371(16):1507–1517

Maude SL, Laetsch TW, Buechner J, Rives S, Boyer M, Bittencourt H et al (2018) Tisagenlecleucel in children and young adults with B-cell lymphoblastic leukemia. N Engl J Med 378(5):439–448

Maus MV (2022) A decade of CAR T cell evolution. Nat Cancer 3(3):270–271

Mavi AK, Gaur S, Gaur G, Jindal P, Kumar N, Kumar U (2023) CAR T-cell therapy: reprogramming patient's immune cell to treat cancer. Cell Signal 105:110638

Mikkilineni L, Kochenderfer JN (2017) Chimeric antigen receptor T-cell therapies for multiple myeloma. Blood 130(24):2594–2602. https://doi.org/10.1182/blood-2017-06-793869

Mitra A, Barua A, Huang L, Feng Q, He B (2023) From bench to bedside: the history and progress of CAR T cell therapy. Front Immunol 14:1188049

Nasta SD, Namoglu EC, Hughes ME, Chong EA, Svoboda J, Ballard HJ et al (2019) Hospitalization patterns with commercial CAR T-cell therapy: a single institution experience. Blood 134:3240

Obaisi O, Fontillas RC, Patel K, Ngo-Huang A (2022) Rehabilitation needs for patients undergoing CAR T-cell therapy. Curr Oncol Rep 24(6):741–749

Oerlemans S, Mols F, Issa DE, Pruijt JHFM, Peters WG, Lybeert M et al (2013) A high level of fatigue among long-term survivors of non-Hodgkin's lymphoma: results from the longitudinal population-based PROFILES registry in the south of the Netherlands. Haematologica 98(3):479

Pulè MA, Straathof KC, Dotti G, Heslop HE, Rooney CM, Brenner MK (2005) A chimeric T cell antigen receptor that augments cytokine release and supports clonal expansion of primary human T cells. Mol Ther 12(5):933–941

Rohaan MW, Wilgenhof S, Haanen JB (2019) Adoptive cellular therapies: the current landscape. Virchows Arch 474(4):449–461

Seimetz D, Heller K, Richter J (2019) Approval of first CAR-Ts: have we solved all hurdles for ATMPs? Cell Med 11:2155179018822781

Skorka K, Ostapinska K, Malesa A, Giannopoulos K (2020) The application of CAR-T cells in haematological malignancies. Arch Immunol Ther Exp 68:1–19

Song DG, Ye Q, Poussin M, Harms GM, Figini M, Powell DJ Jr (2012) CD27 costimulation augments the survival and antitumor activity of redirected human T cells in vivo. Blood, J Am Soc Hematol 119(3):696–706

Sterner RC, Sterner RM (2021) CAR-T cell therapy: current limitations and potential strategies. Blood Cancer J 11(4):69

Su X, Vale R (2018) Mechanisms of chimeric antigen receptor (CAR) signaling during T cell activation. Biophys J 114(3):107a–108a

Teoh PJ, Chng WJ (2021) CAR T-cell therapy in multiple myeloma: more room for improvement. Blood Cancer J 11(4):84

Whitlow M, Bell BA, Feng SL, Filpula D, Hardman KD, Hubert SL et al (1993) An improved linker for single-chain Fv with reduced aggregation and enhanced proteolytic stability. Protein Eng Des Sel 6(8):989–995

Wurdeman SR, Stevens PM, Campbell JH (2018) Mobility Analysis of AmpuTees (MAAT I): quality of life and satisfaction are strongly related to mobility for patients with a lower limb prosthesis. Prosthetics Orthot Int 42(5):498–503. https://doi.org/10.1177/0309364617736089

Zhang X, Zhu L, Zhang H, Xiao Y (2022) CAR-T cell therapy in hematological malignancies: current opportunities and challenges. Front Immunol 13:927153

Zhang N, Wu J, Wang Q, Liang Y, Li X, Chen G et al (2023) Global burden of hematologic malignancies and evolution patterns over the past 30 years. Blood Cancer J 13(1):82

Zhao L, Cao YJ (2019) Engineered T cell therapy for cancer in the clinic. Front Immunol 10:484029

Zhao Z, Chen Y, Francisco NM, Zhang Y, Wu M (2018) The application of CAR-T cell therapy in hematological malignancies: advantages and challenges. Acta Pharm Sin B 8(4):539–551

Zhu F, Wei G, Zhang M, Zhao H, Wu W, Yang L et al (2020) Factors associated with costs in chimeric antigen receptor T-cell therapy for patients with relapsed/refractory B-cell malignancies. Cell Transplant 29:0963689720919434

Part V
Infections in Hematological Patients

Chapter 27
Opportunistic Infection in Hematological Malignancies

Shakti Bedanta Mishra

Learning Points

1. Understand different infectious diseases affecting patients with hematologic malignancies and hematopoietic stem cell transplantation (HSCT).
2. Learn about diagnosis, management, and prevention of viral infections such as cytomegalovirus, herpes simplex virus, varicella-zoster virus, and respiratory viruses.
3. Know about parasitic infections such as toxoplasmosis, strongyloidiasis, and protozoan diseases.
4. Explore new advancements in prophylactic measures and therapeutic options for managing infectious diseases in hematologic and HSCT patients.

27.1 Introduction

The landscape of infectious diseases in patients with hematologic malignancies and those who have undergone hematopoietic stem cell transplantation (HSCT) is both complex and challenging. Within this context, parasitic infections, although less common than their bacterial and viral counterparts, present a significant risk to this immunocompromised population. The prevalence of these infections has been on the rise, attributed in part to the increasing number of HSCT procedures and the global mobility that facilitates the spread of parasitic diseases previously confined to endemic regions (Findlater and Bogoch 2018; Bretagne and Klimko 2020). Moreover, the notable global heterogeneity in the distribution of COVID-19 cases and its association with pre-existing parasitic diseases hint at the complex interplay between infectious diseases and immunocompromised states (Chang et al. 2022).

A. *Prevalence of Parasitic Infections in Hematologic and HSCT Patients*

Parasitic infections in individuals with hematologic malignancies or those who have undergone HSCT are emerging as a concern due to their potential to cause severe complications. These infections, including toxoplasmosis, strongyloidiasis,

S. B. Mishra (✉)
Department of Critical Care Medicine, IMS and SUM Hospital, Bhubaneswar, Odisha, India

S. B. Mishra (ed.), *Critical Care Hematology*,
https://doi.org/10.1007/978-981-97-5565-3_27

and infections caused by protozoans such as Giardia intestinalis and Cryptosporidium spp., can lead to significant morbidity and mortality in this vulnerable patient group. The prevalence rates of these parasitic infections vary widely, influenced by geographic location, environmental exposure, and the intensity of immunosuppressive therapy, among other factors (Durak et al. 2013; Haque et al. 2023).

B. *Comparison with Bacterial and Viral Infections*

While bacterial and viral infections have long been recognized as leading causes of morbidity and mortality in patients with hematologic malignancies and HSCT recipients, parasitic infections have traditionally received less attention. This is despite the fact that the impact of parasitic infections can be equally severe, leading to prolonged hospital stays, increased healthcare costs, and, in some cases, fatal outcomes. The proportion of parasitic infections, though lower than bacterial and viral infections, underscores a crucial gap in the surveillance, diagnosis, and management of infectious diseases in this patient cohort (Machado et al. 2020; Haque et al. 2023).

C. *Importance of Understanding and Managing These Infections*

The complexity of managing parasitic infections in patients with hematologic conditions and HSCT recipients cannot be overstated. These infections often present atypically, complicating diagnosis and delaying appropriate treatment. Understanding the epidemiology, risk factors, and clinical manifestations of parasitic infections is paramount for establishing effective prevention, early detection, and treatment strategies. Moreover, the evolving nature of these infections, with the emergence of drug-resistant parasites and the introduction of new therapeutic agents, highlights the need for ongoing research and education in this area (Sun et al. 2023; Faure et al. 2017). By improving our understanding of these infections, healthcare providers can better navigate the challenges they present, ultimately improving patient outcomes and quality of life for this vulnerable population.

Viral infections in patients with hematologic malignancies and those undergoing HSCT represent a formidable challenge, impacting both clinical outcomes and patient quality of life. The interplay between the weakened immune system in these patients and opportunistic viral pathogens can lead to infections that are severe, recurrent, and sometimes life-threatening.

27.2 Impact on Morbidity and Mortality

The morbidity and mortality associated with viral infections in this patient cohort are substantial. Infections caused by cytomegalovirus (CMV), herpes simplex virus (HSV), varicella-zoster virus (VZV), and others have been linked to significant clinical complications, including but not limited to pneumonitis, hepatitis, encephalitis, and retinitis. These infections can delay or complicate the treatment of the underlying hematologic condition, lead to extended hospital stays, and, in severe cases, result in death. The impact is particularly pronounced in HSCT recipients, where viral infections are a leading cause of post-transplant complications and mortality. The risk is further exacerbated by the fact that these infections can indirectly contribute to other complications, such as graft-versus-host disease (GVHD) in allogeneic transplant recipients (Ottaviano et al. 2020; Gaytán-Morales et al. 2021).

Recent studies and observations emphasize the need for vigilant monitoring and management of these infections to mitigate their impact on this vulnerable population. For instance, the role of γδ T cells in defending against viral infections post-allogeneic stem cell transplantation highlights potential therapeutic strategies to enhance viral control without exacerbating GVHD. Furthermore, delaying transplantation in children with viral respiratory infections has been shown to reduce transplant-related mortality, underlining the importance of timing in transplantation procedures (Ottaviano et al. 2020). The high systemic inflammation associated with episodes of multiple viral detections and an EBV association with elevated IL-1β, IL-8, and GVHD further supports the intricate link between viral infections, immune responses, and transplantation outcomes (Rojas-Rechy et al. 2022).

27.3 Challenges in Defining Incidence and Consequences

Quantifying the true incidence and understanding the full spectrum of consequences of viral infections in patients with hematologic malignancies and HSCT recipients are fraught with challenges. These difficulties stem from several factors, including the variability in surveillance practices across institutions, the evolving nature of diagnostic criteria, and the introduction of new antiviral agents that may alter the natural history of these infections. Furthermore, the incidence and severity of viral infections are influenced by a myriad of patient-specific factors, such as the type and stage of hematologic malignancy, the intensity of chemotherapy or immunosuppression, and the presence of coexisting conditions. This complexity makes it challenging to establish clear epidemiological patterns and directly attribute morbidity and mortality to specific viral infections (Antonova et al. 2021; Cam and Yoruk 2020).

27.4 Role of T-Cell-Mediated Immune Suppression

T-cell-mediated immune suppression plays a central role in the susceptibility to and severity of viral infections in patients with hematologic malignancies and HSCT recipients. The degree of T-cell suppression, whether resulting from the underlying disease, chemotherapy, radiation therapy, or the use of immunosuppressive drugs to prevent or treat GVHD, directly correlates with the risk of viral reactivation and infection. Viruses that establish latency in the host, such as CMV, HSV, and VZV, are particularly adept at exploiting weakened cellular immunity to reactivate and cause disease. The dynamics of T-cell recovery post-transplant or post-therapy are, therefore, critical determinants of the timing and severity of viral infections, underscoring the importance of immune monitoring and targeted prophylaxis in these patients (Kunte et al. 2022).

27.5 Common Viral Infections

Patients with hematologic malignancies and those who have undergone HSCT are particularly vulnerable to a range of viral infections. These infections can complicate treatment protocols, prolong hospitalizations, and significantly affect patient outcomes. Understanding the common viral pathogens, their clinical presentation, diagnostic challenges, recurrence patterns, and management strategies is crucial for optimizing patient care.

Overview of Prevalent Viruses

- Cytomegalovirus (CMV): A latent virus that can cause serious disease in immunocompromised individuals, including pneumonia, gastrointestinal disease, and retinitis (Yang et al. 2024; Uluhan et al. 1995).
- Herpes Simplex Virus (HSV): Known for causing oral and genital lesions, HSV can lead to more severe infections such as encephalitis and systemic disease in immunocompromised patients (Uluhan et al. 1995).
- Varicella-Zoster Virus (VZV): Responsible for chickenpox in primary infection and shingles in reactivation, VZV can cause significant morbidity in hematologic and HSCT patients (Boeckh et al. 2020; Li et al. 2023).
- Respiratory Syncytial Virus (RSV): A major cause of respiratory infections, RSV can lead to severe lower respiratory tract disease in vulnerable populations (Vakil et al. 2018; Baier et al. 2022).
- Parainfluenza Viruses: Cause a spectrum of respiratory illnesses from mild cold-like symptoms to severe pneumonia (Essa et al. 2017; Silvestri et al. 2021).
- Influenza Viruses: Highly contagious viruses causing seasonal outbreaks of flu, with potential for severe complications in immunocompromised patients (Vakil et al. 2018; Baier et al. 2022).

27.6 Presentation and Diagnosis Challenges

The clinical presentation of viral infections in immunocompromised patients can be atypical, complicating the diagnosis. For example, HSV and VZV infections may not present with the classic vesicular rash, and CMV disease can manifest with a range of symptoms depending on the organ system involved. Diagnosis is further complicated by the similarity in symptoms between viral infections and other complications of immunosuppression, such as drug reactions or bacterial infections.

Molecular diagnostic techniques, such as polymerase chain reaction (PCR), have greatly improved the sensitivity and specificity of viral detection. However, the interpretation of these tests requires careful consideration of the clinical context, as detection of viral DNA or RNA does not necessarily indicate active disease (Hijano et al. 2019; Magira et al. 2019) (Fig. 27.1).

27.7 Recurrence and Management Strategies

Recurrence is a significant concern for these infections, particularly for viruses such as HSV and VZV, which establish latency and can reactivate during periods of immune suppression. Management strategies for viral infections in hematologic and HSCT patients include:

- *Prophylaxis*: Antiviral prophylaxis is used to prevent infection or reactivation of viruses such as CMV and HSV. The choice of agent and duration of prophylaxis depend on the patient's risk profile (Lee et al. 2018).
- *Preemptive Therapy*: Monitoring viral loads to initiate treatment before the onset of clinical disease, particularly for CMV.
- *Treatment of Active Infections*: Utilizing antiviral medications tailored to the specific virus and the severity of the infection. For example, ganciclovir or valganciclovir for CMV, acyclovir for HSV and VZV (Szenborn et al. 2016; Bakacs et al. 2023; Grit et al. 2022), and ribavirin for RSV, although treatment efficacy can vary.
- *Immunomodulation*: Adjusting the level of immunosuppression, when possible, to enhance the immune response to the virus while balancing the risk of GVHD in HSCT recipients.

27.8 Emerging Viral Pathogens

The landscape of infectious diseases is continually evolving, with new viral pathogens emerging as significant threats to patients with hematologic malignancies and those undergoing HSCT. The identification of these emerging viruses underscores the need for vigilant surveillance and innovation in both diagnostics and therapeutics (Testi et al. 2021).

Identification of New Viral Threats

- *Human Herpesvirus-6 (HHV-6)*: Known for its potential to cause severe complications such as encephalitis and bone-marrow suppression in immunocompromised individuals.
- *BK Virus*: Primarily associated with nephropathy in kidney transplant recipients, BK virus can also affect HSCT patients, leading to hemorrhagic cystitis and other complications. Studies have highlighted the challenges of BK virus

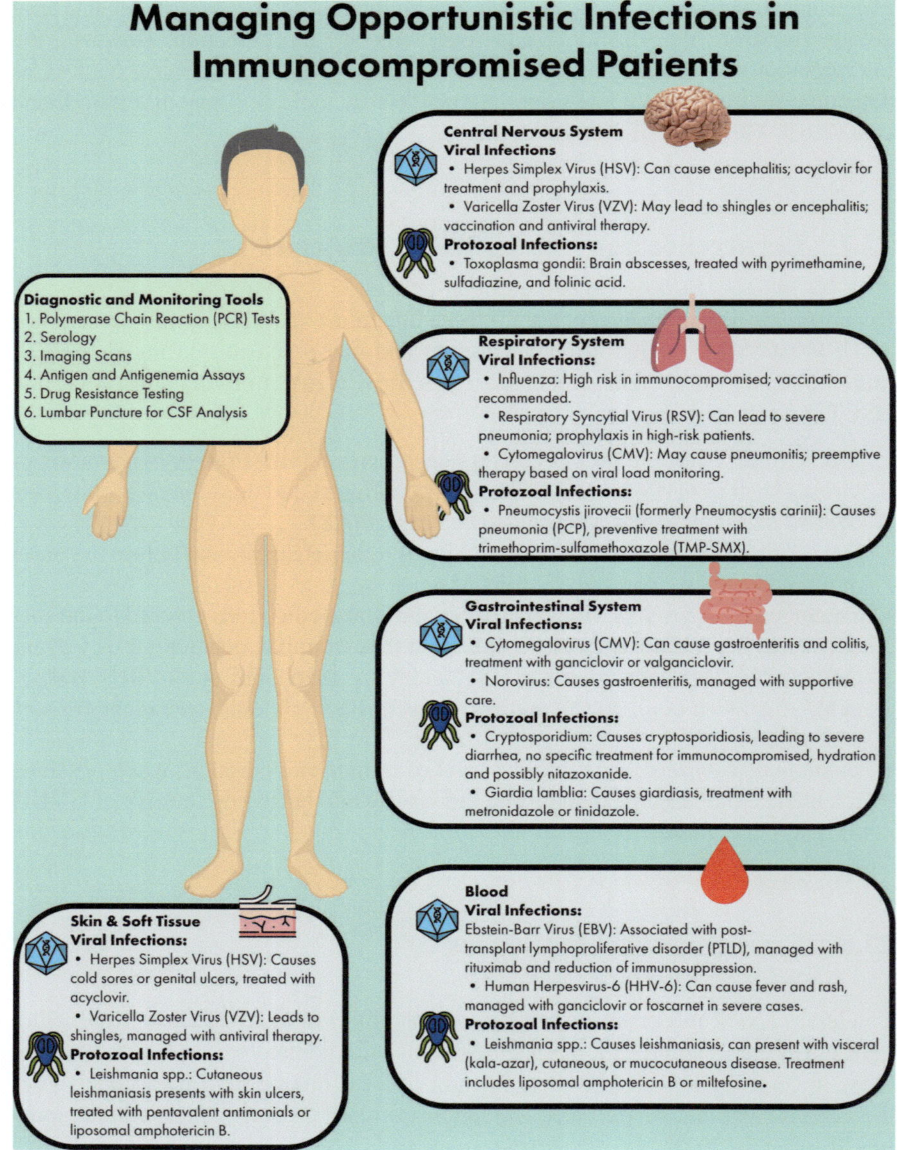

Fig. 27.1 Managing opportunistic infections in immunocompromised patients

nephropathy in post-allogeneic stem cell transplantation, emphasizing its role in renal failure and the complexities of managing this condition (Gutovskaya et al. 2018; Papanicolaou et al. 2013; Burbach et al. 2016).

- *Adenovirus*: Can cause a wide range of diseases, from respiratory infections to gastroenteritis and disseminated disease, particularly severe in immunocompromised hosts. Research underscores the significance of adenovirus infections in both immunocompetent and immunocompromised patients, pointing to the ongoing challenges in diagnostics and treatment (Lion 2014; Cederwall and Påhlman 2019).

- *Human Metapneumovirus*: A cause of respiratory infections with the potential to develop into severe lower respiratory tract diseases in vulnerable populations.

27.9 Implications for Diagnostic and Therapeutic Development

The emergence of these pathogens necessitates the continuous development of diagnostic methods that can accurately and promptly identify these infections. Moreover, there is an urgent need for the development of specific antiviral therapies that are effective against these emerging viruses. The adaptability of these viruses, combined with the specific vulnerabilities of immunocompromised patients, presents a significant challenge in managing these infections effectively (Long et al. 2023; Focosi et al. 2023).

Advances in Molecular Diagnostics
Advancements in molecular diagnostics have revolutionized the detection and management of viral infections in immunocompromised patients, offering improved sensitivity, specificity, and speed over traditional methods.

A. *Improvement in Viral Infection Diagnosis:*

   - The advent of molecular diagnostics has significantly enhanced the ability to diagnose viral infections quickly and accurately, enabling timely initiation of appropriate antiviral therapies and preventive measures.

B. *Techniques:*

   - *Rapid Culture Techniques*: Allow for the faster detection of viruses compared to traditional culture methods, though they are less commonly used with the advent of more advanced techniques.
   - *CMV Antigen Assays*: Provide a direct method for detecting CMV infections, particularly useful for monitoring patients at risk for CMV reactivation.
   - *Polymerase Chain Reaction (PCR) Tests*: The cornerstone of modern viral diagnostics, PCR tests can detect viral DNA or RNA with high sensitivity and specificity, facilitating the diagnosis of active infections even at low viral loads (Marchetti et al. 2011).

27.10 Impact on Patient Management

- Molecular diagnostics have profoundly impacted the management of viral infections in hematologic and HSCT patients.
- Enabling the early detection of viral reactivation or infection, often before the onset of symptoms (Inazawa et al. 2016)

- Allowing for the precise identification of the viral pathogen, thereby guiding targeted antiviral therapy (Stoykova et al. 2023)
- Facilitating the monitoring of viral load during treatment to assess response and guide therapy duration (Winestone et al. 2018)

27.11 New Agents for Prophylaxis and Therapy

The continuous evolution of viral pathogens and the unique vulnerabilities of patients with hematologic malignancies and HSCT recipients necessitate the development of new antiviral agents. These novel therapies not only aim to treat existing infections but also serve as prophylactic measures to prevent the onset of viral diseases.

Introduction of Maribavir and Valganciclovir

- *Maribavir*: An antiviral agent targeting the CMV UL97 kinase, maribavir, has shown promise in treating CMV infections resistant to traditional antivirals. Its mechanism of action differs from that of other antivirals, making it a valuable option for patients who do not respond to or cannot tolerate standard therapies (Schlatzer et al. 2017; Pietersma et al. 2010).
- *Valganciclovir*: A prodrug of ganciclovir and valganciclovir offers improved oral bioavailability, facilitating easier administration and better patient compliance. It is effective against CMV infections and is used both for treatment and prophylaxis in immunocompromised patients (Kang 2013; Omarova et al. 2022).

27.12 Potential Benefits in Reducing Infection-Related Morbidity and Mortality

The introduction of maribavir and valganciclovir represents a significant advancement in the management of viral infections, particularly CMV, in immunocompromised populations. These agents have the potential to:

- Reduce the incidence of CMV reactivation and disease, a common and serious complication in HSCT recipients and patients with hematologic malignancies (Magira et al. 2019).
- Decrease the morbidity associated with CMV infections, including hospitalizations, the need for intravenous treatments, and the impact on quality of life (Gandhi and Kotton 2022).
- Lower the mortality rates associated with severe CMV disease by providing effective treatment options for drug-resistant infections and reducing the overall burden of disease (Kotton and Kamar 2023).

Need for Further Studies
Despite the progress made in the development of antiviral agents and diagnostic techniques, significant gaps remain in our understanding and management of viral infections in immunocompromised patients.

Further studies are needed to clarify the viral infection spectrum, develop effective prevention and treatment strategies, and consider the effects of T-cell depletion. This research will help to optimize the management of CMV and other viral infections in this vulnerable patient population (Chemaly et al. 2014).

- *Clarification of Viral Infection Spectrum*: Comprehensive research is necessary to delineate the full spectrum of viral infections affecting this patient population. This effort should extend beyond merely identifying emerging pathogens to gaining a thorough understanding of their epidemiology, clinical manifestations, and outcomes. Such knowledge is vital for developing more effective diagnostic and management strategies (Hawkinson et al. 2013; Gentry et al. 2023).
- *Development of Effective Prevention and Treatment*: The continuous emergence of viral pathogens underscores the need for novel antiviral agents and preventive measures. Progress in this area depends on sustained research investment aimed at discovering new therapeutics, elucidating mechanisms of antiviral resistance, and refining treatment protocols to enhance patient outcomes (Saha 2022; Moso et al. 2023).
- *Consideration of T-Cell Depletion Effects*: The impact of T-cell depletion—stemming from the underlying disease, therapeutic regimens, or HSCT—on the risk and trajectory of viral infections is a critical area for further study. A deeper understanding of T-cell immunity's role in viral infection dynamics could lead to the development of more effective prophylactic and therapeutic approaches, ultimately improving the prognosis for these at-risk patients (Shahani et al. 2017; Cortes-Penfield et al. 2019).

27.13 Parasitic Infections

Parasitic infections, particularly those caused by protozoans, represent a significant health concern for patients with hematologic malignancies and those undergoing HSCT. These infections can exacerbate the already heightened vulnerability of such patients to infectious diseases, leading to further complications and affecting their overall prognosis.

27.14 Gastrointestinal Protozoan Infections

Gastrointestinal protozoan infections are among the most common parasitic diseases affecting immunocompromised individuals. These infections can lead to severe gastrointestinal symptoms, malabsorption, and weight loss, significantly impacting patient recovery and quality of life.

27.14.1 *Frequency and Factors Affecting Infections*

A landmark study conducted by Łanocha and colleagues aimed to elucidate the frequency of gastrointestinal protozoan infections among patients with hematologic malignancies undergoing intensive hemato-oncological treatment. The research also sought to identify biological factors that might influence the incidence of these infections, providing insights into potential preventive measures and treatment strategies (Łanocha et al. 2022).

27.15 Prevalence in Hematologic Malignancies Versus Control

The study's findings highlighted a higher prevalence of intestinal protozoans in patients with hematologic malignancies compared to a control group of healthy individuals. This increased prevalence underscores the heightened risk that patients with hematologic conditions face regarding parasitic infections, likely due to compromised immune system functions (Łanocha et al. 2022).

Types of Protozoans Identified
Among the protozoans identified in the study were:

- Giardia intestinalis, known to cause giardiasis, characterized by diarrhea, abdominal pain, and malabsorption (Martínez-Gordillo et al. 2014).
- Cryptosporidium spp., associated with cryptosporidiosis, which can lead to severe, life-threatening diarrhea in immunocompromised patients (Lanocha et al. 2022; Yang et al. 2022).
- Potentially pathogenic Blastocystis spp., which can be associated with a range of gastrointestinal symptoms (Tunalı et al. 2018).
- Entamoeba coli, generally considered nonpathogenic but indicative of fecal contamination and potential exposure to other pathogenic organisms (El-Tawel et al. 2020).

27.16 Risk Factors for Infection

The study identified several risk factors for the acquisition of gastrointestinal protozoan infections, including environmental exposure and personal habits. Notably, patients who engaged in gardening without protective gloves or those in close contact with animals were found to have a higher incidence of infection. These findings suggest that lifestyle modifications and increased awareness of potential exposure risks could play a role in reducing the incidence of protozoan infections among patients with hematologic malignancies.

27.17 Toxoplasmosis

Toxoplasmosis, caused by the intracellular protozoan Toxoplasma gondii, poses a significant risk to immunocompromised patients, including those with hematologic malignancies and recipients of HSCT. The disease's transmission dynamics, risk factors, and severe potential outcomes necessitate a comprehensive understanding to effectively manage and mitigate its impact on vulnerable patient populations (Dard et al. 2018).

Transmission and Risk in Immunocompromised Patients: Toxoplasma gondii is typically transmitted to humans through the ingestion of undercooked or raw meat containing tissue cysts, exposure to oocysts in soil contaminated with cat feces, or congenitally from mother to fetus. In immunocompromised patients, toxoplasmosis primarily results from the reactivation of a latent infection. The suppression of the immune system, due to either the underlying disease or the immunosuppressive therapy required for conditions like HSCT, increases the risk of reactivation and symptomatic disease (Dard et al. 2018).

High-Risk Groups Among HSCT Recipients: HSCT recipients at the highest risk for toxoplasmosis include:

- Individuals who are seropositive for Toxoplasma gondii before transplantation.
- Recipients of allogeneic transplants, especially from cord blood, unrelated donors, or those involving T-cell-depleted grafts.
- Patients with a history of high-grade GVHD or those unable to take prophylaxis with trimethoprim–sulfamethoxazole (TMP/SMX), which also offers protection against Toxoplasma gondii (Dard et al. 2018).

Incidence, Prognosis, and Clinical Presentation: Although the incidence of toxoplasmosis in HSCT recipients is relatively low, ranging from 0.3% to 8% depending on the population studied, the disease's prognosis is poor. Mortality rates can reach up to 60%, particularly in cases of disseminated disease, often diagnosed post-mortem. Clinical manifestations vary from asymptomatic seroconversion to severe symptoms, including fever, lymphadenopathy, encephalitis, myocarditis, pneumonitis, and hepatitis. The central nervous system (CNS) is the most commonly affected, leading to neurological symptoms that significantly worsen the prognosis (Dard et al. 2018).

Diagnosis and Preferred Treatment Options: The diagnosis of toxoplasmosis relies on a combination of serological tests, molecular detection of Toxoplasma gondii DNA through PCR, and imaging studies, particularly in cases of CNS involvement. The PCR testing of cerebrospinal fluid is highly specific and valuable for confirming CNS toxoplasmosis. Treatment typically involves a combination of pyrimethamine and sulfadiazine, along with folinic acid to mitigate hematologic toxicity. For patients who cannot tolerate sulfadiazine, clindamycin is an alternative. Prophylaxis with TMP/SMX is effective in preventing reactivation in seropositive patients, particularly those undergoing immunosuppressive therapy or HSCT (Dard et al. 2018).

27.18 Strongyloidiasis

Strongyloidiasis, a parasitic infection caused by Strongyloides stercoralis, a soil-transmitted helminth, poses significant health risks, especially in immunocompromised individuals. Its unique life cycle allows for autoinfection, leading to persistent infections and the potential for a deadly hyperinfection syndrome in vulnerable populations (Czeresnia and Weiss 2022).

27.18.1 Etiology and Endemic Regions

Strongyloides stercoralis is primarily found in tropical and subtropical regions but can also be present in temperate zones. Transmission occurs through direct contact with soil containing infectious larvae, which penetrate human skin. The larvae migrate to the intestines, where they mature and reproduce. The autoinfective cycle of *S. stercoralis* enables it to persist in the host for decades after the initial exposure (Roseman et al. 2013).

27.18.2 Immune Response and Risk of Hyperinfection

The immune system plays a critical role in controlling Strongyloides infection. A robust T-helper 2 (Th2) cell-mediated immune response can limit the parasite's reproduction and dissemination. However, in immunocompromised patients, particularly those with impaired cell-mediated immunity due to chemotherapy, corticosteroid use, or immunosuppressive therapy for transplantation, the autoinfection cycle can escalate, leading to hyperinfection syndrome. This condition is characterized by an overwhelming increase in larval load and dissemination to organs outside the gastrointestinal tract (Salvador et al. 2021).

27.18.3 Clinical Manifestations and Diagnosis

The clinical manifestations of strongyloidiasis range from asymptomatic to severe, life-threatening disease. Symptoms may include abdominal pain, diarrhea, malabsorption, weight loss, cough, and wheezing. Hyperinfection syndrome and disseminated strongyloidiasis can lead to septicemia, meningitis, and respiratory failure.

Diagnosis of strongyloidiasis is challenging due to the wide range of symptoms and the intermittent shedding of larvae in feces. Techniques for diagnosis include microscopic examination of stool for larvae, serological tests for *S. stercoralis* antibodies, and molecular methods such as PCR. The eosinophil count, often elevated in parasitic infections, can be a useful, albeit nonspecific, indicator (Collyer and Anderson 2024).

27.18.4 Treatment Challenges and Recommendations

Ivermectin is the treatment of choice for strongyloidiasis, offering a higher cure rate and fewer side effects than alternative treatments such as albendazole or thiabendazole. Due to the risk of hyperinfection syndrome, particularly in immunocompromised patients, aggressive treatment and sometimes repeated doses of ivermectin are recommended to ensure eradication of the parasite.

Preventing strongyloidiasis in endemic regions includes wearing protective footwear to prevent skin contact with contaminated soil. For individuals with a history of potential exposure who are planning to undergo immunosuppressive therapy or transplantation, screening for *S. stercoralis* and preemptive treatment is crucial to prevent hyperinfection syndrome (Joo et al. 2023).

27.19 Conclusion

The comprehensive examination of viral and parasitic infections in patients with hematologic malignancies and those undergoing HSCT underscores the intricate interplay between immunocompromised states and infectious diseases. These infections pose significant risks, complicating treatment regimens, impacting morbidity and mortality, and necessitating a nuanced approach to prevention, diagnosis, and management.

27.19.1 Summary of Key Findings and Implications for Practice

- *Viral Infections:* The prevalence of viral infections, particularly those caused by CMV, HSV, VZV, and emerging viruses such as BK virus and adenovirus, highlights the necessity for vigilant monitoring and prompt intervention. The development of molecular diagnostic techniques has significantly improved the detection and management of these infections, enabling more targeted and effective treatment strategies (Majewska et al. 2019; Pereira et al. 2019; Harris et al. 2023).
- *Parasitic Infections:* The study of gastrointestinal protozoan infections, toxoplasmosis, and strongyloidiasis reveals the heightened vulnerability of immunocompromised patients to parasitic diseases. The findings emphasize the importance of understanding transmission mechanisms, identifying high-risk populations, and employing appropriate diagnostic and treatment modalities to mitigate the risks associated with these infections (Suputtamongkol et al. 2011; Yates 2021).

Flowchart

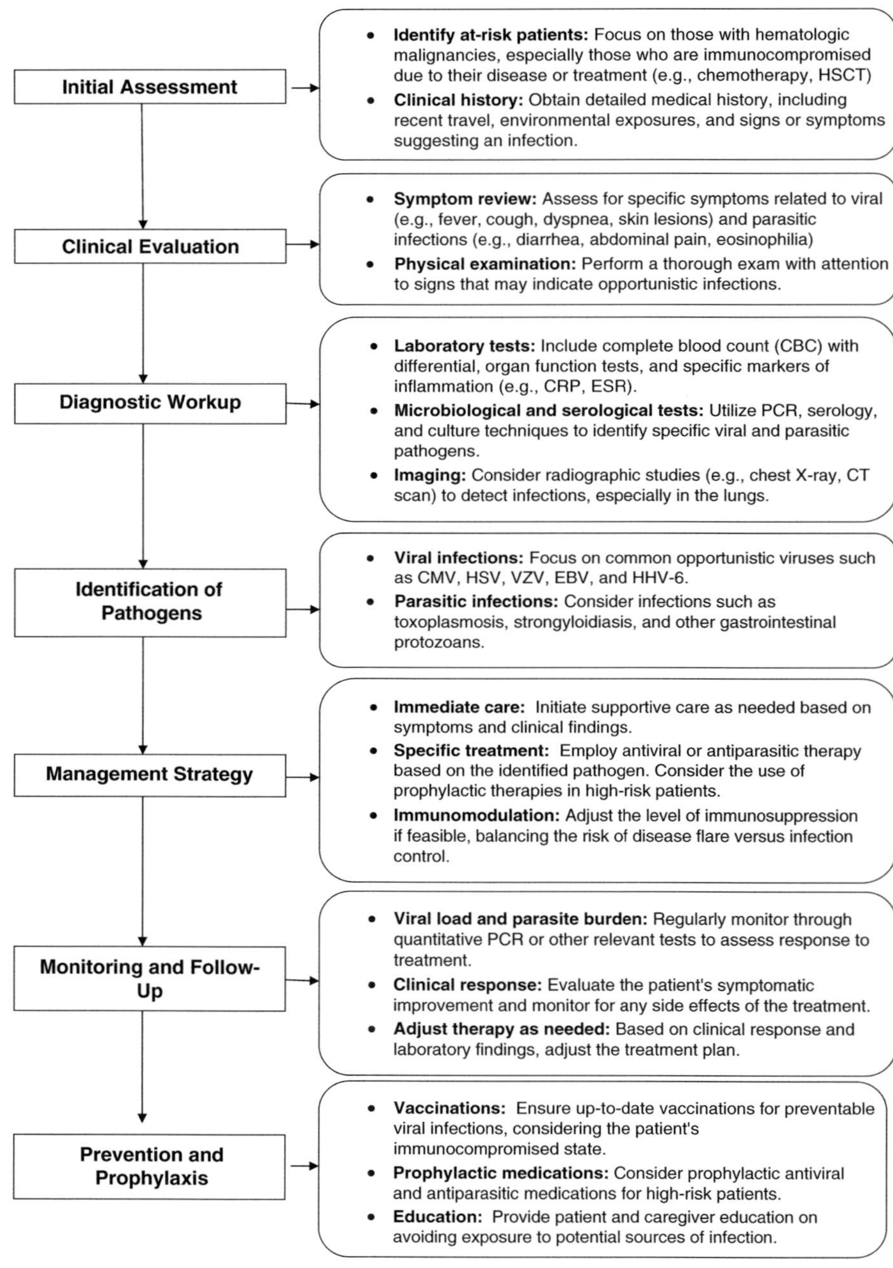

Approach to Opportunistic Viral or Parasitic Infections in Hematologic Malignancies Flowchart

References

Antonova TV, Pobegalova OE, Nozhkin MS, Romanova MA, Gorchakova OV (2021) The impact of viral infections on the results of hemopoietic stem cell transplantation in patients with hematologic malignancies. J Infect 12(5):85–92

Baier C, Huang J, Reumann K, Indenbirken D, Thol F, Koenecke C et al (2022) Target capture sequencing reveals a monoclonal outbreak of respiratory syncytial virus B infections among adult hematologic patients. Antimicrob Resist Infect Control 11(1):88

Bakacs T, Sandig V, Kovesdi I (2023) Combination therapy for the treatment of shingles with an immunostimulatory vaccine virus and acyclovir. Pharmaceuticals 16(2):226

Boeckh MJ, Arvin AM, Mullane KM, Camacho LH, Winston DJ, Morrison VA et al (2020) Immunogenicity of inactivated varicella zoster vaccine in autologous hematopoietic stem cell transplant recipients and patients with solid or hematologic cancer. In: Open Forum infectious diseases, vol 7, No. 7. Oxford University Press, New York, p ofaa172

Bretagne S, Klimko N (2020) Parasitic infections in patients with hematologic malignancies. Hematologic malignancies: parasitic infections

Burbach M, Birsen R, Denis B, Munier AL, Verine J, de Fontbrune FS, Peraldi MN (2016) A case of BK virus nephropathy without hemorrhagic cystitis after hematopoietic stem cell transplantation. Ann Hematol 95:1567–1568

Cam S, Yoruk MA (2020) Alteration in hepatitis B serology in children receiving chemotherapy. Viral Immunol 33(10):628–633

Cederwall S, Påhlman LI (2019) Respiratory adenovirus infections in immunocompetent and immunocompromised adult patients. Epidemiol Infect 147:e328

Chang T, Jung BK, Chai JY, Cho SI (2022) The notable global heterogeneity in the distribution of COVID-19 cases and the association with pre-existing parasitic diseases. PLoS Negl Trop Dis 16(10):e0010826

Chemaly R, Shah D, Boeckh M (2014) Management of respiratory viral infections in hematopoietic cell transplant recipients and patients with hematologic malignancies. Link Missing

Collyer BS, Anderson R (2024) The transmission dynamics of Strongyloides stercoralis and the impact of mass drug administration. Philos Trans R Soc B 379(1894):20220442

Cortes-Penfield NW, Ramani S, Neill F, Ettayebi K, Atmar R, Estes M (2019, October) 2650. Evaluating antiviral agents for human Noroviruses using a human intestinal Enteroid model. In: Open Forum infectious diseases, vol 6, No. Suppl 2. Oxford University Press, p S927

Czeresnia JM, Weiss LM (2022) Strongyloides stercoralis. Lung 200(2):141–148

Dard C, Marty P, Brenier-Pinchart MP, Garnaud C, Fricker-Hidalgo H, Pelloux H, Pomares C (2018) Management of toxoplasmosis in transplant recipients: an update. Expert Rev Anti-Infect Ther 16(6):447–460

Durak F, Dogan M, Atambay M, Özgen Ü, Özen M (2013) Evaluation of the intestinal parasitic infections in children patients with cancer. Turkiye Parazitol Derg 37(3):179

El-Taweel H, Isaa Y, Shehata G, Gaballah A, Lotfy W, Tolba M (2020) Restriction fragment length polymorphism (RFLP) analysis of Blastocystis spp. in symptomatic and asymptomatic individuals from Alexandria, Egypt. Parasitol Unit J 13(3):164–171

Essa S, Al-Tawalah H, AlShamali S, Al-Nakib W (2017) The potential influence of human parainfluenza viruses detected during hospitalization among critically ill patients in Kuwait, 2013–2015. Virol J 14:1–7

Faure E, Lionet A, Kipnis E, Noël C, Hazzan M (2017) Risk factors for Pneumocystis pneumonia after the first 6 months following renal transplantation. Transpl Infect Dis 19(5):e12735

Findlater A, Bogoch II (2018) Human mobility and the global spread of infectious diseases: a focus on air travel. Trends Parasitol 34(9):772–783

Focosi D, Maggi F, D'Abramo A, Nicastri E, Sullivan DJ (2023) Antiviral combination therapies for persistent COVID-19 in immunocompromised patients. Int J Infect Dis 137:55

Gandhi RG, Kotton CN (2022) Evaluating the safety of Maribavir for the treatment of cytomegalovirus. Ther Clin Risk Manag 18:223–232

Gaytán-Morales JF, Castorena-Villa I, Cortés-Flores DC, Avilés-Robles MJ, Sánchez-Huerta JL, Ortiz-Navarrete V et al (2021) Respiratory viral infections in pediatric patients with hematopoietic stem cell transplantation. Bol Med Hosp Infant Mex 78(3):191–199

Gentry CA, Nguyen P, Thind SK, Kurdgelashvili G, Williams RJ (2023) Characteristics and outcomes of US Veterans at least 65 years of age at high risk of severe SARS-CoV-2 infection with or without receipt of oral antiviral agents. J Infect 86(3):248–255

Grit GF, Märtson AG, Knoester M, Toren-Wielema ML, Touw DJ (2022) Shedding a light on Acyclovir pharmacodynamics: a retrospective analysis on Pharmacokinetic/Pharmacodynamic modelling of Acyclovir for the treatment of Varicella Zoster virus infection in immunocompromised patients: a pilot study. Pharmaceutics 14(11):2311

Gutovskaya EI, Tsetlina VA, Mitrofanova AM, Balashov DN (2018) BK-virus nephropathy after allogeneic stem cell transplantation. Pediatr Hematol/Oncol Immunopathol 17(2):107–113

Haque E, Muhsen IN, Rasheed W, Fakih RE, Aljurf M (2023) Parasitic infections in hematopoietic stem cell transplant recipients. Transpl Infect Dis 25:e14160

Harris CE, Vijenthira A, Ong SY, Baden LR, Hicks LK, Baird JH (2023) COVID-19 and other viral infections in patients with hematologic malignancies. Am Soc Clin Oncol Educ Book 43:e390778

Hawkinson D, Hinthorn D, Danziger-Isakov L (2013) Novel antiviral agents for respiratory viral infection in immunocompromised adults. Curr Infect Dis Rep 15:497–503

Hijano DR, Brazelton de Cardenas J, Maron G, Garner CD, Ferrolino JA, Dallas RH et al (2019) Clinical correlation of influenza and respiratory syncytial virus load measured by digital PCR. PLoS One 14(9):e0220908

Inazawa N, Hori T, Yamamoto M, Hatakeyama N, Yoto Y, Nojima M et al (2016) HHV-6 encephalitis may complicate the early phase after allogeneic hematopoietic stem cell transplantation: detection by qualitative multiplex PCR and subsequent quantitative real-time PCR. J Med Virol 88(2):319–323

Joo H, Maskery BA, Alpern JD, Weinberg M, Stauffer WM (2023) Cost-effectiveness of treatment strategies for populations from strongyloidiasis high-risk areas globally who will initiate corticosteroid treatment in the USA. J Travel Med taad054

Kang G (2013) New-generation treatment? Targeted antiviral therapy for rotavirus. Gastroenterology 145(4):711–714

Kotton CN, Kamar N (2023) New insights on CMV management in solid organ transplant patients: prevention, treatment, and management of resistant/refractory disease. Infect Dis Ther 12(2):333–342

Kunte AS, Gagelmann N, Badbaran A, Berger C, Massoud R, Klyuchnikov E et al (2022) Viral reactivation and immune reconstitution after CAR-T cell treatment in patients with hematologic malignancies. Blood 140(Supplement 1):7531–7532

Łanocha A, Łanocha-Arendarczyk N, Wilczyńska D, Zdziarska B, Kosik-Bogacka D (2022) Protozoan intestinal parasitic infection in patients with hematological malignancies. J Clin Med 11(10):2847

Lee YJ, Neofytos D, Kim SJ, Cheteyan L, Huang YT, Papadopoulos EB et al (2018) Efficacy of brincidofovir as prophylaxis against HSV and VZV in hematopoietic cell transplant recipients. Transpl Infect Dis 20(6):e12977

Li P, Li J, Huang H, Chen X, Lin Y, He G, Xu D (2023) The effect of varicella-zoster virus reactivation on the long-term outcomes of patients undergoing allogeneic hematopoietic stem cell transplantation. J Health Popul Nutr 42(1):105

Lion T (2014) Adenovirus infections in immunocompetent and immunocompromised patients. Clin Microbiol Rev 27(3):441–462

Longo BM, Venuti F, Gaviraghi A, Lupia T, Ranzani FA, Pepe A et al (2023) Sequential or combination treatments as rescue therapies in immunocompromised patients with persistent Sars-Cov-2 infection in the omicron era: a case series. Antibiotics 12(9):1460

Machado CM, Kerbauy MN, Colturato I, Arcuri LJ, dos Santos ACF, Silva FR et al (2020) Clinical characteristics and outcomes of COVID-19 in HSCT recipients. Blood 136:19

Magira EE, Chemaly RF, Jiang Y, Tarrand J, Kontoyiannis DP (2019, July) Outcomes in invasive pulmonary aspergillosis infections complicated by respiratory viral infections in patients with hematologic malignancies: a case-control study. In: Open forum infectious diseases, vol 6, No. 7. Oxford University Press, New York, p ofz247

Majewska A, Młynarczyk-Bonikowska B, Malejczyk M, Majewski S, Młynarczyk G (2019) Possibilities of prevention and treatment of human cytomegalovirus infections including new drugs and compounds with potential application. Postępy Mikrobiologii-Adv Microbiol 58(3):291–299

Marchetti S, Santangelo R, Manzara S, D'onghia S, Fadda G, Cattani P (2011) Comparison of real-time PCR and pp65 antigen assays for monitoring the development of Cytomegalovirus disease in recipients of solid organ and bone marrow transplants. Microbiol-Quarter J Microbiol Sci 34(2):157

Martínez-Gordillo MN, Gonzalez-Maciel A, Reynoso-Robles R, Montijo-Barrios E, Ponce-Macotela M (2014) Intraepithelial Giardia intestinalis: a case report and literature review. Medicine 93(29):e277

Moso MA, Sasadeusz J, Morrissey CO, Bond K, Guy S, Slavin MA, Dendle C (2023) Survey of treatment practices for immunocompromised patients with COVID-19 in Australasia. Intern Med J 53(4):619–624

Omarova KG, Balykova LA, Pshenichnaya NY, Zemskov DN, Zaslavskaya KY, Taganov AV, Belyy PA (2022) Feasibility of targeted antiviral therapy for acute respiratory viral infections in the COVID-19 pandemic. Infektsionnye Bolezni 20:104–112

Ottaviano G, Lucchini G, Breuer J, Furtado-Silva JM, Lazareva A, Ciocarlie O et al (2020) Delaying haematopoietic stem cell transplantation in children with viral respiratory infections reduces transplant-related mortality. Br J Haematol 188(4):560–569

Papanicolaou G, Kolitsopoulos Y, Young J, Boruchov A, Sankaranarayanan N, Hull D et al (2013) BK virus-associated nephropathy (BKVN), an under-recognized cause of renal dysfunction in severely immunosuppressed hematopoietic stem cell transplant (HSCT) patients: report of 5 cases of Bkvn and the potential role of CMX001 for treatment. Biol Blood Marrow Transplant 19(2):S302–S303

Pereira MR, Pouch SM, Scully B (2019) Infections in allogeneic stem cell transplantation. In: Principles and practice of transplant infectious diseases. Springer, New York, pp 209–226

Pietersma FL, van Dorp S, Jacobi R, Ran L, Nanlohy NM, Schuurman R et al (2010) High level of perforin expression in T cells: an early prognostic marker of the severity of herpesvirus reactivation after allogeneic stem cell transplantation in adults. Clin Infect Dis 50(5):717–725

Rojas-Rechy MH, Gaytán-Morales F, Sánchez-Ponce Y, Castorena-Villa I, López-Martínez B, Parra-Ortega I et al (2022) Herpesvirus screening in childhood hematopoietic transplant reveals high systemic inflammation in episodes of multiple viral detection and an EBV association with elevated IL-1β, IL-8 and Graft-Versus-Host disease. Microorganisms 10(8):1685

Roseman DA, Kabbani D, Kwah J, Bird D, Ingalls R, Gautam A et al (2013) Strongyloides stercoralis transmission by kidney transplantation in two recipients from a common donor. Am J Transplant 13(9):2483–2486

Saha S (2022) Death and invasive mechanical ventilation risk in hospitalized COVID-19 patients treated with anti-SARS-CoV-2 monoclonal antibodies and/or antiviral agents: a systematic review and network meta-analysis protocol. PLoS One 17(6):e0270196

Salvador F, Lucas-Dato A, Roure S, Arsuaga M, Pérez-Jacoiste A, García-Rodríguez M et al (2021) Effectiveness and safety of a single-dose ivermectin treatment for uncomplicated Strongyloidiasis in immunosuppressed patients (ImmunoStrong study): the study protocol. Pathogens 10(7):812

Schlatzer D, Haqqani AA, Li X, Dobrowolski C, Chance MR, Tilton JC (2017) A targeted mass spectrometry assay for detection of HIV gag protein following induction of latent viral reservoirs. Anal Chem 89(10):5325–5332

Shahani L, Ariza-Heredia EJ, Chemaly RF (2017) Antiviral therapy for respiratory viral infections in immunocompromised patients. Expert Rev Anti-Infect Ther 15(4):401–415

Silvestri F, Lapa D, Ferrara C, Grisolia D, Costantino F, Castilletti C, Tromba V (2021) Parainfluenza viruses: a trigger for type 1 diabetes new onset? New Microbiol 44(4):241–244

Stoykova Z, Kostadinova T, Todorova T, Ivanova L, Kalchev K, Micheva I (2023) Real time quantitative PCR as detection method for CMV reactivation in patients with lymphomas–a single-center experience. Acta Microbiol Bulg 39:162

Sun YQ, Ma R, Huang XJ (2023) Optimizing the treatment of cytomegalovirus infection in allo-HSCT recipients. Expert Rev Clin Immunol 19(2):227–235

Suputtamongkol Y, Premasathian N, Bhumimuang K, Waywa D, Nilganuwong S, Karuphong E et al (2011) Efficacy and safety of single and double doses of ivermectin versus 7-day high dose albendazole for chronic strongyloidiasis. PLoS Negl Trop Dis 5(5):e1044

Szenborn L, Kraszewska-Głomba B, Jackowska T, Duszczyk E, Majda-Stanisławska E, Marczyńska M et al (2016) Polish consensus guidelines on the use of acyclovir in the treatment and prevention of VZV and HSV infections. J Infect Chemother 22(2):65–71

Testi I, Aggarwal K, Jaiswal N, Dahiya N, Thng ZX, Agarwal A et al (2021) Antiviral therapy for varicella zoster virus (VZV) and herpes simplex virus (HSV)-induced anterior uveitis: a systematic review and meta-analysis. Front Med 8:686427

Tunalı V, Öztürk EA, Ünver A, Turgay N (2018) The prevalance of Blastocystosis among patients with gastrointestinal and dermatologic complaints and effects of Blastocystis spp. density on symptomatology. Turkiye Parazitol Derg 42(4):254

Uluhan R, Yaman A, İlkit M, Köksal F, Akan E (1995) Detection of HSV Type-2, CMV and adenovirus lgG antibodies in patients with hematologic and solid organ malignancies. Eur J Therap 6(2):131–136

Vakil E, Sheshadri A, Faiz SA, Shah DP, Zhu Y, Li L, Chemaly RF (2018) Risk factors for mortality after respiratory syncytial virus lower respiratory tract infection in adults with hematologic malignancies. Transpl Infect Dis 20(6):e12994

Winestone LE, Punn R, Tamaresis JS, Buckingham J, Pinsky BA, Waggoner JJ, Kharbanda S (2018) High human herpesvirus 6 viral load in pediatric allogeneic hematopoietic stem cell transplant patients is associated with detection in end organs and high mortality. Pediatr Transplant 22(2):e13084

Yang L, Zhong X, Yang H, Wu Q, Gong Y, Wang B (2022) Pneumatosis cystoides intestinalis associated with etoposide in hematological malignancies: a case report and a literature review. BMC Gastroenterol 22(1):150

Yang J, Kang CI, Lee YH, Ko JH, Huh K, Cho SY, Jung CW (2024) Risk factors and clinical outcomes of cytomegalovirus diseases in hematologic malignancy patients without hematopoietic stem-cell transplantation. Support Care Cancer 32(1):56

Yates J (2021) Parasitic infections: do not neglect Strongyloidiasis. Am Fam Physician 104(2):224–225

Chapter 28
Febrile Neutropenic Patients in Hematological Malignancies

Abhilash Dash

Learning Points

1. Epidemiology and Risk Factors: Neutropenia's prevalence and risk are intricately linked to the type of hematological malignancy and treatment regimens. Understanding these risk factors, including the duration of neutropenia and specific patient characteristics, is pivotal for developing effective management strategies.
2. Diagnostic Protocols: Emphasizes the importance of a thorough diagnostic approach for febrile neutropenia, incorporating laboratory tests, cultures from potential infection sites, and appropriate imaging techniques. This chapter highlights the evolving role of rapid diagnostic tests in enhancing pathogen identification, thereby facilitating targeted therapy.
3. Management and Treatment Strategies: Outlines evidence-based recommendations for empiric antibiotic therapy, stressing the differentiation between high-risk and low-risk patients. It discusses the criteria for choosing appropriate antimicrobial agents, including considerations for antibiotic resistance and the use of hematopoietic growth factors as a preventive measure against neutropenia.
4. Role of Prophylactic Measures: Analyzes the efficacy and clinical relevance of antibiotic, antifungal, and antiviral prophylaxis in neutropenic patients. It underscores the significance of risk stratification in determining the need for prophylaxis and outlines guidelines for its application, aiming to reduce the incidence of febrile episodes and documented infections.

28.1 Introduction

Neutropenia is a critical complication in patients with hematological malignancies, significantly impacting disease management and patient outcomes. The prevalence of neutropenia varies widely among patients undergoing chemotherapy or bone marrow transplantation, with the risk of sepsis or septic shock ranging from 7% to

---

A. Dash (✉)
Critical Care Medicine, IMS & SUM Hospital, Bhubaneswar, India

S. B. Mishra (ed.), *Critical Care Hematology*,
https://doi.org/10.1007/978-981-97-5565-3_28

45% (Situmorang et al. 2022). Proper management of neutropenia is essential due to the high risk of severe infections and other complications, affecting the length of hospital stay and healthcare costs (Rhee et al. 2009). Studies have shown that neutropenia is a common side effect of chemotherapy and a leading cause of severe infections and mortality in patients with hematological malignancies (Asgari et al. 2022).

Research on neutropenia recovery in cancer patients has highlighted associations with deteriorating oxygenation and exacerbation of pulmonary diseases (Rhee et al. 2009). Febrile neutropenia (FN), a common complication in hematology–oncology practice, is often caused by malignancy and cytotoxic therapy, emphasizing the need for specialized care in managing this condition (Situmorang et al. 2022). In addition, the efficacy of antibiotics such as ciprofloxacin in preventing sepsis among patients with chemotherapy-induced neutropenia has been investigated, indicating the importance of infection prevention strategies in this vulnerable population (Asgari et al. 2022).

Neutropenia is a significant risk factor for patients with hematological malignancies, leading to increased susceptibility to bacterial and fungal infections, especially when the absolute neutrophil count (ANC) falls below 500/µL (Sulviani et al. 2007). Prolonged neutropenia exceeding 7 days elevates the risk of bacteremia and other infections (Paolino et al. 2019). Patients with acute leukemia face a higher risk of neutropenia compared to those with other hematological malignancies (Karthaus et al. 1998). Factors such as prior surgical procedures, pre-existing conditions such as diabetes or cardiovascular diseases, and the presence of medical devices such as central venous catheters (CVCs) can further increase the risk of infections in neutropenic patients (Rosa and Goldani 2014).

Biochemical and clinical markers such as elevated procalcitonin levels, high lactate levels, and decreased bicarbonate levels are indicative of sepsis or septic shock in patients with neutropenia, emphasizing the importance of monitoring these parameters for early detection and intervention (Lyman et al. 2005). The duration of neutropenia, type of malignancy, and medical history play crucial roles in determining the risk profile of patients with hematological malignancies, influencing outcomes and the need for specialized care (Hurst et al. 2011).

The Multinational Association for Supportive Care in Cancer (MASCC) Risk Index Score is a well-established tool designed to assess the risk of complications in patients with FN (Kern et al. 2013). This scoring system incorporates various factors such as age, blood pressure, clinical symptoms, medical history, and laboratory parameters to calculate a total score ranging from 0 to 26 (Samoon et al. 2017). A score of 21 or higher is generally indicative of low-risk patients suitable for outpatient management, while a score below 21 suggests a higher risk for severe complications such as septic shock, necessitating inpatient treatment and closer monitoring (Bhardwaj et al. 2021) (Fig. 28.1).

The MASCC score is widely utilized in clinical settings to guide treatment decisions, helping clinicians determine the level of medical intervention required and aiding in the selection of empirical antibiotic therapy (Klastersky and Paesmans 2007). While the MASCC score is valuable, it is essential to note its limitations, as it may not encompass all individual patient factors or rapidly changing clinical statuses (Gunderson et al. 2019). Despite these limitations, the MASCC score remains a valuable and versatile tool in the management of FN, aiding in risk stratification and supporting informed decision-making for patient care (Chaftari et al. 2021).

Components of the MASCC Score

- The score is calculated based on a variety of factors; each assigned a specific point value. These factors include:
- Age
- Blood pressure
- Clinical symptoms such as rigors and dehydration
- Medical history, including chronic obstructive pulmonary disease and other comorbidities
- Laboratory parameters such as hemoglobin level and serum creatinine

Scoring System

- The total score can range from 0 to 26.
- A score of 21 or higher is generally considered low risk, suggesting that the patient may be a candidate for outpatient treatment.

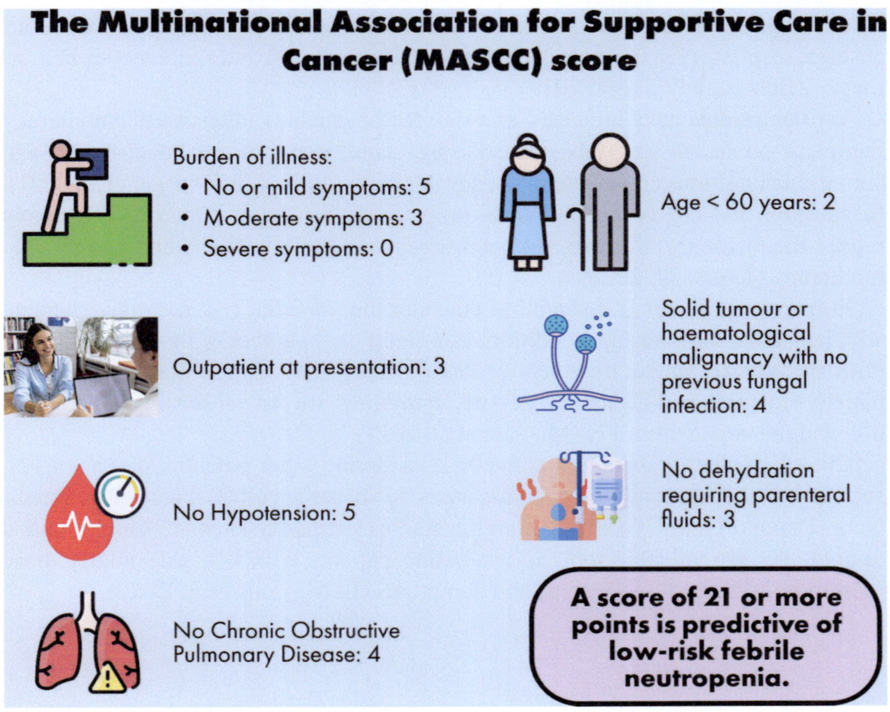

Fig. 28.1 The Multinational Association for Supportive Care in Cancer (MASCC) score

- A score below 21 indicates a higher risk for severe complications such as septic shock, and such patients are usually considered for inpatient treatment and closer monitoring.

Clinical Relevance

- The MASCC score is widely used in clinical settings to tailor treatment plans.
- It helps clinicians decide on the level of medical intervention required, including the choice between inpatient and outpatient care.
- It can also guide the selection of empirical antibiotic therapy.

Limitations

- While the MASCC score is a valuable tool, it is not a substitute for clinical judgment.
- It may not account for all individual patient factors, such as rapidly changing clinical status or specific nuances of the underlying malignancy.

28.2 Clinical Presentation

FN is a critical condition often observed in patients undergoing chemotherapy, characterized by fever as a primary symptom of infection (Zimmer and Freifeld 2019). Other common signs and symptoms include fatigue, oral mucositis, cutaneous abscess, respiratory symptoms, gastrointestinal symptoms, and spontaneous hemorrhage (Zimmer and Freifeld 2019).

Various studies have indicated that risk factors such as intensive chemotherapy regimens, advanced age, advanced disease stage, previous episodes of FN, and comorbid conditions contribute to the development of FN (Merseburger et al. 2021). In addition, the use of pegfilgrastim prophylaxis has been shown to effectively reduce the incidence of grade 3–4 neutropenia and FN in patients undergoing chemotherapy (Jeon et al. 2023).

In managing FN, it is essential to consider the potential risk factors associated with hospitalization for this condition, as a significant number of initial hospitalizations occur early in the treatment cycles (Lyman and Delgado 2003). Moreover, patient education and awareness of early symptoms are crucial for timely intervention and management of FN (Mugada et al. 2017).

Clinicians should also be attentive to considering other potential causes of FN, such as malaria, especially in endemic areas, to ensure accurate diagnosis and treatment (Rapoport and Uys 2008). Imaging studies such as chest X-rays or computed tomography are valuable tools in evaluating patients with FN, particularly those presenting with respiratory signs and symptoms (El Majzoub et al. 2020).

28.3 Diagnostic Approach to Febrile Neutropenia

FN represents a significant clinical challenge, combining the risks of fever with a critically reduced capacity for infection defense due to neutropenia. This section outlines a comprehensive approach to diagnosing FN, emphasizing laboratory tests, physical examinations, additional diagnostic tools, and the role of rapid diagnostic tests (RDTs).

Laboratory Tests

- *CBC with Differential and Platelet Count*

Complete blood count (CBC) with differential and platelet count is indispensable in assessing the patient's hematological status. This test provides essential data on the patient's overall health, revealing anemia, infections, and other potential diseases that could compromise patient care.

- *Serum Levels of Creatinine and Blood–Urea–Nitrogen*

These indicators of renal function are vital, as elevated levels might suggest kidney impairment. Renal function tests, including creatinine and blood–urea–nitrogen levels, offer insights into the patient's kidney health, which can be affected by both disease processes and treatment regimens.

- *Electrolytes, Hepatic Transaminase Enzymes, and Total Bilirubin*

Assessment of hepatic function and electrolyte balance is crucial, especially since severe illness can disrupt these parameters. Tests for electrolytes, hepatic transaminase enzymes, and total bilirubin provide a snapshot of liver health and electrolyte homeostasis.

- *Blood Cultures*

Two Sets Recommended:

For accurate bacterial identification, two sets of blood cultures are recommended: one from each lumen of an existing CVC and another from a peripheral vein. This dual approach ensures comprehensive capture of potential bacteremia.

- *Volume Limitations*

In patients weighing less than 40 kg, care must be taken to limit the volume of blood drawn for cultures to less than 1% of the total blood volume. This consideration helps prevent iatrogenic harm.

- *Other Cultures*

Cultures from any other suspected sites of infection, such as wound swabs, sputum samples, or urine cultures, are crucial for identifying the infection source and tailoring antimicrobial therapy.

Chest Radiograph
A chest X-ray is recommended for patients exhibiting respiratory symptoms or distress to rule out pneumonia and other respiratory conditions.

Physical Examination
- *Detailed History*

A thorough patient history, including any new symptoms, previous infections, antimicrobial prophylaxis, and existing co-morbidities, is essential for a comprehensive diagnostic approach.

- *Careful Examination*

Special attention should be paid to commonly infected sites, including the skin, oropharynx, alimentary tract, lungs, and perineum, to identify potential infection sources.

Additional Diagnostic Tools
- *Radiography:* CT scans of the head, sinuses, abdomen, and pelvis may be required based on clinical indications.
- *Other Laboratory Analysis:* Frequent monitoring, including at least tri-weekly CBC counts, kidney function tests, and weekly liver function tests, is vital, especially under intensive antibiotic therapy.

Serum Markers of Inflammation
Current research does not unequivocally support the routine use of markers such as C-reactive protein or interleukins for guiding antimicrobial therapy due to insufficient data.

Rapid Diagnostic Tests (RDTs)
Advancements in RDTs, such as syndromic polymerase chain reaction (PCR) panels, have revolutionized pathogen identification in FN, significantly reducing diagnosis time.

- *Blood Culture PCR Panels*: These panels have shown efficacy in cancer patients, shortening the pathogen identification timeline, albeit with limited impact on clinical outcomes.
- *Respiratory PCR Panels*: Useful for identifying respiratory viruses, thus enabling targeted therapy and potential antibiotic de-escalation.
- *GI PCR Panels*: These have enhanced the diagnosis of infectious diarrhea in cancer patients but do not differentiate between colonization and active infection.
- *CNS Infections*: The Biofire FilmArray ME PCR panel is widely used for CNS infections, though accuracy concerns remain.
- *MRSA PCR*: This aids in the de-escalation of vancomycin therapy, particularly when MRSA prevalence is low.
- *Fungal Diagnostics*: Biomarkers such as aspergillus galactomannan and 1-3-β-D-glucan play critical roles, despite limitations.

- *Emerging Diagnostics*: Technologies such as T2 magnetic resonance for candidiasis and next-generation sequencing show promise but require further validation.

The diagnostic strategy for FN must be individualized, considering the patient's clinical condition, local epidemiology, and the diagnostic tools available. Rapid diagnostics not only facilitate targeted therapy but also enhance antimicrobial stewardship efforts.

Continue with

- Empiric antibiotic therapy in febrile neutropenic patients
- General considerations for therapy
- Resistance considerations and alternatives for penicillin allergy

28.4 Evidence Summary

The management of FN involves a nuanced approach that considers risk stratification and personalized treatment to prevent morbidity and mortality from bacterial infections (Gea-Banacloche 2013). Empirical antibiotic therapy plays a crucial role in this management, with the selection of antibiotics tailored to local and individual bacterial colonization and resistance patterns (Gea-Banacloche 2013). High-risk patients typically receive broad-spectrum intravenous antibiotics, while low-risk patients may initially be managed with oral broad-spectrum antibiotics (Gea-Banacloche 2013). Special considerations include the judicious use of vancomycin based on specific clinical indicators, careful outpatient management with close monitoring, and the avoidance of fluoroquinolones in initial therapy for patients on fluoroquinolone prophylaxis. The guideline emphasizes the importance of relying on clinical and microbiologic data to modify antibiotic regimens, maintaining initial treatment in stable patients with persistent fever, and tailoring antibiotics to specific infections and organism susceptibilities (Gea-Banacloche 2013). Recommendations include discontinuing gram-positive coverage-like vancomycin if no infection is evident after 2 days, expanding coverage in hemodynamically unstable patients, and simplifying therapy in stable low-risk patients (Gea-Banacloche 2013). For high-risk patients with persistent fever after 4–7 days of broad-spectrum antibiotics, empirical antifungal therapy may be considered (Gea-Banacloche 2013). Therapy duration is determined by factors such as the site of infection, the causative organism, and the duration of neutropenia (Gea-Banacloche 2013). Treatment for unexplained fever continues until marrow recovery, indicated by an ANC over 500 cells/mm^3. Specific approaches are recommended for various infections, including pneumonia, gram-negative and gram-positive bloodstream infections, with an emphasis on early broad-spectrum treatment and appropriate therapy duration based on clinical need and ANC recovery (Gea-Banacloche 2013).

28.5 Antibiotic Prophylaxis in Neutropenic Patients

The management of FN involves a nuanced approach that considers risk stratification and personalized treatment to prevent morbidity and mortality from bacterial infections (Gafter-Gvili et al. 2012). Empirical antibiotic therapy plays a crucial role in this management, with the selection of antibiotics tailored to local and individual bacterial colonization and resistance patterns (Gafter-Gvili et al. 2012). High-risk patients typically receive broad-spectrum intravenous antibiotics. Special considerations include the judicious use of vancomycin, careful outpatient management with close monitoring (Gafter-Gvili et al. 2012). The guideline emphasizes the importance of relying on clinical and microbiologic data to modify antibiotic regimens, maintaining initial treatment in stable patients with persistent fever, and tailoring antibiotics to specific infections, and organism susceptibilities (Gafter-Gvili et al. 2012). Recommendations include discontinuing gram-positive coverage-like vancomycin if no infection is evident after 2 days, expanding coverage in hemodynamically unstable patients, and simplifying therapy in stable low-risk patients (Gafter-Gvili et al. 2012). Therapy duration is determined by factors such as the site of infection, the causative organism, and the duration of neutropenia (Gafter-Gvili et al. 2012). Specific approaches are recommended for various infections, including pneumonia, gram-negative, and gram-positive bloodstream infections, with an emphasis on early broad-spectrum treatment and appropriate therapy duration based on clinical need and ANC recovery (Gafter-Gvili et al. 2012; Nakamura et al. 2010).

28.6 Antifungal Management in Neutropenic Patients

Antifungal prophylaxis in FN is a critical aspect of management, especially for high-risk patients with prolonged neutropenia (Cornely et al. 2009). Initiating empirical antifungal treatment is advisable for high-risk neutropenic patients experiencing sustained or recurring fever after 4–7 days on antibiotics and expecting neutropenia to exceed 7 days (Cornely et al. 2009). Preemptive antifungal therapy may be considered for certain high-risk patients meeting specific criteria (Cornely et al. 2009). In contrast, routine initiation of empirical antifungal treatment is not recommended for low-risk patients (Cornely et al. 2009).

Clinical evidence supports the use of empirical antifungal treatment to target suspected hidden fungal infections in cases where neutropenic fever persists despite empirical antibacterial therapy (Cornely et al. 2009). Pre-emptive therapy, which combines clinical observation, serologic tests, and imaging studies, has shown effectiveness in certain cases (Cornely et al. 2009).

Guidelines recommend antifungal prophylaxis for high-risk groups such as allogeneic hematopoietic stem cell transplant recipients or acute leukemia patients undergoing intense chemotherapy (Cornely et al. 2009; Karthaus and Hentrich 2011). Various antifungal agents such as Fluconazole, Itraconazole, Voriconazole,

Posaconazole, Micafungin, and Caspofungin are recommended for prophylaxis against Candida infections (Cornely et al. 2009). Posaconazole is advised for Aspergillus prophylaxis in specific patient populations (Cornely et al. 2009). Prophylaxis is generally not recommended for patients with an expected short neutropenia period (less than 7 days) (Cornely et al. 2009).

28.7 Antiviral Prophylaxis and Management

Antiviral prophylaxis in FN is a crucial aspect of management, especially for high-risk patients with expected durations of prolonged and profound neutropenia (Droubi et al. 2022). HSV-seropositive individuals undergoing allogeneic HSCT or leukemia induction are recommended to receive acyclovir for prophylaxis (Droubi et al. 2022). Clinical or laboratory confirmation of active HSV or VZV infection warrants antiviral treatment (Droubi et al. 2022). Yearly influenza vaccination is advocated for all cancer patients, and influenza infections should be treated with neuraminidase inhibitors if the viral strain is susceptible (Droubi et al. 2022).

28.8 Utilization of Hematopoietic Growth Factors

Utilization of hematopoietic growth factors in the management of FN is a critical consideration in clinical practice. Prophylactic application of myeloid colony-stimulating factors (CSFs) is recommended for patients with over a 20% anticipated risk of fever and neutropenia, while the use of CSFs is generally not recommended for managing established fever and neutropenia. Neutropenia severity, duration, acute leukemia, and prolonged hospital stay are key risk factors for FN, emphasizing the importance of risk stratification tools such as the MASCC Score alongside clinical judgment. Diagnostic essentials include CBC, creatinine levels, and blood cultures, with emerging roles for rapid PCR panels in the diagnosis of FN. Empiric antibiotic therapy varies based on risk level, with high-risk patients requiring IV antibiotics and prophylaxis advised for specific cases. Antifungal and antiviral treatments are considered based on patient risk and specific clinical conditions, with hematopoietic growth factors serving as a potential prophylactic option. Primary hematopoietic growth factor prophylaxis is recommended for the safe administration of adjuvant FEC-D chemotherapy, aligning with international oncology guidelines (Madarnas et al. 2011).

Flowchart

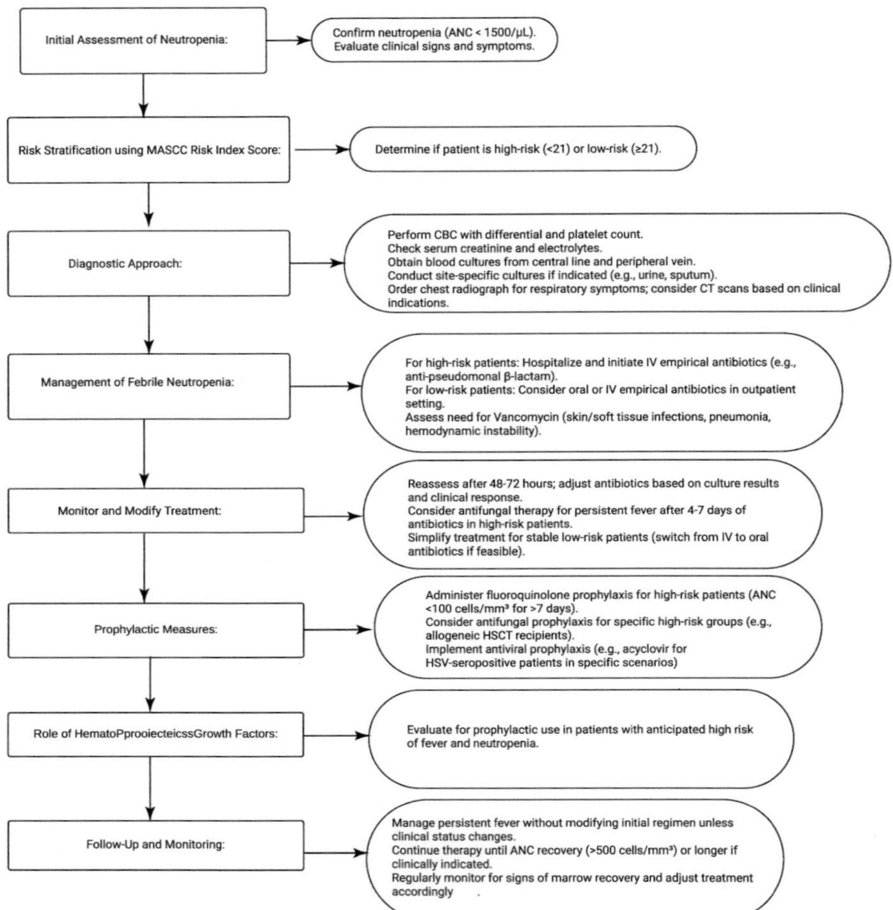

References

Asgari A, Qaletaaki R, Ranjbar H, Jalaeikhoo H, Hamidi-Farahani R, Kazemi-Galougahi MH, Soleiman-Meigooni S (2022) Efficacy of ciprofloxacin in prevention of sepsis among the patients with chemotherapy-induced neutropenia: a randomized double-blind clinical trial in a university hospital in Tehran, Iran. Ann Milit Health Sci Res 20(3):e130618

Bhardwaj PV, Emmich M, Knee A, Ali F, Walia R, Roychowdhury P et al (2021) Use of MASCC score in the inpatient management of febrile neutropenia: a single-center retrospective study. Support Care Cancer 29:5905–5914

Chaftari P, Chaftari AM, Hachem R, Yeung SCJ, Dagher H, Jiang Y et al (2021) The role of procalcitonin in identifying high-risk cancer patients with febrile neutropenia: a useful alternative to the multinational association for supportive care in cancer score. Cancer Med 10(23):8475–8482

Cornely OA, Böhme A, Buchheidt D, Einsele H, Heinz WJ, Karthaus M et al (2009) Primary prophylaxis of invasive fungal infections in patients with hematologic malignancies. Recommendations of the Infectious Diseases Working Party of the German Society for Haematology and Oncology. Haematologica 94(1):113

Droubi S, Shastri P, Yared N, Ibrahim D, Elsaghir H, Ibrahim DY (2022) Herpes simplex virus Esophagitis as a presentation of febrile Neutropenia: a case report. Cureus 14(11):e31280

El Majzoub I, El Zakhem A, Cheaito R, Cheaito MA, Kaddoura R, Alkozah M, Zgheib H (2020) The utility of chest X-ray vs. computed tomography in febrile neutropenia patients presenting to the emergency department. J Infect Dev Countr 14(10):1178–1184

Gafter-Gvili A, Fraser A, Paul M, Vidal L, Lawrie TA, van de Wetering MD et al (2012) Antibiotic prophylaxis for bacterial infections in afebrile neutropenic patients following chemotherapy. Cochrane Database Syst Rev 1:CD004386

Gea-Banacloche J (2013) Evidence-based approach to treatment of febrile neutropenia in hematologic malignancies. Hematol Am Soc Hematol Educ Program Book 2013(1):414–422

Gunderson CC, Erickson BK, Wilkinson-Ryan I, Vesely SK, Leath CA III, Gehrig PA, Moore KN (2019) Prospective evaluation of Multinational Association of Supportive Care in cancer risk index score for gynecologic oncology patients with febrile neutropenia. Am J Clin Oncol 42(2):138–142

Hurst FP, Belur P, Nee R, Agodoa LY, Patel P, Abbott KC, Jindal RM (2011) Poor outcomes associated with neutropenia after kidney transplantation: analysis of United States Renal Data System. Transplantation 92(1):36–40

Jeon Y, Yang DH, Oh SJ, Park JH, Kim JA, Kim SY et al (2023) Effectiveness of pegfilgrastim prophylaxis in preventing febrile neutropenia during R-FC chemoimmunotherapy for chronic lymphocytic leukemia: a multicenter prospective phase II study. Front Oncol 13:998014

Karthaus M, Hentrich M (2011) Wait and see or rush and switch? New questions for the management of patients with febrile neutropenia receiving antifungal prophylaxis. Mycoses 54:1–6

Karthaus M, Carratala J, Jürgens H, Ganser A (1998) New strategies in the treatment of infectious complications in haematology and oncology: is there a role for out-patient antibiotic treatment of febrile neutropenia? Chemotherapy 44(6):427–435

Kern W, Marchetti O, Drgona L, Akan H, Aoun M, Akova M et al (2013) Oral antibiotics for fever in low-risk neutropenic patients with cancer: a double-blind, randomized, multicenter trial comparing single daily moxifloxacin with twice daily ciprofloxacin plus amoxicillin/clavulanic acid combination therapy-EORTC infectious diseases group trial XV. J Clin Oncol 31(9):1149

Klastersky J, Paesmans M, Institut Jules Bordet, Centre des Tumeurs de l'Université Libre de Bruxelles (2007) Risk-adapted strategy for the management of febrile neutropenia in cancer patients. Support Care Cancer 15:477–482

Lyman GH, Delgado DJ (2003) Risk and timing of hospitalization for febrile neutropenia in patients receiving CHOP, CHOP-R, or CNOP chemotherapy for intermediate-grade non-Hodgkin lymphoma. Cancer 98(11):2402–2409

Lyman GH, Lyman CH, Agboola O, ANC Study Group (2005) Risk models for predicting chemotherapy-induced neutropenia. Oncologist 10(6):427–437

Madarnas Y, Dent SF, Husain SF, Robinson A, Alkhayyat S, Hopman WM et al (2011) Real-world experience with adjuvant fec-d chemotherapy in four Ontario regional cancer centres. Curr Oncol 18(3):119–125

Merseburger AS, Geiges G, Klier J, Wiesholzer M, Pichler P (2021) Pooled analysis on the effectiveness and safety of lipegfilgrastim in patients with urological malignancies in the real-world setting. Front Oncol 11:655355

Mugada V, Ramineni H, Padala D (2017) 5-Fluorouracil induced severe febrile neutropenia and death. J Young Pharm 9(1):133

Nakamura A, Sugimoto Y, Ohishi K, Sugawara Y, Fujieda A, Monma F et al (2010) Diagnostic value of PCR analysis of bacteria and fungi from blood in empiric-therapy-resistant febrile neutropenia. J Clin Microbiol 48(6):2030–2036

Paolino J, Mariani J, Lucas A, Rupon J, Weinstein H, Abrams A, Friedmann A (2019) Outcomes of a clinical pathway for primary outpatient management of pediatric patients with low-risk febrile neutropenia. Pediatr Blood Cancer 66(7):e27679

Rapoport BL, Uys A (2008) Malaria parasitemia associated with febrile neutropenia in African patients undergoing chemotherapy for haematological malignancies: a report of three patients. Chemotherapy 54(2):117–119

Rhee CK, Kang JY, Kim YH, Kim JW, Yoon HK, Kim SC et al (2009) Risk factors for acute respiratory distress syndrome during neutropenia recovery in patients with hematologic malignancies. Crit Care 13:1–8

Rosa RG, Goldani LZ (2014) Factors associated with hospital length of stay among cancer patients with febrile neutropenia. PLoS One 9(10):e108969

Samoon Z, Beg M, Moosajee MS, Kamran M, Masood N, Asghar A, Ahmed A (2017) Applying Multinational Association of Supportive Care of cancer index score for identifying Febrile Neutropenia patients at high risk of complications at Tertiary Care Hospital, Pakistan. Open J Epidemiol 7(02):159

Situmorang AGM, Wardhani P, Ugrasena IDG (2022) Clinical and hematological profile of Febrile Neutropenia in pediatric patients who suffered from malignancy at Dr. Soetomo General Academic Hospital Surabaya. Int J Res Publ 92(1):7–7

Sulviani R, Idjradinata P, Raspati H (2007) The risk factors for febrile neutropenia during chemotherapy in children with malignancy. Paediatr Indones 47(2):83–87

Zimmer AJ, Freifeld AG (2019) Optimal management of neutropenic fever in patients with cancer. J Oncol Pract 15(1):19–24

Chapter 29
Invasive Fungal Infection in Hematological Malignancies

Rupali Patnaik

Learning Points

1. IFIs are increasingly common in patients with hematological malignancies. They are associated with significant mortality.
2. Risk factors for IFIs are multifactorial and include treatment-related, patient-related, and hospital-related factors.
3. A comprehensive diagnostic approach is necessary for accurate diagnosis of IFIs. This includes microscopic examination, culturing techniques, imaging, endoscopic procedures, and specialized diagnostic methods.
4. Antifungal agents, prophylactic measures, and organ biopsies are key components of a holistic treatment strategy that balances efficacy and cost.

29.1 Introduction

Invasive fungal infections (IFIs) pose a significant challenge in managing patients with hematological malignancies due to their immunosuppressed state, often exacerbated by aggressive treatments. The incidence of IFIs in this patient population has been increasing, with mortality rates ranging from 30% to 60%, highlighting the critical need for effective prevention, early diagnosis, and treatment strategies. Studies have identified Candida and Aspergillus species as the most common types of IFIs in these patients, with mortality rates reported as high as 37.2%. Risk factors for IFIs in patients with hematological malignancies include male gender, higher ECOG scores, specific immunosuppressive treatments, and in-hospital transfers. Antifungal prophylaxis has consistently proven effective in reducing the prevalence of IFIs in patients with hematological malignancies, underscoring its importance in patient management.

While Candida and Aspergillus species are predominant, other clinically significant fungi such as Cryptococcus, Fusarium, and Mucorales also warrant attention. Despite advancements in antifungal treatments, breakthrough invasive mold

R. Patnaik (✉)
Critical Care Medicine, IMS & SUM Hospital, Bhubaneswar, India
e-mail: rupali.patnaik87@gmail.cm

S. B. Mishra (ed.), *Critical Care Hematology*,
https://doi.org/10.1007/978-981-97-5565-3_29

infections still occur in a subset of patients, necessitating ongoing vigilance. The epidemiology of IFIs in patients with hematological malignancies is a multifaceted and evolving area, with studies indicating high prevalence rates and concerning mortality rates. Healthcare professionals in hematology and critical care settings require a comprehensive understanding of IFIs to enhance the diagnosis and management of these complex infections. The increasing incidence of IFIs highlights the importance of vigilant monitoring, timely interventions, and the consideration of antifungal prophylaxis as a cornerstone in patient management.

29.2 Risk Factor

The risk factors for IFIs in individuals with hematological cancers are multifaceted and encompass various aspects related to treatment, patient characteristics, and medical care provision (De Pauw et al. 2008). Treatment-related factors, such as the use of targeted drugs and specific immunosuppressive medications, significantly increase the risk of IFIs, with incidence rates reported as high as 30% (De Pauw et al. 2008). In addition, the duration of neutropenia resulting from chemotherapy is directly associated with higher IFI rates, emphasizing the importance of monitoring this aspect of patient care (De Pauw et al. 2008). Patient-related risk factors include genetic predispositions, gender, ECOG scores, and the specific type of hematological malignancy (De Pauw et al. 2008). Male patients and those with higher ECOG scores are at a greater risk of developing IFIs, with certain types of leukemia, such as acute myeloid leukemia (AML), carrying a higher prevalence of IFIs compared to others (De Pauw et al. 2008). Understanding these patient-related factors is crucial for tailored prevention, early diagnosis, and management strategies. Antifungal prophylaxis has been shown to significantly reduce the prevalence of IFIs in patients with hematological malignancies, underscoring its importance in patient care (De Pauw et al. 2008). Studies have highlighted the effectiveness of antifungal prophylaxis in reducing IFI prevalence, with a notable p value of 0.004 (De Pauw et al. 2008). These findings emphasize the critical role of preventive measures in reducing the burden of IFIs in this vulnerable patient population. In conclusion, a comprehensive understanding of the risk factors associated with IFIs in individuals with hematological cancers is essential for effective prevention, early detection, and management of these infections. Treatment-related factors, patient characteristics, and the use of antifungal prophylaxis all play crucial roles in mitigating the risk of IFIs and improving patient outcomes in this susceptible population.

29.3 Microscopic Examination and Culturing Techniques

29.3.1 Microscopic Examination

Microscopic examination is a crucial tool in diagnosing invasive fungal diseases (IFDs) by enabling the visualization of fungal elements in clinical samples. However, the accurate identification of fungal structures can be challenging due to potential confusion with artifacts. To address this issue, specialized fungal stains such as periodic acid–Schiff (PAS), Grocott's methenamine silver (GMS), and Calcofluor white are commonly used to enhance the visibility of fungal elements (Shalin et al. 2020). Each of these stains serves a specific purpose in highlighting different components of fungal structures, aiding in their identification under the microscope (Schnietz and Wilson 2018). For example, PAS stain is effective in highlighting fungal cell walls and capsules, making them more distinguishable against the background tissue, while GMS stain is useful in visualizing fungal structures, such as hyphae and spores, providing additional clarity in identifying fungal elements (Schnietz and Wilson 2018). Calcofluor white stain is particularly valuable in detecting fungal cell walls, especially in cases where other stains may not be as effective (Shalin et al. 2020).

By utilizing these specialized fungal stains during microscopic examination, healthcare professionals can overcome the challenges associated with accurately identifying fungal elements in clinical samples, thereby enhancing the diagnostic accuracy of IFDs. These stains play a crucial role in differentiating fungal structures from artifacts, enabling more precise identification and diagnosis of fungal infections (Reisberger et al. 2003). The use of PAS and GMS staining has been extensively studied and proven to be effective in dermatopathology, providing valuable insights into skin and nail biopsies (Shalin et al. 2020). Moreover, combining staining methods like PAS with Wright–Giemsa staining has been shown to be a simple and rapid technique that contributes to the effective identification of various pathogens, further emphasizing the importance of specialized staining techniques in diagnostic procedures (Qin et al. 2015).

29.3.2 Culturing Techniques

The type of culturing technique used varies depending on the suspected fungal pathogen, highlighting the importance of tailoring culturing methods to the specific infection (Einsele et al. 1997). Isolating molds from clinical samples is generally more challenging compared to Candida species, emphasizing the need for specialized techniques in fungal identification (Gülmez et al. 2020). Blood cultures are commonly used for detecting fungaemia; however, they may not capture all types of fungal pathogens, necessitating the use of alternative culturing methods when blood cultures are insufficient (Wilson 2020; De et al. 2014). Special media supplemented with antibiotics, such as Sabouraud with 2% glucose, are often utilized for culturing, enhancing the growth of fungal pathogens (Ntusi et al. 2010).

Identification of Candida isolates down to the species level is crucial for effective treatment planning, underscoring the significance of accurate fungal identification in clinical practice (Farmakiotis et al. 2015). Given the limitations of individual methods, a comprehensive approach that combines microscopic examination with various culturing techniques is often the most effective diagnostic strategy for IFDs (Girmenia et al. 2001). This integrated approach allows for a more thorough assessment of fungal infections, leading to improved diagnostic accuracy and patient outcomes.

29.4 Imaging and Endoscopic Procedures

29.4.1 Imaging Procedures

Imaging plays a crucial role in the early detection and monitoring of IFDs, especially in high-risk patients (Patterson et al. 2016). High-resolution computed tomography (HRCT) is often preferred over traditional chest X-rays and is primarily utilized for diagnosing pulmonary IFDs. HRCT provides detailed images that assist in early detection and accurate diagnosis, with specific signs such as the halo sign and hypodense sign serving as indicators, although not exclusive to fungal infections (Ullmann et al. 2018). Magnetic resonance imaging (MRI) is recommended for fungal diseases affecting the central nervous system, sinuses, and eyes, offering superior soft tissue contrast ideal for detecting subtle abnormalities. MRI is particularly useful in diagnosing fungal meningitis, sinusitis, and ocular infections (Donnelly et al. 2020).

By incorporating HRCT and MRI in the diagnostic process, clinicians can improve their ability to detect and monitor IFDs effectively. These imaging modalities offer valuable insights into the presence and progression of fungal infections in various anatomical locations, contributing to more accurate diagnoses and treatment planning.

29.4.2 Endoscopic Procedures

Endoscopy is a crucial tool in diagnosing IFDs as it allows for the collection of tissue samples to confirm the presence of fungal elements (Memoli et al. 2012). Bronchoscopy with bronchoalveolar lavage (BAL) is a common procedure for diagnosing pulmonary IFDs, involving the collection of alveolar fluid through a bronchoscope. While this method enables direct examination and culturing of respiratory secretions, its sensitivity may be limited, necessitating the use of additional diagnostic methods (Ruhnke et al. 2018). Esophagogastroduodenoscopy is recommended for cases of esophagitis that do not respond to antifungal therapy, facilitating the examination of the esophagus, stomach, and upper part of the small intestine to obtain tissue samples for histological examination and culturing (Fanelli et al. 2020).

Incorporating endoscopic procedures such as bronchoscopy and esophagogastroduodenoscopy in the diagnostic pathway enhances the ability to confirm IFDs through direct visualization and sampling of affected tissues. These techniques offer valuable insights into the presence of fungal elements in specific anatomical sites, aiding in precise diagnosis and the development of targeted treatment strategies.

29.5 Specialized Diagnostic Methods

29.5.1 Lysis Centrifugation

Lysis centrifugation is a method that enhances the sensitivity of fungal detection in clinical samples by breaking down cellular components to release fungal elements, followed by centrifugation to concentrate the sample (Einsele et al. 1997). This technique increases the likelihood of detecting low-abundance fungal elements, providing a valuable tool for accurate diagnosis of fungal infections. However, one drawback of lysis centrifugation is the potential for false positives due to the high sensitivity of the method (Bougoure et al. 2014).

In clinical practice, lysis centrifugation serves as a valuable approach to improve the detection of fungal pathogens in various sample types. By utilizing this method, healthcare professionals can enhance the diagnostic accuracy of fungal infections, particularly in cases where traditional culturing methods may have limitations.

29.5.2 Cerebrospinal Fluid (CSF) Culturing and Antigen Testing

Cerebrospinal fluid (CSF) culturing and antigen testing are essential diagnostic methods primarily used for detecting *Cryptococcus neoformans* in suspected cases of cryptococcal meningitis. The procedure involves culturing CSF in specialized media designed for fungal growth while simultaneous antigen tests are conducted to confirm the presence of specific fungal elements. This approach is highly indicative and often considered a gold standard in diagnosing cryptococcal meningitis.

By utilizing CSF culturing and antigen testing, healthcare providers can accurately diagnose cryptococcal meningitis, enabling timely and targeted treatment interventions to improve patient outcomes.

This comprehensive review covers the epidemiology, clinical manifestations, diagnosis, and treatment of cryptococcosis, providing valuable insights into the management of this fungal infection.

29.5.3 Polymerase Chain Reaction (PCR)

Polymerase chain reaction (PCR) is a valuable tool used for the molecular identification of fungal pathogens. There are different types of PCR techniques employed in fungal diagnostics, including genus-specific PCR that targets genomic sequences unique to specific fungal genera and multiple-copy genes PCR that focuses on genes present in multiple copies to enhance detection sensitivity. The sensitivity and specificity of PCR vary depending on the approach, with species-specific nested PCR achieving up to 89% specificity. Real-time PCR is particularly useful as it allows for the quantification of fungal burden, providing insights into the severity of the infection. When it comes to sample types, BAL samples often yield higher sensitivity and specificity compared to blood samples. However, PCR has its limitations, such as the lack of standardization across laboratories and the possibility of positive results despite treatment, which may indicate breakthrough infections or insufficient therapeutic response.

By leveraging the capabilities of PCR in fungal diagnostics, healthcare professionals can enhance the accuracy and efficiency of identifying fungal pathogens, leading to improved patient care and outcomes (Fig. 29.1).

29.6 Antigen and Antibody Detection in IFD Diagnosis

29.6.1 Cryptococcal Antigen Detection

Cryptococcal antigen detection is essential in diagnosing cryptococcal meningitis, particularly in patients with AIDS and those receiving hemato-oncological treatments. The common methodologies for detection include latex agglutination or enzyme immunoassays, which are used to identify cryptococcal antigens in blood and/or CSF (Ganiem et al. 2014). These tests have demonstrated high sensitivity and specificity, typically exceeding 95%, making them highly reliable for diagnosing cryptococcal infections (Tanner et al. 1994). A positive test result often prompts immediate antifungal therapy and further diagnostic investigations (Pujari et al. 2020).

Research has emphasized the importance of cryptococcal antigen detection in various contexts. For example, in Indonesia, asymptomatic cryptococcal antigenemia has been linked to mortality among HIV-positive individuals, underscoring the significance of early detection (Ganiem et al. 2014). In addition, studies have

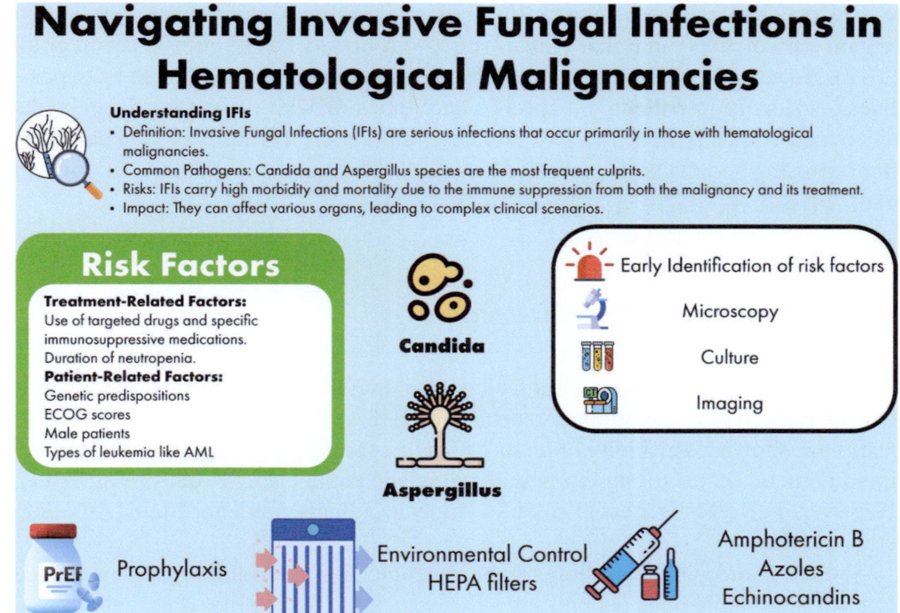

Fig. 29.1 Navigating invasive fungal infections in hematological malignancies

indicated that directly determining cryptococcal antigen in transthoracic needle aspirate can assist in diagnosing pulmonary cryptococcosis (Liaw et al. 1995).

Moreover, the efficacy of different assays for detecting cryptococcal antigen has been assessed, with studies comparing the performance of various tests in serum and CSF samples (Binnicker et al. 2012). These evaluations are crucial for ensuring precise and dependable diagnostic results. In addition, the development of new lateral flow immunoassays for detecting cryptococcal antigen has shown promise in enhancing the rapid diagnosis of cryptococcosis (Huang et al. 2015).

29.6.2 Aspergillus Antigen (Galactomannan, GM) Detection

Aspergillus antigen (Galactomannan, GM) detection is crucial for the early diagnosis and monitoring of invasive aspergillosis, especially in high-risk patient populations (Yoshimura et al. 2018). The detection of GM typically involves the use of enzyme-linked immunosorbent assay (ELISA) to identify GM in serum or BAL fluid (Husain et al. 2004). These tests have shown a sensitivity ranging from 80% to 100% and a specificity ranging from 90% to 100%, making them highly reliable for diagnosing invasive aspergillosis (Almeida-Paes et al. 2022). It is recommended to perform these tests at least twice a week for high-risk patients to ensure timely detection and monitoring (Haynes and Rogers 1994).

The predictive value of Aspergillus antigen detection is significant, with a high negative predictive value that aids in ruling out invasive aspergillosis (Oren et al. 2012). However, it is essential to consider the limitations associated with false positives, especially in patients on specific antibiotics or with other fungal infections (Swoboda-Kopeć et al. 2015). Despite these limitations, the utility of GM detection in diagnosing and managing invasive aspergillosis remains substantial (Huurneman et al. 2016).

29.6.3 Candida Antigen Detection

Candida antigen detection is a valuable tool in diagnosing Candida infections, primarily through latex agglutination tests and ELISA (Kahn and Jones 1986). These tests have shown a sensitivity of up to 70% and a specificity of around 88%, making them particularly useful in non-granulocytopenic patients (Al-Kasaby et al. 2017). However, their effectiveness in granulocytopenic patients is still uncertain (Arendrup et al. 2010).

While Candida antigen testing can be beneficial, it is not routinely recommended for hemato-oncological patients due to its variable sensitivity (Pasqualotto and Denning 2005). False positives are a concern, especially in patients on specific antibiotics or with other fungal infections, emphasizing the need for cautious result interpretation (Bougnoux et al. 1990). Despite these limitations, Candida antigen detection remains a valuable diagnostic approach in specific clinical contexts.

29.6.4 Beta-D-Glucans (BG) Detection

Beta-D-glucans (BG) are utilized for detecting various types of IFIs due to their clinical relevance (Pham et al. 2020). While BG assays exhibit higher sensitivity than GM in certain studies, they may lack the ability to differentiate between fungal species (Wright et al. 2011). However, it is crucial to note that factors such as plastic tubes, water, or dust can interfere with the BG test, impacting its accuracy (Wright et al. 2011). In clinical settings, BG detection may be recommended for routine screening in high-risk hematological patients (Wright et al. 2011).

The immunomodulatory properties of beta-glucans are well-documented, with their ability to modulate immune functions, possess anti-cancer and antibiotic properties, and impact blood pressure or cholesterol levels (Bergandi et al. 2021). Moreover, beta-glucans have been associated with the activation of immune responses and are recognized by the reticuloendothelial system (Swift et al. 2019).

In the context of pharmaceutical products, beta-glucan contamination has been a concern, with studies detecting contamination in various solutions (Barton et al. 2016). In addition, the presence of beta-glucans in house dust has been linked to airway hyperresponsiveness and atopic asthma in adolescents (Maheswaran et al. 2014).

29.6.5 General Recommendations for Antigen and Antibody Detection

By incorporating antigen and antibody detection methods into the diagnostic algorithm, clinicians can achieve a more accurate and timely diagnosis, thereby facilitating prompt and effective treatment. These tests should be used complementarily with other diagnostic methods for a comprehensive diagnosis (Guimarães et al. 2006). The choice of test should be guided by the suspected fungal infection and the patient's clinical status (Martinez et al. 1998). Some tests like GM are useful for both initial diagnosis and treatment monitoring, making them valuable in patient management (Markovic et al. 2002). However, it is essential to consider the limitations of each test, such as false positives and variable sensitivity, when interpreting results (Hartfield et al. 2014).

Antigen detection can be particularly useful in acute disease, especially in individuals also infected with HIV, who frequently have the disseminated form of histoplasmosis without detectable antibodies to the fungus (Guimarães et al. 2006). Fungal antigens may stimulate specific cell-mediated and humoral immune responses (Martinez et al. 1998). Antibodies promote the opsonization of fungi and their phagocytosis, complement activation, and antibody-dependent cell toxicity (Elluru et al. 2015). In the context of fungal infections, the detection of antibodies against different Candida antigens may aid in the diagnosis (Laín et al. 2008).

29.6.6 Organ Biopsies in the Diagnosis of IFD

Organ biopsies are essential in diagnosing IFDs due to their high diagnostic accuracy and detailed histopathological analysis capabilities (Lawal et al. 2021). When combined with other diagnostic methods such as imaging and serology, these biopsies offer a comprehensive approach to confirming the presence of fungal elements and identifying the specific type of fungus involved (Cao et al. 2017).

Various types of organ biopsies, including pulmonary, liver, gastrointestinal, and CNS biopsies, serve specific diagnostic purposes in IFDs (He et al. 2021). For example, pulmonary biopsies guided by CT scans are particularly useful in diagnosing pulmonary aspergillosis, with a diagnostic yield of up to 80% (Zhang et al. 2020). Liver biopsies are valuable in cases of hepatosplenic candidosis, especially within the first 3 week post-granulocytopenia (Otto and Green 2020). Gastrointestinal biopsies can aid in diagnosing invasive mycoses that may lead to fatal bowel necrosis, while CNS biopsies are considered in suspected fungal meningitis or brain abscess cases (Boch et al. 2015).

The methodology for organ biopsies involves sample preparation, mycological culture, molecular analysis, and histopathological processing to provide definitive evidence of IFD (Pana et al. 2017). However, challenges such as invasiveness, risk of complications, timing considerations, and the need for an interdisciplinary approach must be carefully addressed (Zhao et al. 2015).

Recommendations for organ biopsies in IFDs emphasize clinical feasibility, complementary diagnostics, obtaining informed consent, and post-procedure monitoring to ensure patient safety and optimal management. By integrating organ biopsies into the diagnostic regimen for IFDs, clinicians can enhance diagnostic certainty, leading to more targeted and effective treatment strategies.

29.7 Diagnostic Schedules for IFD Management

29.7.1 Baseline Screening Before Infection Manifestation

Diagnostic schedules for IFD management are crucial in high-risk patients to detect pre-existing fungal manifestations early. Routine surveillance cultures are generally not recommended, but baseline screening with abdominal ultrasound and chest X-ray is advised for initial screening. Serological and PCR tests, although optional, can offer early indicators of fungal infection. Establishing regular screening programs for high-risk patients is essential to enhance early detection and management of IFDs.

29.7.2 General Recommendations for Diagnostic Schedules

A comprehensive diagnostic approach involving multiple facets is vital for accurate and early diagnosis of IFDs. Tailoring the diagnostic schedule to the patient's clinical context and risk factors is crucial for effective management. Diagnostic strategies should be dynamic, allowing flexibility and adaptation based on the patient's response to treatment. Interdisciplinary collaboration among microbiologists, radiologists, and clinicians is necessary for optimal diagnosis and management of IFDs. Regular follow-up tests and imaging studies are indispensable for monitoring treatment efficacy and identifying any complications.

29.7.2.1 Antifungal Prophylaxis

Antifungal prophylaxis plays a critical role in managing IFDs, particularly in patients undergoing targeted therapies for hematological malignancies. Fluconazole and voriconazole are commonly used for prophylaxis due to their effectiveness and oral administration, which enhances patient compliance. Little et al highlighted the significance of prophylaxis in reducing the incidence of IFIs, emphasizing its standard recommendation in treatment protocols. Monitoring liver function is essential during antifungal therapy to detect hepatotoxicity early, and attention to potential drug interactions is crucial, especially in patients with complex medication regimens.

Posaconazole, a triazole antifungal agent, plays a significant role in the management of IFDs in high-risk patients, particularly those with hematological malignancies. Studies have shown that posaconazole prophylaxis effectively reduces the rate and probability of IFDs in high-risk patients. It has been demonstrated to prevent IFIs more effectively than other antifungal agents such as fluconazole or itraconazole, leading to improved overall survival.

Novel formulations of posaconazole, including gastro-resistant tablets and intravenous solutions, have been approved for prophylaxis and therapy of IFDs, highlighting its versatility in different clinical settings. Despite relatively low serum concentrations, posaconazole prophylaxis has proven highly effective in preventing IFIs. In real-world clinical conditions, patient education about correct intake has been shown to impact the plasma concentrations and effectiveness of posaconazole oral suspension.

Posaconazole has emerged as a preferred choice for antifungal prophylaxis, especially in patients with AML and those undergoing induction/reinduction chemotherapy for hematologic malignancies. It is considered the most efficacious azole for antifungal prophylaxis, particularly in patients with AML. In addition, posaconazole has been found to be clinically superior to other triazoles in preventing IFIs, especially aspergillosis.

The choice of antifungal agent should be based on the specific fungal pathogen identified through diagnostic tests, as emphasized by Ruiz-Camps and Aguilar-Company. Antifungal susceptibility testing is recommended, particularly for isolates from sterile sites, to ensure the most effective treatment against the specific pathogen. In cases of treatment failure or drug resistance, switching to another class of antifungal agents may be necessary. Combination antifungal therapy is considered for severe or refractory cases, although its long-term benefits and risks are still under investigation.

Cost considerations are crucial in antifungal treatment, especially with newer patented medications, and cost-effectiveness analyses can provide insights into the long-term economic impact of different treatment options. Antifungal stewardship programs aim to optimize antifungal agent use by balancing efficacy and cost.

Monitoring and follow-up are essential components of IFD management, with therapeutic drug monitoring increasingly used to optimize dosing and minimize toxicity. Imaging studies and follow-up diagnostic tests are crucial for assessing treatment effectiveness and confirming successful eradication of the infection.

Flowchart

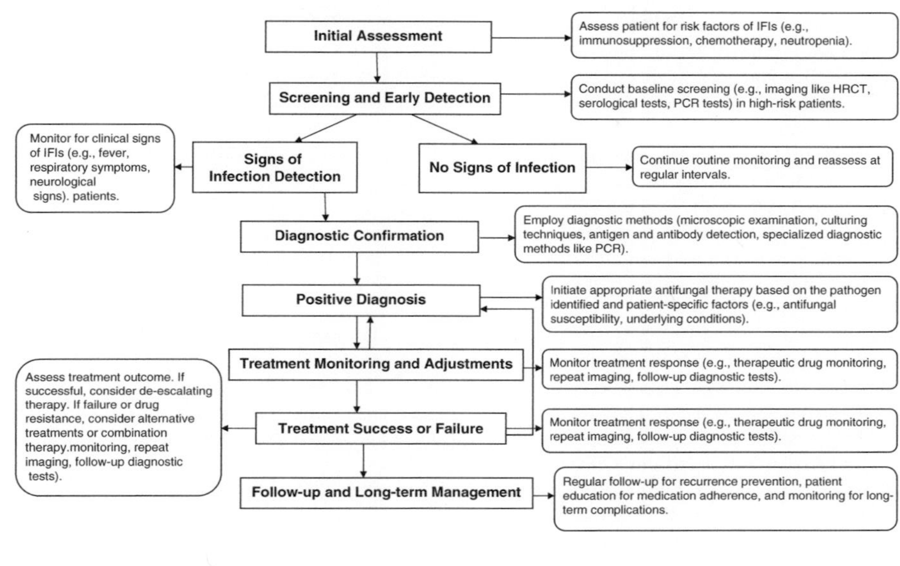

Invasive Fungal Infection in Hematological Malignancies Flowchart

References

Al-Kasaby NM, Abou El Kheir N, Mefreh M, Zaki MES (2017) Evaluation of semi-nested polymerase chain reaction (PCR) and mannan antigen detection compared to blood culture for diagnosis of candidemia. Afr J Microbiol Res 11(26):1061–1068

Almeida-Paes R, Almeida MDA, de Macedo PM, Caceres DH, Zancopé-Oliveira RM (2022) Performance of two commercial assays for the detection of serum Aspergillus galactomannan in non-neutropenic patients. J Fungi 8(7):741

Arendrup MC, Bergmann OJ, Larsson L, Nielsen HV, Jarløv JO, Christensson B (2010) Detection of candidaemia in patients with and without underlying haematological disease. Clin Microbiol Infect 16(7):855–862

Barton C, Vigor K, Scott R, Jones P, Lentfer H, Bax HJ et al (2016) Beta-glucan contamination of pharmaceutical products: how much should we accept? Cancer Immunol Immunother 65:1289–1301

Bergandi L, Apprato G, Silvagno F (2021) Vitamin D and beta-glucans synergically stimulate human macrophage activity. Int J Mol Sci 22(9):4869

Binnicker MJ, Jespersen DJ, Bestrom JE, Rollins LO (2012) Comparison of four assays for the detection of cryptococcal antigen. Clin Vaccine Immunol 19(12):1988–1990

Boch T, Reinwald M, Postina P, Cornely OA, Vehreschild JJ, Heussel CP et al (2015) Identification of invasive fungal diseases in immunocompromised patients by combining an Aspergillus specific PCR with a multifungal DNA-microarray from primary clinical samples. Mycoses 58(12):735–745

Bougnoux ME, Hill C, Moissenet D, Feuilhade de Chauvin M, Bonnay M, Vicens-Sprauel I et al (1990) Comparison of antibody, antigen, and metabolite assays for hospitalized patients with disseminated or peripheral candidiasis. J Clin Microbiol 28(5):905–909

Bougoure J, Ludwig M, Brundrett M, Cliff J, Clode P, Kilburn M, Grierson P (2014) High-resolution secondary ion mass spectrometry analysis of carbon dynamics in mycorrhizas formed by an obligately myco-heterotrophic orchid. Plant Cell Environ 37(5):1223–1230

Cao GJ, Xing ZF, Hua L, Ji YH, Sun JB, Zhao Z (2017) Evaluation of the diagnostic performance of panfungal polymerase chain reaction assay in invasive fungal diseases. Exp Ther Med 14(5):4208–4214

De Pauw B, Walsh TJ, Donnelly JP, Stevens DA, Edwards JE, Calandra T et al (2008) Revised definitions of invasive fungal disease from the European organization for research and treatment of cancer/invasive fungal infections cooperative group and the national institute of allergy and infectious diseases mycoses study group (EORTC/MSG) consensus group. Clin Infect Dis 46(12):1813–1821

De SK, Shetty N, Kelsey M (2014) How to use… blood cultures. Arch Dis Child Educ Pract 99(4):144–151

Donnelly JP, Chen SC, Kauffman CA, Steinbach WJ, Baddley JW, Verweij PE et al (2020) Revision and update of the consensus definitions of invasive fungal disease from the European Organization for Research and Treatment of Cancer and the Mycoses Study Group Education and Research Consortium. Clin Infect Dis 71(6):1367–1376

Einsele H, Hebart HOLGER, Roller GOTTFRIED, Löffler J, Rothenhofer I, Müller CA et al (1997) Detection and identification of fungal pathogens in blood by using molecular probes. J Clin Microbiol 35(6):1353–1360

Elluru SR, Kaveri SV, Bayry J (2015) The protective role of immunoglobulins in fungal infections and inflammation. In: Seminars in immunopathology, vol 37. Springer, Berlin Heidelberg, pp 187–197

Fanelli U, Iannarella R, Meoli A, Gismondi P, Cella S, Vincenzi F, Esposito S (2020) An unusual dysphagia for solids in a 17-year-old girl due to a lusoria artery: a case report and review of the literature. Int J Environ Res Public Health 17(10):3581

Farmakiotis D, Kyvernitakis A, Tarrand JJ, Kontoyiannis DP (2015) Early initiation of appropriate treatment is associated with increased survival in cancer patients with Candida glabrata fungaemia: a potential benefit from infectious disease consultation. Clin Microbiol Infect 21(1):79–86

Ganiem AR, Indrati AR, Wisaksana R, Meijerink H, van der Ven A, Alisjahbana B, van Crevel R (2014) Asymptomatic cryptococcal antigenemia is associated with mortality among HIV-positive patients in Indonesia. J Int AIDS Soc 17(1):18821

Girmenia C, Nucci M, Martino P (2001) Clinical significance of Aspergillus fungaemia in patients with haematological malignancies and invasive aspergillosis. Br J Haematol 114(1):93–98

Guimarães AJ, Nosanchuk JD, Zancopé-Oliveira RM (2006) Diagnosis of histoplasmosis. Braz J Microbiol 37:1–13

Gülmez DOLUNAY, Alp S, Gursoy G, Ayaz CM, Dogan O, Arikan-Akdagli S, Akova M (2020) Mixed fungaemia: an 18-year report from a tertiary-care university hospital and a systematic review. Clin Microbiol Infect 26(7):833–841

Hartfield JN, Grooters AM, Waite KJ (2014) Development and evaluation of an ELISA for the quantitation of anti-Lagenidium giganteum forma caninum antibodies in dogs. J Vet Intern Med 28(5):1479–1484

Haynes K, Rogers TR (1994) Retrospective evaluation of a latex agglutination test for diagnosis of invasive aspergillosis in immunocompromised patients. Eur J Clin Microbiol Infect Dis 13:670–674

He Z, Zhu XL, Chan TMD, Cheung CYT, Ng HK, Mok CTV, Poon WS (2021) The diagnostic accuracy and era for improvement for frameless stereotactic brain biopsy: a series of 109 procedures and a systemic review. Research Square

Huang HR, Fan LC, Rajbanshi B, Xu JF (2015) Evaluation of a new cryptococcal antigen lateral flow immunoassay in serum, cerebrospinal fluid and urine for the diagnosis of cryptococcosis: a meta-analysis and systematic review. PLoS One 10(5):e0127117

Husain S, Kwak EJ, Obman A, Wagener MM, Kusne S, Stout JE et al (2004) Prospective assessment of Platelia™ Aspergillus galactomannan antigen for the diagnosis of invasive aspergillosis in lung transplant recipients. Am J Transplant 4(5):796–802

Huurneman LJ, Neely M, Veringa A, Docobo Pérez F, Ramos-Martin V, Tissing WJ et al (2016) Pharmacodynamics of voriconazole in children: further steps along the path to true individualized therapy. Antimicrob Agents Chemother 60(4):2336–2342

Kahn FW, Jones JM (1986) Latex agglutination tests for detection of Candida antigens in sera of patients with invasive candidiasis. J Infect Dis 153(3):579–585

Laín A, Elguezabal N, Amutio E, Fernández de Larrinoa I, Moragues MD, Pontón J (2008) Use of recombinant antigens for the diagnosis of invasive candidiasis. J Immunol Res 2008:721950

Lawal IO, Mokoala KM, Kgatle MM, Dierckx RA, Glaudemans AW, Sathekge MM, Ankrah AO (2021) Radionuclide imaging of invasive fungal disease in immunocompromised hosts. Diagnostics 11(11):2057

Liaw YS, Yang PC, Yu CJ, Chang DB, Wang HJ, Lee LN et al (1995) Direct determination of cryptococcal antigen in transthoracic needle aspirate for diagnosis of pulmonary cryptococcosis. J Clin Microbiol 33(6):1588–1591

Maheswaran D, Zeng Y, Chan-Yeung M, Scott J, Osornio-Vargas A, Becker AB, Kozyrskyj AL (2014) Exposure to Beta-(1, 3)-D-glucan in house dust at age 7–10 is associated with airway hyperresponsiveness and atopic asthma by age 11–14. PLoS One 9(6):e98878

Markovic VL, Stummer BE, Hill AS (2002) Immunodetection and characterization of antigens expressed by Uncinula necator. J Phytopathol 150(11–12):663–673

Martínez JP, Gil ML, López-Ribot JL, Chaffin WL (1998) Serologic response to cell wall mannoproteins and proteins of Candida albicans. Clin Microbiol Rev 11(1):121–141

Memoli JSW, Nietert PJ, Silvestri GA (2012) Meta-analysis of guided bronchoscopy for the evaluation of the pulmonary nodule. Chest 142(2):385–393

Ntusi N, Aubin L, Oliver S, Whitelaw A, Mendelson M (2010) Guideline for the optimal use of blood cultures: guideline. S Afr Med J 100(12):839–843

Oren I, Avidor I, Sprecher H (2012) Lack of intra-laboratory reproducibility in using Platelia Aspergillus enzyme immunoassay test for detection of Aspergillus galactomannan antigen. Transpl Infect Dis 14(1):107–109

Otto WR, Green AM (2020) Fungal infections in children with haematologic malignancies and stem cell transplant recipients. Br J Haematol 189(4):607–624

Pana ZD, Roilides E, Warris A, Groll AH, Zaoutis T (2017) Epidemiology of invasive fungal disease in children. J Pediatr Infect Dis Soc 6(suppl_1):S3–S11

Pasqualotto AC, Denning DW (2005) Diagnosis of invasive fungal infections–current limitations of classical and new diagnostic methods. Eur Oncol Rev 11

Patterson TF, Thompson GR III, Denning DW, Fishman JA, Hadley S, Herbrecht R et al (2016) Practice guidelines for the diagnosis and management of aspergillosis: 2016 update by the Infectious Diseases Society of America. Clin Infect Dis 63(4):e1–e60

Pham KN, Nhut ND, Cuong NM (2020) New method for preparing purity β-D-glucans (beta-Glucan) from baker's yeast (Saccharomyces cerevisiae). Sci Technol Dev J 23(3):678–683

Pujari S, Arjunwadkar V, Sangle S, Kagal A, Bharadwaj R, Karyakarte R (2020) Cryptococcal Antigenemia in HIV-infected patients with CD4+ T-cell count≤ 200 cells/µl: a study from a tertiary care hospital. Int J Contemp Med Res 7:B1–B4

Qin L, Zhao L, Tan C, Chen XU, Yang Z, Mo W (2015) A novel method of combining Periodic Acid Schiff staining with Wright-Giemsa staining to identify the pathogens Penicillium marneffei, Histoplasma capsulatum, Mucor and Leishmania donovani in bone marrow smears. Exp Ther Med 9(5):1950–1954

Reisberger EM, Abels C, Landthaler M, Szeimies RM (2003) Histopathological diagnosis of onychomycosis by periodic acid–Schiff-stained nail clippings. Br J Dermatol 148(4):749–754

Ruhnke M, Behre G, Buchheidt D, Christopeit M, Hamprecht A, Heinz W et al (2018) Diagnosis of invasive fungal diseases in haematology and oncology: 2018 update of the recommendations of the infectious diseases working party of the German society for hematology and medical oncology (AGIHO). Mycoses 61(11):796–813

Schnietz R, Wilson ML (2018) Grocott methenamine silver and periodic acid-Schiff positivity in cutaneous Mycobacterium avium complex infection. J Cutan Pathol 45(7):551–553

Shalin SC, Ferringer T, Cassarino DS (2020) PAS and GMS utility in dermatopathology: review of the current medical literature. J Cutan Pathol 47(11):1096–1102

Swift O, Vilar E, Farrington K (2019) Unexplained inflammation in end-stage kidney disease: is the combination of enhanced gastrointestinal permeability and reticuloendothelial dysfunction its cause? Semin Dial 32(5):417–423

Swoboda-KopEć E, Gołaś M, PisKorsKa K, Dąbkowska M, Niecwietajewa I, Pączek L, Sikora M (2015) Aspergillus galactomannan detection in comparison to a real-time PCR assay in serum samples from a high-risk group of patients. Centr Eur J Immunol 40(4):454–460

Tanner DC, Weinstein MP, Fedorciw B, Joho KL, Thorpe JJ, Reller L (1994) Comparison of commercial kits for detection of cryptococcal antigen. J Clin Microbiol 32(7):1680–1684

Ullmann AJ, Aguado JM, Arikan-Akdagli S, Denning DW, Groll AH, Lagrou K et al (2018) Diagnosis and management of Aspergillus diseases: executive summary of the 2017 ESCMID-ECMM-ERS guideline. Clin Microbiol Infect 24:e1–e38

Wilson ML (2020) Development of new methods for detecting bloodstream pathogens. Clin Microbiol Infect 26(3):319–324

Wright WF, Overman SB, Ribes JA (2011) (1–3)-β-D-glucan assay: a review of its laboratory and clinical application. Lab Med 42(11):679–685

Yoshimura K, Suzuki Y, Inoue Y, Nishimoto K, Mori K, Karayama M et al (2018) Utility of serum Aspergillus-galactomannan antigen to evaluate the risk of severe acute exacerbation in chronic obstructive pulmonary disease. PLoS One 13(6):e0198479

Zhang J, Cui N, Wang H, Han W, Li Y, Xiao M, Liu D (2020) Invasive fungal disease in critically ill patients at high risk: usefulness of lymphocyte subtyping. J Intensive Care Med 35(9):909–918

Zhao D, Qiu G, Luo Z, Zhang Y (2015) Platelet parameters and (1, 3)-β-D-glucan as a diagnostic and prognostic marker of invasive fungal disease in preterm infants. PLoS One 10(4):e0123907

Part VI
Critical Care Pathways and Prognosis

Chapter 30
Early Care of Unstable Hematologic Malignancies Patients: Preventing Admission into ICU

Indubala Maurya, Umadri Singh, Shreyas H. Gutte, and Mohan Gurjar

Learning Points

1. Early Recognition of Symptoms: Understanding the early signs of neurological, cardiovascular, and respiratory complications in patients with hematological malignancies is crucial for timely intervention and preventing progression that requires ICU care.
2. Ward-based Management: Implementing effective ward-based interventions, such as using noninvasive diagnostic tools and immediate pharmacological treatments, can significantly reduce ICU admissions and improve patient outcomes.
3. Interdisciplinary Approach: Coordination between hematologists, oncologists, and critical care specialists is vital for the early identification of at-risk patients and the implementation of organ support strategies to prevent critical complications.
4. Education and Training: Ensuring that ward staff are well-trained in recognizing the early signs of organ dysfunction and are equipped with the knowledge and tools to perform necessary interventions can lead to better management of hematological malignancies in a non-ICU setting.

I. Maurya
Anaesthesiology, Kalyan Singh Super Specialty Cancer Institute,
Lucknow, Uttar Pradesh, India

U. Singh · S. H. Gutte · M. Gurjar (✉)
Critical Care Medicine, Sanjay Gandhi Postgraduate Institute of Medical Sciences,
Lucknow, Uttar Pradesh, India
e-mail: mohan@sgpgi.ac.in

S. B. Mishra (ed.), *Critical Care Hematology*,
https://doi.org/10.1007/978-981-97-5565-3_30

30.1 Introduction

Patients with hematologic malignancy may develop systemic or organ-specific dysfunction due to the primary disease progression, its ongoing treatment (chemotherapy and radiotherapy), or new deterioration in coexisting illness during the current hospitalization. These clinical deteriorations, expected or unexpected, alert the treating team and prompt them to triage for timely intensive care unit (ICU) admission for better clinical outcomes. However, the decision to admit an unstable patient with hematologic malignancy in ICU depends on the patient's or caregiver's preference, risk–benefit assessment of invasive or intensive treatments, and unavailability of ICU beds (Ferreyro et al. 2021; Vijenthira et al. 2020). An oncologist must triage these patients for ICU admission, thus reducing the burden on already resource-constrained ICUs. Hematologists/oncologists can coordinate with Critical care outreach services in the early identification of at-risk patients and organ support strategies to prevent critical complications. As the majority of related topics have been covered in various chapters of this book, this chapter aims to provide an overview of early recognition of organ dysfunction in patients with hematologic malignancy, ward-based standard treatment, and strategies to minimize these varieties of organ failure (Table 30.1).

Table 30.1 Overview of strategies reducing ICU admissions for hematologic malignancies patients

Identify the category of patient	Strategies to prevent ICU admission
High-risk group Patients having malignancies with a known higher incidence of expected clinical issues or complication	Baseline clinical scoring (if available), investigations Frequent monitoring (clinical/laboratory) Early arrangement of therapeutic options/ discussion with the relevant medical team, etc. Consider discussing expected issues/ complications in advance with family members Always review for timely admission to the ICU
Low-risk group Patients having malignancies with lower incidence or unexpected clinical issues or complication	Early identification of issue/complication by clinical, laboratory, imaging, etc., to measure severity Start initial management at bedside itself, including intervention (if feasible) and enhance monitoring Plan for specific management for that particular issue/complication Always review for timely admission to the ICU

ICU Intensive care unit

30.2 Central Nervous System

Neurological complications in hematologic patients may have a fatal course and catastrophic and long-term consequences if not recognized. Although the involvement of the peripheral nervous system is more common in illnesses involving plasma cells, involvement of the central nervous system (CNS) by lymphoma or leukemia is more common after a relapse. At the same time, it can occur at any point during the disease. Infections, vascular and paraneoplastic complications can all indirectly impact the central nervous system (CNS) and peripheral nervous system (PNS). It is essential to recognize neurological complications of cancer promptly and establish appropriate distinctions between symptoms directly related to cancer and those associated with other neurological illnesses or cancer treatment to avert disastrous consequences. Meningeal leukemia, raised intracranial pressure, spinal cord compression, CNS infection, status epilepticus, hyperviscosity, etc., are only a few examples of the spectrum of signs that could occur (de la Fuente et al. 2020). Table 30.2 thoroughly overviews common CNS signs and symptoms that can be life-threatening.

30.2.1 Leukemic Deposits

Depending on the site and severity of infiltration, leukemic deposits can affect any part of the central nervous system and cause a variety of signs and symptoms (Sussman and Davies-Jones 2014). Headaches, nausea, and vomiting are the most common symptoms. These symptoms may also be accompanied by irritability, lethargy, stiff neck, somnolence, coma, and convulsions (Blumenthal and Glenn 2002). Diffuse meningeal infiltration reduces cerebral spinal fluid (CSF) flow, which can result in communicative hydrocephalus. Papilledema is the most common sign. The leukemic deposits have the potential to spread between the nerve fibers and compress or invade the spinal nerve roots or cranial nerves.

Hypothalamic and pituitary dysfunction may be associated with hydrocephalus. CSF examination shows meningeal leukemia in approximately 90% of the cases. There may be a reduction in glucose concentration and typically a rise in CSF pressure (Sussman and Davies-Jones 2014). Therefore, such nonspecific complaints by a leukemic patient in the ward that are not relieved on standard medications should prompt the clinician to rule out leukemic deposits for early diagnosis and management, precluding ICU admission.

Table 30.2 Approach to common signs and symptoms of central nervous system (CNS) for underlying life-threatening conditions

Sign/symptom	Differential diagnosis	Initial diagnostic Work-up	Primary management
Headache	Leukemic deposits Meningitis Hyperviscosity syndrome Elevated intracranial pressures	**Clinical** Characterize headaches in details Look for other associated signs/symptoms like vomiting, photophobia, blurred vision, and dizziness Examine and assess in detail including GCS, consciousness, orientation to time, place person, pupil size (asymmetry, pinpoint, dilated, reacting or not), AVPU score if not able to assess GCS, facial asymmetry, any weakness in all four limbs, neck rigidity, noninvasive blood pressure, oxygen saturation if any altered pattern of respiration is seen, temperature, ONSD if raised ICP, is suspected, fundoscopy if raised blood pressure **Laboratory and imaging** Serum sodium, serum BUN, serum blood glucose level, serum osmolarity, hemoglobin, total leucocyte count, platelet count, INR, serum ammonia, CSF (if meningitis is suspected), procalcitonin and blood culture if meningitis suspected Appropriate brain imaging like CT scan/MRI brain	**General** If symptoms are severe but conscious and there is no neurological deficit, then consider stopping oral feed provide appropriate analgesic till further evaluation If associated with compromise in airway. Breathing and/or circulation (ABC), then resuscitate accordingly Prepare for intubation trolley, vasoactive drugs Seek urgent neurology consultation **Issue specific** **Meningitis** Isolation for neutropenic patients. Perform imaging (NCCT head)-if there are no contraindications to LP → CSF analysis and differential counts, biochemistry, culture, microscopy for opportunistic infections. Initiate targeted antimicrobial therapy according to sensitivity profile. **Elevated intracranial pressures** NCCT head, ONSD monitoring for objectivity, neuroprotective measures, hyperosmotic agents, and dexamethasone for vasogenic edema. Treat the underlying cause. **Hyperviscosity syndrome** Consider leukapheresis, plateletpheresis, or plasmapheresis; if APML gives ATRA **Leukemic deposits** Symptomatic treatment followed by targeted therapy with chemotherapeutic agents

Neurological deficits (altered sensorium/ neuromuscular weakness)	Cerebrovascular complications Spinal cord compression (leukemic deposits or metastasis)	**Clinical** First, look for any compromises in the airway, breathing, and/or circulation (ABC) Assess detailed examination of neurological deficit including GCS, consciousness, orientation to time, place person, pupil size (asymmetry, pinpoint, dilated, reacting, or not), AVPU score if not able to assess GCS, facial asymmetry, any weakness in all four limbs, neck rigidity, noninvasive blood pressure, oxygen saturation if any altered pattern of respiration is seen, temperature, ONSD if raised ICP, is suspected, fundoscopy if raised blood pressure **Laboratory and imaging** Serum sodium, serum BUN, serum blood glucose level, serum osmolarity, hemoglobin, total leucocyte count, platelet count, INR, serum ammonia, CSF (if meningitis is suspected), procalcitonin and blood culture if meningitis suspected Appropriate brain imaging like CT scan/MRI brain/ spine Neurophysiological studies include nerve conduction study and electromyography.	**General** If associated with compromise in airway, breathing, and/or circulation (ABC), then resuscitate accordingly Prepare for intubation trolley, vasoactive drugs Seek urgent neurology and intensive care consultation **Issue specific** **Cerebrovascular complications** Objective monitoring with ONSD, fundoscopy, and NCCT head to treat the precipitating cause (depending upon ischemic or hemorrhagic presentation) Chemotherapy-related endothelial injury ➔ withhold chemotherapy. **Spinal cord compression** Symptomatic treatment for pain and sensory symptoms is dexamethasone therapy. Targeted therapy with chemotherapeutic agents or surgery.

APML Acute promyelocytic leukemia, *ATRA* all trans-retinoic acid, *AVPU* Alert, voice, pain, unresponsive, *BUN* Blood urea nitrogen, *CSF* cerebrospinal fluid, *GCS* Glasgow coma scale, *ICP* intracranial pressure, *INR* International normalized ratio, *NCCT* noncontrast CT, *ONSD* Optic nerve sheath diameter

30.2.2 Raised Intracranial Pressure

Raised intracranial pressure (ICP) is an emergency in hematologic malignancy, which can lead to irreversible neurological injury and death if not addressed immediately. Primary and secondary brain tumors can cause increased blood-brain barrier permeability, leading to extravasation of proteins, electrolytes, and water into the extracellular space. Patients with strokes, status epilepticus, and meningoencephalitis, have fluid accumulation in the intracellular space, causing cytotoxic edema. Although management of raised intracranial pressure mandates intensive care admission, mitigation, and early intervention in raised ICP can have favorable outcomes and prevent ICU admission. Raised ICP usually presents as headache, nausea or vomiting as the first symptom. Associated cranial CN VI palsies can cause diplopia. Patients may also experience lethargy, stupor, or coma (de la Fuente et al. 2020).

Papilledema, commonly seen in raised ICP, can be recognized by a simple bedside fundus examination showing optic disc swelling. Bedside ultrasound-guided optic nerve sheath diameter (ONSD) measurement can triage patients who need urgent intensive care management (Montorfano et al. 2021). Early brain imaging, such as noncontrast computed tomography (NCCT), will help to identify at-risk patients. Treatment strategies for raised ICP depend on the underlying etiology. Dexamethasone is the first line of treatment for a mass lesion with vasogenic edema. Hypertonic saline and mannitol, which leads to an osmotic gradient across the blood-brain barrier (BBB), are helpful for treatment. Obstructive or noncommunicating hydrocephalus should be treated immediately with a ventriculoperitoneal shunt (VPS) or third ventriculostomy, followed by specialized treatment for the obstructing lesion if possible (de la Fuente et al. 2020).

30.2.3 Spinal Cord Compression

Spinal cord compression (SCC) may affect 2–10% of cancer patients; hematologic malignancies contribute to 10% of these incidents. Patients with multiple myeloma (MM) are most likely to develop SCC (8%).In solid tumors, SCC arises when spinal metastases migrate dorsally, resulting in epidural SCC. Epidural SCC is most common in the thoracic spinal cord (60%) but may develop as low as L1-L2. Malignant epidural disease compresses nerve roots below the L1-L2 level, causing cauda equina syndrome.

Pain is the initial and most common presenting symptom, subsequently followed by weakness, sensory loss, and autonomic dysfunction (de la Fuente et al. 2020). High cervical cord compression may result in respiratory impairment and autonomic dysreflexia, leading to bradycardia and hypertension (Sussman and Davies-Jones 2014). MRI may show the degree of severity of SCC, the presence of cord edema, and ischemia.

On early recognition, a bolus of dexamethasone should be administered, followed by 4 mg every 6 h or 8 mg every 12 h. When SCC is recognized and treated early, most patients retain or regain their capacity to walk and control sphincters (de la Fuente et al. 2020).

30.2.4 Status Epilepticus

Status epilepticus (SE) can occur either continuously or intermittently, with no recovery of consciousness between episodes. They can be convulsive (CSE) or non-convulsive (NCSE).It may arise due to neurological complications from a brain tumor or its therapy, metabolic disorders caused by hematologic malignancies, or meningoencephalitis. Temporal trends in seizure incidence may shed light on the underlying cause. Seizures that occur shortly after or during the initial course of cancer chemotherapeutic therapy are likely drug-induced. Seizures triggered by intracranial metastases or CNS infections occur later in the disease's course (de la Fuente et al. 2020). Posterior reversible encephalopathy syndrome, caused by drugs such as cyclophosphamide, cisplatin, gemcitabine, and L-asparaginase, is a further possibility that might cause high blood pressure, headaches, altered mental status, and cortical blindness (Floeter et al. 2017). The prevention of SE should be targeted in at-risk patients. Avoiding chemotherapeutic agents known to reduce the seizure threshold, use of prophylactic antiseizure medications with chemotherapeutic agents known to cause seizures, and timely correction of metabolic derangements can prevent the occurrence of status epilepticus, thus reducing the disease burden (de la Fuente et al. 2020).

30.2.5 Neurovascular Complications

It can occur in the form of either intracranial hemorrhage or thrombosis. Intracerebral hemorrhage (ICH) is the second most frequent neurological complication encountered in adult patients with hematologic malignancies. The highest risk is in acute leukemia (20%), with a high mortality rate (20%). It may occur as a result of disseminated intravascular coagulopathy (DIC), which is common in acute promyelocytic leukemia (APL), thrombocytopenia, blast crisis, or hyperleukocytosis (more than 300×10^9 cells/l) and Chemotherapy-related endothelial injury (Ferreyro et al. 2021; de la Fuente et al. 2020). Thrombocytopenia can occur as a complication of the underlying hematologic malignancy, immune-mediated platelet destruction, or result from chemotherapy. A new headache with an altered level of consciousness must be monitored closely or may require imaging, especially with a background of thrombocytopenia or DIC (Sussman and Davies-Jones 2014; Blumenthal and Glenn 2002). With the advent of bedside ultrasonography, ONSD can help triage patients requiring urgent intensive care management.

Neurovascular complications are emergencies that require intensive care management, but with prevention and targeted management of at-risk patients, such emergencies can be avoided. Thrombocytopenia and coagulopathy should be optimized with suitable blood products using platelets, fresh frozen plasma (FFP), etc. Raised blood pressure in patients with coagulation abnormalities should be identified and treated early.

Invasive procedures (e.g., lumbar puncture) should be avoided since they could result in a spinal subdural hematoma leading to spinal cord compression or cauda equine syndrome. Drugs like Ibrutinib have been linked to CNS hemorrhage, with subdural hematomas being the most prevalent; thus, these should be avoided in high-risk patients (de la Fuente et al. 2020).

Similarly, patients with hematologic malignancies are also susceptible to intracranial thrombosis, which may be triggered due to hypercoagulability, heparin-induced thrombocytopenia, and L-asparaginase treatment. Presentation is usually in the form of headaches, focal neurological deficits, seizures, and other signs of raised ICP, which should prompt the clinician for an early or more frequent CT/MRI monitoring as well as administration of anticoagulants (heparin or LMWH), blood products to prevent the progression and hence curb the poor outcomes. In L-asparaginase-associated venous sinus thrombosis cases, therapy with the antithrombin concentrate and cryoprecipitate is suggested to maintain antithrombin III > 60 u/ml and fibrinogen >1.0 g/l, respectively (de la Fuente et al. 2020).

30.2.6 CNS Infection

CNS infection is an infrequent complication of cancer. Recognizing and treating these conditions is challenging as the traditional triad of fever, neck stiffness, and altered mental status is uncommon (de la Fuente et al. 2020). Other illnesses like metabolic abnormalities or chemotherapy side effects might conceal or mimic symptoms. With the frequent administration of corticosteroids, chemotherapy, and broad-spectrum antibiotics, it is reasonable to expect CNS involvement with rare or nonpathogenic organisms (Vijenthira et al. 2020). Atypical presentations such as multifocal strokes secondary to small or large vessel vasculopathy caused by varicella zoster reactivation in immunocompromised patients with hematologic malignancy are also possible (Saito et al. 2021). Patients undergoing allogeneic hematopoietic stem cell transplantation (allo-HSCT) are at the highest risk of CNS infections, with an incidence of up to 15%. Patients who get alemtuzumab-based conditioning before allo-HSCT pose an elevated risk of developing viral CNS infections. Hence, early recognition is critical to diagnose and treat immediately with antimicrobial and antiviral drugs (Schmidt-Hieber et al. 2016). Patients with neutropenia and hypogammaglobulinemia require isolation with good hand hygiene practices and barrier nursing. Invasive procedures should be avoided if possible. Patients who require central venous or intracerebral devices may benefit from antimicrobial-coated catheters, which have a lower infection rate than ordinary catheters.

Primary and secondary antimicrobial prophylaxis should be considered and administered on time to at-risk patients (Nucci and Anaissie 2018).

30.2.7 Cellular Hyperviscosity

Hyperleucocytosis, commonly seen in leukemia, causes an increase in blood viscosity (Bewersdorf and Zeidan 2020). Symptoms can appear in myelogenous leukemia, even at lower leucocyte counts, due to the larger cell size (Sussman and Davies-Jones 2014). Elevated serum immunoglobulin levels in Waldenstrom macroglobulinemia can also lead to acute hyperviscosity syndrome due to increased blood viscosity, causing decreased tissue perfusion. The traditional triad of hyperviscosity involves visual problems, neurological abnormalities, and mucosal hemorrhage. The severity of the symptoms depends on the degree of tissue hypoperfusion and can progress to life-threatening conditions such as heart failure and pulmonary hypertension; consequently, people at risk should be recognized and treated as soon as possible (Aliyeva 2021). Frequent blood transfusions should be avoided in such patients as they may further elevate viscosity. Further treatment options are leukapheresis and plasmapheresis.

30.3 Cardiovascular System

Cardiovascular involvement in patients with hematologic malignancies may develop as a part of the disease progression itself or secondary to the chemotherapeutic agents. The manifestations may range from subclinical electrocardiogram (ECG) changes to life-threatening emergencies. Hence, cardiovascular screening should be routine care for high-risk groups. Such fatal emergencies can be missed easily if one is not cautious in picking up the subtle signs at the bedside. Several cardiac complications reported are shock, pericardial diseases, cardiac infiltration, superior vena cava syndrome, vaso-occlusion/vasospasm causing angina/myocardial infarction, and drug/radiation-induced cardiac toxicity (Allegra et al. 2010). Most cardiovascular complications mandate intensive care management, but early intervention with simple diagnostic approaches and prompt treatment may prevent further organ dysfunction. Table 30.3 comprehensively overviews common cardiovascular signs and symptoms for life-threatening illnesses.

Table 30.3 Approach to common signs and symptoms of cardiovascular system (CVS) for underlying life-threatening conditions

Sign/ symptom	Differential diagnosis	Initial diagnostic work-up	Primary management
Hypotension (circulatory shock)	Cardiogenic shock Obstructive shock Hypovolemic shock Vasodilatory shock	**Clinical** Identify signs of early organ dysfunction due to hypoperfusion like altered mental status, oliguria, tachypnoea, tachycardia, cold clammy (hyperemic skin in early distributive shock), or cyanotic skin. Examine and assess for GCS, noninvasive blood pressure, capillary refill time, JVP, auscultation-crepitations(cardiogenic), and altered pattern of respiration. **Laboratory and imaging** ABG (look for metabolic acidosis, hyperlactatemia) ECG (look for arrhythmias, STEMI, low QRS complexes, electrical alternans (pericardial tamponade), etc.) Cardiac biomarkers (cardiogenic shock) Echocardiography Intravascular volume assessment by bedside USG CBC, chest X-ray, blood cultures (sepsis) Pulmonary angiography, if pulmonary embolism suspected	**General** Asses and stabilize airway, breathing, and/or circulation (ABC), then resuscitate accordingly, while the initial diagnostic work-up is ongoing Peripheral (14/16G) or central venous access(vasoactive agents) Consider volume resuscitation, if no contraindications Use crystalloid fluids, can prefer a balanced salt solution Use norepinephrine as a choice of vasopressor Prepare for intubation trolley, vasoactive drugs Early risk stratification and seek urgent consultation from intensive care outreach team Always suspect the possibility of the co-existence of two types of shock **Issue specific** **Cardiogenic shock** ***Tamponade:*** POCUS—Systolic atrial collapse, diastolic ventricle collapse. Immediate pericardiocentesis, maintain preload. ***MI:*** POCUS-RWMA, reduced contractility, raised cardiac biomarkers, ruled out hyperviscosity syndrome. Manage with oxygen, nitrates, anticoagulation, pain relief, and coronary revascularization. **Obstructive shock** ***Pulmonary embolism:*** POCUS—Dilated RA, RV and IVC. Early thrombolysis, regular DVT screening, routine thromboprophylaxis for prevention. **Hypovolemic shock** POCUS IVC diameter reduced with respirophasic changes, PLRT-increase in systolic pressure by 20 mmhg suggests fluid responsiveness. POCUS guided fluid therapy, source control; hemorrhagic shock ➔ FAST scan(if positive-early surgical intervention) followed by blood and blood products transfusion **Vasodilatory shock** ***Sepsis:*** Rule out clinical signs of sepsis, low diastolic pressure, increased pulse pressure, CBC-increased total leucocyte counts, and raised procalcitonin. POCUS hyper-dynamic heart functions. Treat according to the surviving sepsis guidelines: Early fluid therapy, send pan cultures, empirical antibiotic therapy ***Anaphylaxis:*** Inj epinephrine 0.3–0.5 mg of 1:1000 IM

Palpitation	Cardiomyopathy/arrhythmias secondary to cardiac infiltration of the malignant cells, drug toxicity, etc.	**Clinical** Complaints of palpitations, altered mental status, chest pain. Look for signs of congestive cardiac failure-hypotension, hypertension, arrhythmias, and ischemia; look for temporal association with drug initiation. **Laboratory and imaging** ECG—Arrhythmia, low QRS voltage with left ventricular hypertrophy, POCUS—Systolic or diastolic dysfunction (restrictive/constrictive cardiomyopathy) Noninvasive blood pressure Oximetry Echocardiography Cardiac biomarkers Serum electrolytes, CBC	**General** Asses and stabilize airway, breathing, and/or circulation (ABC) Peripheral (14/16G) or central venous access(vasoactive agents) Prepare for intubation trolley, vasoactive drugs Monitor strictly the fluid balance Early risk stratification-seek urgent consultation from intensive care outreach team **Issue specific** Arrhythmias ➔ specific antiarrhythmic according to ACLS. Cardiomyopathy ➔ preload dependent-maintain intravascular volume. Judicious use of diuretics. ACE inhibitors and beta blockers for early disease states. If suspecting drug toxicity-reduction of dosage/discontinuation of the drug, use of diuretics and ACE inhibitors in case of left ventricular dysfunction.

ABG Arterial blood gas analysis, *ACE inhibitors* Angiotensin converting enzyme inhibitors, *ACLS* Advanced cardiac life support, *CBC* complete blood count, *FAST* focused assessment with sonography in trauma, *GCS* Glasgow coma scale, *IVC* Inferior vena cava, *JVP* Jugular venous pressure, *POCUS* Point of care ultrasound, *PLRT* Passive leg raising test, *RA* Right atrium, *RV* Right ventricle, *RWMA* Regional wall motion abnormality, *STEMI* ST-elevation myocardial infarction

30.3.1 Circulatory Shock

Broadly, shock in any patient can be hypovolemic, vasodilatory, cardiogenic, or obstructive (Vincent and De Backer 2013). Often, two of these situations may coexist. Hypovolemic shock can be treated effectively even outside the ICU if diagnosed in time. It can be caused by inadequate oral intake due to the ailment or in the face of diarrhea or polyuria induced by chemotherapeutic agents. After the clinical analysis for signs of dehydration and the input and output balance, simple bedside tests such as a passive leg raise test or bedside point-of-care ultrasound (POCUS) can be performed to assess for fluid responsiveness. The bedside ultrasound assessment methods laid out by the RUSH and FALLS protocols provide a step-wise, concise approach to ruling out the various causes of shock and can be easily mastered (Ait-Hamou et al. 2019). Another bedside technique, that is, the shock index, is a commonly used perfusion index to look for fluid responsiveness. It is the heart rate to systolic blood pressure ratio, with an average measurement ranging from 0.5 to 0.7 bpm/mmHg. It can be used as a tool for risk evaluation to identify changes in hemodynamic parameters before systemic hypotension or cardiorespiratory collapse occurs (Liu et al. 2012). Vasodilatory shock occurs most commonly due to sepsis. The at-risk population, especially neutropenic patients, should be identified, isolated, and started on prophylactic antibiotics in order to prevent sepsis. Signs of sepsis may be obscured in such patients; therefore, vigilance is advised. According to Surviving sepsis guidelines (SSG), early antibiotic therapy and fluid resuscitation should be initiated.

Even in septic shock, a shock index of <=1 has a negative predictive value of 88% for hemodynamic improvement after fluid resuscitation, indicating the need for early vasopressor medication (Al Aseri et al. 2020). Cardiogenic shock and obstructive shocks are emergencies that obligate intensive care management. Early diagnosis can be performed with POCUS at the bedside by looking at the cardiac functions in cardiogenic shock or right atrial, right ventricle dilatation, and deep vein thrombosis to rule out obstructive causes of shock, hence further limiting organ dysfunction by establishing early ICU care.

30.3.2 Cardiac Parenchyma Infiltration

A large number of hematologic malignancies are known to infiltrate the heart but have minimal impact clinically. The pattern of involvement is also different with each type of malignancy. Primary cardiac lymphoma is a non-Hodgkin lymphoma that affects solely the heart and pericardium. It may cause pericardial effusion, arrhythmias, or heart failure. Pericardial involvement is mainly due to lymphatic or hematogenous metastasis. It may be clinically silent or may lead to pericardial tamponade. Patients with multiple myeloma may develop heart failure as a result of metastatic heart disease, myocardial amyloidosis, hyperviscosity syndrome, or coexisting coronary artery disease. Initially, the cardiac functions are preserved due to myocardial hypertrophy; however, as the condition progresses, the myocardium's function declines, and the left atrium and ventricle may dilate. Cardiac amyloidosis causes restrictive cardiomyopathy and causes heart failure. A low QRS voltage on electrocardiography and left ventricular hypertrophy on two-dimensional echocardiography may not correlate. Natriuretic peptide (B-type) testing and cardiac magnetic resonance imaging can be beneficial in distinguishing between constrictive pericarditis and restrictive cardiomyopathy. Bedside echocardiography may diagnose systolic or diastolic dysfunction due to cardiac infiltration. Most of these patients are preload dependent. Hence, optimal fluid balance should be achieved. Judicious use of diuretics is the mainstay treatment. Angiotensin-converting enzyme (ACE) inhibitors and beta-blockers in low doses may also help during the early stages of the disease but may exacerbate symptoms in advanced phases (Allegra et al. 2010).

30.3.3 Malignant Pericardial Effusion and Cardiac Tamponade

Pericardial involvement can be in the form of pericarditis, pericardial effusion, and pericardial tamponade, which is a life-threatening complication (Shenoy et al. 2017). Pericardial involvement may result from hematogenous spread, lymphatic invasion, or direct malignant invasion. Pericardial effusions resulting from malignancies may also be caused by radiation, chemotherapy, and opportunistic infections. Symptoms may be mild, such as cough, chest pain, and dyspnea on exertion. With disease progression, there may be symptoms of heart failure as well (Halfdanarson et al. 2017). Pericardial tamponade is a medical emergency and mandates ICU admission, but sometimes, there may not be enough time for transport; therefore, early diagnosis with definitive management at the bedside will mitigate damage. Bedside Doppler echocardiography will show diastolic collapse of the right atrium (high sensitivity) and ventricle (high specific sign) due to pericardial fluid accumulation. Assessment for hypovolemia should be done simultaneously as these patients are preload dependent. Intubation should be reserved only for impending respiratory failure. Inotropes can be used as adjunctive therapy, but their use is controversial. Definitive management with pericardiocentesis with a catheter should be performed at the earliest. Patients with malignant pericardial involvement have a poor prognosis even with appropriate treatment. In as many as 85% of cases, the cause of death in individuals with malignant pericardial effusion was the development of tamponade (Shenoy et al. 2017).

30.3.4 Hyperviscosity Syndrome

It occurs due to increased viscosity secondary to hyperleukocytosis, such as in leukemia and myeloproliferative disorders, and increased circulating proteins, such as monoclonal gammopathies (Shenoy et al. 2017). This may lead to impaired blood flow, causing relative end-organ hypoperfusion, including in the heart, and ischemia (Shenoy et al. 2017; Halfdanarson et al. 2017). The presentation may vary according to the organ involved, but cardiac involvement occurs mainly in thromboembolic events, which may mimic angina, myocardial ischemia, and thrombosis of both arteries and veins. The clinical diagnosis of hyperviscosity syndrome (HVS) requires a high level of clinical suspicion. There may be chest pain, mucosal, or skin bleeding, or peripheral gangrenous changes. Cardiovascular manifestations and signs of reduced perfusion in other organs may also give a clue in favor of HVS. Fundoscopy may show retinal venous engorgement ("string of sausages"). Serum viscosity and erythrocyte sedimentation rate should be measured as soon as possible; values higher than four centipoises indicate the possibility of HVS. Albumin or fresh frozen plasma is used in plasmapheresis; typically, 2–3 cycles are needed, and the procedure is continued until symptomatic relief is seen. Targeted therapy with chemotherapy of the underlying disease is the definitive management (Shenoy et al. 2017).

30.3.5 Drug or Radiation-Induced Cardiac Toxicity

Chemotherapy used in several hematologic malignancies may lead to cardiac toxicity, ranging from asymptomatic subclinical abnormalities such as ECG changes to a decline in left ventricle ejection fraction decline (Allegra et al. 2010). Common anticancer drugs known to cause cardiac toxicity include Anthracycline, Cisplatin, tyrosine kinase inhibitors, Arsenic Trioxide, Bortezomib, Monoclonal Antibodies, etc. Symptoms may include congestive heart failure, cardiomyopathy, blood pressure changes, arrhythmias, and even ischemia. Management includes the administration of diuretics and ACE inhibitors in case of evidence of impaired left ventricular function in 2D echo. In case of persistent heart failure, oral digoxin therapy may be considered. Cardiac arrhythmias should be treated with appropriate antiarrhythmics, and other factors, such as electrolytes, should be optimized. Most of the time, symptoms are dose-dependent and hence may be reduced with dose reduction or withdrawal of the offending agent (Shenoy et al. 2017).

30.4 Respiratory System

Acute respiratory failure affects 10–20% of patients with acute lymphoma or leukemia and approximately 50% of patients undergoing hematopoietic stem cell transplantation with neutropenia (Vadde and Pastores 2016). It occurs most commonly due to pneumonia, acute respiratory distress syndrome (ARDS), pulmonary edema, venous thromboembolism, pulmonary hemorrhage, and drug-induced lung toxicity (Fizza Haider et al. 2023). A comprehensive approach to signs and symptoms of the respiratory system for life-threatening conditions is listed in the table below (Table 30.4).

30.4.1 Pneumonia

Poor immunity makes these patients highly susceptible to pathogens (bacteria, fungi, and viruses). Factors responsible for the high risk of pulmonary infection include deranged humoral/cell-mediated immunity, neutropenia, corticosteroid treatment, exposure to multiple antibiotics, and prolonged hospitalization (Aleem et al. 2020). Patients may present with the typical signs and symptoms of infection. Early diagnosis can be made by nasal swabs, sputum analysis, or bronchoalveolar lavage (BAL) through a fiber-optic bronchoscope; however, these techniques might not be safe outside of ICU (Vadde and Pastores 2016; Fizza Haider et al. 2023). Bedside evaluation through point-of-care ultrasound may reveal dynamic air bronchograms or shreds' signs (liver-like "tissue sign") (Bhoil et al. 2021). It will help distinguish between the various respiratory emergencies, reducing the time for implementation of targeted therapy and further preventing the need for ICU admission. According to the clinical judgment, empirical broad-spectrum antimicrobial should be initiated in patients with suspected pulmonary infection and later de-escalated according to the culture results. According to surviving sepsis guidelines, procalcitonin can be used to guide antibiotic therapy in patients with sepsis, especially for de-escalation of therapy (Evans et al. 2021). Patients with a high infection risk should be considered for prophylactic antimicrobial therapy (Vadde and Pastores 2016).

30.4.2 Acute Respiratory Distress Syndrome

Management of acute respiratory distress syndrome (ARDS) requires specific therapeutic interventions, which may not be possible in the ward. However, early diagnosis and intervention may prevent worsening and reduce the need for ICU. Patients usually present with worsening hypoxemia and bilateral chest infiltrates. In order to manage such patients in the ward, the frequency of monitoring, such as pulse oximetry, ABG, and POCUS, should be increased. In many settings, ABG is unavailable for PaO_2 assessment; alternatively, the SpO_2 /FiO_2 ratio can be considered a surrogate marker (Catoire et al. 2021). In ARDS patients, POCUS will reveal heterogeneous B lines and subpleural consolidation; in severe cases, even lung sliding may be absent (Baston and West 2016). Treatment of ARDS should be done according to the ARDS net protocol. For treatment for mild ARDS, supplemental oxygen therapy

Table 30.4 Approach to common signs and symptoms of respiratory system (RS) for underlying life-threatening conditions

Sign/symptom	Differential diagnosis	Initial diagnostic work-up	Primary management
Dyspnea—Sudden onset	Pulmonary embolism Pulmonary edema Pulmonary hemorrhage	**Clinical** Do detailed respiratory examination, altered pattern of respiration, SpO_2, ABG calculate A-a gradient, PaO_2/FiO_2 or SpO_2/FiO_2 ratio, Identify signs of volume overload—Auscultation-crepitations, generalized edema. Examine and assess for associated tachycardia, pleuritic chest pain, hypotension, GCS-confusion, somnolence **Laboratory and imaging** ABG—Respiratory alkalosis, type 1 or 2 respiratory failure POCUS including lung ultrasonography Chest X-ray, CT pulmonary angiography ECG-arrhythmias, cardiac biomarkers trop I, NT-pro-BNP Echocardiography D-dimer, CBC	**General** Asses and stabilize airway. Breathing and/or circulation (ABC), oxygen therapy (NIV/HFNC for mild to moderate respiratory failure P/F < 200) Enhance cardiorespiratory monitoring ABG analysis for underlying cause Start nebulization with salbutamol/ipratropium/budecortisone in case of spasm due to airway irritation induced by pulmonary hemorrhage Peripheral (14/16G) or central venous access (vasoactive agents) Prepare for intubation trolley, vasoactive drugs Strict fluid intake-output monitoring, Early risk stratification and seek urgent consultation from the intensive care outreach team and pulmonology teamsters **Issue specific** **Pulmonary embolism** Early transfer to ICU Invasive hemodynamic monitoring Optimize oxygen therapy Therapeutic anticoagulation therapy Tareted therapy—Thrombolysis, catheter-based therapies, and surgical embolectomy **Pulmonary edema** Optimize oxygen therapy Consider for noninvasive ventilation Diuretic support, renal replacement therapy Strict fluid intake-output monitoring, **Pulmonary hemorrhage** Optimize oxygen therapy/ventilation Correct underlying coagulopathy, if present Diagnose and treat underlying disease

Dyspnea—Gradual onset	Pneumonia and pleural effusion Acute respiratory distress syndrome (ARDS) Transfusion-related acute lung injury (TRALI) Drug-induced pulmonary toxicity	**Clinical** Characterize dyspnea with clinical details Do detailed respiratory examination, altered pattern of respiration, SpO_2, ABG calculate A-a gradient, PaO_2/FiO_2 or SpO_2/FiO_2 ratio Look and assess for features suggestive of infection Look for temporal association with drug initiation or blood and blood product transfusion **Laboratory and imaging** ABG analysis POCUS including lung ultrasonography Chest X-ray, HRCT thorax Echocardiography Sputum analysis, broncho-alveolar lavage (BAL) Pleural fluid analysis Routine blood investigations	**General** Asses and stabilize airway. Breathing and/or circulation (ABC), oxygen therapy (NIV/HFNC for mild to moderate respiratory failure P/F < 200) Enhance cardiorespiratory monitoring ABG analysis for underlying cause Start nebulization, if bronchospasm present Prepare for intubation trolley, vasoactive drugs Strict fluid intake-output monitoring Early risk stratification and seek urgent consultation from the intensive care outreach team and pulmonology teamsters **Issue specific** **Pneumonia and pleural effusion** Optimize oxygen therapy/ventilation Early empirical antimicrobial therapy followed by targeted therapy guided by sensitivity profile once culture reports available **Acute respiratory distress syndrome** Optimize oxygen therapy/ventilation including NIV or HFNC Follow ARDS net protocol (with lung protective strategy) Consider prone ventilation Strict fluid intake-output monitoring Treat underlying cause **Transfusion-related acute lung injury (TRALI)** Management same as mentioned above for ARDS **Drug-induced pulmonary toxicity** Management same as mentioned above for ARDS

ABG Arterial blood gas analysis, *A-a gradient* Alveolar arterial gradient, *CBC* complete blood count, FiO_2 Fraction of inspired oxygen, *GCS* Glasgow coma scale, *HFNC* high-frequency nasal cannula, *NIV* Noninvasive ventilation, PaO_2 Partial pressure of oxygen, *POCUS* Point of care ultrasound, *Pro-BNP* pro-brain natriuretic peptide, SpO_2 Saturation pressure of oxygen can be provided via an oxygen mask and a nonrebreathing mask with a reservoir (Jiang et al. 2021). Oxygen therapy should always be humidified to reduce the drying of secretions, which causes sputum retention and atelectasis (Cuquemelle et al. 2012). Strict input and output monitoring should be done to maintain an equal to negative balance. Higher FiO_2 ranges can be achieved by HFNC, which can be easily used at the bedside in the ward (Mendil et al. 2021). Noninvasive ventilation (NIV) can be delivered via continuous positive airway pressure (CPAP) and bilevel positive airway pressure (BIPAP). They may help in lung recruitment and hence preclude the requirement of invasive mechanical ventilation. Lastly, precipitating factors for ARDS, such as pneumonia, should also be treated to prevent progression (Vadde and Pastores 2016). Patients with severe hypoxemia may require ICU admission and invasive ventilation; however, it is associated with poor prognosis, with mortality exceeding 75% for those who develop ARDS. Hence, invasive ventilation should be prevented and avoided as much as possible (Jiang et al. 2021).

30.4.3 Pulmonary Edema

It is a common noninfectious respiratory complication occurring in patients with hematologic malignancies. It may occur due to cardiac dysfunction, acute kidney injury, fluid overload secondary to a large amount of blood product administration, intravenous fluid required for multiple antibiotics, parenteral nutrition, or cytotoxic drugs. Patients may present with respiratory distress, which may progress fast, causing hypoxemia. A general examination may reveal bilateral crepitations or other signs of fluid overload, such as generalized edema. Initial management is to restrict intake, use diuretics, and limit blood transfusions. The use of NIV can alleviate hypoxemia. In the case of cardiogenic pulmonary edema, NIV will help in the improvement of cardiovascular physiology as well by decreasing venous return and reducing afterload and transmural pressures, increasing the myocardial oxygen supply/ demand ratio (Vadde and Pastores 2016).

30.4.4 Drug-Induced Lung Toxicity

Anticancer therapies associated with pulmonary toxicities and diagnosis require a thorough history, imaging, or biopsy. At-risk patients should undergo frequent screening with general physical examination for signs of hypoxemia, respiratory examination, and imaging (X-ray and HRCT thorax). Most of the time, symptoms may be reduced with cessation of the offending agent. However, supplemental oxygen therapy may be required initially. While treating any patients with bleomycin-induced lung, oxygen therapy should be administered carefully (Sears et al. 2020). Early recognition and intervention in case of drug-induced lung injury may decrease the progression and prevent ICU admission.

30.4.5 *Others*

Patients with acute leukemia and HSCT often experience pulmonary hemorrhage, which is due to thrombocytopenia, coagulopathy, and infectious diseases. Management usually includes early diagnosis with the help of imaging (X-ray and HRCT thorax), oxygen support to prevent hypoxemia, and blood and blood product transfusion (Chan et al. 2020; Cairo et al. 2010). Another common entity seen in these patients receiving multiple transfusions is transfusion-related acute lung injury (TRALI). Diagnosis is made by exclusion, which can be managed by supplemental oxygen therapy and the judicious use of diuretics. Most patients may recover within 3–4 days (Vadde and Pastores 2016).

30.5 Renal System

At least 30% of adults hospitalized with newly diagnosed hematologic malignancies are known to have acute kidney damage (AKI). The malignancies at higher risk of developing AKI are leukemia, lymphomas, and multiple myeloma (May et al. 2021). According to the RIFLE classification, worsening of renal function can range from impending risk of renal dysfunction, injury to the kidney, failure of kidney function, loss, and end-stage kidney disease (Bellomo et al. 2004). The symptomatology may range from subclinical AKI to overt acute tubular injury, tubulointerstitial nephritis, etc. In order to avoid intensive care admission, our aim should be to recognize and target the patients who are at risk or have sustained injury to the kidney to avoid further deterioration into failure. Patients with hematologic malignancies may be at risk of acute kidney injury due to shock, nephrotoxic drugs, or tumor lysis syndrome. At-risk patients, that is, patients with malignancies who have a high risk of AKI (leukemia, lymphomas, and multiple myeloma) or other risk factors such as advanced age, CKD, diabetes, etc., should be triaged early. The use of nephrotoxic drugs such as diuretics, ARBs or intravenous contrast agents should be avoided (Gupta et al. 2022). Prevention and management of shock, as well as tumor lysis syndrome (TLS), have been covered in this chapter. The aim is to maintain a mean arterial pressure >65 mmHg to maintain renal perfusion and avoid nephrotoxic agents. Strategies to avoid tumor lysis syndrome during the initiation phase of chemotherapy should be in place (Halfdanarson et al. 2017). With frequent monitoring of input-output balance and investigations, we can begin our preventive therapies earlier and avoid failure and loss of kidney function.A comprehensive approach to common signs and symptoms of the renal system for life-threatening conditions is listed (Table 30.5).

Table 30.5 Approach to common signs and symptoms of renal system for underlying life-threatening conditions

Sign/symptom	Differential diagnosis	Initial diagnostic work-up	Primary management
Decreased urine output	AKI due to shock Nephrotoxic drugs Tumor lysis syndrome	**Clinical** Identify at-risk patients-k/c/o CKD, age, and diabetes. Assess for hematuria, oliguria/anuria, edema, hypertension, altered mental functions(uremia). Examine for signs of hypovolemia/ hypotension(prerenal AKI), and drug rash(AIN), auscultation, noninvasive blood pressure (MAP). Look for drugs causing AKI, for example, ARBs, ACEi, and NSAIDS. **Laboratory and imaging** Kidney function tests, serum electrolytes(K^+, PO_4^-, ca^{++}), complete urine routine(albuminuria, abnormal urine sediments), serum uric acid, and kidney biopsy. POCUS(volume assessment), chest X-ray, renal ultrasound, CT, MRI.	**General** Asses and stabilize: Airway, breathing, and/or circulation (ABC) Peripheral (14/16G) or central venous access(vasoactive agents) Prepare for intubation trolley, vasoactive drugs Prevent and manage shock early, frequent monitoring of input and output balance Avoid use of nephrotoxic drugs Early risk stratification-seek urgent consultation from the intensive care outreach team and nephrology team **Issue specific** **AKI due to shock** Avoid hypotension, maintain MAP>65 mmhg, fluid resuscitation (hypovolemia) consider vasoactive agents over fluid resuscitation to maintain MAP if hypervolemic. **Nephrotoxic drugs-** Avoid the use of nephrotoxic drugs in at-risk patients. Discontinue drugs causing AKI. **Tumor lysis syndrome** Prevent exacerbations, fluid management and hydration, use of hypouricemic agents, electrolyte optimization, RRT

ABG Arterial blood gas analysis, *ACE* i-Angiotensin converting enzyme inhibitors, *AIN* Acute interstitial nephritis; AKI-Acute kidney injury, *CKD* chronic kidney disease, *MAP* Mean arterial pressure, *NSAIDS* Nonsteroidal anti-inflammatory drugs converting enzyme inhibitors, *POCUS* Point of care ultrasound, *RRT* Renal replacement therapy, K^+ Potassium, PO_4^- Phosphorus, Ca^{++} Calcium

30.6 Coagulation System

Hemostasis abnormalities can lead to hemorrhagic and thrombotic complications in hematologic malignancy. The pathogenesis of the coagulation abnormalities in these patients includes tumor cell-derived procoagulants, angiogenesis, etc. The 10-year absolute risk for thromboembolic or bleeding complication in a cohort of 32,141 patients with hematologic malignancy was 19%. The bleeding complications requiring hospital admission were higher for myelodysplastic syndrome, myeloproliferative neoplasms, and chronic myeloid leukemia, while it was lowest for Hodgkin lymphoma. The gastrointestinal tract accounted for 47% of the clinical signs of bleeding problems, followed by the respiratory tract (20%), urinary tract (16%), brain (12%), and anemia (5%) (Adelborg et al. 2019).

Bleeding is a common problem in patients with acute leukemia. Patients may present with clinical features of petechiae, epistaxis, hemoptysis, hematemesis, melena, or hematuria. Skin or submucosal bleeding is present in about 40–70% of patients with acute leukemia. A hemorrhagic complication is a common cause of mortality in acute promyelocytic leukemia (APL). These patients may present with features of intracranial bleeding. Ongoing Radiation therapy and chemotherapies increase the risk of bleeding. Platelet abnormalities (thrombocytopenia or platelet dysfunction), preexisting coagulation factor deficiencies, Liver dysfunction, vitamin K deficiency, hemorrhagic disseminated intravascular coagulation, infections, concomitant use of antiplatelet or anticoagulants, L-asparaginase, stem cell transplantation, etc., are major causes of bleeding complications (Franchini et al. 2013; Kuter 2015).

Hematologic malignancy with a higher risk of bleeding complications should be monitored closely and considered for serial investigation accordingly. Complete blood counts, peripheral blood smears, coagulation tests (PT, PTT, D dimers, and fibrinogen level), liver function tests, kidney function tests, and urine examinations should be considered for patients with bleeding complications. Besides this, the viscoelastic test (rotational thromboelastometry, thromboelastography) seems beneficial and provides a global assessment for coagulation, fibrinolysis process, and platelet function. It helps in an individualized approach to diagnosing and treating bleeding complications. Selected patients may need bone marrow examination. The clinician must search for any precipitating factors, for example, sepsis. Remove any culprit drug from the prescription if possible. Dose/frequency reduction or change in the regimen for ongoing chemotherapy may be considered if possible. However, bleeding complications due to chemotherapy are transient and responsive to standard treatments (Walsh et al. 2019).

Primary treatment can be given to patients with bleeding complications and managed in the ward /HDU. Treating bleeding manifestations in patients with hematologic malignancy includes platelet concentrates, fresh frozen plasma, and cryoprecipitate. Any patients with platelet counts $<10 \times 10^9$/L should receive prophylactic platelet transfusion to reduce the risk of bleeding complications (Table 30.6). However, if patients have any signs of active bleeding, hyperleukocytosis, showing a falling trend in platelet count, or coagulation abnormalities, they can receive platelet concentrate at a higher platelet count. In case of refractoriness to platelet transfusion, consider HLA-A and HLA-B antigens histocompatible platelet concentrate (Schiffer et al. 2018).

Antifibrinolytics such as tranexamic acid and epsilon amino caproic acid can be used instead of prophylactic platelet transfusions for high-risk patients. This group of drugs is also helpful if fibrinolysis is a primary cause of bleeding. Recombinant activated factor VII (rFVIIa) and thrombopoietin receptor agonists (eltrombopag

Table 30.6 Approach to common signs and symptoms of coagulation complications for underlying life-threatening conditions

Sign/symptom	Differential diagnosis	Initial diagnostic work-up	Primary management
Bleeding	Platelet abnormalities Preexisting coagulation factor deficiencies Von Willebrand disease Liver dysfunction Vitamin K deficiency Hemorrhagic disseminated intravascular coagulation Side effects of drugs: L-asparaginase, NSAIDS, anticoagulants	**Clinical** Petechiae, epistaxis, hemoptysis, hematemesis, melena, hematuria Intracranial bleeding: Altered sensorium, feature of raised ICP **Laboratory and imaging** Complete blood counts, peripheral blood smears, coagulation tests (PT, PTT, D dimers, fibrinogen level), liver function tests, renal function tests, and urine examination, viscoelastic test CT-head (patients with CNS symptoms) Bone marrow examination (in selected patients)	**General:** With CNS symptoms: Prepare for intubation and urgent neurology consultation Significant blood volume loses: Consider fluid resuscitation and vasopressor support Consider to give vitamin K injection **Issue specific** Platelet counts $<10 \times 10^9$/L: Prophylactic platelet transfusion Patients with any signs of active bleeding, hyperleukocytosis, showing a falling trend in platelet count, or coagulation abnormalities: Give platelet concentrate at a higher platelet count Refractoriness to platelet transfusion: Histocompatible platelet concentrate Fibrinolysis: Tranexamic acid, epsilon aminocaproic acid Refractory to standard treatment: Recombinant activated factor VII and thrombopoietin receptor agonists (eltrombopag and romiplostim)

(continued)

Table 30.6 (continued)

Sign/symptom	Differential diagnosis	Initial diagnostic work-up	Primary management
Thrombosis	Paraproteinemia-associated hyper-viscosity syndromes Chemotherapy and hormonal therapy Infections Immobility Central venous catheters	**Clinical:** Leg pain and swelling Acute right ventricular failure Hypoxia, tachycardia, and arrhythmias. **Laboratory and imaging:** Coagulation tests (PT, PTT, D dimers, fibrinogen level) Regular bedside compression ultrasonography and transthoracic echocardiography	**General:** Support to hemodynamic and respiratory instability Consider fluid, vasopressor, and oxygen therapy **Issue specific** Mechanical prophylaxis (bedridden patient) unless contraindicated. Consider anticoagulation only if the platelet count is more than 50×10^9/L. Dalteprin, enoxaparin, fondaparinux, and unfractionated heparin.

NSAIDS Nonsteroidal anti-inflammatory drugs, *ICP* Intra Cranial Pressure, *PT* Prothrombin Time, *PPT* Partial thromboplastin time, *CNS* Central Nervous System

and romiplostim) might prove beneficial in bleeding, which is refractory to standard treatment (Estcourt et al. 2016; Antun et al. 2013; Ghanima et al. 2019).

Hematological patients are not only at risk of bleeding complications but also venous thromboembolism (VTE) complications. The 10-year risk of VTE in hematologic malignancy is 5%. Multiple myeloma and myeloproliferative neoplasms had the highest risk of VTE, whereas AML had the lowest risk. Patients with CLL had the highest 10-year risks of myocardial infarction in cases of hematologic malignancy (5%), whereas patients with myeloproliferative neoplasms had the highest 10-year risks of ischemic stroke (7%) (Adelborg et al. 2019).

The specific type of hematologic malignancy, for example, aggressive lymphomas, ongoing chemotherapy or hormonal therapy (L-asparaginase, platinum compounds, immune-modulatory agents, VEGF inhibitors, thalidomide, Selective estrogen receptor modulators, and progestins), paraproteinemia-associated hyperviscosity syndromes, history of DVT, immobility, central venous catheters, associated comorbidities and obesity are the important cause for VTE. In hospitals, patients on chemotherapy are at the highest risk for VTE, followed by sepsis and pneumonia (Colombo et al. 2014; Kekre and Connors 2019; Liu et al. 2021).

Many VTE risk prediction models are being used to predict the risk of VTE in oncological patients, such as the Khorana scoring system, Vienna CATS score, and PROTECHT score (prophylaxis thromboembolic event chemotherapy). The Khorana scoring system considers the site of cancer, platelet count, hemoglobin, treatment with erythropoiesis-stimulating agents, leucocyte count, and body mass index. Biomarkers (soluble P-selectin and D-dimer) and platinum- or gemcitabine-based treatment were added to modify this score. However, the use of these scoring systems for hematological malignancy has still not been validated. Patients with hematologic malignancies were under-represented in the scoring system. The hematologic malignancies present disorders with various underlying pathological conditions; each disease carries a different risk of VTE (Mulder et al. 2019; Sanfilippo 2022; van Es et al. 2017; Chan et al. 2020).

However, the NCCN Guidelines Panel for Cancer-Associated Venous Thromboembolic Disease was described using the Khorana risk score for medical oncology outpatients (Streiff et al. 2021).

Prophylactic treatment for VTE complications in hematologic malignancies is challenging because these patients are also at high risk of hemorrhagic complications. Concurrent thrombocytopenia in these patients is caused by suppression or involvement of the bone marrow. As anticoagulant or antiplatelet therapy can cause bleeding, VTE prophylaxis in patients with hematologic malignancies is still controversial (Sorigue et al. 2020).

A platelet count of more than 50×10^9/L is usually sufficient for full-dose VTE anticoagulation. However, the platelet count used for prophylaxis varies slightly. The NCCN recommendation applies the same 50×10^9/L cut-off to prophylactic and therapeutic anticoagulation. Apart from thrombocytopenia, deranged renal function, concomitant antiplatelet therapy, etc., can also make patients susceptible to bleeding complications during VTE prophylaxis or treatment (Streiff et al. 2021; Rank et al. 2020; Farge et al. 2019).

Mechanical prophylaxis should be considered in all bedridden patients unless contraindicated, such as arterial insufficiency, large hematoma, and skin ulceration Dalteparin, enoxaparin, fondaparinux, and unfractionated heparin are recommended for VTE prophylaxis for hospitalized medical oncology patients. Regular bedside compression ultrasonography and transthoracic echocardiography help in the early and quick identification of thrombosis in high-risk patients. The patients may also have clinical features of acute right ventricular failure, hypoxia, tachycardia, and arrhythmias. Immediate support for hemodynamic and respiratory instability using fluid, vasopressor, and oxygen therapy should be considered. An individualized approach to therapeutic anticoagulation is needed in patients with hematologic malignancy (Table 30.6) (Streiff et al. 2021).

30.7 Metabolic Homeostasis

Patients with hematological malignancy are at risk of developing several metabolic complications, which may complicate the disease course. The common metabolic complications are tumor lysis syndrome (TLS), hypercalcemia, hyponatremia, etc. (Higdon et al. 2018).

30.7.1 Tumor Lysis Syndrome

Tumor lysis syndrome (TLS) is a clinical condition caused due to tumor cell lysis triggered by chemotherapy or spontaneously. Tumor cell lysis releases massive amounts of potassium, phosphate, and uric acid, which enter the bloodstream and result in hyperkalemia, hyperphosphatemia, hyperuricemia, and secondary hypocalcemia. Diagnosis of TLS is made using the Cairo-Bishop definition, which includes two or more laboratory changes (Increase in >25% of baseline uric acid, potassium, phosphorus, or calcium level) within three days or seven days after starting chemotherapy. It also includes a grading system (on a scale from zero to five) to define the TLS severity based on the serum creatinine level, cardiac arrhythmia, and seizures.

High-grade non-Hodgkin lymphoma and acute lymphoblastic leukemia (Burkitt's lymphoma/leukemia) are most frequently associated with TLS. Besides the type of malignancy, patients' clinical conditions, such as advanced age, history of hyperuricemia or hyperphosphatemia, preexisting renal insufficiency, dehydration, etc., can predispose them to TLS during chemotherapy. A risk stratification system for TLS is based on the type of malignancy, disease burden, ongoing therapy, and renal dysfunction, which also provides a guide for prevention and treatment (Durani and Hogan 2020, Cairo et al. 2010).

High risk (>5% risk of TLS): CLL treated with venetoclax and lymph node≥10 cm, or lymph node ≥5 cm and absolute lymphocyte count ≥25 × 10^9/L and elevated baseline uric acid, AML and WBC ≥100 × 10^9/L, all Burkitt's leukemia and Burkitt lymphoma stage III/IV.

Intermediate risk group (1–5% risk of TLS): CLL treated with fludarabine, rituximab, or lenalidomide, or venetoclax and lymph node ≥5 cm or absolute lymphocyte count ≥25 × 10^9/L, and/or those with high WBC ≥50 × 10^9/L, AML with WBC 25 to 100 × 10^9/L, Burkitt lymphoma and LDH <2x Upper normal limit.

Low-risk group (<1% risk of TLS): Multiple myeloma and chronic myelogenous leukemia, indolent non-Hodgkin lymphomas, Hodgkin lymphomas, CLL, and WBC <50 × 10^9/L treated only with alkylating agents.

The TLS clinical features primarily reflect the associated metabolic abnormalities such as hyperkalemia, hyperphosphatemia, and hypocalcemia. This clinical feature includes nausea, vomiting, diarrhea, lethargy, hematuria, ECG changes, seizures, muscle cramps, syncope etc. Patients may develop acute kidney injury. The prophylaxis measures are generally selected based on the estimated risk of TLS. Identifying high-risk patients and early preventive measures are the best ways to minimize complications due to TLS, thus reducing the need for ICU admission. (Cairo et al. 2010; Matuszkiewicz-Rowinska and Malyszko 2020; Jones et al. 2015).

Preventive measures include:

- Close monitoring of fluid intake and urine output.
- Serial measurement of potassium, phosphate, calcium, renal function test.

- Eliminating/avoiding nephrotoxic medications.
- Volume expansion: It will maintain renal perfusion and glomerular filtration rate (GFR) while improving uric acid, potassium, and phosphate excretion. Intravenous fluid hydration should be initiated before starting chemotherapy. The urine output for all high or intermediate risk should be at least 80–100 mL/ m^2 per hour. If required, consider loop diuretics such as Furosemide.
- Consider hypouricemic Agents (allopurinol, febuxostat, and rasburicase) in high-risk patients.

Despite appropriate preventive measures, if patients develop TLS, they should receive supportive care with continuous urine output and hemodynamic monitoring. Repeat laboratory investigation of electrolytes, creatinine, and uric acid every 4–6 h and treat specific electrolyte abnormalities. Early hydration with or without loop diuretics and using hypouricemic agents can defer the need for renal replacement therapy. However, patients must undergo renal replacement therapy if they develop severe oliguria and refractory hyperkalemia (Table 30.7).

Table 30.7 Approach to common signs and symptoms of metabolic complications for underlying life-threatening conditions

Sign/symptom	Differential diagnosis	Initial diagnostic work-up	Primary management
Nonspecific gastrointestinalor neurological Symptoms	Tumor lysis syndrome Hyponatremia Hypercalcemia	**Clinical** Nausea, vomiting, diarrhea, lethargy, seizures, muscle cramp, syncope, decreased urine output **Laboratory and imaging** Complete blood count, lipid profile, serial electrolyte level (sodium, potassium, calcium, phosphate level), uric acid level Urine osmolality, urine sodium and potassium Renal function test Arterial blood gas analysis ECG monitoring	**General:** Hemodynamic monitoring Input/output charting **Issue specific** **Tumor lysis syndrome** Eliminate nephrotoxins medications Volume expansion Consider hypouricemic agents (allopurinol, febuxostat, and rasburicase) Renal replacement therapy **Hypercalcemia** Maintain hydration Judicious use of furosemide Consider bisphosphonate, calcitonin, corticosteroids, and denusumab **Hyponatremia** Asymptomatic /mild symptom: Isotonic (0.9%) saline or balanced crystalloid solution Symptomatic: Hypertonic (3%) saline solution

30.7.2 Hypercalcemia

Hypercalcemia is a life-threatening metabolic disorder in advanced-stage cancers commonly encountered in patients with multiple myeloma, Hodgkin, and non-Hodgkin lymphoma. The most common mechanisms of hypercalcemia in this group of patients are parathyroid hormone-related protein, local osteoclastic activity, and excess production of 1,25-hydroxyvitamin D. Patients present with elevated calcium levels and are severely symptomatic. Serum calcium >14 mg/dL or 3.5 mmol/L is nearly always symptomatic. Clinical symptoms of hypercalcemia include neurologic, gastrointestinal, renal, cardiac, and bone-related issues. Patients may show nonspecific symptoms, including malaise, lethargy, confusion, muscle weakness, constipation, anorexia, and nausea. ECG may show QT interval shortening and dysrhythmias. It may also cause nephrogenic diabetic insipidus, which results in decreased concentrating ability.

Oncologists must evaluate for other common correctable causes of hypercalcemia, including thiazide diuretics, calcitriol, vitamin D supplementation, and any other exogenous sources of calcium. Identifying high-risk groups of patients and maintaining adequate hydration and judicious use of furosemide, bisphosphonate, calcitonin, corticosteroids, and denusumab helps to prevent critical conditions due to hypercalcemia (Asonitis et al. 2019; Sternlicht and Glezerman 2015).

30.7.3 Hyponatremia

Hyponatremia is one of the most prevalent electrolyte imbalances seen in patients with hematologic cancers. Ectopic ADH secretion, leading to a syndrome of inappropriate antidiuretic hormone (SIADH) secretion, is the most common mechanism in this patient population. Besides the side effects of chemotherapeutic drugs, concomitant renal impairment, heart failure, hypovolemia, and infections may be associated with hyponatremia. Mild hyponatremia (serum Na: 130–134 mEq/L) is a very common hematologic malignancy. All hospitalized patients should be regularly monitored for electrolytic disturbances, especially if patients show neurological or gastrointestinal symptoms. Consider laboratory tests of serum and urine osmolarities, urine Na + and K+, uric acid, lipid profile, complete blood count, and phosphate levels. Before starting hyponatremia therapy in these individuals, the possibility of pseudohyponatremia caused by hyperglobulinemia must be ruled out. In asymptomatic or minimally symptomatic individuals with hypovolemic hyponatremia, administer isotonic (0.9%) saline or balanced crystalloid solution at 0.5–1.0 mL/kg/h. Symptomatic individuals with hypovolemic hyponatremia require hypertonic (3%) saline solution at a rate of 1–2 mL per kg (Table 30.7) (Doshi et al. 2012; Workeneh et al. 2020).

30.7.4 *Lactic Acidosis*

B-type lactic acidosis is an uncommon, life-threatening complication of Hodgkin's, non-Hodgkin's, and acute lymphocytic leukemia. The postulated mechanism for type B lactic acidosis in hematologic malignancies is the "Warburg effect," or aerobic glycolysis, characterized by increased glucose uptake and lactate generation even in the presence of adequate oxygen. These tumor microenvironments rarely cause systemic effects. However, concomitant nutritional deficiency, for example, thiamine deficiency, decreased lactate clearance due to renal or liver impairment or high proliferative cancer, can cause lactic acidosis.

These patients develop unexplained anion gap acidosis without signs of organ hypoperfusion or show deterioration of the respiratory system without apparent cause. It represents the aggressive nature of the disease. These patients are prone to hypoglycemia. Always exclude other causes of lactic acidosis and initiate treatment for malignancy. Consider all supporting management for respiratory compromise, cardiovascular instability, and electrolyte imbalance. An urgent simultaneous treatment of the underlying malignancy and the metabolic derangements may improve outcomes. Early renal replacement therapy may be considered (Claudino et al. 2015; Brault et al. 2018).

30.8 Superior Vena Cava Syndrome

Lymphoma, especially non-Hodgkin's lymphoma, can have features of superior vena cava syndrome (SVCS). Clinical symptoms can range from exercise intolerance or orthopnea headache, facial edema, hemoptysis, cough, neurological deterioration, and cardiorespiratory compromise. CT chest with contrast should be considered for imaging. Early supportive management in the ward for early mild symptoms includes a propped-up position, supplemental oxygen, and diuretics. However, patients should be closely monitored for respiratory compromise and the need for mechanical ventilation. Chemotherapy and/or radiotherapy are the definitive treatment for SVCS. Early recognition and timely intervention are essential for better outcomes (Patriarcheas et al. 2022; Besteiro et al. 2021).

30.9 Summary

To ensure better patient outcomes and prevent ICU admission, the ward or high-dependency team must ensure early recognition of high-risk patients, close vital sign monitoring, and identification of organ dysfunction. However, oncologists must also recognize the need for ICU care when aggressive management is impossible in ward settings (Fig. 30.1).

Preventing ICU Admissions in Hematological Malignancies

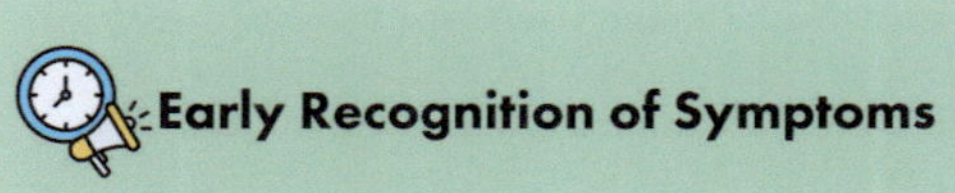

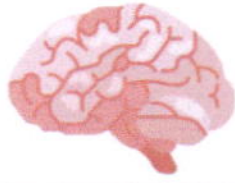	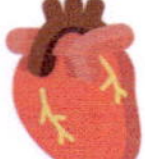	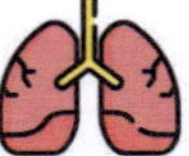
Early Signs: • Headaches, nausea, vomiting • Altered mental status or confusion • Visual disturbances like papilledema • Seizures or focal neurological deficits	**Early Signs:** • Chest pain, palpitations • Signs of hypoperfusion such as cold extremities, altered mental status • Dyspnea or tachypnea • Hypotension or shock	**Early Signs:** • Increased work of breathing, use of accessory muscles • Hypoxemia or cyanosis • Rapid onset of fatigue or altered level of consciousness • Cough, possibly productive of frothy sputum if pulmonary edema is present
Recommended Non-Invasive Diagnostics: • Bedside fundus examination to check for papilledema indicating raised intracranial pressure. • MRI or CT scans if available to assess for CNS lesions or hemorrhage. • Lumbar puncture for CSF analysis, avoided in cases of raised intracranial pressure but considered under controlled settings to diagnose meningitis or leukemic infiltration.	**Simple Bedside Tests:** • ECG to detect arrhythmias, ischemia, or other cardiac abnormalities. • Bedside echocardiogram to evaluate cardiac function and structure, looking for signs of pericardial effusion or wall motion abnormalities. • Measurement of lactate levels as an indicator of tissue hypoperfusion.	**Point-of-Care Tools:** • Pulse oximetry for continuous monitoring of oxygen saturation. • Bedside ultrasound (lung ultrasound) • Capnography for monitoring CO2 levels.
Immediate Treatments: • Administration of corticosteroids like dexamethasone to reduce CNS inflammation and swelling. • Mannitol or hypertonic saline for cases of acute raised intracranial pressure. • Antiepileptic drugs for seizure control. • Prompt referral to neurology or neurosurgery if mechanical interventions are required.	**Initial Pharmacological Actions:** • IV fluids for volume resuscitation in cases of hypovolemic shock. • Vasopressors (e.g., norepinephrine) for septic or cardiogenic shock if there is no response to fluid resuscitation. • Antiarrhythmic medications for new or worsening arrhythmias. • Consideration of non-invasive positive pressure ventilation if cardiac function is compromised but does not yet require invasive support.	**Supportive Treatments Without ICU:** • Oxygen therapy, adjusting the modality based on severity (nasal cannula, face mask, non-rebreather mask). • Non-invasive ventilation (NIV) such as CPAP or BiPAP for patients with moderate respiratory distress not improving with simple oxygen delivery. • Conservative fluid management if ARDS is suspected to avoid exacerbating pulmonary edema. • Empirical antibiotics if an infectious etiology like pneumonia is suspected.

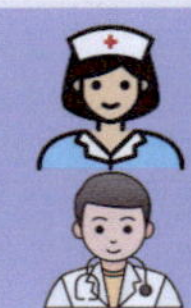

Training and Workshops to sensitise nurses and juinior doctors for early recognition & intervention

Fig. 30.1 Preventing ICU admissions in hematological malignancies

References

Adelborg K, Corraini P, Darvalics B, Frederiksen H, Ording A, Horváth-Puhó E et al (2019) Risk of thromboembolic and bleeding outcomes following hematological cancers: a Danish population-based cohort study. J Thromb Haemost 17(8):1305–1318

Ait-Hamou Z, Teboul JL, Anguel N, Monnet X (2019) How to detect a positive response to a fluid bolus when cardiac output is not measured? Ann Intensive Care 9:1–9

Al Aseri Z, Al Ageel M, Binkharfi M (2020) The use of the shock index to predict hemodynamic collapse in hypotensive sepsis patients: a cross-sectional analysis. Saudi J Anaesth 14(2):192–199

Aleem MS, Sexton R, Akella J (2020) Pneumonia in an immunocompromised patient

Aliyeva GD (2021) Rapid response situations: management in adult and geriatric hospitalist medicine. Elsevier Health Sciences

Allegra A, Alonci A, Russo S, Cannavò A, Penna G, D'Angelo A et al (2010) Cardiac involvement in patients with hematologic malignancies. J Investig Med 58(7):859–874

Antun AG, Gleason S, Arellano M, Langston AA, McLemore ML, Gaddh M et al (2013) Epsilon aminocaproic acid prevents bleeding in severely thrombocytopenic patients with hematological malignancies. Cancer 119(21):3784–3787

Asonitis N, Angelousi A, Zafeiris C, Lambrou GI, Dontas I, Kassi E (2019) Diagnosis, pathophysiology and management of hypercalcemia in malignancy: a review of the literature. Horm Metab Res 51(12):770–778

Baston C, West TE (2016) Lung ultrasound in acute respiratory distress syndrome and beyond. J Thorac Dis 8(12):E1763

Bellomo R, Ronco C, Kellum JA, Mehta RL, Palevsky P, ADQI workgroup. (2004) Acute renal failure–definition, outcome measures, animal models, fluid therapy and information technology needs: the second international consensus conference of the Acute Dialysis Quality Initiative (ADQI) Group. Crit Care 8:1–9

Besteiro B, Teixeira C, Gullo I, Pereira S, Almeida M, Almeida J (2021) Superior vena cava syndrome caused by mediastinal lymphoma: a rare clinical case. Radiol Case Rep 16(4):929–933

Bewersdorf JP, Zeidan AM (2020) Hyperleukocytosis and leukostasis in acute myeloid leukemia: can a better understanding of the underlying molecular pathophysiology lead to novel treatments? Cells 9(10):2310

Bhoil R, Ahluwalia A, Chopra R, Surya M, Bhoil S (2021) Signs and lines in lung ultrasound. J Ultrasonogr. 21(86):225–233

Blumenthal DT, Glenn MJ (2002) Neurologic manifestations of hematologic disorders. Neurol Clin 20(1):265–281

Brault C, Zerbib Y, Delette C, Marc J, Gruson B, Marolleau JP, Maizel J (2018) The Warburg effect as a type B lactic acidosis in a patient with acute myeloid leukemia: a diagnostic challenge for clinicians. Front Oncol 8:232

Cairo MS, Coiffier B, Reiter A, Younes A, TLS Expert Panel (2010) Recommendations for the evaluation of risk and prophylaxis of tumour lysis syndrome (TLS) in adults and children with malignant diseases: an expert TLS panel consensus. Br J Haematol 149(4):578–586

Catoire P, Tellier E, de La Rivière C, Beauvieux MC, Valdenaire G, Galinski M et al (2021) Assessment of the SpO2/FiO2 ratio as a tool for hypoxemia screening in the emergency department. Am J Emerg Med 44:116–120

Chan TSY, Hwang YY, Tse E (2020) Risk assessment of venous thromboembolism in hematological cancer patients: a review. Expert Rev Hematol 13(5):471–480

Claudino WM, Dias A, Tse W, Sharma VR (2015) Type B lactic acidosis: a rare but life threatening hematologic emergency. A case illustration and brief review. Am J Blood Res 5(1):25

Colombo R, Gallipoli P, Castelli R (2014) Thrombosis and hemostatic abnormalities in hematological malignancies. Clin Lymphoma Myeloma Leuk 14(6):441–450

Cuquemelle E, Pham T, Papon JF, Louis B, Danin PE, Brochard L (2012) Heated and humidified high-flow oxygen therapy reduces discomfort during hypoxemic respiratory failure. Respir Care 57(10):1571–1577

de la Fuente MI, Alderuccio JP, Lossos IS (2020) Central nervous system emergencies in haematological malignancies. Br J Haematol 189(6):1028–1037

Doshi SM, Shah P, Lei X, Lahoti A, Salahudeen AK (2012) Hyponatremia in hospitalized cancer patients and its impact on clinical outcomes. Am J Kidney Dis 59(2):222–228

Durani U, Hogan WJ (2020) Emergencies in haematology: tumour lysis syndrome. Br J Haematol 188(4):494–500

Estcourt LJ, Desborough M, Brunskill SJ, Doree C, Hopewell S, Murphy MF, Stanworth SJ (2016) Antifibrinolytics (lysine analogues) for the prevention of bleeding in people with haematological disorders. Cochrane Database Syst Rev 3

Evans L, Rhodes A, Alhazzani W, Antonelli M, Coopersmith CM, French C et al (2021) Surviving sepsis campaign: international guidelines for management of sepsis and septic shock 2021. Crit Care Med 49(11):e1063–e1143

Farge D, Frere C, Connors JM, Ay C, Khorana AA, Munoz A et al (2019) 2019 international clinical practice guidelines for the treatment and prophylaxis of venous thromboembolism in patients with cancer. Lancet Oncol 20(10):e566–e581

Ferreyro BL, Scales DC, Wunsch H, Cheung MC, Gupta V, Saskin R et al (2021) Critical illness in patients with hematologic malignancy: a population-based cohort study. Intensive Care Med 47:1104–1114

Fizza Haider S, Sloss R, Jhanji S, Nicholson E, Creagh-Brown B (2023) Management of adult patients with haematological malignancies in critical care. Anaesthesia 78(7):874–883

Floeter AE, Patel A, Tran M, Chamberlain MC, Hendrie PC, Gopal AK, Cassaday RD (2017) Posterior reversible encephalopathy syndrome associated with dose-adjusted EPOCH (etoposide, prednisone, vincristine, cyclophosphamide, doxorubicin) chemotherapy. Clin Lymphoma Myeloma Leuk 17(4):225–230

Franchini M, Frattini F, Crestani S, Bonfanti C (2013) Bleeding complications in patients with hematologic malignancies. In: Seminars in thrombosis and hemostasis, Vol. 39, No. 01. Thieme Medical Publishers, pp 094–100

Ghanima W, Cooper N, Rodeghiero F, Godeau B, Bussel JB (2019) Thrombopoietin receptor agonists: ten years later. Haematologica 104(6):1112

Gupta S, Gudsoorkar P, Jhaveri KD (2022) Acute kidney injury in critically ill patients with cancer. Clin J Am Soc Nephrol 17(9):1385–1398

Halfdanarson TR, Hogan WJ, Madsen BE (2017) Emergencies in hematology and oncology. In: Mayo clinic proceedings, Vol. 92, No. 4. Elsevier, pp 609–641

Higdon ML, Atkinson CJ, Lawrence KV (2018) Oncologic emergencies: recognition and initial management. Am Fam Physician 97(11):741–748

Jiang L, Wan Q, Ma H (2021) Management strategy for hematological malignancy patients with acute respiratory failure. Eur J Med Res 26:1–8

Jones GL, Will A, Jackson GH, Webb NJ, Rule S (2015) Guidelines for the management of tumour lysis syndrome in adults and children with haematological malignancies on behalf of the British Committee for Standards in Haematology. Br J Haematol 169(5)

Kekre N, Connors JM (2019) Venous thromboembolism incidence in hematologic malignancies. Blood Rev 33:24–32

Kuter DJ (2015) Managing thrombocytopenia associated with cancer chemotherapy. Oncology 29(4):282–282

Liu YC, Liu JH, Fang ZA, Shan GL, Xu J, Qi ZW et al (2012) Modified shock index and mortality rate of emergency patients. World J Emerg Med 3(2):114

Liu S, Wu X, Zhang Y, Yin J (2021) Comparison of clinical features in hematologic-malignancy patients and tumor patients developing pulmonary embolism

Matuszkiewicz-Rowinska J, Malyszko J (2020) Prevention and treatment of tumor lysis syndrome in the era of onco-nephrology progress. Kidney Blood Press Res 45(5):645–660

May HP, Barreto EF, Mara KC, McCullough KB, Patnaik MS, Leung N, Habermann TM (2021) Risk for significant kidney function decline after acute kidney injury in adults with hematologic malignancy. Kidney Int Rep 6(4):1050–1057

Mendil NÖA, Temel Ş, Yüksel RC, Gündoğan K, Eser B, Kaynar L, Sungur M (2021) The use of high-flow nasal oxygen vs. standard oxygen therapy in hematological malignancy patients with acute respiratory failure in hematology wards. Turkish J Med Sci 51(4):1756–1763

Montorfano L, Yu Q, Bordes SJ, Sivanushanthan S, Rosenthal RJ, Montorfano M (2021) Mean value of B-mode optic nerve sheath diameter as an indicator of increased intracranial pressure: a systematic review and meta-analysis. Ultrasound J 13:1–12

Mulder FI, Candeloro M, Kamphuisen PW, Di Nisio M, Bossuyt PM, Guman N et al (2019) The Khorana score for prediction of venous thromboembolism in cancer patients: a systematic review and meta-analysis. Haematologica 104(6):1277

Nucci M, Anaissie EJ (2018) Prevention of infections in patients with hematological malignancies. In: Neoplastic diseases of the blood, pp 1047–1062

Patriarcheas V, Grammoustianou M, Ptohis N, Thanou I, Kostis M, Gkiozos I et al (2022) Malignant superior vena cava syndrome: state of the art. Cureus 14(1)

Rank CU, Lynggaard LS, Als-Nielsen B, Stock W, Toft N, Nielsen OJ et al (2020) Prophylaxis of thromboembolism during therapy with asparaginase in adults with acute lymphoblastic leukaemia. Cochrane Database Syst Rev 10

Saito M, Kawano H, Amano T, Hirano T (2021) Acute stroke caused by progressive intracranial artery stenosis due to varicella zoster virus vasculopathy after chemotherapy for malignant lymphoma. Intern Med 60(11):1769–1773

Sanfilippo KM (2022) Venous thromboembolism and risk stratification in hematological malignancies. Thromb Res 213:S16–S21

Schiffer CA, Bohlke K, Delaney M, Hume H, Magdalinski AJ, McCullough JJ et al (2018) Platelet transfusion for patients with cancer: American Society of Clinical Oncology clinical practice guideline update. J Clin Oncol 36(3):283–299

Schmidt-Hieber M, Silling G, Schalk E, Heinz W, Panse J, Penack O et al (2016) CNS infections in patients with hematological disorders (including allogeneic stem-cell transplantation)—guidelines of the Infectious Diseases Working Party (AGIHO) of the German Society of Hematology and Medical Oncology (DGHO). Ann Oncol 27(7):1207–1225

Sears SP, Carr G, Bime C (2020) Acute and chronic respiratory failure in cancer patients. Oncologic Critical Care:445–475

Shenoy S, Shetty S, Lankala S, Anwer F, Yeager A, Adigopula S (2017) Cardiovascular oncologic emergencies. Cardiology 138(3):147–158

Sorigue M, Cañamero E, Siguenza P, Nomdedeu M, López-Núñez JJ (2020) Recent developments and persisting challenges in the prevention and treatment of venous thromboembolism in patients with hematological malignancies. Leuk Lymphoma 61(6):1277–1291

Sternlicht H, Glezerman IG (2015) Hypercalcemia of malignancy and new treatment options. Ther Clin Risk Manag:1779–1788

Streiff MB, Holmstrom B, Angelini D, Ashrani A, Elshoury A, Fanikos J et al (2021) Cancer-associated venous thromboembolic disease, version 2.2021, NCCN clinical practice guidelines in oncology. J Natl Compr Cancer Netw 19(10):1181–1201

Sussman JD, Davies-Jones GAB (2014) Neurologic manifestations of hematologic disorders. In: Aminoff's neurology and general medicine. Academic, pp 505–537

Vadde R, Pastores SM (2016) Management of acute respiratory failure in patients with hematological malignancy. J Intensive Care Med 31(10):627–641

van Es N, Di Nisio M, Cesarman G, Kleinjan A, Otten HM, Mahé I et al (2017) Comparison of risk prediction scores for venous thromboembolism in cancer patients: a prospective cohort study. Haematologica 102(9):1494

Vijenthira A, Chiu N, Jacobson D, Freedman Z, Cheung MC, Goddard S et al (2020) Predictors of intensive care unit admission in patients with hematologic malignancy. Sci Rep 10(1):21145

Vincent JL, De Backer D (2013) Circulatory shock. N Engl J Med 369(18):1726–1734

Walsh M, Moore EE, Moore H, Thomas S, Lune SV, Zimmer D et al (2019, June) Use of viscoelastography in malignancy-associated coagulopathy and thrombosis: a review. In: Seminars in thrombosis and hemostasis, Vol. 45, No. 04. Thieme Medical Publishers, pp 354–372

Workeneh BT, Jhaveri KD, Rondon-Berrios H (2020) Hyponatremia in the cancer patient. Kidney Int 98(4):870–882

Chapter 31
Decision for Intensity of Treatment for Onco-patients After ICU Admission

Afzal Azim and Jitendra Singh Chahar

Learning Points

1. Factors Influencing ICU Admission Decisions: Understanding the clinical criteria that guide the admission of oncology patients to the ICU, including the severity of their condition, potential for recovery, and the specific complications associated with their cancer treatment.
2. Prognostication and Treatment Intensity: Evaluating the prognostic tools and scores that help predict outcomes for cancer patients in the ICU and how these predictions influence the aggressiveness of the treatment administered.
3. Management of Organ Failures: Insight into the approaches to managing organ failures in oncology patients, which are comparable to those used in general ICU patients, and how the presence of organ failures affects survival outcomes.
4. Ethical Considerations and End-of-Life Care: Discussion on the ethical considerations in providing intensive care to oncology patients, including when to limit treatment and how to approach end-of-life care decisions with a multidisciplinary team.

31.1 Introduction

Cancer patients may account for up to 15% of all admissions to ICU, and 5% of them may require ICU admission (Azoulay et al. 2017; Puxty et al. 2015). These frequencies are constantly growing due to the rising global burden of cancer worldwide. The analysis also shows that a higher percentage of admitted cancer patients survive ICU discharge (Puxty et al. 2015; Shimabukuro-Vornhagen et al. 2016). The 5-year survival rate is close to 41% after ICU discharge in these patients, and hence, reluctance to admit them to the ICU must be avoided from clinical practice (Bos et al. 2015). Factually, the most recent evidence supports an increased ICU admission because of the availability of advanced ICU comprehensive care, which leads to better ICU and hospital outcomes. In the past few decades, there has been

A. Azim (✉) · J. S. Chahar
Critical Care Medicine, Sanjay Gandhi Postgraduate Institute of Medical Sciences, Lucknow, Uttar Pradesh, India

S. B. Mishra (ed.), *Critical Care Hematology*,
https://doi.org/10.1007/978-981-97-5565-3_31

accelerating progress in therapies for cancer patients, with an increased number of patients benefiting from life-supportive therapies for infective or toxicity related to chemotherapy (Wigmore and Farquhar-Smith 2016; Torres et al. 2016). In the early nineties, these patients were considered as less likely to benefit from ICU admission, but recently, there has been a paradigm shift in the approach of the intensivists for triaging for ICU admission. The factors contributing to better survival include early ICU admission, advancements in ICU therapies, timely advanced monitoring, and use of minimally-invasive diagnostic and therapeutic strategies (Lengliné et al. 2012; Hanzelka et al. 2013; Song et al. 2012). Studies reveal that timely ICU admission for these patients is associated with better survival rates. Critical care utilization for these patients is generally required at different time points depending on the disease trajectory and often serves as a bridge to definitive therapy (Larché et al. 2003). In the last 25 years, hospital mortality has decreased to less than 40% in patients with hematologic malignancies and is almost comparable to general ICU patients (Azoulay et al. 2013).

The objective of this chapter is to give an insight to critical care clinicians regarding an overview of relevant and current information on the need of cancer patients requiring ICU admission and if admitted to ICU, then what should be the aggressiveness of management and when to limit the therapy.

31.2 Indications for ICU Admission

The main indications for ICU admission are post-surgical care, acute respiratory failure (ARF) requiring oxygen therapy or ventilation therapy, and sepsis related to infections. Other than these they are also predisposed to certain clinical situations arising out of hospital admission and therapies administered to them. These clinical situations can be related to cardiac complications, neurologic issues, acute kidney injury, bleeding, and certain oncologic emergencies (Soubani 2017). Mucositis, acute graft-versus-host disease, acute alveolar hemorrhage, hypertension with cardiac dysfunction, and hepatic venoocclusive disease are other presentations of these patients requiring ICU admission (Biskup et al. 2017). These are presented below in a tabulated form (Fig. 31.1).

31.2.1 Assessment of Severity at Admission

The reluctance to admit cancer patients to intensive care units (ICU) for advanced life-support therapies is increasingly being viewed as unjustified, particularly when the decision is solely based on the cancer diagnosis (Paz et al. 1993). Numerous scoring systems exist to assess severity and predict outcomes for cancer patients in need of ICU admission (Beniwal et al. 2022). These include the Acute Physiology and Chronic Health Evaluation (APACHE) II, the Sequential Organ Failure

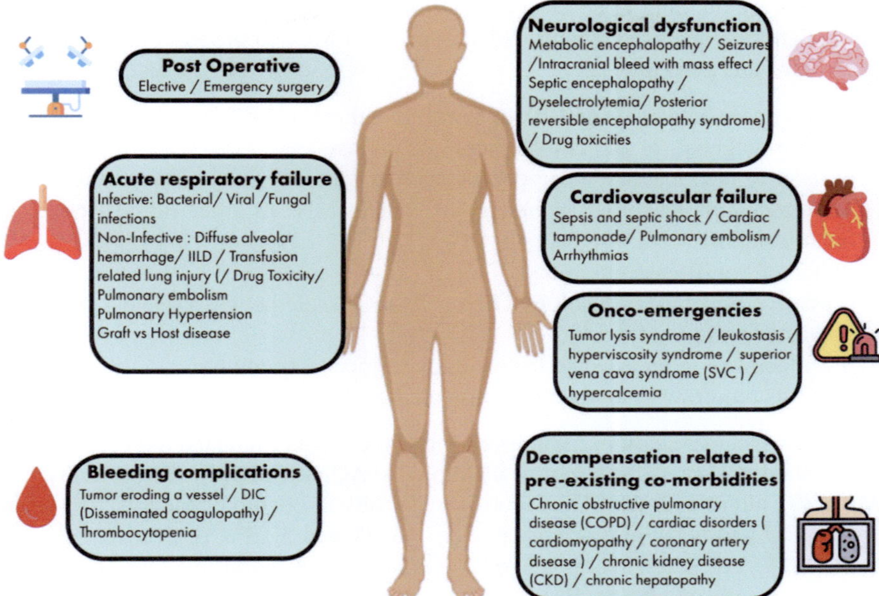

Fig. 31.1 Indications for ICU admission

Assessment (SOFA) score, the Simplified Acute Physiology Score (SAPS) II, and the Mortality Probability Models (MPM). Notably, severity illness scores like APACHE II and the SOFA score, typically used for general ICU patients, are also effective for cancer patients (Reichner et al. 2006). These systems are valuable tools for medical professionals to assess patient conditions, guide treatment strategies, and estimate prognoses. Each system has its limitations, and the final decision to transfer a patient to the ICU depends on the clinical judgment of the treating team, in conjunction with family consent.

Research indicates that certain scores, such as APACHE III and SAPS II, when assessed at admission, may correlate with poorer outcomes. However, their reliability is less certain in patients post-hematopoietic cell transplant. Studies involving patients with solid and hematologic malignancies have revealed a higher mortality rate associated with increased SOFA scores (odds ratio [OR] 1.25, 95% confidence interval [CI] 1.17–1.34), compared to the less frequently used ICU score, the logistic organ dysfunction score (hazard ratio 1.19, 95% CI 1.08–1.32).

An analysis within the Sepsis Occurrence in Acutely Ill Patients (SOAP) study, a large prospective cohort involving 198 ICUs across 24 European countries, focused on ICU and hospital mortality rates at 60 days post-admission. This study found that these mortality rates were similar in patients with solid tumors and those without cancer, supporting the case for ICU admission and care for cancer patients (Taccone et al. 2009).

Efforts are ongoing to develop criteria for guiding ICU admissions and predicting patient outcomes. Namendys-Silva et al. from Mexico proposed the following criteria for this purpose:

- SOFA score between 7 and 10, or fewer than three organ failures.
- Recent diagnosis of an onco-hematologic disease.
- Cancer-related medical emergencies, such as tumor lysis syndrome, pulmonary infiltrates in leukemia patients, or leukostasis as the initial leukemia manifestation.
- Potential for disease cure.
- Eastern Cooperative Oncology Group (ECOG) scale between 0 and 2 (with the total scale ranging from 0 to 5).
- Postoperative intensive care for complex surgical procedures.
- Patients requiring hemodynamic monitoring and/or ventilatory support.

A retrospective study in India involving 400 patients evaluated the performance of standard ICU prediction scores, including APACHE II, III, IV, SAPS II, III, and MPM II0, along with the SOFA score, in critically ill oncology patients. The study found ICU and hospital mortality rates of 43.5% and 57.8%, respectively (Suhag et al. 2014). All seven scores tended to underestimate mortality, with MPM II0's predicted death rate being closest to the actual mortality, followed by APACHE II. Given the negligible differences in efficacy and performance among these scores, the study suggests that the selection of a scoring system should be based on clinician preference and local practices (Ñamendys-Silva et al. 2015).

31.2.2 The Concept of ICU Trial

In the context of ICU admission for oncology patients, intensivists often face challenging decisions regarding the appropriateness of admitting a patient for intensive care. In situations with uncertainty about the potential benefit of ICU care, a trial period of ICU management is recommended. This approach ensures that patients are not prematurely denied the opportunity to recover from an acute medical event.

A typical period for this ICU trial is suggested to be between 3 and 5 days of aggressive ICU management. This trial period allows for comprehensive and holistic ICU care, including full support and intervention for any organ failures. During this time, the patient's clinical status is closely monitored and reassessed. This approach is often referred to as "full-code status," encompassing a range of treatments such as cancer chemotherapy, antibiotics, and other life-sustaining therapies.

Following the initial 3–5 days of intensive management, the patient's response to treatment is evaluated. Improvement in the severity of organ failures suggests that life-supporting treatment should be continued. Conversely, a deteriorating clinical status, characterized by an increase in the number or severity of organ failures, should prompt immediate discussion regarding the suitability of continuing aggressive treatment.

There are specific clinical scenarios, such as tumor lysis syndrome, neoplasm-related pulmonary or renal involvement, associated sepsis from obstructive pneumonia, or cancer-related ureteric compression, where aggressive supportive treatment may be necessary for an extended period, potentially beyond 5–7 days. This extended period allows time for cancer chemotherapy and other treatments to take effect (Schnell et al. 2013).

The process of ICU triage and admission, particularly for oncology patients, is dynamic and requires a careful, patient-specific approach. Decisions should be made collaboratively, involving a multidisciplinary team and considering the unique aspects of each patient's condition and prognosis. The concept of ICU triage and admission for these patients is shown in Fig. 31.2 (Thiéry et al. 2005).

31.3 Respiratory Support

Respiratory failure stands as a primary reason for admitting oncology patients to the Intensive Care Unit (ICU), and it is also a significant factor contributing to mortality in this patient group. The most prevalent cause of respiratory failure is pneumonia, although other etiologies, unique to oncology patients, may be present concurrently. These include complications arising from immunosuppression, adverse effects of

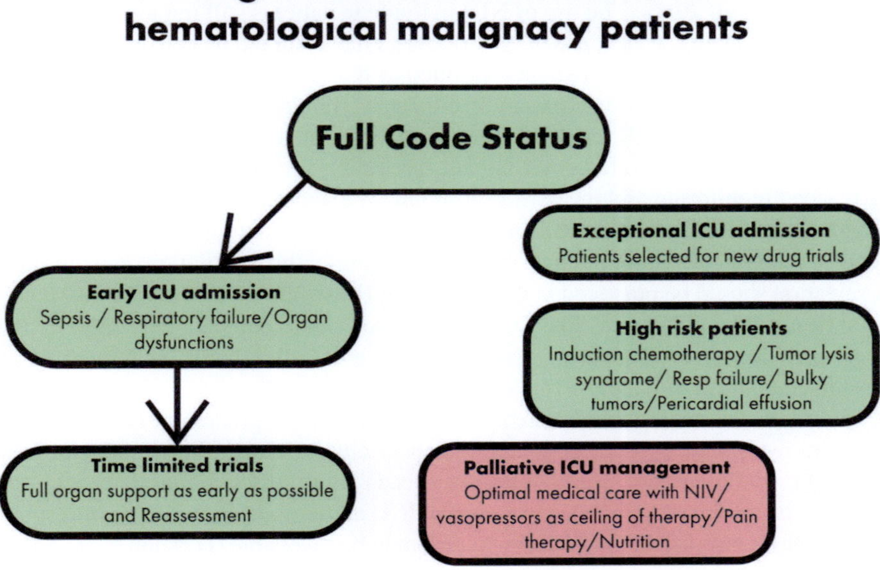

Fig. 31.2 ICU Triage and admission decisions in cancer patients

chemotherapy and radiation therapy, and post-hematopoietic stem cell transplant (HCT) complications (Contejean et al. 2016).

Management of respiratory failure in oncology patients focuses on supportive care alongside targeted treatment for the specific underlying cause. In the context of Acute Respiratory Failure (ARF) in cancer patients, diagnostic procedures are critically important. These procedures entail a comprehensive analysis of the patient's oncologic history, evaluation of immunosuppression mechanisms, and assessment of antineoplastic and antimicrobial therapies used both for treatment and prophylaxis. Diagnostic strategies should be tailored to identify not only common hospital-acquired infections but also pathogens that are particularly prevalent among immunocompromised individuals. The prompt initiation of suitable therapy is crucial in influencing the overall outcome for these patients (Bartlett et al. 1986).

The diagnostic tests include sputum assessment, bronchoalveolar lavage, transbronchial biopsy, blood serology and polymerase chain reaction (PCR), and urinary antigens with the purpose of diagnosing the reason for respiratory failure which can be of bacterial, viral, fungal or atypical origin (Azoulay et al. 2010). Chemotherapeutic agents and their influence on the lungs should also be kept in mind when deciding on treatment regimens for these patients. A detailed review of prior chemotherapy regimens, as well as past and current medications, is mandatory. While a single-center randomized controlled trial suggested the benefit of NIV over the use of conventional oxygen therapy in hematologic patients in avoiding intubation and better survival rates, successive studies showed conflicting results (Hilbert et al. 2001, Westhoff 2013). A meta-analysis of 2380 hematologic patients shows the advantage of NIV as an initial ventilator strategy in reducing mortality. However, it could be just an association and can be taken as a good clinical practice (Amado-Rodriguez et al. 2016). The use of NIV in hypoxic patients still remains an issue of debate. As a matter of fact, use of NIV or even HFNO should be considered in these patients, similar to general patients admitted to ICU with similar contraindications. Early switch to invasive ventilation, if indicated, should be done because it has an influence on outcome (Depuydt et al. 2004; Groeger et al. 1999). It is also advisable to use NIV in a controlled environment, preferably in an ICU with facilities for advanced monitoring and invasive ventilation. The approach to invasive ventilation focuses on ARDS management protocol and guidelines similar to those for non-cancer respiratory failure patients utilizing lung protective ventilation, and the same escalation should be practiced in these patients. However, intensivists are still reluctant to use rescue therapies like ECMO in this cohort of patients. Few adult oncology patients have also shown good survival even after being ventilated for a prolonged period (typically >14 days) (Hauser et al. 1982).

In a few cases, lung involvement occurs due to a high-grade non-Hodgkin lymphoma, hyperleukocytosis, ongoing anticancer chemotherapy, immunochemotherapy, or radiotherapy. Such patients need joint discussions between the hemato-oncologist and intensivist to assure ICU admission and initiation of respiratory support because the respiratory failure may be reversible (Darmon et al. 2005).

31.4 Other Organs Support

Patients admitted to the ICU for multiorgan dysfunction or failure present a challenging clinical scenario. The decision to provide ICU services to these patients, particularly those with oncologic conditions, is a subject of ongoing debate. The intensity and extent of the therapy provided in these cases are contingent upon the progression of organ failures. A brief trial of optimal organ support (full-code status) may be considered in certain situations.

Multiple organ dysfunction syndromes in the ICU are indicative of a poor prognosis, with mortality rates escalating as the number of organ failures increases. The prognosis becomes particularly dire when four or more organ systems fail, with mortality rates approaching 100%. Research focusing on critically ill oncology patients indicates that the concurrent occurrence of specific organ failures is associated with a higher mortality rate. These include:

- Respiratory failure
- Renal failure
- The need for vasopressor support
- Hepatic failure

Literature reviews and studies provide insight into how organ failures impact outcomes in oncology patients. For instance, a prospective multicentric study in a mixed adult critically ill cancer patient population revealed that mortality rates for patients with septic shock requiring vasopressors or those needing renal replacement therapy were comparable to those suffering from respiratory failure alone (58% and 59% versus 61%). This finding suggests that the presence of septic shock or the need for renal replacement therapy should not preclude ICU care.

When considering renal replacement therapy, nephrology services should be consulted. The factors contributing to renal failure should be evaluated, and the choice of renal replacement therapy should align with the standards applied to general ICU patients.

An observational study involving 100 adult patients with solid and hematologic malignancies reported that patients in septic shock and those with hepatic failure had significantly higher odds of mortality. The presence of hepatic failure, especially in cancer patients, may further elevate the risk of mortality, considering its already high mortality rate in non-oncologic ICU patients.

A retrospective study on critically ill adult patients with hematologic malignancies identified several variables independently associated with mortality in the ICU. These include the requirement for vasopressor support, a BUN level of >34 mg/dL, and leukopenia. The presence of these conditions, especially when combined, may limit the feasibility of continuing aggressive ICU therapy if they do not resolve after initial treatment.

Furthermore, a retrospective analysis of 139 adult lung cancer patients in the ICU identified two independent predictors of mortality: the need for vasopressors and the presence of two or more organ failures. These findings underscore the complexity of managing critically ill oncology patients in the ICU and highlight the need for individualized, evidence-based approaches to care (Adam and Soubani 2008).

31.5 Septic Shock

Sepsis, a critical health concern, is particularly prevalent among oncology patients. However, the research specifically addressing sepsis and septic shock within this demographic remains limited. Despite advancements over the past decade that have improved the overall outcomes of critically ill cancer patients, research consistently indicates a higher mortality rate in these patients compared to those without cancer (Moore et al. 2018).

Sepsis-related circulatory, metabolic, and cellular abnormalities are linked to a high mortality rate in general ICU patients, with figures ranging from 40% to 60%. A significant study in this field, involving 1408 patients, was conducted at a cancer center in Jordan. The study revealed that 67.8% of these patients had solid malignancies, and 28.6% had undergone chemotherapy within the month preceding their ICU admission. Notably, 42% required invasive ventilation, and acute kidney injury was present at admission in 41% of the cases. Additional complications included hyperbilirubinemia in 13.8% of patients and hyperlactatemia in 65.2%. Furthermore, 59.4% of the patients, or 836 individuals, presented positive cultures predominantly for Gram-negative pathogens. The study reported ICU and hospital mortality rates of 48.9% and 64.9%, respectively. Factors such as the need for mechanical ventilation, thrombocytopenia, elevated total bilirubin and lactic acid levels, the presence of positive cultures, and an Apache II admission score greater than 23 were significantly associated with both ICU and hospital mortality (Benoit et al. 2003).

It is important to acknowledge the limitations of this study, including its retrospective nature and the fact that it was conducted at a single center, which may affect the generalizability of its findings (Awad et al. 2021).

31.6 Transition to End-of-Life Care

The reassessment of prognosis at regular, short intervals is crucial in the management of ICU patients, especially those with oncologic conditions. This reassessment should specifically focus on the emergence or progression of multiple organ dysfunctions. In cases where the prognosis appears poor during the ICU admission, such as in hematopoietic cell transplantation (HCT) recipients with multiorgan failure, early discussions and counseling with caregivers and family members are vital. These discussions might lead to considerations of early withdrawal of care (Rubenfeld and Crawford 1996).

Research has consistently indicated that life expectancy often declines for patients once discharged from the ICU. This decline is particularly noted in patients who are bedridden, those without treatment options that extend life, individuals over 70 years of age, and those with altered performance status or allogeneic stem cell transplantation complicated by uncontrolled graft-versus-host disease (GVHD).

It is important to counsel patients or their families/caregivers about the likelihood of progression of an untreatable malignancy during critical illness and that, despite optimal management, death from the underlying cancer may be imminent. In scenarios where post-discharge survival is expected to be poor, initiating early discussions about palliative and end-of-life care can address the family's concerns regarding re-admission to the ICU and facilitate the transition to palliative care in the event of another life-threatening episode (Gade et al. 2008).

The shift from intensive care, aimed at saving or prolonging life, to end-of-life care (EOLC) can be challenging for clinicians, patients, and families. Clinical indicators that signify a patient's likely transition to EOLC during their ICU stay can be difficult to define (Sprung et al. 2003).

The principles of palliative care and EOL management in cancer patients are similar to those in general critically ill patients. However, the approach may be influenced by the patient's wishes, the presence of progressive organ failure despite aggressive ICU management without prospects for reversibility, or the rapid progression of cancer without further treatment options.

Effective communication between the oncology and intensive care teams is crucial, particularly since the ICU team may not be fully aware of the current treatment status and estimated prognosis of cancer patients. Therefore, consulting with an oncologist is highly recommended for such patients. ICU admissions can represent an additional burden for patients and families in situations where optimal cure is not an option. Proficient communication skills are essential to align patient and family preferences with EOL care. Literature suggests that EOL decisions are often delayed, and early comprehensive discussions with an interdisciplinary palliative care team can lead to fewer ICU admissions. Moreover, the implementation of proactive palliative care in ICUs, including palliative care rounds, has been shown to reduce the length of ICU and hospital stays (Rady and Johnson 2004).

31.7 Anticancer Therapy During ICU

In certain scenarios, such as patients with pulmonary complications from high-grade non-Hodgkin lymphoma or hyperleukocytosis, ICU supportive care alone may not suffice. These patients may require the initiation or completion of anticancer therapies, including chemotherapy, immunochemotherapy, or radiotherapy, to improve their clinical condition. This necessitates a collaborative approach between the primary treating hemato-oncologist and the intensivist.

The decision to initiate anticancer therapy in the ICU setting is complex, acting as a double-edged sword. While such therapy can exacerbate or precipitate sepsis, its timely administration can also lead to the reversal of conditions necessitating ICU admission. Consequently, the authors advocate for joint assessments of these patients by cancer specialists and the critical care team, emphasizing the need for integrated day-to-day management.

Incorporating the fundamental principles of caring for critically ill cancer patients into the educational curricula of both cancer specialists and intensivists is crucial. This integration ensures a comprehensive understanding and a collaborative approach to the management of these complex cases, ultimately aiming to enhance patient outcomes (Ostermann et al. 2017).

31.8 Conclusion

The appropriateness of ICU admission is generally contingent on the potential benefits of intensive care treatment, typically for patients with conditions deemed potentially reversible. In the realm of oncology, patients, particularly those with advanced cancer, are often perceived as irreversibly ill. However, it's important to recognize that patients with chronic illnesses considered "irreversible," such as chronic obstructive pulmonary disease (COPD) or heart failure, are routinely admitted to ICUs. These admissions occur despite awareness of the challenges these patients and their families may face due to post-ICU syndrome.

This perspective necessitates a critical approach toward the ICU admission of cancer patients. The decision-making process should involve a thorough evaluation of the patient's overall condition and prognosis. The extent and intensity of the measures applied in the ICU should be carefully individualized for each patient, considering their specific clinical scenario. This individualized approach ensures that the treatment aligns with the patient's health status and potential for benefit from intensive care, thereby optimizing patient outcomes and respecting their unique healthcare needs.

<a href="https://www.flaticon.com/free-icons/emergency" title="emergency icons">Emergency icons created by pojok d - Flaticon</a>

<a href="https://www.flaticon.com/free-icons/lung-cancer" title="lung cancer icons">Lung cancer icons created by surang - Flaticon</a>

Flowchart

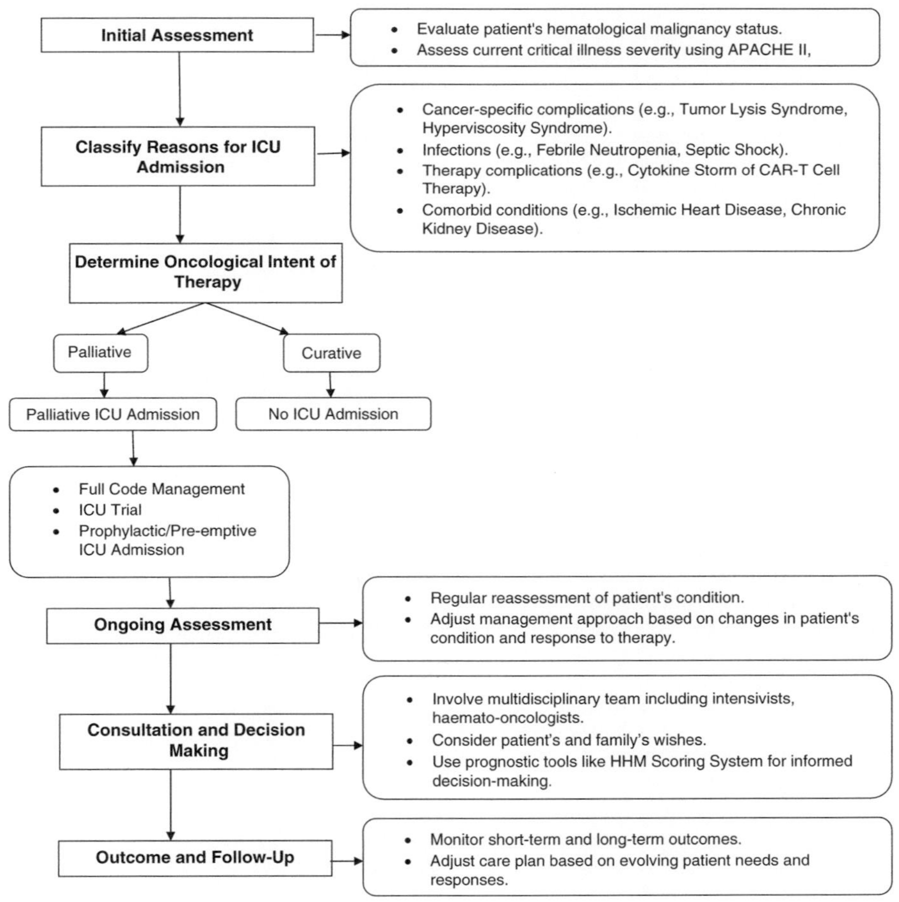

Decision for intensity of treatment for Onco-patients after ICU admission Flowchart

References

Adam AK, Soubani AO (2008) Outcome and prognostic factors of lung cancer patients admitted to the medical intensive care unit. Eur Respir J 31(1):47–53

Amado-Rodriguez L, Bernal T, Lopez-Alonso I, Blazquez-Prieto J, Garcia-Prieto E, Albaiceta GM (2016) Impact of initial ventilatory strategy in hematological patients with acute respiratory failure: a systematic review and meta-analysis. Crit Care Med 44(7):1406–1413

Awad WB, Nazer L, Elfarr S, Abdullah M, Hawari F (2021) A 12-year study evaluating the outcomes and predictors of mortality in critically ill cancer patients admitted with septic shock. BMC Cancer 21:1–7

Azoulay É, Mokart D, Lambert J, Lemiale V, Rabbat A, Kouatchet A et al (2010) Diagnostic strategy for hematology and oncology patients with acute respiratory failure: randomized controlled trial. Am J Respir Crit Care Med 182(8):1038–1046

Azoulay E, Mokart D, Pène F, Lambert J, Kouatchet A, Mayaux J et al (2013) Outcomes of critically ill patients with hematologic malignancies: prospective multicenter data from France and Belgium—a groupe de recherche respiratoire en reanimation onco-hematologique study. J Clin Oncol 31(22):2810–2818

Azoulay E, Schellongowski P, Darmon M, Bauer PR, Benoit D, Depuydt P et al (2017) The intensive care medicine research agenda on critically ill oncology and hematology patients. Intensive Care Med 43:1366–1382

Bartlett RH, Morris AH, Fairley HB, Hirsch R, O'Connor N, Pontoppidan H (1986) A prospective study of acute hypoxic respiratory failure. Chest 89(5):684–689

Beniwal A, Juneja D, Singh O, Goel A, Singh A, Beniwal HK (2022) Scoring systems in critically ill: which one to use in cancer patients? World J Critic Care Med 11(6):364

Benoit DD, Vandewoude KH, Decruyenaere JM, Hoste EA, Colardyn FA (2003) Outcome and early prognostic indicators in patients with a hematologic malignancy admitted to the intensive care unit for a life-threatening complication. Crit Care Med 31(1):104–112

Biskup E, Cai F, Vetter M, Marsch S (2017) Oncological patients in the intensive care unit: prognosis, decision-making, therapies and end-of-life care. Swiss Med Wkly 147(3132):w14481–w14481

Bos MM, Verburg IW, Dumaij I, Stouthard J, Nortier JW, Richel D et al (2015) Intensive care admission of cancer patients: a comparative analysis. Cancer Med 4(7):966–976

Contejean A, Lemiale V, Resche-Rigon M, Mokart D, Pène F, Kouatchet A et al (2016) Increased mortality in hematological malignancy patients with acute respiratory failure from undetermined etiology: a Groupe de Recherche en Réanimation Respiratoire en Onco-Hématologie (Grrr-OH) study. Ann Intensive Care 6:1–9

Darmon M, Thiery G, Ciroldi M, de Miranda S, Galicier L, Raffoux E et al (2005) Intensive care in patients with newly diagnosed malignancies and a need for cancer chemotherapy. Crit Care Med 33(11):2488–2493

Depuydt PO, Benoit DD, Vandewoude KH, Decruyenaere JM, Colardyn FA (2004) Outcome in noninvasively and invasively ventilated hematologic patients with acute respiratory failure. Chest 126(4):1299–1306

Gade G, Venohr I, Conner D, McGrady K, Beane J, Richardson RH et al (2008) Impact of an inpatient palliative care team: a randomized controlled trial. J Palliat Med 11(2):180–190

Groeger JS, White P Jr, Nierman DM, Glassman J, Shi W, Horak D, Price K (1999) Outcome for cancer patients requiring mechanical ventilation. J Clin Oncol 17(3):991–991

Hanzelka KM, Yeung SCJ, Chisholm G, Merriman KW, Gaeta S, Malik I, Rice TW (2013) Implementation of modified early-goal directed therapy for sepsis in the emergency center of a comprehensive cancer center. Support Care Cancer 21:727–734

Hauser MJ, Tabak J, Baier H (1982) Survival of patients with cancer in a medical critical care unit. Arch Intern Med 142(3):527–529

Hilbert G, Gruson D, Vargas F, Valentino R, Gbikpi-Benissan G, Dupon M et al (2001) Noninvasive ventilation in immunosuppressed patients with pulmonary infiltrates, fever, and acute respiratory failure. N Engl J Med 344(7):481–487

Larché J, Azoulay É, Fieux F, Mesnard L, Moreau D, Thiery G et al (2003) Improved survival of critically ill cancer patients with septic shock. Intensive Care Med 29:1688–1695

Lengliné E, Raffoux E, Lemiale V, Darmon M, Canet E, Boissel N et al (2012) Intensive care unit management of patients with newly diagnosed acute myeloid leukemia with no organ failure. Leuk Lymphoma 53(7):1352–1359

Moore JX, Akinyemiju T, Bartolucci A, Wang HE, Waterbor J, Griffin R (2018) A prospective study of cancer survivors and risk of sepsis within the REGARDS cohort. Cancer Epidemiol 55:30–38

Ñamendys-Silva SA, Plata-Menchaca EP, Rivero-Sigarroa E, Herrera-Gómez A (2015) Opening the doors of the intensive care unit to cancer patients: a current perspective. World J Critic Care Med 4(3):159

Ostermann M, Ferrando-Vivas P, Gore C, Power S, Harrison D (2017) Characteristics and outcome of cancer patients admitted to the ICU in England, Wales, and Northern Ireland and national trends between 1997 and 2013. Crit Care Med 45(10):1668–1676

Paz HL, Crilley P, Weinar M, Brodsky I (1993) Outcome of patients requiring medical ICU admission following bone marrow transplantation. Chest 104(2):527–531

Puxty K, McLoone P, Quasim T, Sloan B, Kinsella J, Morrison DS (2015) Risk of critical illness among patients with solid cancers: a population-based observational study. JAMA Oncol 1(8):1078–1085

Rady MY, Johnson DJ (2004) Admission to intensive care unit at the end-of-life: is it an informed decision? Palliat Med 18(8):705–711

Reichner CA, Thompson JA, O'Brien S, Kuru T, Anderson ED (2006) Outcome and code status of lung cancer patients admitted to the medical ICU. Chest 130(3):719–723

Rubenfeld GD, Crawford SW (1996) Withdrawing life support from mechanically ventilated recipients of bone marrow transplants: a case for evidence-based guidelines. Ann Intern Med 125(8):625–633

Schnell D, Mayaux J, Lambert J, Roux A, Moreau AS, Zafrani L et al (2013) Clinical assessment for identifying causes of acute respiratory failure in cancer patients. Eur Respir J 42(2):435–443

Shimabukuro-Vornhagen A, Boell B, Kochanek M, Azoulay E, von Bergwelt-Baildon MS (2016) Critical care of patients with cancer. CA Cancer J Clin 66(6):496–517

Song JU, Suh GY, Park HY, Lim SY, Han SG, Kang YR et al (2012) Early intervention on the outcomes in critically ill cancer patients admitted to intensive care units. Intensive Care Med 38:1505–1513

Soubani AO (2017) Critical care prognosis and outcomes in patients with cancer. Clin Chest Med 38(2):333–353

Sprung CL, Sjokvist P, Hovilehto S, Wennberg E (2003) End-of-life practices in European intensive care units-reply. JAMA 290(22):2939–2940

Suhag V, Sunita BS, Sarin A (2014) Intensive care for cancer patients: an overview. Asian Austral J Anim 13:193–201

Taccone FS, Artigas AA, Sprung CL, Moreno R, Sakr Y, Vincent JL (2009) Characteristics and outcomes of cancer patients in European ICUs. Crit Care 13:1–10

Thiéry G, Azoulay É, Darmon M, Ciroldi M, De Miranda S, Lévy V et al (2005) Outcome of cancer patients considered for intensive care unit admission: a hospital-wide prospective study. J Clin Oncol 23(19):4406–4413

Torres VB, Vassalo J, Silva UV, Caruso P, Torelly AP, Silva E et al (2016) Outcomes in critically ill patients with cancer-related complications. PLoS One 11(10):e0164537

Westhoff M (2013) Implementation of the German S3-guideline of non-invasive ventilation for acute respiratory failure in daily practice. Deutsche Medizinische Wochenschrift (1946) 138(16):825–830

Wigmore T, Farquhar-Smith P (2016) Outcomes for critically ill cancer patients in the ICU: current trends and prediction. Int Anesthesiol Clin 54(4):e62–e75

Chapter 32
Assessing Goals of Care in ICU with Short-Term and Long-Term Outcomes in Hematologic Malignancies

Jasper Rathinam J and Thomas Isiah Sudarsan

Learning Points

1. Complexity in Decision-Making: ICU admissions for patients with hematologic malignancies are highly complex, requiring multidimensional assessments that include patient-related factors (such as age and comorbidities), disease-related factors (such as type and stage of malignancy), and critical illness-related factors (such as the need for mechanical ventilation and severity scores like APACHE II and SOFA).
2. Impact of Early ICU Admission: Early ICU admission can potentially reduce mortality among patients with hematologic malignancies. This is crucial since these patients can deteriorate rapidly due to their immunocompromised status.
3. Importance of Combined Decision-Making: The need for combined decision-making involving both intensivists and haemato-oncologists is emphasized, along with incorporating the patient's and family's wishes.
4. Role of Prognostic Indicators: Identifying accurate prognostic indicators is critical for guiding ICU admission and management decisions. Factors such as the APACHE II score, disease stability post-therapy, and comorbidities play significant roles in predicting short-term outcomes.

J. Rathinam J (✉) · T. I. Sudarsan
Medical ICU, Division of Critical Care, Christian Medical College, Vellore, Tamil Nadu, India

S. B. Mishra (ed.), *Critical Care Hematology*,
https://doi.org/10.1007/978-981-97-5565-3_32

32.1 Epidemiology

Intensive care admissions happen in about 10% of patients with hematologic malignancies (Vijenthira et al. 2020). The annual incidence of critical illness requiring ICU admission was 13.9% in a large population-based cohort study in Canada. This varies widely between different hematologic malignancies, ranging from 22.5% in acute myeloid leukemia to 7.5% in low-grade lymphoma (Ferreyro et al. 2021). The timing of ICU admissions since the diagnosis also varies widely between hematologic malignancies, with the median ranging from close to a month in acute leukemias and high-grade NHLs and up to 10 weeks in low-grade lymphomas (Azoulay et al. 2021).

The reasons for ICU admissions also vary widely (Schellongowski et al. 2016). They can be classified into four groups:

S.No.	Group	Common clinical diagnoses
1	Cancer-specific complications	Tumor Lysis syndrome (Mirrakhimov et al. 2015) Hyperviscosity syndrome Large tumor burden-related metabolic or pressure-related complications Pulmonary embolism Bleeding manifestations due to thrombocytopenia caused by marrow involvement Disseminated intravascular coagulation caused by the malignancy (Hambley et al. 2021)
2.	Infections due to immunosuppressed state due to the disease and due to chemotherapy	Extensive list including febrile neutropenia Commonly Present as Acute Hypoxemic Respiratory Failure or septic shock.(Kochanek et al. 2019)
3	Complications of therapy	Drug reactions Chemotherapy related complications Differentiation syndrome of APML (Reyhanoglu et al. 2020) Cytokine storm of CAR-T cell therapy Stem cell Transplantation-related complications (Stephens 2020) like graft versus host disease and peri-engraftment syndrome.
4	Problems not pertinent to cancer or therapy but pertinent to their comorbidities	Ischemic heart disease Chronic kidney disease Chronic liver disease Chronic obstructive pulmonary disease Diabetes mellitus Systemic hypertension Other common unrelated disease conditions require ICU admissions (Azoulay et al. 2021).

However, the important thing to consider is that the clinical outcome is majorly influenced by the underlying hematologic condition, even when the admission diagnosis may not be related to the hematologic condition.

32.2 Importance of Decision-Making in ICU Admission

Identifying patients who would benefit from ICU admission and critical care services is very challenging in patients with hematologic malignancies. The reason for this is the difficulty of prognosticating these patients accurately. There can be two extremes of inappropriate decision-making with consequent poor outcomes. One is aggressive, irrational ICU admissions for patients who may not be good candidates, which can lead to unnecessary emotional and physical suffering at the end of life. The other extreme would be a delay in ICU admissions in view of the background of a malignancy and losing out on valuable time where appropriate therapy may have provided good short-term or long-term outcomes for some patients.

Early ICU admission may potentially reduce mortality in these patients. In a post hoc analysis that was done on a prospective multinational cohort of cancer patients, the unadjusted analysis showed a mortality benefit with early admission (Hourmant et al. 2021). And the fact that these patients are immunocompromised and may deteriorate very rapidly might make hematologists adapt a preemptive approach toward early ICU transfer (Desprez et al. 2023). This type of decision-making without a proper prognostication at the time of clinical worsening may lead to unwarranted ICU admissions for the wrong subset of patients.

32.3 Prediction of Outcome in Patients Requiring ICU Admission in Hematologic Malignancy

Before identifying the goals of therapy, we must be able to make a prediction of prognosis and outcome as accurately as possible for the critically ill patient with underlying hematologic malignancy. The overall outcomes for this subgroup are worse compared to the patients with solid cancers and also the general ICU population without cancers in a large observational cohort of European ICUs. In-hospital mortality was 58% in patients with hematologic malignancy but only 27% in those with solid cancers and 23% in those without cancer (Taccone et al. 2009). And it is also worthwhile to remember the fact that outcomes in specific set of these patients have improved in the past few years with advancement in cancer therapy and critical care services (de Vries et al. 2018).

There are two different facets to outcomes as well. The short-term outcomes are going to depend on the severity and nature of the acute event that is bringing the patient to the ICU with the background illness and therapy playing a pretty significant role in their chances to recovery. The long-term outcome is going to depend more on the nature of the underlying hematologic condition and its response to therapy, with the comorbidities and age playing a significant role. These factors are not mutually exclusive and have significant overlap. The intensivist may have a deeper understanding of the severity of the current acute illness, and the haemato-oncologist may have a deeper understanding of the underlying malignancy and chances of cure and survival. Hence, a combined discussion and decision-making session would be vital to do the best for the patient. Along with this, the individual's wishes and current and expected quality of life should all be included in the decision-making process. Limitation of resources and ICU beds may also play a part in decision-making in developing nations.

32.4 Prognostic Indicators of Short-Term Outcomes

Predictors of short-term outcomes could be classified into three groups—Patient-related factors, disease-related factors and critical illness-related factors.

32.4.1 Patient-Related Factors

The age of the patient was shown to correlate with hospital mortality (Hampshire et al. 2009). Charlson's comorbidity index and ECOG scores failed to show a significant association, probably because of less admission to ICU of patients with poor functional status (Rawson et al. 2019). Sex did not have an effect on the outcome. APACHE II score, which also includes the chronic health of the patient, was found to be a significant predictor of mortality in most studies (Hampshire et al. 2009; Rawson et al. 2019, Chen et al. 2023; Tridente et al. 2023).

32.4.2 Disease-Related Factors

The grade of hematologic malignancy/diagnosis was a predictor of mortality. (Rawson et al. 2019; Chen et al. 2023) Stable clinical status of the malignancy after therapy—if the disease is in complete response, partial response, or stable disease showed better outcomes compared to progressive/refractory disease or non-evaluable disease (Chen et al. 2023). Post stem cell transplant status was also a predictor of mortality among critically ill patients with hematologic malignancy (Rawson et al. 2019, Al-Zubaidi et al. 2018). Patients admitted to the ICU postoperatively had good short-term outcomes compared to the other critically ill patients admitted with organ failures for supportive care (Cornish et al. 2016). The diagnoses of febrile neutropenia or neutropenia at admission were not associated with poor outcomes (Hampshire et al. 2009; Cornish et al. 2016; Awad et al. 2021). Hence, neutropenia should not be a factor we look at when deciding on ICU admission and outcomes. However, the presence of thrombocytopenia was a predictor of mortality in critically ill cancer patients with septic shock (Awad et al. 2021). Most studies in hematologic malignancy have not looked at thrombocytopenia because of the higher prevalence of thrombocytopenia.

32.4.3 Critical Illness-Related Factors

The need for mechanical ventilation has been shown as a strong predictor of short-term outcomes in the critically ill with hematologic malignancy (Chen et al. 2023; Tridente et al. 2023; Al-Zubaidi et al. 2018; Cornish et al. 2016). However, the thing to note is that this may not always be available before ICU admission to help us in decision-making. The requirement of vasopressor therapy, the requirement of renal replacement therapy, and prolonged ICU stay, which are all indicators of severe organ failure but may not be available information at the time of deciding on ICU admission, have been shown to predict mortality (Chen et al. 2023; Cornish et al. 2016; Kalicińska et al. 2021). Scoring systems for assessing the severity of illness have also been shown to predict mortality. APACHE 2 at admission has been shown as a reliable predictor of mortality (Chen et al. 2023; Tridente et al. 2023). Other scores like SOFA and SAPS were also shown to significantly predict mortality in some studies (Hampshire et al. 2009; Chen et al. 2023). Other factors like the lowest P/F ratio and the presence of ICU-acquired infections were also associated with poor outcomes (Chen et al. 2023; Tridente et al. 2023).

32.5 Factors Specific to Post-Stem Cell Transplant Patients

Among post stem cell transplant patients, factors affecting outcomes were quite similar. High APACHE score at admission, requirement of mechanical ventilation and older age were associated with poor outcomes. The other factors which are specific to these patients associated with high mortality were the presence of severe GVHD (grade 3 or 4), acute GVHD and active GVHD in various studies. ICU admission during conditioning regime was also associated with poor outcome (Saillard et al. 2016; McArdle 2009).

32.6 Scoring Systems for Short-Term Outcomes

APACHE II score, ICNARC score, and SAPS II score were shown to predict hospital mortality in a large study, with ICNARC performing the best (Hampshire et al. 2009). SOFA score also was shown to predict mortality in another study (Chen et al. 2023). These scoring systems are for general ICU patients and not specific for patients with hematologic malignancy.

A scoring system has been suggested by Chen et al. called the HHM scoring system with the following components:

S.No.	Prognostic factor	Score
1	Relapsed or refractory disease	2 points
2	Non-evaluable disease status	1 point
3	Invasive mechanical ventilation	2 points
4	Renal replacement therapy initiation in ICU	2 points
5	SOFA score ≥11	1 point
6	ICU acquired infection	1 point
	Total	9 points

HHM Score—Prediction of Hospital Mortality

0–1	≤20%
≥3	>48%
≥5	>80%
≥7	100%

This HHM score had an AUROC of 0.81 in predicting mortality, and a score of >5 was associated with 80% mortality. However, the drawbacks of this scoring system are that some of the components may not be available at admission, and it has not been validated externally in other populations yet.

32.7 Prognostic Indicators of Long-Term Outcomes

There is paucity of data especially on the long-term outcomes of critically ill patients with hematologic malignancy. One-year mortality was also looked at in a large cohort in the United Kingdom and showed no factors that predicted long-term outcomes in a multivariate analysis (Tridente et al. 2023). Another large observational study data showed that the need for mechanical ventilation and multi-organ failure were associated with poor outcomes (de Vries et al. 2019). Post-operative status, post-bone marrow transplant status, and multiple myeloma were good prognostic features (Cornish et al. 2016). HRQOL, which is health-related quality of life, was poor in patients with hematologic malignancy requiring ICU admission at 3 months and 1 year (Ehooman et al. 2019).

The overall impression we get by looking at the current data is that ICU admission affects short-term outcomes and also seems to have an effect on quality of life. There is evidence to support that the survivors of ICU admission have comparable long-term outcomes with those without ICU admission in a large cohort of AML patients from Europe (Schellongowski et al. 2011). And it is not wise to compare data on long-term outcomes in ICU patients with the overall cohort of patients with the same diagnosis. This is due to the fact that the starting point for most non-ICU data is the time of diagnosis, whereas, in studies of ICU patients, it is the time of ICU admission.

32.8 Choosing the Goals of Therapy and Code of ICU Management

A review by Azoulay et al. gives a detailed description of the possible codes or types of ICU admissions (Azoulay et al. 2011). Our decision-making will be discussed based on these codes. And the intent of therapy can be either curative or palliative.

1. *Full Code Management*

This is when we do everything possible for the patient when they are admitted to the ICU. Mostly, the intent of therapy is curative. This includes mechanical ventilation, vasoactive agent support, renal replacement therapy, invasive monitoring, blood product support, and other possible life support therapies. Chemotherapy may also be administered if indicated. This type of management is selected for the following patients:

- Most patients are at the initial stage of presentation when the intent of therapy is curative.
- Before an accurate diagnosis is established and when accurate prognostication is not possible(factors like response to therapy are unknown).
- Malignancies have good long-term prognosis like multiple myeloma, CLL, and low-grade lymphomas.
- Good premorbid physical status with a disease that has considerably good outcomes.
- Acute stage of hematopoietic stem cell transplant (which is always done with a curative intent) during its conditioning regime and pre-engraftment state.

Decision-making in ICU for these patients is similar to the patients without the underlying hematologic malignancy. Also, discussing with the patient and his/her family their wishes for care including mechanical ventilation and their expectations should be asked and incorporated into decision-making at admission. We also ought to remember that we do encounter scenarios where we reach futility of care and adverse outcomes as well in these patients quite often. That's where the severity of the current illness and clinical progress should help us in further reassessment of goals.

2. *ICU Trial*

This is full code management for a limited duration of time followed by a reassessment of goals of therapy. This concept was introduced in 2007 based on an observational study (Lecuyer et al. 2007) where it was noted that patients who had to be initiated on more organ support after 3 days had very high mortality. The subgroup surviving 5 days in ICU had a much higher hospital survival than the overall survival (40% vs. 21%) favoring the concept of ICU trial. Hence, a trial duration of 3–5 days was suggested. RCTs to decide the ideal duration of ICU trial may not be ethical, and hence, we are forced to make decisions with the limited information we have. The ideal duration still remains unclear. Another study that used design analysis based on microsimulation suggested shorter ICU trials of 1–4 days in patients with poor prognosis and longer trials of 10–12 days in patients who were relatively less sick with lower SOFA scores (Shrime et al. 2016). After a 3-day ICU trial, regular discussions among the clinicians can even be done daily and goals of therapy can be re-assessed and re-defined when the outcomes become more obvious and predictable. In very sick patients' these decisions can be taken earlier with a shorter trial as well. Conflicts in opinion among intensivists and hematologists can also be solved by a short ICU trial where things become more obvious.

32.9 Other Special Occasions

- Exceptional ICU Admission: This is when a new life saving therapy/trial drug which is available now for an advanced malignancy where intent of therapy would otherwise be palliative.
- Heroic ICU Admission: This is when the haemato-oncologist and intensivist think the ICU admission would be futile but the patient and family want to continue full code management.
- ICU admission with palliative intent:

(i) Palliative ICU admission: Non-invasive strategies only with ceiling in terms of mechanical ventilation and invasive therapies.
(ii) In ICU but non-ICU care: Admission in ICU with no life-sustaining therapies and only optimal comfort care.
(iii) Terminal ICU Admission: ICU admission just to provide optimal palliative care and symptom control.

ICU admissions with palliative intent remain controversial, especially in resource-limited settings where there may be ICU beds non-availability for patients with treatable conditions. It does raise an ethical dilemma when an elderly patient with refractory AML is receiving palliative care in the ICU, and a young pregnant lady with a complicated UTI in septic shock does not have an ICU bed.

1. *No ICU Admission*

   This may be chosen in patients with advanced refractory disease with short life expectancy or poor baseline functional status and when no further life-extending anti-cancer therapies are available. And it can also be considered for advanced refractory GVHD post-BMT. When these patients develop major critical illnesses with high severity scores (like APACHE 2 and SOFA) with multi-organ failure, it is the right time to consider this type of decision to avoid futile invasive therapies at the end of life. A patient wishing against ICU admission would be another scenario where such a decision is taken.
2. *Prophylactic/Preemptive ICU Admission*

   Prophylactic ICU admission is done in high-risk patients to avoid the development of organ failures. Clinical scenarios where this could be applicable are anticipated tumor lysis in high-risk malignancies with massive tumor burden at the initiation of chemotherapy post-operative or post-procedure monitoring.

   Preemptive ICU admission is anticipating organ failure based on the patient's clinical picture and shifting to ICU for aggressive and early life-saving interventions and keeping them in a monitored environment where life-sustaining therapies could be initiated without delay. Shifting to ICU early in neutropenic sepsis at the onset of Fever and Tachycardia may help in aggressive resuscitation, early blood culture, early antibiotics administration, and source control and can help in adhering to various bundles of care that may improve outcomes. There is promising data from observational studies to show the benefit of early ICU admission (Lengliné et al. 2012). A preemptive strategy has been propagated by intensivists around the world to improve outcomes (Azoulay et al. 2021), and its impact on overall clinical outcomes will soon be appreciated.

32.10 Decision-Making

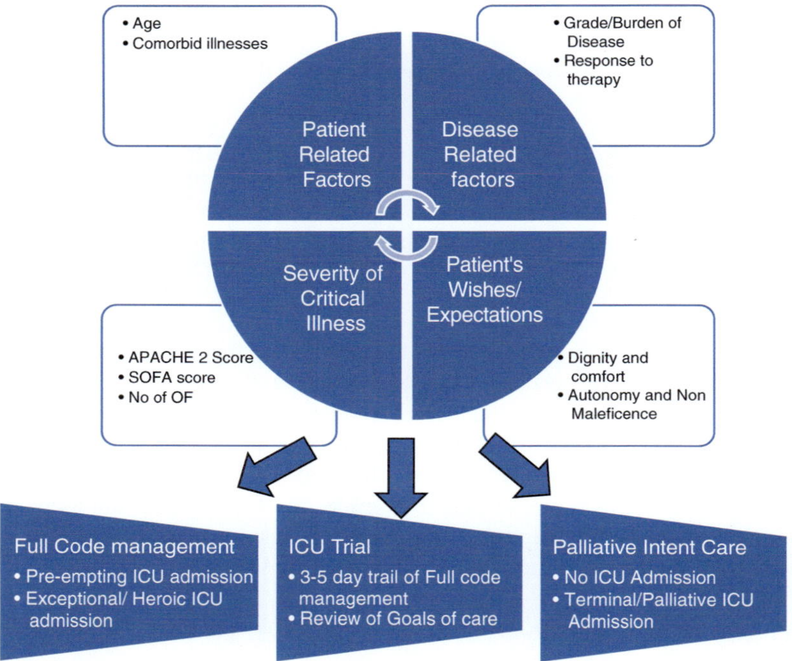

Intensive care admission decision-making is not something that can be done with a simple formula. Even in the age of AI-based tools, combined decision-making with open lines of communication would be vital to helping us make these decisions. Three categories of factors need to be looked at. Patient-related involving their age, baseline status, and comorbid illnesses. Disease related—nature of disease and stage and expected survival, and the severity and nature of the critical illness bringing the patient to ICU. Oncological intent of therapy, if it's curative or palliative should also be weighed in. Adding to this, the patient's and family's wishes, the clinical course of the patient, and the response to therapy would guide us in decision-making in critically ill patients with hematologic malignancies. Healthy communication, both among the healthcare team and with the patient and family, will come a long way in facilitating ICU decision-making.

References

Al-Zubaidi N, Shehada E, Alshabani K, ZazaDitYafawi J, Kingah P, Soubani AO (2018) Predictors of outcome in patients with hematologic malignancies admitted to the intensive care unit. Hematol Oncol Stem Cell Ther 11(4):206–218

Awad WB, Nazer L, Elfarr S, Abdullah M, Hawari F (2021) A 12-year study evaluating the outcomes and predictors of mortality in critically ill cancer patients admitted with septic shock. BMC Cancer 21:1–7

Azoulay E, Soares M, Darmon M, Benoit D, Pastores S, Afessa B (2011) Intensive care of the cancer patient: recent achievements and remaining challenges. Ann Intensive Care 1:1–13

Azoulay É, Soares M, Lengliné É (2021) Preempting critical care services for patients with hematological malignancies. Intensive Care Med:1–4

Chen CL, Wang ST, Cheng WC, Wu BR, Liao WC, Hsu WH (2023) Outcomes and prognostic factors in critical patients with hematologic malignancies. J Clin Med 12(3):958

Cornish M, Butler MB, Green RS (2016) Predictors of poor outcomes in critically ill adults with hematologic malignancy. Can Respir J 2016

de Vries VA, Müller MC, Sesmu Arbous M, Biemond BJ, Blijlevens NM, Kusadasi N et al (2018) Time trend analysis of long term outcome of patients with haematological malignancies admitted at dutch intensive care units. Br J Haematol 181(1):68–76

de Vries VA, Mueller MC, Arbous MS, Biemond BJ, Blijlevens NM, Kusadasi N et al (2019) Long-term outcome of patients with a hematologic malignancy and multiple organ failure admitted at the intensive care. Crit Care Med 47(2):e120–e128

Desprez C, Kouatchet A, Marchand T, Mear JB, Tadié JM, Peterlin P et al (2023) Outcome of patients with newly diagnosed AML admitted to the ICU, including preemptive admission–a multi-center study. Ann Hematol 102(6):1383–1393

Ehooman F, Biard L, Lemiale V, Contou D, de Prost N, Mokart D et al (2019) Long-term health-related quality of life of critically ill patients with haematological malignancies: a prospective observational multicenter study. Ann Intensive Care 9:1–10

Ferreyro BL, Scales DC, Wunsch H, Cheung MC, Gupta V, Saskin R et al (2021) Critical illness in patients with hematologic malignancy: a population-based cohort study. Intensive Care Med 47:1104–1114

Hambley BC, Tomuleasa C, Ghiaur G (2021) Coagulopathy in acute promyelocytic leukemia: can we go beyond supportive care? Front Med 8:722614

Hampshire PA, Welch CA, McCrossan LA, Francis K, Harrison DA (2009) Admission factors associated with hospital mortality in patients with haematological malignancy admitted to UK adult, general critical care units: a secondary analysis of the ICNARC Case Mix Programme Database. Crit Care 13:1–17

Hourmant Y, Kouatchet A, Lopez R, Mokart D, Pene F, Mayaux J et al (2021) Impact of early ICU admission for critically ill cancer patients: post-hoc analysis of a prospective multicenter multinational dataset. J Crit Care 62:6–11

Kalicińska E, Kuszczak B, Dębski J, Szukalski Ł, Wątek M, Strzała J et al (2021) Hematological malignancies in Polish population: what are the predictors of outcome in patients admitted to Intensive Care Unit? Support Care Cancer 29:323–330

Kochanek M, Schalk E, von Bergwelt-Baildon M, Beutel G, Buchheidt D, Hentrich M et al (2019) Management of sepsis in neutropenic cancer patients: 2018 guidelines from the Infectious Diseases Working Party (AGIHO) and Intensive Care Working Party (iCHOP) of the German Society of Hematology and Medical Oncology (DGHO). Ann Hematol 98:1051–1069

Lecuyer L, Chevret S, Thiery G, Darmon M, Schlemmer B, Azoulay É (2007) The ICU trial: a new admission policy for cancer patients requiring mechanical ventilation. Crit Care Med 35(3):808–814

Lengliné E, Raffoux E, Lemiale V, Darmon M, Canet E, Boissel N et al (2012) Intensive care unit management of patients with newly diagnosed acute myeloid leukemia with no organ failure. Leuk Lymphoma 53(7):1352–1359

McArdle JR (2009) Critical care outcomes in the hematologic transplant recipient. Clin Chest Med 30(1):155–167

Mirrakhimov AE, Voore P, Khan M, Ali AM (2015) Tumor lysis syndrome: a clinical review. World J Critic Care Med 4(2):130

Rawson JL, Fagan FM, Burrough GC, Tang HM, Cuncannon MA, Ellem KL, Enjeti AK (2019) Intensive care unit outcomes in patients with hematological malignancy. Blood Sci 1(03):189–193

Reyhanoglu G, Hughes B, King KE, Cambridge R (2020) Differentiation syndrome, a side effect from the therapy of acute promyelocytic leukemia. Cureus 12(12)

Saillard C, Blaise D, Mokart D (2016) Critically ill allogeneic hematopoietic stem cell transplantation patients in the intensive care unit: reappraisal of actual prognosis. Bone Marrow Transplant 51(8):1050–1061

Schellongowski P, Staudinger T, Kundi M, Laczika K, Locker GJ, Bojic A et al (2011) Prognostic factors for intensive care unit admission, intensive care outcome, and post-intensive care survival in patients with de novo acute myeloid leukemia: a single center experience. Haematologica 96(2):231

Schellongowski P, Sperr WR, Wohlfarth P, Knoebl P, Rabitsch W, Watzke HH, Staudinger T (2016) Critically ill patients with cancer: chances and limitations of intensive care medicine—a narrative review. ESMO Open 1(5):e000018

Shrime MG, Ferket BS, Scott DJ, Lee J, Barragan-Bradford D, Pollard T et al (2016) Time-limited trials of intensive care for critically ill patients with cancer: how long is long enough? JAMA Oncol 2(1):76–83

Stephens RS (2020) ICU complications of hematopoietic stem cell transplant, including graft vs host disease. In: Evidence-based critical care: A case study approach. Springer, Cham, pp 599–609

Taccone FS, Artigas AA, Sprung CL, Moreno R, Sakr Y, Vincent JL (2009) Characteristics and outcomes of cancer patients in European ICUs. Crit Care 13:1–10

Tridente A, Dempsey NC, Khalifa M, Goddard J, Shuker K, Hall J et al (2023) Predicting outcomes of hematological malignancy patients admitted to critical care. Front Hematol 2:1127322

Vijenthira A, Chiu N, Jacobson D, Freedman Z, Cheung MC, Goddard S et al (2020) Predictors of intensive care unit admission in patients with hematologic malignancy. Sci Rep 10(1):21145

Chapter 33
Management of Postoperative Bleeding Patient

Shakti Bedanta Mishra

Learning Points

- Comprehensive Management Approach: Understanding the multifaceted approach to managing postoperative bleeding, which includes assessment, monitoring, and intervention strategies tailored to individual patient needs.
- Specific Patient Considerations: Recognizing the importance of specialized treatments for patients on anticoagulants or with inherited platelet disorders and how to navigate these complexities.
- Emerging Trends: Keeping abreast of current trends in postoperative bleeding management, including the utilization of goal-directed therapy and the implications of new research findings.
- Optimizing Patient Outcomes: Implementing best practices and evidence-based guidelines to minimize complications, ensure patient safety, and improve overall outcomes in the ICU setting.

33.1 Introduction

Postoperative bleeding management in the intensive care unit (ICU) is a critical aspect of patient care following surgical procedures. Patients with significant bleeding complications require close monitoring and prompt interventions to optimize outcomes (Ghallab 2018). The ICU plays a crucial role in providing the necessary setting for managing postoperative bleeding, which can lead to hemodynamic instability, necessitating timely and appropriate management strategies to prevent further complications and ensure patient safety (Wassef et al. 2001).

Effective management of postoperative bleeding in the ICU involves a comprehensive approach that includes assessment, monitoring, and tailored treatment strategies for critically ill patients (Crochemore et al. 2024). Understanding the causes and risk factors associated with postoperative bleeding is essential, as it impacts patient recovery and poses challenges in the ICU setting (Crochemore et al. 2024). Assessment techniques, monitoring parameters, and various management strategies

S. B. Mishra (✉)
Department of Critical Care Medicine, IMS and SUM Hospital, Bhubaneswar, Odisha, India

S. B. Mishra (ed.), *Critical Care Hematology*,
https://doi.org/10.1007/978-981-97-5565-3_33

such as fluid resuscitation, blood product transfusion, pharmacological interventions, and the use of vasopressors play a crucial role in stabilizing patients with postoperative bleeding (Crochemore et al. 2024).

According to, the overall incidence of postoperative bleeding in adult tonsillectomy and day care surgery patients was 1.95% (Verma et al. 2007) found that in laser hemorrhoidoplasty patients, the bleeding incidence was highest at 1-week postoperatively (17.1%), decreasing to 1.3% at 6-weeks (Lim et al. 2022) reported a 14% overall incidence of bleeding in medical ICU patients not receiving prophylaxis, with a 6% incidence of "overt bleeding"(Bresalier 1990) focused on aspirin administration after surgery and found no significant differences in post-aspirin bleeding, blood product usage, or incidences of re-operation for bleeding control between groups (Nouraei et al. 2015) observed that 16% of children following cardiac surgery involving cardiopulmonary bypass experienced severe bleeding in the first 24 h postoperatively (Bartucca et al. 2023).

Specific considerations in managing postoperative bleeding patients in the ICU, such as those on anticoagulants or with inherited platelet disorders, require specialized treatments like desmopressin and prothrombin complex concentrate (Akinwale et al. 2016). Addressing complications and special situations related to postoperative bleeding, such as heparin-induced thrombocytopenia, is vital to equip healthcare providers with the necessary knowledge to handle complex scenarios effectively (Akinwale et al. 2016).

By synthesizing evidence-based practices and clinical guidelines, healthcare professionals in the ICU can deliver optimal care and improve patient outcomes (Hof et al. 2021). This chapter serves as a valuable resource, offering insights into best practices, emerging trends, and recommendations for the optimal management of postoperative bleeding patients in the critical care setting (Hof et al. 2021).

33.2 Understanding Postoperative Bleeding

33.2.1 Causes and Risk Factors for Postoperative Bleeding

Postoperative bleeding can arise from various factors related to the surgical procedure, patient characteristics, and underlying health conditions. Surgical causes may include inadequate hemostasis, vessel injury, or complications like anastomotic leaks (Nouraei et al. 2015). Patient-related factors such as coagulopathies, platelet disorders, and anticoagulant use significantly increase the risk of postoperative bleeding (Russell et al. 2017). Highly invasive surgical procedures with substantial blood loss potential inherently pose a heightened risk of postoperative bleeding (Ñamendys-Silva et al. 2017). Hemoglobin abnormalities, anemia, and platelet disorders can further exacerbate bleeding risk in surgical patients (Lim et al. 2022).

33.2.2 *Impact of Postoperative Bleeding on Patient Outcomes*

Postoperative bleeding can have significant implications for patient outcomes, leading to hemodynamic instability, increased transfusion requirements, prolonged hospital stays, and elevated morbidity and mortality rates (Jensen et al. 2019). In critically ill patients, active bleeding can worsen hemostatic defects and contribute to disseminated intravascular coagulation (DIC) (Lin et al. 2021). Effective management of postoperative bleeding is crucial to avert adverse outcomes and ensure patient safety. Timely recognition and appropriate interventions can aid in stabilizing patients, optimizing hemostasis, and enhancing overall recovery. Understanding the causes and risk factors for postoperative bleeding is essential for tailoring management strategies and mitigating the impact of bleeding on patient outcomes in the ICU setting.

33.3 Assessment and Monitoring

A. Hemodynamic monitoring plays a crucial role in the management of postoperative bleeding patients, especially in the intensive care unit (ICU). Continuous assessment of hemodynamic parameters such as blood pressure, heart rate, central venous pressure, and cardiac output is essential for early detection of hemodynamic instability and guiding resuscitative efforts (Schefold et al. 2019). Monitoring these parameters allows healthcare providers to promptly identify changes in the patient's condition and adjust treatment strategies accordingly.
B. Laboratory tests are vital for evaluating coagulopathy in postoperative bleeding patients. Common tests include prothrombin time (PT), activated partial thromboplastin time (aPTT), platelet count, and fibrinogen levels. These tests help assess the patient's coagulation status, identify abnormalities in the clotting cascade, and guide the administration of blood products or coagulation factors as needed. Additionally, specific tests like thromboelastography (TEG) or rotational thromboelastometry (ROTEM) provide a more comprehensive assessment of hemostasis and guide individualized treatment strategies (Lins et al. 2018).
C. Serial monitoring of laboratory test results is essential for tracking changes in coagulation parameters over time in postoperative bleeding patients. Serial studies enable healthcare providers to assess the effectiveness of interventions, monitor the progression of coagulopathy, and adjust treatment plans accordingly (Bartucca et al. 2023). By conducting serial tests at regular intervals, clinicians can identify trends, anticipate potential complications, and optimize the management of postoperative bleeding in the ICU setting.

Proper assessment and monitoring of hemodynamic parameters and coagulation status through laboratory tests and serial studies are critical components of the comprehensive care provided to postoperative bleeding patients in the ICU, ensuring timely interventions and improved patient outcomes.

33.4 Management Strategies

33.4.1 Fluid Resuscitation and Avoidance of Over-Resuscitation

In the management of postoperative bleeding patients, a balanced approach to fluid resuscitation is crucial to maintain hemodynamic stability and prevent complications. Aggressive fluid resuscitation can lead to increased bleeding and mortality, highlighting the importance of avoiding over-resuscitation (Krausz 2006). Monitoring parameters like central venous pressure and urine output can guide fluid management to optimize patient outcomes (Miller et al. 2016).

33.4.2 Use of Blood Products and Transfusion Guidelines

The use of blood products, guided by specific transfusion thresholds based on hemoglobin levels and coagulation parameters, is essential in correcting coagulopathies and restoring hemostasis in postoperative bleeding patients (Kaafarani and Velmahos 2014). Transfusion guidelines aim to prevent unnecessary transfusions and associated risks, emphasizing the importance of judicious use of blood products (Kaafarani and Velmahos 2014). Transfusion of blood and blood products is a critical intervention in emergency and intensive care settings for managing critically ill patients (Lu et al. 2018). The decision to transfuse involves clinical judgment, laboratory findings, and evidence-based guidelines to balance benefits against risks such as transfusion reactions or infections. Different blood products serve specific purposes in patient care:

- Packed Red Blood Cells (PRBCs) are commonly used to increase oxygen-carrying capacity in patients with anemia or acute blood loss, guided by hemoglobin levels and clinical symptoms (Karanjkar et al. 2019).
- Fresh Frozen Plasma (FFP) is essential for treating coagulation disorders and reversing warfarin therapy, indicated in patients with coagulation factor deficiencies or significant bleeding (Devaney et al. 2023).
- Platelets are transfused to prevent or treat bleeding in patients with platelet deficiencies based on platelet counts and bleeding risk (Parker et al. 2023).
- Cryoprecipitate, rich in various factors, treats fibrinogen deficiencies seen in conditions like disseminated intravascular coagulation (DIC) (Baysinger et al. 2016) (Fig. 33.1).

Studies have shown that the implementation of perioperative point-of-care coagulation management algorithms can reduce transfusion requirements for various blood products and the incidence of massive transfusion (Palmieri et al. 2011). While blood product transfusion is crucial, it is associated with adverse effects, emphasizing the need to weigh the benefits against the risks (Görlinger et al. 2012). Additionally, inappropriate use of blood products, such as FFP and cryoprecipitate, has been reported, highlighting the importance of judicious transfusion practices (Yoon et al. 2011).

Transfusion of blood and its components plays a crucial role in managing critically ill patients, with decisions guided by clinical judgment and evidence-based guidelines. Recent guidelines advocate for a conservative approach to transfusions, recommending transfusion only when necessary to minimize transfusion-related complications. Carson et al. (2016).

Specific guidelines suggest transfusion when hemoglobin levels fall below 7–8 g/dL in stable, critically ill adults, with variations based on patient conditions(Carson et al. 2023; J. L. 2023; Du Pont-Thibodeau et al. 2014):—General ICU Patients: Transfusion is recommended when hemoglobin levels fall below 7 g/dL, aiming for a posttransfusion hemoglobin level of 7–9 g/dL.—Patients with Cardiovascular Disease: Higher thresholds (around 8 g/dL) may be considered for those with cardiovascular disease to prevent myocardial ischemia.

Active Bleeding and Massive Transfusion: Decisions in cases of massive bleeding rely on clinical judgment, considering bleeding rate, hemodynamic stability, and coagulation status. While hemoglobin thresholds provide guidance, transfusion decisions should consider patient-specific factors like symptoms of anemia, underlying conditions, and volume status. The decision to transfuse should not solely rely on laboratory values but also on individual patient needs and clinical context. (Rao et al. 2004).

33.5 Risks and Benefits

The decision to transfuse blood products in critically ill patients must carefully balance the immediate necessity against potential risks. Transfusion can be life-saving, restoring hemodynamic stability and improving oxygen delivery to tissues. However, it also carries risks that can adversely affect patient outcomes. Understanding these risks and benefits is paramount in making informed transfusion decisions.

Understanding the Balance Between the Necessity and Risks of Transfusion Benefits

- *Restores Blood Volume*: Crucial in patients with significant blood loss, improving circulatory volume and preventing hypovolemic shock.
- *Improves Oxygen Delivery*: By increasing the hemoglobin level, transfusions enhance the oxygen-carrying capacity of the blood, crucial for tissue repair and function.

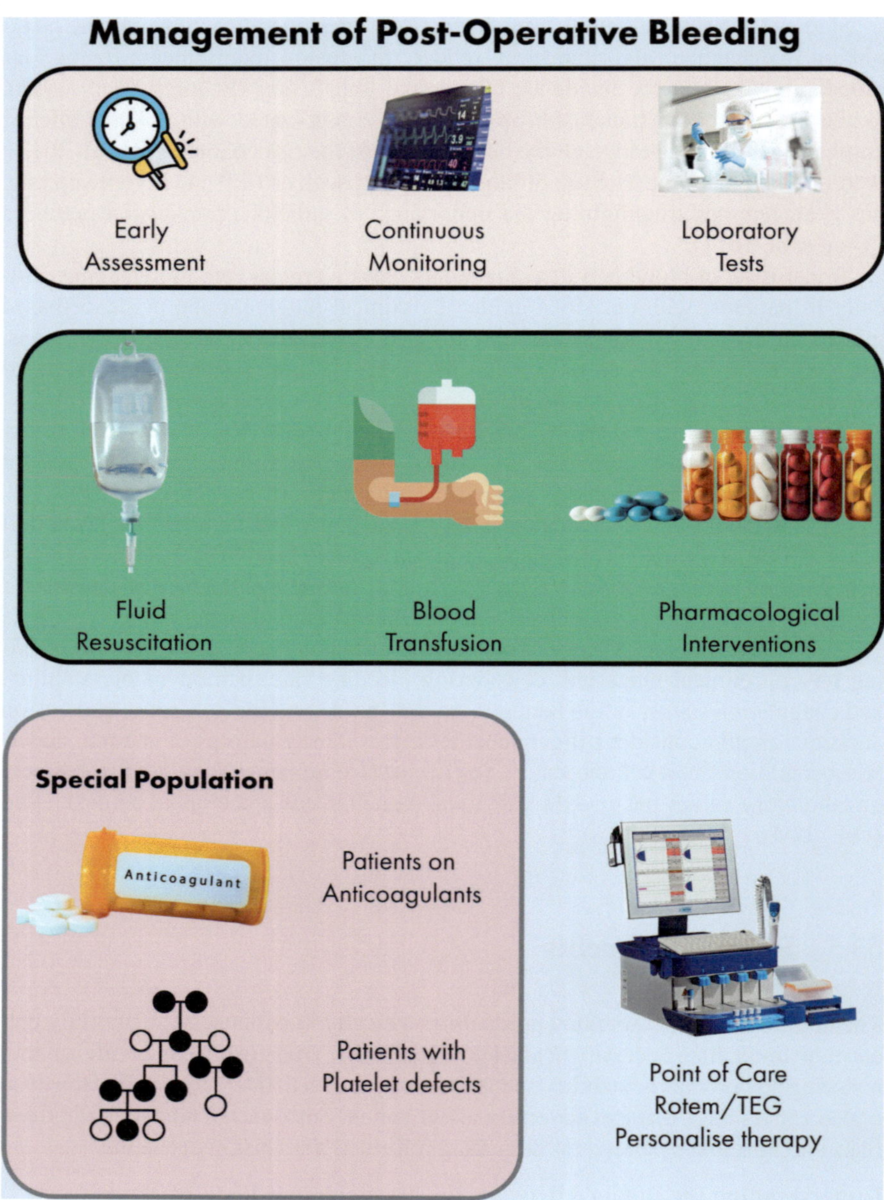

Fig. 33.1 Management of post-operative bleeding

- *Corrects Coagulopathies*: Transfusing components like fresh frozen plasma and platelets can correct coagulation disorders, reducing the risk of hemorrhage.

Risks

- *Transfusion-Related Acute Lung Injury (TRALI)*: A leading cause of transfusion-related mortality, TRALI is characterized by acute lung injury occurring within 6 hours of transfusion. It is thought to be immune-mediated, involving donor antibodies against recipient leukocytes.
- *Transfusion-Associated Circulatory Overload (TACO)*: TACO results from the volume of transfused blood products exceeding the circulatory system's capacity, leading to acute pulmonary edema and heart failure (Page et al. 2013).
- *Alloimmunization*: The development of antibodies in response to transfused blood products can lead to difficulties in finding compatible blood, delayed hemolytic transfusion reactions, and complications in pregnancies (Ali et al. 2014).

33.6 Blood Conservation Strategies

Given the risks associated with transfusions, blood conservation strategies are employed to minimize blood loss and reduce the need for transfusions. These strategies are integral to patient blood management programs, aiming to improve patient outcomes through the judicious use of transfusions and enhancement of patient's own blood (Godet et al., n.d.).

Techniques to Minimize Blood Loss and the Need for Transfusion

- *Minimally Invasive Surgical Techniques*: Reduces surgical blood loss compared to traditional open surgery.
- *Point-of-Care Testing*: Allows for rapid, bedside testing of coagulation profiles, enabling targeted correction of coagulopathies.
- *Pharmacologic Agents*: Antifibrinolytics such as tranexamic acid reduce bleeding in various surgical and trauma settings.

The Role of Autologous Transfusion and Normovolemic Hemodilution

- *Autologous Transfusion*: Involves collecting and reinfusing the patient's own blood. This can be done pre-operatively or intraoperatively using cell salvage techniques. It eliminates the risks associated with allogeneic blood transfusions (Kurlander et al. 2020).
- *Normovolemic Hemodilution*: This technique involves the removal of blood from the patient immediately before surgery, replacing it with volume expanders to maintain blood pressure and flow. The collected blood, rich in red cells, is then reinfused during or after surgery. This approach reduces the need for allogeneic transfusions and preserves the patient's own blood components for critical times (Chen et al. 2015).

33.7 Pharmacological Interventions for Coagulopathy

1. **Understanding Coagulopathy in Critically Ill Patients: Pathophysiology of Coagulopathy in Trauma, Surgery, and Critical Illness**

Coagulopathy in critically ill patients can arise from multiple etiologies, often presenting as a complex interplay between bleeding and thrombosis. In trauma and surgery, tissue injury and inflammation initiate coagulation pathways, leading to the consumption of clotting factors and platelets. This can be compounded by dilutional coagulopathy from fluid resuscitation. Critical illnesses, including sepsis and liver disease, further disrupt coagulation through impaired synthesis of coagulation factors, endothelial dysfunction, and activation of fibrinolysis.

Disseminated Intravascular Coagulation (DIC) exemplifies coagulopathy's complexity in critical illness, where systemic activation of coagulation leads to microvascular thrombosis, organ dysfunction, and secondary fibrinolytic bleeding.

The Importance of Early Identification and Treatment

Early recognition and treatment of coagulopathy are pivotal to preventing progression to uncontrolled bleeding or thrombotic complications. Timely interventions, guided by clinical assessment and coagulation tests, can mitigate the risk of severe hemorrhage and organ failure. Strategies include the administration of blood products, correction of underlying conditions, and pharmacological agents to stabilize the patient's coagulation status.

2. **Antifibrinolytic Agents**

Antifibrinolytic agents play a critical role in managing bleeding by inhibiting the breakdown of fibrin clots. They are especially beneficial in conditions where hyperfibrinolysis contributes to coagulopathy.

Mechanism of Action

- *Tranexamic Acid (TXA)* and *ε-Aminocaproic Acid (EACA)* are synthetic analogs of the amino acid lysine. They exert their antifibrinolytic effects by competitively inhibiting plasminogen activation and plasmin binding to fibrin, thereby stabilizing the fibrin clot.(Schober et al. 2022).
- By preventing the degradation of fibrin, antifibrinolytics reduce bleeding and the need for transfusions in various clinical settings.

Clinical Use

- *TXA* and *EACA* are widely used in trauma, surgical procedures, and conditions associated with increased risk of bleeding. Their use has been extensively studied in orthopedic surgery, cardiac surgery, traumatic bleeding, and obstetric hemorrhage (Ng et al. 2015).
- The administration of TXA within 3 h of traumatic injury has been shown to reduce mortality due to bleeding in the CRASH-3 trial. Similarly, in surgical settings, these agents have demonstrated efficacy in reducing blood loss and transfusion requirements (Crash 2019).

Evidence Supporting the Use of Antifibrinolytics

- CRASH-3 and World Maternal Antifibrinolytic Network (WOMAN) trials underscored the life-saving potential of TXA in trauma and postpartum hemorrhage, respectively, highlighting its role in global health settings. (Shakur et al. 2017).
- Meta-analyses and systematic reviews have consistently supported the use of TXA and EACA in reducing perioperative blood loss across a range of surgical specialties. (O O'Donnell et al. 2024).
- The safety profile of antifibrinolytics, particularly concerning thrombotic events, has been favorable, with large-scale studies showing no significant increase in thrombotic complications.

3. **Procoagulant Agents**

Procoagulant agents are essential in the management of bleeding, especially in patients with coagulopathy, where rapid correction of the coagulation defect is critical. These agents include prothrombin complex concentrates (PCC), recombinant Factor VIIa (rFVIIa), and fibrinogen concentrates.

Prothrombin Complex Concentrates (PCC)

- *Mechanism*: PCCs contain a combination of vitamin K-dependent factors (II, VII, IX, and X), sometimes including proteins C and S. They work by replenishing deficient coagulation factors to promote clot formation (Carrick et al. 2016).
- *Indications*: Used for the rapid reversal of vitamin K antagonists (e.g., warfarin) and in the treatment of bleeding associated with factor deficiencies when specific coagulation factor concentrates are not available.
- *Dosing*: Depends on the severity of bleeding, the patient's weight, and the specific PCC product used. A typical dose for warfarin reversal might range from 25 to 50 IU/kg, adjusted based on initial International Normalized Ratio (INR).
- *Considerations*: Risk of thrombosis requires careful patient selection, especially in those with a history of thromboembolic events.

Recombinant Factor VIIa (rFVIIa)

- *Mechanism*: rFVIIa directly activates Factor X on the surface of activated platelets, leading to localized thrombin generation and clot formation, bypassing the need for factors VIII and IX.
- *Indications*: Approved for hemophilia A or B patients with inhibitors, acquired hemophilia, and Factor VII deficiency. Off-label uses include uncontrolled bleeding in trauma or surgical settings.
- *Dosing*: Typically administered as an intravenous bolus of 90 μg/kg, repeated every 2–3 h as needed, based on the clinical response.
- *Considerations*: The off-label use requires a careful risk-benefit assessment due to the potential for thrombotic complications.

Fibrinogen Concentrates

- *Mechanism*: Directly increases plasma fibrinogen levels, a critical component of clot formation.

- *Indications*: Used for bleeding patients with hypofibrinogenemia, such as those seen in DIC, massive transfusion, or hereditary fibrinogen deficiencies.
- *Dosing*: This depends on the fibrinogen levels and clinical scenario, and it is often initiated with a dose of 70 mg/kg.
- *Considerations*: Monitoring of fibrinogen levels is recommended to guide therapy and avoid complications associated with excessive fibrinogen replacement.

33.8 Hemostatic Agents in Specific Conditions

The application of hemostatic agents needs to be tailored to the specific clinical scenario, taking into account the underlying condition, the mechanism of coagulopathy, and the risk profile of each agent.

Liver Transplantation

- Coagulopathy in liver transplantation is complex, involving both bleeding and thrombotic risks. Fibrinogen concentrates and PCCs may be used to correct specific factor deficiencies. rFVIIa is reserved for refractory bleeding, given the risk of thromboembolic events. (Akamatsu et al. 2015; Stellingwerff et al. 2012).

Cardiopulmonary Bypass (CPB)

- CPB surgery is associated with dilutional coagulopathy and platelet dysfunction. Antifibrinolytics like tranexamic acid are commonly used to reduce bleeding. PCCs and fibrinogen concentrates may be employed to correct specific coagulation factor deficiencies (Kunduz et al. 2019; Nishiguchi et al. 2020).

Traumatic Bleeding

- Trauma-induced coagulopathy (TIC) may benefit from early administration of tranexamic acid to inhibit hyperfibrinolysis. Fibrinogen concentrates are used in the presence of hypofibrinogenemia, and PCCs may be considered for rapid correction of coagulopathy, especially in warfarin-associated bleeding.

33.9 Monitoring and Complications

Effective management of bleeding and coagulopathy in critically ill patients requires vigilant monitoring to assess the effectiveness of pharmacological interventions and to identify potential side effects promptly. Additionally, procoagulant therapies, while life-saving, carry a risk of thrombosis, necessitating strategies to mitigate this risk (Møller et al. 2022).

Strategies for Monitoring Effectiveness and Side Effects

- *Laboratory Testing*: Regular monitoring of coagulation parameters (e.g., PT, aPTT, INR, and fibrinogen levels) and complete blood counts can guide therapy and detect early signs of overcorrection or adverse effects.

- *Clinical Assessment*: Continuous evaluation of bleeding sites, wound healing, and any new symptoms suggestive of thrombosis (e.g., swelling, pain, or discoloration in limbs) is essential.
- *Therapeutic Drug Monitoring*: For certain agents, such as antifibrinolytics, monitoring plasma levels could be helpful in adjusting dosages to optimize efficacy and minimize toxicity, although this practice is more theoretical and not widely adopted due to practical limitations (Kwon and MacLaren 2016).

Managing Thrombotic Risk Associated with Procoagulant Therapy

- *Risk Assessment*: Before initiating procoagulant therapy, assess each patient's risk of thrombosis by considering history, comorbidities, and the current clinical situation.(Rech et al. 2023).
- *Dose Minimization*: Use the lowest effective dose of procoagulant agents to achieve hemostatic control, reducing the potential for thrombotic complications (Al Sulaiman et al. 2021).
- *Duration of Therapy*: Limit the duration of procoagulant therapy to the shortest period necessary to manage the bleeding risk.
- *Thromboprophylaxis*: In patients at high risk of thrombosis, consider the use of mechanical or pharmacological thromboprophylaxis, balancing the risk of bleeding with the benefit of preventing thrombotic events.

Future Directions

The field of hemostasis and management of bleeding in critically ill patients is rapidly evolving, with ongoing research promising to bring new therapies and improve existing treatment paradigms.

Emerging Therapies

- *Novel Antifibrinolytics*: Research into new antifibrinolytic agents aims to provide more targeted control of fibrinolysis with fewer side effects.
- *Gene Therapy*: For hereditary bleeding disorders, gene therapy offers the potential for long-term correction of the underlying defect.
- *Recombinant Coagulation Factors*: Development of new recombinant factors, including modified versions with extended half-lives or enhanced activity, could improve the management of coagulopathy.
- *Hemostatic Agents*: Exploration of new hemostatic agents that can be applied locally to bleeding sites, including biologically active materials that promote clot formation and stability.

Ongoing Research

- *Personalized Medicine*: Advances in genomics and pharmacogenetics may allow for personalized therapy in coagulopathy, tailoring treatment based on individual genetic profiles and responses to therapy (Zhang et al. 2020).
- *Biomarkers*: Identification and validation of biomarkers for early detection of coagulopathy and prediction of response to therapy could improve outcomes by allowing earlier and more targeted interventions.

- *Clinical Trials*: Large-scale, multicenter trials are essential to evaluate the efficacy and safety of emerging therapies and to refine the use of existing treatments in diverse patient populations.

Role of Vasopressors and Inotropic Agents
In cases of severe postoperative bleeding and hemodynamic instability, the strategic use of vasopressors and inotropic agents is necessary to support cardiovascular function and maintain tissue perfusion (Zhang et al. 2022). These agents help optimize blood pressure and cardiac output, especially in patients with ongoing bleeding, to prevent further deterioration and improve outcomes (Zhang et al. 2022).

Overall, effective management strategies in postoperative bleeding patients require a multidisciplinary approach that integrates fluid resuscitation, appropriate use of blood products, pharmacological interventions, and the strategic use of vasopressors and inotropic agents to optimize patient care and outcomes in the ICU setting (Zhang et al. 2022).

33.10 Specific Considerations

33.10.1 Management of Patients on Anticoagulants

In the management of postoperative bleeding, tailored approaches are essential for patients on anticoagulants to balance bleeding risks with the need for anticoagulation therapy. Strategies may involve the use of reversal agents like prothrombin complex concentrate (PCC) for vitamin K antagonists or specific antidotes for direct oral anticoagulants (DOACs) (Tanzi 2018). Close monitoring of coagulation parameters and individualized treatment plans are crucial to optimize outcomes in these patients (Tanzi 2018).

Management strategies for bleeding in postoperative patients on anticoagulants involve a multifaceted approach that includes pharmacological interventions and clinical considerations. Key strategies include discontinuation of anticoagulants for high-risk procedures, use of antifibrinolytic agents guided by viscoelastic monitoring, and consideration of damage control surgery if bleeding persists (Tran et al. 2014). For patients on new oral anticoagulants (NOACs) like rivaroxaban and apixaban, managing bleeding may involve assessing renal function, using prothrombin complex concentrates, and considering hemodialysis for dabigatran (Van Ryn et al. 2010). However, the lack of specific reversal agents for NOACs like dabigatran, rivaroxaban, and apixaban poses challenges in managing bleeding complications (Lauer et al. 2013).

In cases of severe bleeding, interventions such as blood component replacement, vitamin K administration for coumadin patients, idarucizumab for dabigatran, and andexanet alfa for apixaban and rivaroxaban are recommended (Koscielny et al.

2020). The approach to severe bleeding in postoperative patients on direct oral anticoagulants (DOACs) involves assessing the balance between bleeding and thrombosis risks to determine the level of anticoagulant reversal needed, including the use of hemostatic agents, specific reversal agents, transfusions, supportive management, and potentially surgery in critical events (Masotti et al. 2013).

The management of bleeding in patients on anticoagulants necessitates a careful and individualized approach, considering the specific anticoagulant used, the severity of bleeding, and the patient's overall clinical condition (Tran et al. 2014). Reversal strategies for anticoagulants like warfarin may involve vitamin K administration, while for DOACs, options like idarucizumab and andexanet alfa are available (Lauer et al. 2013). Overall, a comprehensive understanding of the pharmacology of anticoagulants and their reversal strategies is crucial for optimal management of bleeding in postoperative patients on anticoagulants (Tran et al. 2014).

33.10.2 Treatment of Patients with Inherited Platelet Disorders

Managing bleeding in postoperative patients with inherited platelet disorders requires a comprehensive approach that integrates prophylactic, pre-operative pro-hemostatic treatments, and personalized interventions based on the specific type and severity of the disorder. Prophylactic treatments are essential for reducing bleeding risks during surgery, with desmopressin being particularly effective in minimizing bleeding rates (Bunimov et al. 2013). Managing anticoagulation in these patients is complex, necessitating a careful balance between bleeding and thrombotic risks, highlighting the importance of individualized treatment plans (Nurden et al. 2021).

Various strategies are recommended for the management of inherited platelet disorders. Desmopressin and antifibrinolytic agents are crucial for controlling bleeding in different platelet disorders (Bariana et al. 2017). While platelet transfusions are commonly utilized, their efficacy may be limited in conditions like Glanzmann's thrombasthenia due to competition between transfused and endogenous platelets (Israels et al. 2010). Recombinant activated factor VII has demonstrated efficacy in managing bleeding in specific disorders such as Glanzmann's thrombasthenia and platelet refractoriness (Boeckelmann et al. 2021). Moreover, the use of autologous platelet-rich clots in combination with tranexamic acid has been shown to effectively prevent blood loss and facilitate rapid healing in certain surgical procedures (Bolton-Maggs et al. 2006).

Understanding the specific inherited platelet disorder is crucial for selecting the most appropriate treatment strategy to mitigate bleeding risks and address the unique challenges associated with the underlying disorder (James et al. 2020). By tailoring interventions to the individual's condition, healthcare providers can optimize outcomes and enhance patient safety during surgical procedures.

33.10.3 Guidelines for Fibrinogen Levels and Platelet Count

Maintaining optimal fibrinogen levels and platelet count is crucial in managing postoperative bleeding. Monitoring these parameters allows healthcare providers to assess coagulation status, guide transfusion decisions, and prevent excessive bleeding (Hashem 2015). Adherence to established guidelines for fibrinogen replacement and platelet transfusion based on specific thresholds and clinical indications is essential for appropriate postoperative bleeding management and improved patient outcomes (Hashem 2015).

Incorporating these specific considerations into the management of postoperative bleeding patients, including those on anticoagulants with inherited platelet disorders, utilizing pharmacological interventions, and following guidelines for fibrinogen levels and platelet count, is essential for providing individualized and effective care in the ICU setting.

33.11 Complications and Special Situations

33.11.1 Recognition and Management of Heparin-Induced Thrombocytopenia

In the management of postoperative bleeding, addressing complications like heparin-induced thrombocytopenia (HIT) is crucial. HIT is characterized by a decrease in platelet count due to heparin exposure and can lead to thrombotic complications (Ahmed et al. 2007). Prompt recognition of HIT is essential to prevent thrombosis, and management involves discontinuation of heparin and initiation of alternative anticoagulation strategies, such as direct thrombin inhibitors, to mitigate the risk of thrombosis in affected patients (Ahmed et al. 2007).

33.11.2 Addressing Complications Like Hyponatremia and Arterial Thrombosis

Complications such as hyponatremia and arterial thrombosis can also arise in postoperative bleeding patients and require timely intervention. Hyponatremia, often due to fluid shifts and inappropriate fluid management, should be corrected cautiously to prevent osmotic demyelination syndrome (Grouzi et al. 2010). Arterial thrombosis, a potential consequence of hypercoagulability in bleeding patients, may necessitate anticoagulation therapy or surgical intervention to prevent ischemic complications (Grouzi et al. 2010).

33.11.3 Legal Considerations and Documentation in Postoperative Bleeding Cases

Legal considerations and documentation are essential in postoperative bleeding cases to ensure comprehensive patient care. Accurate and detailed documentation of the clinical course, interventions performed, and patient responses is crucial for legal and quality assurance purposes (Mehdizade et al. 2021). Adherence to established documentation standards and protocols is vital in mitigating legal risks and ensuring accountability in postoperative bleeding cases (Mehdizade et al. 2021).

Recognition and proactive management of complications like HIT, hyponatremia, and arterial thrombosis, along with meticulous legal considerations and documentation practices, are integral components of the comprehensive care provided to postoperative bleeding patients in the ICU setting, ensuring optimal patient outcomes and legal compliance.

33.12 Future Directions and Conclusion

33.12.1 Emerging Trends in Postoperative Bleeding Management

During the Hyperthermic Intraperitoneal Chemotherapy (HIPEC) phase, heated chemotherapy can lead to vasodilation and hyperdynamic circulation (Ryu and Koo 2021).

Postoperative variables such as creatinine levels, duration of postoperative mechanical ventilation, length of stay in the intensive care unit and hospital, as well as the incidence of acute kidney injury, pneumonitis, and vasospasm were found to be similar between groups in a study comparing goal-directed fluid therapy to conventional fluid therapy during craniotomy and clipping of cerebral aneurysm (Bloria et al. 2022).

In the context of Enhanced Recovery After Surgery (ERAS), it is recommended that all patients avoid excessive crystalloid administration (Miller et al. 2016).

The modalities of fluid administration during the early phase of septic shock have been a topic of significant debate (Malbrain et al. 2018).

A study on goal-directed fluid therapy based on stroke volume variations in patients undergoing major orthopedic surgery found improvements in intraoperative organ perfusion, hemodynamic parameters, hospitalization, postoperative complications, and mortality (Peng et al. 2014).

Perioperative goal-directed fluid therapy (GDFT) involves the tailored optimization of hemodynamics and oxygen delivery through intravenous fluid and/or vasoactive infusions (Manning et al. 2017).

33.12.2 Summary of Key Points and Recommendations for Optimal Patient Care

In conclusion, the optimal management of postoperative bleeding requires a multidisciplinary approach that integrates fluid resuscitation, judicious use of blood products, pharmacological interventions, and meticulous monitoring of coagulation parameters. Key recommendations include maintaining minimally acceptable preload and blood pressure, adopting Patient Blood Management (PBM) pathways to reduce transfusion rates, and utilizing pharmacological agents like prothrombin complex concentrate (PCC) for specific coagulopathies. Furthermore, close attention to emerging trends in postoperative bleeding management, such as the use of IV iron perioperatively, can further enhance patient care and outcomes.

As the field of postoperative bleeding management continues to advance, healthcare providers must stay abreast of emerging trends and evidence-based practices to deliver optimal care to patients. By incorporating key recommendations and embracing innovative strategies, healthcare teams can effectively navigate the complexities of postoperative bleeding, improve patient outcomes, and ensure the highest standards of care in the ICU setting.

References

Ahmed I, Majeed A, Powell R (2007) Heparin induced thrombocytopenia: diagnosis and management update. Postgrad Med J 83(983):575–582

Akamatsu N, Sugawara Y, Nakazawa A, Nishioka Y, Kaneko J, Aoki T et al (2015) Hemostatic status in liver transplantation: association between preoperative procoagulants/anticoagulants and postoperative hemorrhaging/thrombosis. Liver Transpl 21(2):258–265

Akinwale MO, Sanusi AA, Adebayo OK (2016) Typhoid perforation: post-operative intensive care unit care and outcome. Afr J Paediatr Surg 13(4):175–180

Al Sulaiman K, Al Mutairi M, Al Harbi O, Al Duraihim A, Aldosary S, Al Khalil H et al (2021) Appropriateness of using vitamin K for the correction of INR elevation secondary to hepatic disease in critically ill patients: an observational study. Clin Appl Thromb Hemost 27:10760296211050923

Ali L, Jagadish MB, Jamgond S (2014) Blood conservation techniques in surgical patients: a review article. J Evol Med Dent Sci 3(61):13588–13602

Bariana TK, Ouwehand WH, Guerrero JA, Gomez K, BRIDGE Bleeding, Thrombotic and Platelet Disorders and ThromboGenomics Consortia (2017) Dawning of the age of genomics for platelet granule disorders: improving insight, diagnosis and management. Br J Haematol 176(5):705–720

Bartucca LM, Shaykh R, Stock A, Dayton JD, Bacha E, Haque KD, Nellis ME (2023) Epidemiology of severe bleeding in children following cardiac surgery involving cardiopulmonary bypass: use of Bleeding Assessment Scale for critically Ill Children (BASIC). Cardiol Young 33(10):1913–1919

Baysinger K, Barnett ME, Ott M, Bromberg W, McBride K, Thompson L et al (2016) What's in the box? The effectiveness of a low-volume massive transfusion protocol. Am Surg 82(7):602–607

Bloria SD, Panda NB, Jangra K, Bhagat H, Mandal B, Kataria K et al (2022) Goal-directed fluid therapy versus conventional fluid therapy during craniotomy and clipping of cerebral aneurysm: a prospective randomized controlled trial. J Neurosurg Anesthesiol 34(4):407–414

Boeckelmann D, Glonnegger H, Sandrock-Lang K, Zieger B (2021) Pathogenic aspects of inherited platelet disorders. Hamostaseologie 41(06):460–468

Bolton-Maggs PH, Chalmers EA, Collins PW, Harrison P, Kitchen S, Liesner RJ et al (2006) A review of inherited platelet disorders with guidelines for their management on behalf of the UKHCDO. Br J Haematol 135(5):603–633

Bresalier RS (1990) Prophylaxis of stress-related gastric mucosal hemorrhage: a critical appraisal. J Intensive Care Med 5(1):5–6

Bunimov N, Fuller N, Hayward CP (2013, March) Genetic loci associated with platelet traits and platelet disorders. In: Seminars in thrombosis and hemostasis. Thieme Medical Publishers, pp 291–305

Carrick MM, Leonard J, Slone DS, Mains CW, Bar-Or D (2016) Hypotensive resuscitation among trauma patients. BioMed Res Int 2016:8901938

Carson JL, Guyatt G, Heddle NM, Grossman BJ, Cohn CS, Fung MK et al (2016) Clinical practice guidelines from the AABB: red blood cell transfusion thresholds and storage. JAMA 316(19):2025–2035

Carson JL, Stanworth SJ, Guyatt G, Valentine S, Dennis J, Bakhtary S et al (2023) Red blood cell transfusion: 2023 AABB international guidelines. JAMA 330(19):1892–1902

Chen JH, Fang DZ, Tim Goodnough L, Evans KH, Lee Porter M, Shieh L (2015) Why providers transfuse blood products outside recommended guidelines in spite of integrated electronic best practice alerts. J Hosp Med 10(1):1–7

CRASH, T. (2019) Effects of tranexamic acid on death, disability, vascular occlusive events and other morbidities in patients with acute traumatic brain injury (CRASH-3): a randomised, placebo-controlled trial. Lancet 394(10210):1713–1723

Crochemore T, Görlinger K, Lance MD (2024) Early goal-directed hemostatic therapy for severe acute bleeding management in the intensive care unit: a narrative review. Anesth Analg 138(3):499–513

Devaney GL, Tarrant SM, Weaver N, King KL, Balogh ZJ (2023) Major pelvic ring injuries: fewer transfusions without deaths from bleeding during the last decade. World J Surg 47(5):1136–1143

Du Pont-Thibodeau G, Harrington K, Lacroix J (2014) Anemia and red blood cell transfusion in critically ill cardiac patients. Ann Intensive Care 4:1–11

Ghallab ET (2018) Post-operative bleeding and its management. Egypt J Hosp Med 70(9):1480–1483

Görlinger K, Fries D, Dirkmann D, Weber CF, Hanke AA, Schöchl H (2012) Reduction of fresh frozen plasma requirements by perioperative point-of-care coagulation management with early calculated goal-directed therapy. Transfus Med Hemother 39(2):104–113

Grouzi E, Kyriakou E, Panagou I, Spiliotopoulou I (2010) Fondaparinux for the treatment of acute heparin-induced thrombocytopenia: a single-center experience. Clin Appl Thromb Hemost 16(6):663–667

Hashem S (2015) The impact of clinical pharmacist managed anticoagulation management service versus routine medical care on the clinical outcome of atrial fibrillation patients: an Egyptian pilot study. Al-Azhar J Pharm Sci 52(2):57–81

Hof L, Choorapoikayil S, Meybohm P, Zacharowski K (2021) Patient blood management in intensive care patients. Curr Opin Crit Care 27(6):709–716

Israels SJ, El-Ekiaby M, Quiroga T, Mezzano D (2010) Inherited disorders of platelet function and challenges to diagnosis of mucocutaneous bleeding. Haemophilia 16:152–159

James TW, Thomson BJ, Naumann DN, Stevenson DS (2020) Platelet function testing in patients with post-operative tonsillectomy bleeding may be a useful early identifier of inherited platelet function disorders. J Laryngol Otol 134(10):882–886

Jensen MM, Marker S, Do HQ, Perner A, Møller MH (2019) Stress ulcer prophylaxis in critically ill children: protocol for a systematic review. Acta Anaesthesiol Scand 63(7):966–972

Kaafarani HMA, Velmahos GC (2014) Damage control resuscitation in trauma. Scand J Surg 103(2):81–88

Karanjkar A, Kapoor PM, Sharan S, Bhardwaj V, Malik V, Hasija S et al (2019) A prospective randomized clinical trial of efficacy of algorithm-based point of care guided hemostatic therapy in cyanotic congenital heart disease surgical patients. J Cardiac Critic Care TSS 3(01):08–16

Koscielny J, Rutkauskaite E, Sucker C, Von Heymann C (2020) How do I reverse oral and parenteral anticoagulants? Hamostaseologie 40(02):201–213

Krausz MM (2006) Initial resuscitation of hemorrhagic shock. World J Emerg Surg 1:1–5

Kunduz E, Dinçer ZA, Şeker B, Saylak HK, Demir O, Akbulut H, Ayşan E (2019) A novel herbal extract medicine for liver hemostasis: an experimental animal study. J Istanbul Fac Med 82(3):156–161

Kurlander DE, Ascha M, Marshall DC, Wang D, Ascha MS, Tripi PA et al (2020) Impact of multidisciplinary engagement in a quality improvement blood conservation protocol for craniosynostosis. J Neurosurg Pediatr 26(4):406–414

Kwon JO, MacLaren R (2016) Comparison of fresh-frozen plasma, four-factor prothrombin complex concentrates, and recombinant factor VII a to facilitate procedures in critically ill patients with coagulopathy from liver disease: a retrospective cohort study. Pharmacotherapy 36(10):1047–1054

Lauer A, Pfeilschifter W, Schaffer CB, Lo EH, Foerch C (2013) Intracerebral haemorrhage associated with antithrombotic treatment: translational insights from experimental studies. Lancet Neurol 12(4):394–405

Lim SY, Rajandram R, Roslani AC (2022) Comparison of post-operative bleeding incidence in laser hemorrhoidoplasty with and without hemorrhoidal artery ligation: a double-blinded randomized controlled trial. BMC Surg 22(1):146

Lin SL, Gao PT, Ni WK, Li QL, Chen WF, Zhang YQ et al (2021) Controlled hypertension under hemostasis prevents post-gastric endoscopic submucosal dissection bleeding: a prospective randomized controlled trial. Surg Endosc 35:1–11

Lins RC, Rolim Filho EL, Oliveira FDSC, Santos SMD, Rolim TLV, Kreimer F (2018) Estudo prospectivo da aspirina como profilaxia do tromboembolismo em artroplastia total do quadril. Acta Ortopédica Brasileira 26(2):86–90

Lu Q, Zhang J, Gao WM, Lv Y, Zhang XF, Liu XM (2018) Intraoperative blood transfusion and postoperative morbidity following liver resection. Med Sci Monit 24:8469

Malbrain ML, Van Regenmortel N, Saugel B, De Tavernier B, Van Gaal PJ, Joannes-Boyau O et al (2018) Principles of fluid management and stewardship in septic shock: it is time to consider the four D's and the four phases of fluid therapy. Ann Intensive Care 8:1–16

Manning MW, Dunkman WJ, Miller TE (2017) Perioperative fluid and hemodynamic management within an enhanced recovery pathway. J Surg Oncol 116(5):592–600

Masotti L, Landini G, Panigada G (2013) The practical management of bleedings during treatment with direct oral anticoagulants: the emergency reversal therapy. Ital J Med 7(s8):48–58

Mehdizade T, Kelahmetoglu O, Gurkan V, Çetin G, Guneren E (2021) Early suspicion of heparin-induced thrombocytopenia for successful free flap salvage: reports of two cases. J Hand Microsurg 13(03):178–180

Miller TE, Bunke M, Nisbet P, Brudney CS (2016) Fluid resuscitation practice patterns in intensive care units of the USA: a cross-sectional survey of critical care physicians. Perioper Med 5:1–13

Møller MH, Sigurðsson MI, Olkkola KT, Rehn M, Yli-Hankala A, Chew MS (2022) Transfusion strategies in bleeding critically ill adults: a clinical practice guideline from the European Society of Intensive Care Medicine: endorsement by the Scandinavian Society of Anaesthesiology and Intensive Care Medicine. Acta Anaesthesiol Scand 66(5):638–639

Ñamendys-Silva SA, Ruiz-Beltran AM, Barragán-Dessavre M, Bautista-Ocampo AR, Meneses-García A, González-Chon O, Herrera-Gómez A (2017) Clinical characteristics of critically ill cancer patients who are undergoing isolated limb perfusion. Mol Clin Oncol 7(5):747–750

Ng WCK, Jerath A, Wasowicz M (2015) Tranexamic acid: a clinical review. Anaesthesiol Intensive Ther 47(4):339–350

Nishiguchi A, Kurihara Y, Taguchi T (2020) Hemostatic, tissue-adhesive colloidal wound dressing functionalized by UV irradiation. ACS Appl Bio Mater 3(3):1705–1711

Nouraei SM, Baradari AG, Zeydi AE (2015) Does early post-operative administration of aspirin influence the risk of bleeding after coronary artery bypass graft surgery? A prospective observational study. Med Arch 69(6):381

Nurden P, Stritt S, Favier R, Nurden AT (2021) Inherited platelet diseases with normal platelet count: phenotypes, genotypes and diagnostic strategy. Haematologica 106(2):337

O'Donnell O, Gallagher C, Davey MG, Coulter J, Regan M (2024) A systematic review and meta-analysis assessing the use of tranexamic acid (TXA) in acute gastrointestinal bleeding. Ir J Med Sci 193:705–719

Page C, Retter A, Wyncoll D (2013) Blood conservation devices in critical care: a narrative review. Ann Intensive Care 3:1–6

Palmieri TL, Sen S, Falwell K, Greenhalgh DG (2011) Blood product transfusion: does location make a difference? J Burn Care Res 32(1):61–65

Parker MJ, Crowder EW, Miles MVP, Harrell KN, Maxwell RA (2023) Hypofibrinogenemic massive transfusion trauma patients experience worse outcomes. Am Surg 89(8):3423–3428

Peng K, Li J, Cheng H, Ji FH (2014) Goal-directed fluid therapy based on stroke volume variations improves fluid management and gastrointestinal perfusion in patients undergoing major orthopedic surgery. Med Princ Pract 23(5):413–420

Rao SV, Jollis JG, Harrington RA, Granger CB, Newby LK, Armstrong PW et al (2004) Relationship of blood transfusion and clinical outcomes in patients with acute coronary syndromes. JAMA 292(13):1555–1562

Rech MA, Gilbert BW, Nei S, Garg R, Brown CS (2023) The clot thickens: how to use viscoelastic testing in critical illness. J Am College Clin Pharm 6(8):954–963

Russell L, Holst LB, Kjeldsen L, Stensballe J, Perner A (2017) Risks of bleeding and thrombosis in intensive care unit patients with haematological malignancies. Ann Intensive Care 7:1–11

Ryu JH, Koo CH (2021) Anesthetic concerns during cytoreductive surgery with hyperthermic intraperitoneal chemotherapy. Korean J Anesthesiol 74(2):89

Schefold JC, Krag M, Marker S, Perner A, Wetterslev J, Wise MP et al (2019) Outcomes of prophylactic pantoprazole in adult intensive care unit patients receiving dialysis: results of a randomized trial. Am J Nephrol 50(4):312–319

Schober P, Loer SA, Schwarte LA (2022) Antifibrinolytics in the treatment of traumatic brain injury. Curr Opin Anesthesiol 35(5):583–592

Shakur H, Roberts I, Fawole B, Chaudhri R, El-Sheikh M, Akintan A et al (2017) Effect of early tranexamic acid administration on mortality, hysterectomy, and other morbidities in women with post-partum haemorrhage (WOMAN): an international, randomised, double-blind, placebo-controlled trial. Lancet 389(10084):2105–2116

Stellingwerff M, Brandsma A, Lisman T, Porte RJ (2012, February) Prohemostatic interventions in liver surgery. In: Seminars in thrombosis and hemostasis, vol 38. Thieme Medical Publishers, pp 244–249

Tanzi MG (2018) New guidance for managing bleeding in patients on oral anticoagulants. Pharm Today 24(2):2

Tran H, Joseph J, Young L, McRae S, Curnow J, Nandurkar H et al (2014) New oral anticoagulants: a practical guide on prescription, laboratory testing and peri-procedural/bleeding management. Intern Med J 44(6):525–536

Van Ryn J, Stangier J, Haertter S, Liesenfeld KH, Wienen W, Feuring M, Clemens A (2010) Dabigatran etexilate–a novel, reversible, oral direct thrombin inhibitor: interpretation of coagulation assays and reversal of anticoagulant activity. Thromb Haemost 103(06):1116–1127

Verma A, Al Nabhani S, Al-Khabori M (2007) Adult tonsillectomy and day care surgery. Indian J Otolaryngol Head Neck Surg 59:341–345

Wassef W, Obando J, Sharma A (2001) Upper gastrointestinal bleeding of nonvariceal origin in the ICU setting. J Intensive Care Med 16(3):105–113

Yoon S, Park AJ, Kim HO (2011) Clinical observation study of massive blood transfusion in a tertiary care hospital in Korea. Yonsei Med J 52(3):469

Zhang R, Dahl AB, Marchant B, Jackups RR Jr, Karnes HE, Shah P et al (2020) Optimizing management of replacement fluids for therapeutic plasma exchange: use of an automated mathematical model to predict post-procedure fibrinogen and antithrombin levels in high-risk patients. J Clin Apher 35(1):41–49

Zhang J, Han D, Zhang K, Guan W, Li L, Gu Z (2022) Observation on the effectiveness and safety of sodium bicarbonate Ringer's solution in the early resuscitation of traumatic hemorrhagic shock: a clinical single-center prospective randomized controlled trial. Trials 23(1):825

Chapter 34
Acute Respiratory Failure in Hematological Malignancies

Banani Poddar and Nilanchal Chakraborty

Learning Points

- The significance of ARF as a risk factor for ICU admission in patients with hematological malignancies.
- The various etiologies of ARF in this patient group and their respective diagnostic approaches.
- Management strategies for ARF, including criteria for choosing between noninvasive and invasive respiratory support.
- Prognostic factors affecting the outcomes of hematological patients with ARF, with a focus on intervention timing and patient-specific considerations.
- Future directions for research and potential improvements in the management of ARF in the context of hematological malignancies.

34.1 Introduction

Acute respiratory failure (ARF) presents a significant challenge in managing patients with hematological malignancies, often resulting in intensive care unit (ICU) admissions. The management of ARF in this patient population, including leukemia, lymphoma, and multiple myeloma, necessitates early recognition, precise diagnosis, and a comprehensive treatment approach (Vadde and Pastores 2016). The etiological spectrum of ARF in these patients varies from cancer invasion to infectious complications and treatment-induced pulmonary toxicity, highlighting the necessity for a multidisciplinary strategy (Lemiale et al. 2015). Studies have indicated that ARF is a common cause of ICU admissions in patients with hematologic malignancies and is linked to high mortality rates (Na et al. 2018; Seong et al. 2020; Horster et al. 2012).

The literature supports the integration of invasive and noninvasive ventilation strategies to improve patient outcomes (Fujiwara et al. 2016). Noninvasive

B. Poddar (✉)
Department of Critical Care Medicine, SGPGIMS, Lucknow, Uttar Pradesh, India

N. Chakraborty
Critical Care Medicine, Apollo Multispeciality Hospitals, Kolkata, West Bengal, India

S. B. Mishra (ed.), *Critical Care Hematology*,
https://doi.org/10.1007/978-981-97-5565-3_34

ventilation has demonstrated effectiveness in managing respiratory failure in patients with hematologic malignancies, potentially enhancing outcomes by avoiding endotracheal intubation. Moreover, the use of noninvasive ventilation, particularly CPAP or BiPAP, has been suggested as an initial treatment for ARF in these patients (Fujiwara et al. 2016).

Additionally, the presence of respiratory failure in patients with hematologic malignancies has been associated with increased ICU mortality, underscoring the critical need for early intervention and appropriate management strategies (Horster et al. 2012). Predictors of poor outcomes in critically ill patients with hematologic malignancies often include respiratory distress and hemodynamic instability, emphasizing the importance of promptly recognizing and addressing these factors (Yeo et al. 2012).

34.2 Etiology and Pathogenesis

Respiratory failure in patients with hematological malignancies is a multifaceted condition with various contributing factors. Infections, particularly pneumonia, are prevalent in cancer patients, with bacterial pneumonia being a primary cause of acute respiratory failure. Besides infections, the cancer itself can directly invade the lungs, leading to pulmonary dysfunction. Moreover, treatments such as chemotherapy (Table 34.1) and radiation can harm the lungs, exacerbating respiratory issues. Complications like graft-versus-host disease (GVHD) post-stem cell transplant can further compromise breathing. Other factors like pulmonary embolism, blood transfusion complications, pulmonary hemorrhage, heart failure, and airway obstructions due to fluid accumulation or mechanical blockages can also contribute to respiratory failure (Fujiwara et al. 2016; Martino et al. 2003; Ewig et al. 1998).

Managing respiratory failure in patients with hematological malignancies requires a comprehensive approach. Timely diagnosis and assessment are critical, involving vigilant monitoring of vital signs, oxygen levels, and respiratory function to detect respiratory distress early. Effective treatment and improved patient outcomes hinge on accurately identifying the specific causes of respiratory failure (Fujiwara et al. 2016; Martino et al. 2003; Ewig et al. 1998).

Research indicates that patients with hematological malignancies requiring mechanical ventilation for respiratory failure often experience unfavorable outcomes (Fujiwara et al. 2016). Patients with hematologic malignancies are predisposed to more complications compared to those with solid tumors, underscoring the necessity for tailored management strategies (Martino et al. 2003). Additionally, the use of noninvasive ventilation has been proposed as an initial treatment for acute respiratory failure in these patients, potentially averting the need for invasive interventions (Ewig et al. 1998).

Detailed Patient Evaluation A thorough patient history, physical examination, and assessment of recent treatments provide context for current symptoms. Acute

Table 34.1 Chemotherapeutic drugs and their pulmonary side effects

Drugs	Associated pulmonary complications
Bleomycin	Interstitial infiltrates, eosinophilic pneumonia, organizing pneumonia, pulmonary fibrosis, and acute interstitial pneumonia
Methotrexate	Interstitial infiltrates, nonspecific interstitial pneumonia, hypersensitivity pneumonitis, and organizing pneumonia
Taxanes	Interstitial infiltrates
Platin	Interstitial infiltrates and pulmonary hemorrhage
Rituximab	Interstitial infiltrates, diffuse alveolar damage, eosinophilic pneumonia, and hypersensitivity pneumonitis
Gemcitabine	Capillary leak syndrome, eosinophilic pneumonia, and diffuse alveolar damage
5-FU	Pulmonary fibrosis, and pulmonary edema
Bevacizumab	Pulmonary hemorrhage and pulmonary arterial hypertension
Carfilzomib	ARDS and diffuse alveolar damage
Carmustin	Pulmonary fibrosis, ARDS, and pleural effusion
Cyclophosphamide	Organizing pneumonia, pulmonary fibrosis, and ARDS
Doxorubicin	Organizing pneumonia and pulmonary fibrosis
Etoposide	ARDS, bronchospasm, and angioedema
Fludarabine	Eosinophilic pneumonia, organizing pneumonia, ARDS, and DAH
Ifosfamide	Interstitial pneumonitis and pulmonary fibrosis
Melphalan	Interstitial pneumonitis and pulmonary fibrosis
Paclitaxel	ARDS and acute interstitial pneumonia
Pemetrexed	Organizing pneumonia, pulmonary edema, pulmonary embolism, and pulmonary arterial hypertension
Thalidomide	Cryptogenic organizing pneumonia and pulmonary embolism
Vincristine	Cellular NSIP and laryngospasm
Nivolumab	Pulmonary sarcoid and sarcoid-like reaction and NSIP

respiratory failure in cancer patients can be intricately linked to both the stage of the disease and the type of therapy they are undergoing. In the early stages of cancer, respiratory failure is often a direct result of the tumor itself, such as through airway obstruction or the involvement of lung parenchyma. As the disease progresses or during active chemotherapy, the etiology may shift toward chemotherapy-induced complications like pneumonitis or opportunistic infections due to immunosuppression. In advanced stages, complications such as lymphangitic spread or treatment-related toxicities like radiation pneumonitis become more prevalent. Additionally, post-therapy stages may involve complications related to bone marrow transplantation, such as graft-versus-host disease, which can also impact respiratory function. Understanding this dynamic relationship between the disease stage, therapy, and respiratory failure etiology is crucial for timely diagnosis and appropriate management of these patients.

The course of hematological malignancies presents a varying landscape of etiological agents responsible for complications at different time points. In the early phase, immediately following chemotherapy or bone marrow transplantation, patients are predominantly susceptible to bacterial infections due to neutropenia. Common pathogens include Gram-positive bacteria like *Staphylococcus aureus* and Gram-negative bacteria such as *Pseudomonas aeruginosa*. As the patient progresses into the intermediate phase, typically one to 6 months post-transplant, opportunistic infections become more common. This period is marked by a higher risk of viral infections, particularly from cytomegalovirus (CMV) and fungal infections like *Aspergillus*. In the late phase, more than 6 months after therapy, the patient's immune system starts to recover. However, they remain at risk for encapsulated bacterial infections due to ongoing immunosuppressive therapy or graft-versus-host disease. This evolving pattern of etiological agents necessitates a tailored approach to prophylactic and therapeutic strategies throughout the different stages of treatment and recovery in hematological malignancy patients.

Radiological Investigations: Initial imaging, often with chest X-rays, helps assess lung condition and guide further diagnostic steps (Vadde and Pastores 2016).

Identifying the Cause: DIRECT Approach (Fig. 34.1)

D (Delay): Time since the hematological malignancy diagnosis or stem cell transplantation, influencing potential complications.

I (Immune Deficiency Pattern): Evaluate the specific immune deficiencies caused by the malignancy or its treatment, impacting susceptibility to infections.

R (Radiological Evaluation—Chest Radiography): Initial imaging to assess lung conditions and identify possible complications.

E (Experience): Utilize clinical expertise to interpret findings and integrate patient history with current clinical presentations.

C (Clinical Picture): Comprehensive assessment of the patient's current health status, symptoms, and medical history to guide further testing.

T (Tomography—CT): Advanced imaging to provide detailed views of the lungs, crucial for identifying specific pathologies not visible on chest X-rays.

Pulmonary complications are a significant concern in the administration of common chemotherapeutic drugs used in chemotherapy agents like bleomycin. Chemotherapeutic agents, while central to cancer management, can lead to a variety of pulmonary issues (Azoulay and Lemiale 2012). Drugs like bleomycin, busulfan, and carmustine are known to potentially cause conditions such as interstitial pneumonitis and pulmonary fibrosis. Other agents, including cyclophosphamide and methotrexate, may result in acute pneumonitis (Huprikar et al. 2019). Furthermore, the advent of newer targeted therapies has introduced additional pulmonary side effects. Medications like bevacizumab and rituximab, for example, are associated with complications including hypertension and interstitial lung disease. It is crucial for healthcare providers to be cognizant of these risks and to diligently monitor patients receiving these drugs for any signs of respiratory distress or changes in lung function (Fujiwara et al. 2016). This vigilance is key in promptly identifying and addressing pulmonary complications, thereby ensuring better outcomes for patients undergoing cancer therapy (Wohlfarth et al. 2014).

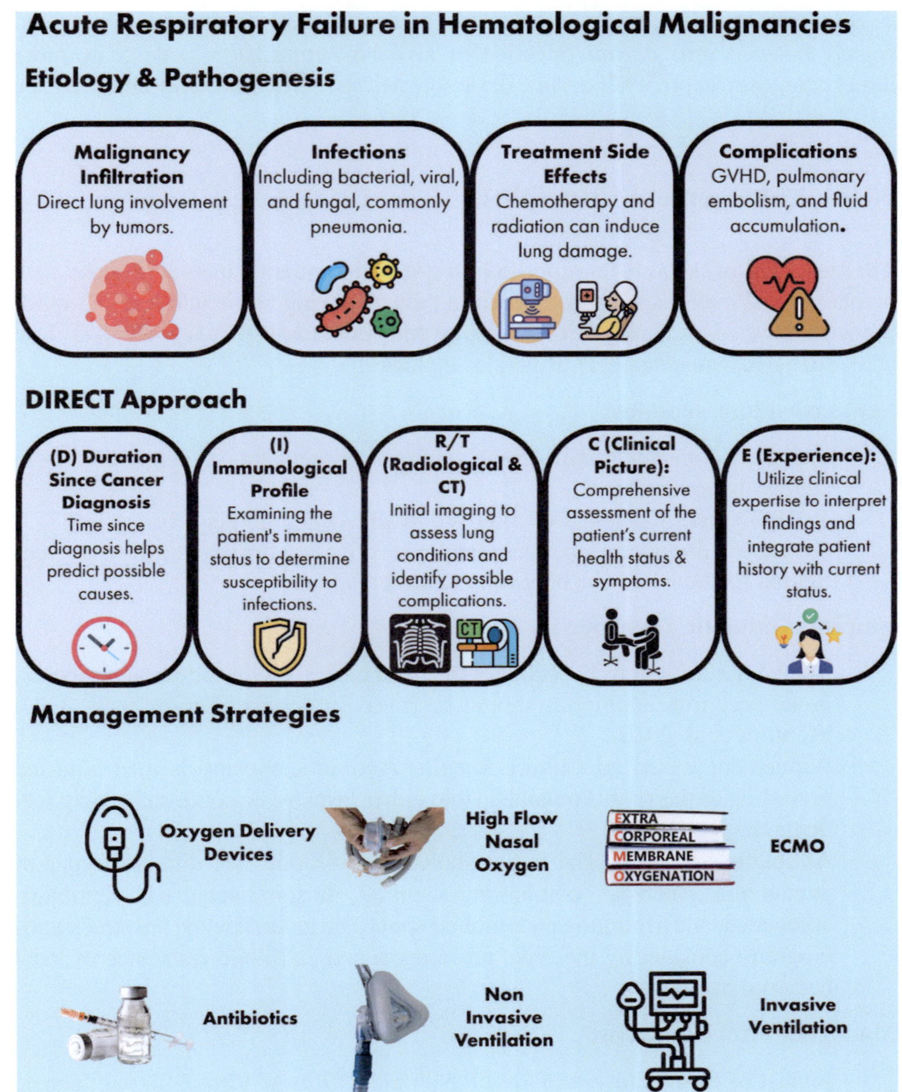

Fig. 34.1 Acute respiratory failure in hematological malignancies etiology and pathogenesis

34.2.1 Navigating Advanced Diagnostic Procedures

Balancing Risk and Necessity: Invasive procedures like bronchoscopic lavage are reserved for when noninvasive methods are inconclusive, considering the risks involved (Tyngkan et al. 2023).

Specific Conditions Requiring Invasive Testing: Certain scenarios, such as suspected *Pneumocystis carinii* infection or alveolar hemorrhage, necessitate more direct diagnostic approaches despite the associated risks (Medarov and Challa 2011).

34.3 Management Principles

The treatment of acute respiratory failure (ARF) in patients, including those with hematological malignancies, is tailored to the underlying cause while also providing supportive care to enhance oxygenation and ventilation (Renda et al. 2021; Frat et al. 2015). Key management principles include:

Supportive Interventions:

Oxygen Supplementation: Administering supplemental oxygen is crucial to address hypoxemia.
Use of Diuretics: These are employed to alleviate pulmonary congestion.
Ventilatory Support: Depending on the severity, noninvasive or invasive ventilation methods may be necessary to aid breathing.

Empiric Antibiotic Therapy:

Immediate Initiation: Especially critical in patients with febrile neutropenia, broad-spectrum antibiotics should be started promptly (Kruser et al. 2023; Montrief et al. 2020).
Refinement Based on Culture Results: Antibiotic therapy is then adjusted according to the results obtained from either invasive or noninvasive diagnostic methods.
Antibiotic Selection: The initial choice of antibiotics for different types of pneumonia (such as community-acquired, hospital-acquired, ventilator-associated, and aspiration pneumonia) should be guided by the hospital's antibiogram, considering the type, prevalence, and antibiotic resistance of local bacterial pathogens.

Managing Viral Infections:

Impact of Community-Acquired Respiratory Viruses: Viruses like influenza, respiratory syncytial virus (RSV), and parainfluenza can cause severe pneumonia, often accompanied by bacterial or fungal co-infections (Lapinsky et al. 2009; Suárez-Sipmann et al. 2018).
Advanced Diagnostic Techniques: PCR-based molecular diagnostics have become the preferred method for identifying viral infections, replacing older techniques like viral culture and serologic testing, especially in allogeneic hematopoietic stem cell transplant (HSCT) recipients.
Tailored Viral Management: The specific antiviral treatment depends on the type of viral infection identified.

34.4 Management of Noninfectious Causes of ARF

The management of noninfectious causes of acute respiratory failure (ARF) in patients with hematological malignancies involves addressing a variety of conditions, each requiring specific interventions (Wilson and Matthay 2014; Lazzarini et al. 2022). These noninfectious causes include:

- Cardiogenic Pulmonary Edema (CPE): Treatment focuses on reducing heart strain and fluid buildup in the lungs.
- Pulmonary Hemorrhage: Management involves stabilizing the patient and addressing the underlying cause of bleeding.
- Aspiration Pneumonitis: Treatment typically includes supportive care and sometimes interventions to clear the aspirated material.
- Radiation-Induced Pneumonitis: Management may involve corticosteroids and symptomatic treatment (Lecuyer et al. 2008; Schnell et al. 2013).
- Venous Thromboembolism: Anticoagulation therapy is the mainstay of treatment.
- Transfusion-Related Acute Lung Injury (TRALI): Supportive care, including oxygen therapy and mechanical ventilation, is essential.
- Retinoic Acid Syndrome: This condition often requires corticosteroids and supportive measures.
- Leukemic Pulmonary Leukostasis: Treatment focuses on reducing leukocyte counts and improving oxygenation.
- Leukemic Pulmonary Infiltrates: Management includes treating the underlying leukemia and supportive respiratory care.
- Pulmonary Lysis Syndrome: This involves careful management of metabolic complications and supportive respiratory care (Flowchart 1).

34.5 Comprehensive Approach to Ventilatory Management in Acute Respiratory Failure (ARF) for Patients with Hematological Malignancies

The management of acute respiratory failure in patients with hematological malignancies necessitates a nuanced understanding of various ventilatory support strategies. This approach is critical for optimizing patient outcomes while minimizing the risks associated with prolonged mechanical ventilation (Wright et al. 2017) The following outlines the key aspects of ventilatory management in this patient cohort (Flowchart 2).

- **Conventional Oxygen Therapy:**

  Modes of Delivery: This includes the use of Venturi masks, partial rebreathing masks, or non-rebreathing masks, which are essential tools in the initial management of hypoxemia (Cortegiani et al. 2018; Yigenoglu et al. 2021).

Limitations: While these methods are widely accessible and easy to implement, they are constrained by a maximum flow rate of 15 L/min and do not facilitate alveolar recruitment. Additionally, there is a potential risk of oxygen toxicity, particularly affecting the tracheobronchial tree.

- **Noninvasive Ventilation (NIV):**

  Mechanism and Benefits: NIV operates by providing continuous positive airway pressure, augmenting breaths with added pressure to enable alveolar recruitment, which can be crucial in the early stages of respiratory compromise.
  Clinical Outcomes: The timely application of NIV in patients with hematological malignancies has been associated with improved survival outcomes. However, its efficacy can vary between individuals, and failure of NIV is often linked with a higher mortality rate.
  Indicators of NIV Failure: Factors such as an elevated respiratory rate during NIV use, delayed initiation following ICU admission, and the need for concurrent vasopressors or renal replacement therapy can be predictive of NIV failure.
  Considerations for Early Intubation: In scenarios where patients exhibit persistent tachypnea or significant hypoxemia despite NIV, early intubation should be considered to avert further respiratory deterioration.

- **High-Flow Nasal Cannula (HFNC):**

  Mechanism and Advantages: HFNC delivers heated, humidified oxygen at high-flow rates (40–60 L/min), offering advantages such as improved mucociliary clearance, reduction in dead space, and provision of a small degree of positive end-expiratory pressure (PEEP).
  Clinical Evidence: Studies have demonstrated that HFNC can reduce the need for intubation compared to conventional oxygen therapy and NIV in immunocompromised patients with ARF. However, its impact on mortality rates remains a subject of ongoing research.
  Indicators of HFNC Failure: Clinicians should be vigilant for signs such as a high heart rate following an hour of HFNC treatment, which may necessitate the consideration of intubation.
  Individualized Patient Care: The decision regarding the choice of ventilatory support should be guided by the specific needs of each patient, their clinical response, and the evolving dynamics of their respiratory status (Hilbert et al. 2004; Rhee et al. 2009). Figure 34.1 provides a visual guide to aid in this decision-making process.

34.6 Weaning from Ventilatory Support in Patients with Hematological Malignancies Experiencing Acute Respiratory Failure

In the critical care management of acute respiratory failure (ARF) in patients with hematological malignancies, weaning from ventilatory support constitutes a pivotal phase. This process must be meticulously managed, balancing the delicate state of immunocompromised patients with the necessity of reducing ventilator-associated complications.

Considerations for Ventilator-Associated Pneumonia Risk: Patients who are immunocompromised and intubated for ARF are at an increased risk of developing ventilator-associated pneumonia. This risk is further compounded by the potential development of specific, high-mortality fungal infections.

Approach To Noninvasive Ventilation (NIV): The early application of NIV is crucial in the management of ARF. However, it's imperative to recognize the signs of NIV failure, such as persistent tachypnea, tachycardia, or increased work of breathing. Delayed intubation after the failure of NIV has been associated with increased mortality rates.

Criteria for Invasive Mechanical Ventilation (IMV): IMV should be considered in cases of escalating respiratory or hemodynamic instability or neurological deterioration. Parameters warranting the initiation of IMV include a significant decrease in the PaO_2/FiO_2 ratio, an increase in $PaCO_2$, or signs of respiratory muscle fatigue (Gristina et al. 2011).

Prophylactic Use of NIV: Initially, NIV was popularly used prophylactically to avoid intubation due to the high infection risks in these patients. However, its effectiveness has been found to be variable and may be more beneficial in controlled environments with experienced medical teams.

Weaning from IMV to NIV: Recent studies suggest that transitioning patients from IMV to NIV can increase the number of IMV-free days. This strategy does not appear to affect overall mortality rates or the incidence of complications.

34.7 Advanced Techniques for Refractory Cases

In severe cases unresponsive to standard measures, advanced techniques such as prone positioning, high-frequency oscillatory ventilation, recruitment maneuvers, vasodilator treatment, the use of Extracorporeal Membrane Oxygenation (ECMO), and neuromuscular blocking agents may be considered, akin to the strategies employed in immunocompetent patients.

Role of ECMO: ECMO has emerged as a potential option for patients with ARDS who are unresponsive to conventional ventilation strategies. While preliminary studies show promise, its application in patients with hematologic malignancies remains limited due to concerns like severe thrombocytopenia and increased bleeding risks (Tathineni et al. 2020; Brodie et al. 2019).

34.8 Integration of Research Findings in Ventilatory Management

Clinical Outcomes from Various Studies: A body of research indicates that the early utilization of NIV in the management of ARF can lead to improved patient outcomes. In contrast, the High-Flow Nasal Cannula (HFNC) has been found to reduce the need for intubation compared to both conventional oxygen therapy and NIV, presenting a viable alternative in certain clinical scenarios (Roca and Masclans 2015; Lindenauer et al. 2014).

Insights from the FLORALI Trial: The FLORALI trial, a significant study in this domain, demonstrated that HFNC reduced 90-day mortality rates in comparison to NIV and conventional oxygen therapy in a general ICU population. Subsequent analyses focusing on immunocompromised patients have suggested a continued benefit of HFNC over NIV in this specific cohort (Lemiale et al. 2015).

Implications of IMV to NIV Transition Studies: Research exploring the transition from IMV to NIV has revealed that this approach can lead to an increase in the number of days patients spend off IMV. Importantly, these studies indicate that such a transition does not adversely affect overall mortality rates or increase complication rates.

34.9 Outcome and Prognosis

The prognosis and outcomes for patients with hematologic malignancies who develop acute respiratory failure (ARF), especially those undergoing hematopoietic stem cell transplantation (HSCT), have evolved but remain challenging (Fujiwara et al. 2016).

Historical Mortality Rates: In the late 1990s and early 2000s, ICU and hospital mortality rates for these patients ranged significantly, with particularly poor 3- to 5-year survival rates, especially when mechanical ventilation was needed.

Risk Factors Influencing Mortality: Demographic factors like race (higher mortality in African Americans and Hispanics), comorbid conditions, and functional status significantly impact mortality.

Clinical factors include the severity of illness upon ICU admission, indicated by high SAPS II scores and elevated C-reactive protein levels.

Specific complications like treatment-refractory graft-versus-host disease (GVHD), NIV failure in ARDS, invasive fungal infections requiring IMV, and unidentified etiology of ARF are linked to higher mortality.

The presence of acute lung injury/ARDS, shock requiring vasopressors, the need for renal replacement therapy (RRT), and prolonged IMV duration are critical indicators of poor prognosis.

Impact of HSCT: Patients receiving autologous or allogeneic HSCT do not necessarily have higher hospital mortality compared to non-transplant patients when adjusted for various factors, as shown in a post hoc analysis of the EFRAIM study.

ICU Admission Timing and Duration: Early ICU admission (within 24 hours) and shorter ICU stays are associated with better outcomes. Prolonged ICU stays, particularly beyond 2 days, correlate with poorer prognoses.

Advancements and Improvements: Progress in noninvasive ventilation techniques, lung-protective ventilation strategies, and advancements in antimicrobial treatments have contributed to improved mortality rates in recent years.

HSCT Recipients with ARF: The in-hospital mortality rate for HSCT recipients who develop ARF is around 50%. The need for IMV in this group significantly worsens outcomes, with mortality rates soaring to 90–97% in the presence of neutropenia.

Current Understanding of Mortality Determinants: Recent studies indicate that ICU mortality is more closely associated with the severity and reversibility of the ARF episode rather than the characteristics of the underlying hematologic disease.

34.10 Conclusion

Acute respiratory failure is encountered often in patients with hematological malignancies who need to be admitted to the ICU and infection (pneumonia) is the most common underlying cause. Achieving adequate oxygenation and ventilation are important goals apart from treatment for the etiology of respiratory failure. Patients in whom the cause remains undetermined even after workup fare badly. Aggressive management and early referral have improved the prognosis, though the overall outcome is not comparable to patients without malignancy.

<a href="https://www.flaticon.com/free-icons/tumor" title="tumor icons">Tumor icons created by Freepik - Flaticon</a>

<a href="https://www.flaticon.com/free-icons/chemotherapy" title="chemotherapy icons">Chemotherapy icons created by Eucalyp - Flaticon</a>

<a href="https://www.flaticon.com/free-icons/infection" title="Infection icons">Infection icons created by Freepik - Flaticon</a>

<a href="https://www.flaticon.com/free-icons/complications" title="complications icons">Complications icons created by juicy_fish - Flaticon</a>

<a href="https://www.flaticon.com/free-icons/clock" title="clock icons">Clock icons created by Freepik - Flaticon</a>

<a href="https://www.flaticon.com/free-icons/broken-shield" title="broken shield icons">Broken shield icons created by Freepik - Flaticon</a>

<a href="https://www.flaticon.com/free-icons/ct-scan" title="CT scan icons">CT scan icons created by Freepik - Flaticon</a>

<a href="https://www.flaticon.com/free-icons/xray" title="xray icons">Xray icons created by Nadiinko - Flaticon</a>

<a href="https://www.flaticon.com/free-icons/hospital" title="hospital icons">Hospital icons created by Prosymbols Premium - Flaticon</a>

<a href="https://www.flaticon.com/free-icons/experience" title="experience icons">Experience icons created by Dewi Sari - Flaticon</a>

Flowcharts

Flowchart 1

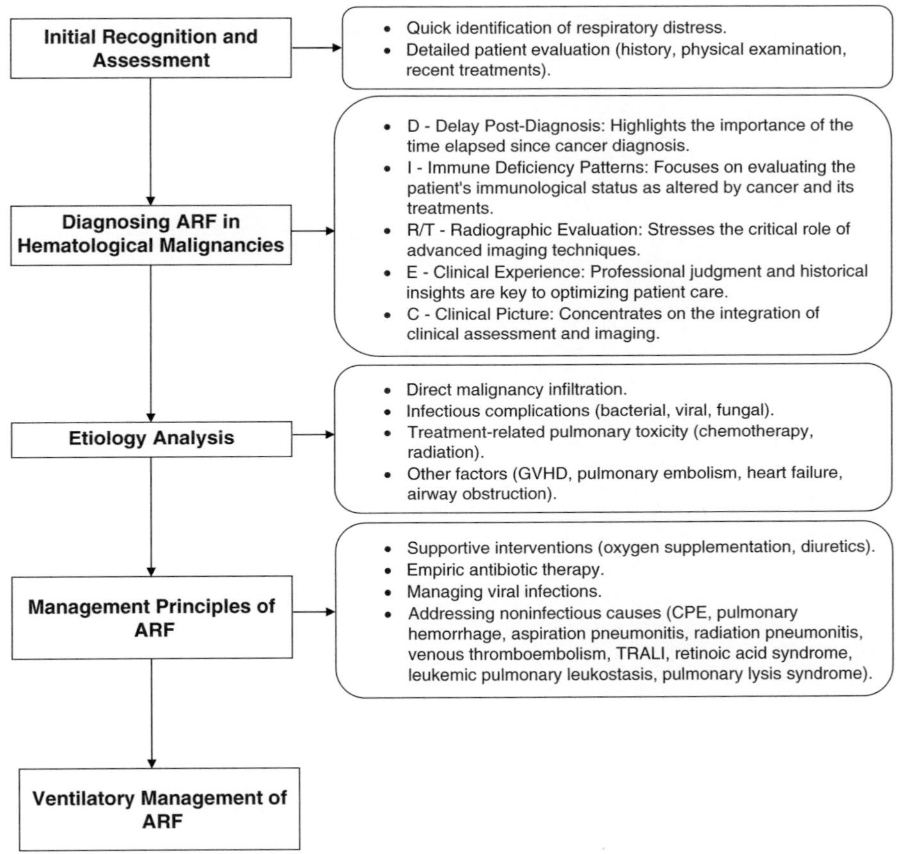

Flowchart 2

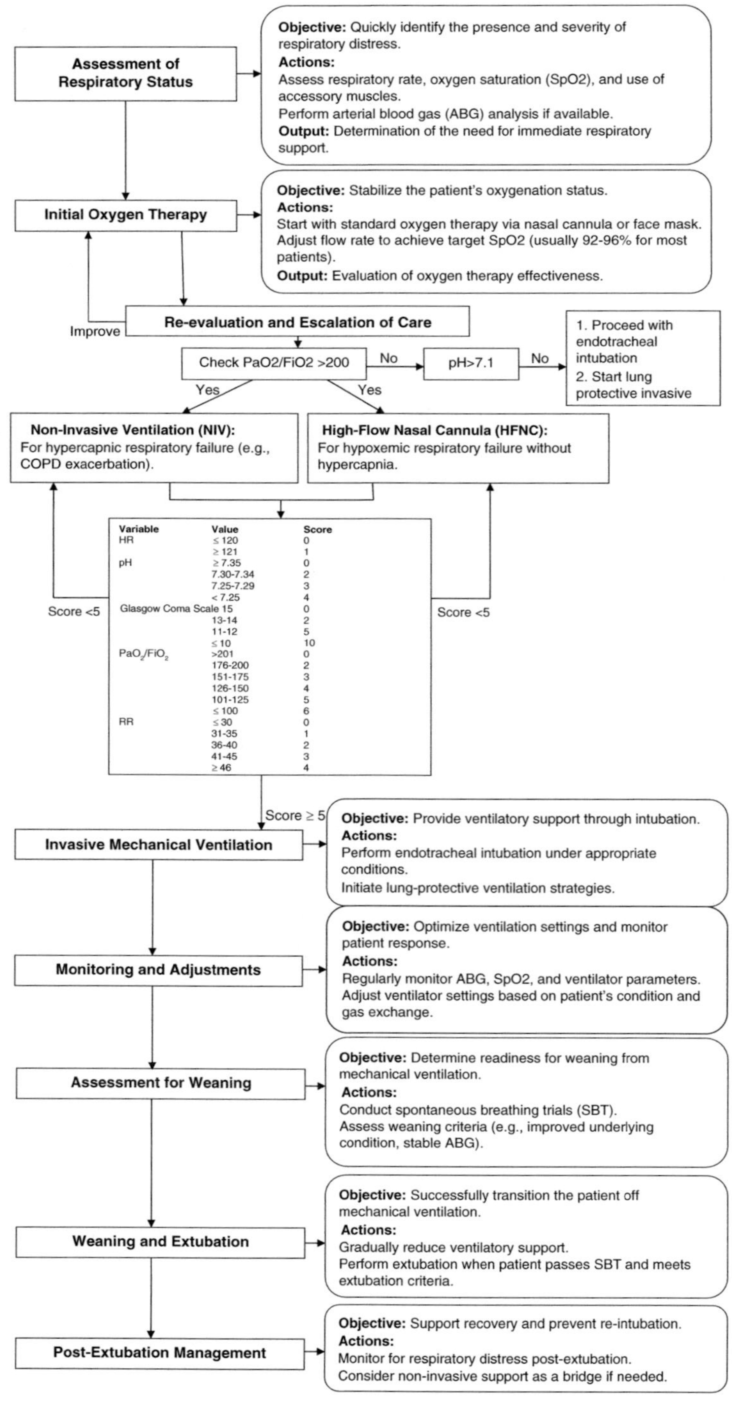
Assessment of Respiratory Status
Objective: Quickly identify the presence and severity of respiratory distress.
Actions:
Assess respiratory rate, oxygen saturation (SpO2), and use of accessory muscles.
Perform arterial blood gas (ABG) analysis if available.
Output: Determination of the need for immediate respiratory support.
Initial Oxygen Therapy
Objective: Stabilize the patient's oxygenation status.
Actions:
Start with standard oxygen therapy via nasal cannula or face mask.
Adjust flow rate to achieve target SpO2 (usually 92-96% for most patients).
Output: Evaluation of oxygen therapy effectiveness.
Improve
Re-evaluation and Escalation of Care
Check PaO2/FiO2 >200
No
pH>7.1
No
1. Proceed with endotracheal intubation
2. Start lung protective invasive
Yes
Yes
Non-Invasive Ventilation (NIV): For hypercapnic respiratory failure (e.g., COPD exacerbation).
High-Flow Nasal Cannula (HFNC): For hypoxemic respiratory failure without hypercapnia.
Score <5
Score <5
Variable Value Score
HR ≤ 120 0
≥ 121 1
pH ≥ 7.35 0
7.30-7.34 2
7.25-7.29 3
< 7.25 4
Glasgow Coma Scale 15 0
13-14 2
11-12 5
≤ 10 10
PaO2/FiO2 >201 0
176-200 2
151-175 3
126-150 4
101-125 5
≤ 100 6
RR ≤ 30 0
31-35 1
36-40 2
41-45 3
≥ 46 4
Score ≥ 5
Invasive Mechanical Ventilation
Objective: Provide ventilatory support through intubation.
Actions:
Perform endotracheal intubation under appropriate conditions.
Initiate lung-protective ventilation strategies.
Monitoring and Adjustments
Objective: Optimize ventilation settings and monitor patient response.
Actions:
Regularly monitor ABG, SpO2, and ventilator parameters.
Adjust ventilator settings based on patient's condition and gas exchange.
Assessment for Weaning
Objective: Determine readiness for weaning from mechanical ventilation.
Actions:
Conduct spontaneous breathing trials (SBT).
Assess weaning criteria (e.g., improved underlying condition, stable ABG).
Weaning and Extubation
Objective: Successfully transition the patient off mechanical ventilation.
Actions:
Gradually reduce ventilatory support.
Perform extubation when patient passes SBT and meets extubation criteria.
Post-Extubation Management
Objective: Support recovery and prevent re-intubation.
Actions:
Monitor for respiratory distress post-extubation.
Consider non-invasive support as a bridge if needed.

References

Azoulay E, Lemiale V (2012) Non-invasive mechanical ventilation in hematology patients with hypoxemic acute respiratory failure: a false belief? Bone Marrow Transplant 47(4):469–472

Brodie D, Slutsky AS, Combes A (2019) Extracorporeal life support for adults with respiratory failure and related indications: a review. JAMA 322(6):557–568

Cortegiani A, Madotto F, Gregoretti C, Bellani G, Laffey JG, Pham T et al (2018) Immunocompromised patients with acute respiratory distress syndrome: secondary analysis of the LUNG SAFE database. Crit Care 22:1–15

Ewig S, Torres A, Riquelme R, El-Ebiary M, Rovira M, Carreras E et al (1998) Pulmonary complications in patients with haematological malignancies treated at a respiratory ICU. Eur Respir J 12(1):116–122

Frat JP, Thille AW, Mercat A, Girault C, Ragot S, Perbet S et al (2015) High-flow oxygen through nasal cannula in acute hypoxemic respiratory failure. N Engl J Med 372(23):2185–2196

Fujiwara Y, Yamaguchi H, Kobayashi K, Marumo A, Omori I, Yamanaka S et al (2016) The therapeutic outcomes of mechanical ventilation in hematological malignancy patients with respiratory failure. Intern Med 55(12):1537–1545

Gristina GR, Antonelli M, Conti G, Ciarlone A, Rogante S, Rossi C et al (2011) Noninvasive versus invasive ventilation for acute respiratory failure in patients with hematologic malignancies: a 5-year multicenter observational survey. Crit Care Med 39(10):2232–2239

Hilbert G, Gruson D, Vargas F (2004) Noninvasive mechanical ventilation in immunocompromised patients. Clin Pulm Med 11(3):175–182

Horster S, Stemmler HJ, Mandel PC, Mück A, Tischer J, Hausmann A et al (2012) Mortality of patients with hematological malignancy after admission to the intensive care unit. Oncol Res Treat 35(10):556–561

Huprikar NA, Peterson MR, DellaVolpe JD, Sams VG, Lantry JH, Walter RJ et al (2019) Salvage extracorporeal membrane oxygenation in induction-associated acute respiratory distress syndrome in acute leukemia patients: a case series. Int J Artif Organs 42(1):49–54

Kruser JM, Sharma K, Holl JL, Nohadani O (2023) Identifying patterns of medical intervention in acute respiratory failure: a retrospective observational study. Critic Care Explor 5(10):e0984

Lapinsky SE, Posadas-Calleja JG, McCullagh I (2009) Clinical review: ventilatory strategies for obstetric, brain-injured and obese patients. Crit Care 13:1–7

Lazzarini LM, Werner JM, Perez IA, Seruya M, Ramos-Platt L, Tiongson E, Keens TG (2022) Does acute flaccid myelitis cause respiratory failure in children? Pediatr Pulmonol 57(3):682–685

Lecuyer L, Chevret S, Guidet B, Aegerter P, Martel P, Schlemmer B, Azoulay E (2008) Case volume and mortality in haematological patients with acute respiratory failure. Eur Respir J 32(3):748–754

Lemiale V, Resche-Rigon M, Mokart D, Pène F, Rabbat A, Kouatchet A et al (2015) Acute respiratory failure in patients with hematological malignancies: outcomes according to initial ventilation strategy. A groupe de recherche respiratoire en reanimation onco-hematologique (Grrr-OH) study. Ann Intensive Care 5:1–9

Lindenauer PK, Stefan MS, Shieh MS, Pekow PS, Rothberg MB, Hill NS (2014) Outcomes associated with invasive and noninvasive ventilation among patients hospitalized with exacerbations of chronic obstructive pulmonary disease. JAMA Intern Med 174(12):1982–1993

Martino M, Morabito F, Console G, Irrera G, Messina G, Pucci G et al (2003) Differences in transplant-related complications between hematologic malignancies and solid tumors receiving high-dose chemotherapy and autologous peripheral blood stem cell transplantation. Tumori J 89(4):385–390

Medarov B, Challa TR (2011) Short-term mortality among patients with non–small cell lung cancer and respiratory failure: a retrospective study. Chest Dis Rep 1(1):e7–e7

Montrief T, Ramzy M, Long B, Gottlieb M, Hercz D (2020) COVID-19 respiratory support in the emergency department setting. Am J Emerg Med 38(10):2160–2168

Na SJ, Ha TS, Koh Y, Suh GY, Koh SO, Lim CM et al (2018) Characteristics and clinical outcomes of critically ill cancer patients admitted to Korean intensive care units. Acute Critic Care 33(3):121

Renda T, Scala R, Corrado A, Ambrosino N, Vaghi A, Scientific Group on Respiratory Intensive Care of the Italian Thoracic Society (ITS-AIPO) (2021) Adult pulmonary intensive and intermediate care units: the Italian Thoracic Society (ITS-AIPO) position paper. Respiration 100(10):1027–1037

Rhee CK, Kang JY, Kim YH, Kim JW, Yoon HK, Kim SC et al (2009) Risk factors for acute respiratory distress syndrome during neutropenia recovery in patients with hematologic malignancies. Crit Care 13:1–8

Roca O, Masclans JR (2015) High-flow nasal cannula oxygen therapy: innovative strategies for traditional procedures. Crit Care Med 43(3):707–708

Schnell D, Mayaux J, Lambert J, Roux A, Moreau AS, Zafrani L et al (2013) Clinical assessment for identifying causes of acute respiratory failure in cancer patients. Eur Respir J 42(2):435–443

Seong GM, Lee Y, Hong SB, Lim CM, Koh Y, Huh JW (2020) Prognosis of acute respiratory distress syndrome in patients with hematological malignancies. J Intensive Care Med 35(4):364–370

Sipmann FS, Santos A, Tusman G (2018) Heart-lung interactions in acute respiratory distress syndrome: pathophysiology, detection and management strategies. Ann Transl Med 6(2)

Tathineni P, Pandya M, Chaar B (2020) The utility of extracorporeal membrane oxygenation in patients with hematologic malignancies: a literature review. Cureus 12(7)

Tyngkan L, Singh V, Mathew V, Laharwal MA (2023) Posttraumatic retropharyngeal pseudomeningocele—a case report. Indian J Neurotrauma 20(01):041–044

Vadde R, Pastores SM (2016) Management of acute respiratory failure in patients with hematological malignancy. J Intensive Care Med 31(10):627–641

Wilson JG, Matthay MA (2014) Mechanical ventilation in acute hypoxemic respiratory failure: a review of new strategies for the practicing hospitalist. J Hosp Med 9(7):469–475

Wohlfarth P, Ullrich R, Staudinger T, Bojic A, Robak O, Hermann A et al (2014) Extracorporeal membrane oxygenation in adult patients with hematologic malignancies and severe acute respiratory failure. Crit Care 18:1–8

Wright CJ, Allan RM, Gillon SA (2017) Medical high dependency unit series, article 3: respiratory support in the MHDU. Acute Med 16(3):115–122

Yeo CD, Kim JW, Kim SC, Kim YK, Kim KH, Kim HJ et al (2012) Prognostic factors in critically ill patients with hematologic malignancies admitted to the intensive care unit. J Crit Care 27(6):739–7e1

Yigenoglu TN, Ata N, Altuntas F, Bascı S, Dal MS, Korkmaz S et al (2021) The outcome of COVID-19 in patients with hematological malignancy. J Med Virol 93(2):1099–1104

Chapter 35
End-of-Life Care and Palliative Care of Hematologic Malignancies

Biswajit Bhuyan

Learning Points

1. Palliative care should be integrated early for patients with hematologic malignancies to manage symptoms, support them psychologically, and enhance their quality of life.
2. Involve patients and their families in care decisions to ensure treatments align with their values and preferences.
3. Address the unique challenges of hematologic malignancies, including fluctuating prognoses and intense symptomatology, with personalized care strategies.
4. Overcome barriers to palliative care access, such as misperceptions about its scope, communication gaps regarding prognosis, and dependency on hematologists due to prolonged duration of chemotherapy treatments.

35.1 Introduction

The World Health Organization (WHO), defines palliative care as "an approach that improves the quality of life of patients and their families facing the problem associated with life-threatening illness, through the prevention and relief of suffering by means of early identification and impeccable assessment and treatment of pain and other problems, physical, psychosocial, and spiritual" (World Health Organization et al. 2002). End-of-life care, as the name suggests, refers to the care provided to individuals who are in the final stages of their disease and approaching death. Hospice care seeks to support dignified dying or a good death experience for those with terminal illness. Palliative care is a broad term encompassing both end-of-life care and hospice care (Fig. 35.1). Palliative care is an integrated component of comprehensive cancer care to ensure optimal outcomes and patient-centered care. In the United States, hematologic malignancies comprising leukemia, lymphomas, and myeloma account for approximately 9.7% of all newly diagnosed cancer cases (Siegel et al. 2018). These groups of malignancies are known for their

B. Bhuyan (✉)
Clinical Hematology, KIMS and PBMH Hospital, Bhubaneswar, Odisha, India
e-mail: biswajit.bhuyan@kims.ac.in

S. B. Mishra (ed.), *Critical Care Hematology*,
https://doi.org/10.1007/978-981-97-5565-3_35

heterogeneous nature, unpredictable clinical courses, and transfusion dependence. It is important to integrate palliative care early in the disease course in hematologic malignancies as in solid tumors. In the context of hematologic malignancies, end-of-life care and palliative care require a tailored and individualized approach. The disease-specific characteristics, including the potential for rapid disease progression, treatment-related toxicities, and the impact on blood counts and immune function, necessitate specialized expertise and collaborative efforts between hematologists, oncologists, palliative care specialists, and supportive care teams.

35.2 Current Situation of Palliative Care and Clinical Implications in Hematologic Malignancies

Access to palliative care for patients with hematologic malignancies is often limited. Various studies published have shown the underutilization of palliative care services in hematologic malignancies as compared to non-hematologic malignancies. Howell et al. in a systematic review and meta-analysis, found out significantly reduced number of patients availing palliative care services in hematologic malignancies vs other solid malignancies (risk ratio 0.46 [95% CI 0.42–0.50]) (Howell et al. 2011; Wang et al. 2017; LeBlanc et al. 2015). Furthermore, patients with hematologic malignancies have more inpatient and ICU admissions and are more likely to die in the hospital as compared to those with non-hematologic malignancies, as reported by Kirtane et al. 2018. The biology, clinical course, and presentation of hematologic malignancies, especially leukemia and lymphoma, differ considerably as compared to non-hematologic malignancies which necessitates

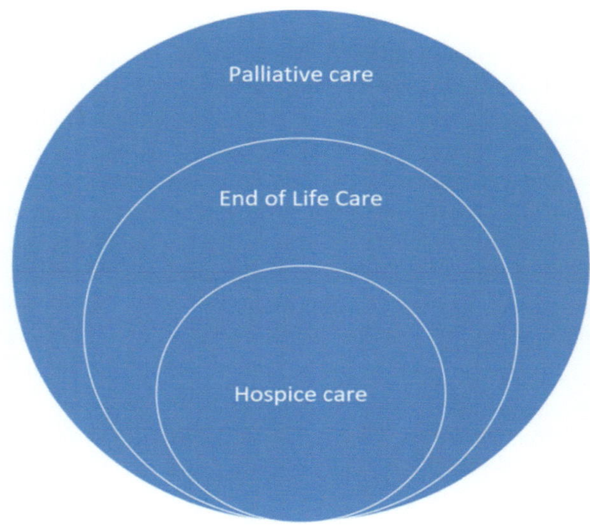

Fig. 35.1 Terms commonly used in palliative care medicine

modification of the conventional approach used in non-hematologic malignancies which is summarized in Table 35.1 (Wang et al. 2017; Odejide et al. 2016; Button et al. 2017).

35.3 Indications for PC in Hematologic Malignancies

There is no general consensus about the timing of referral to specialized palliative care services in hematologic malignancies due to the paucity of data available. However, a list of clinical scenarios that may consider the treating hematologists to refer to specialized palliative care services is provided in Table 35.2. It is important to note that these indications have been taken primarily from studies in solid tumors and have been extrapolated to hematologic malignancies (LeBlanc et al. 2015).

Table 35.1 Biology, clinical course, and palliative care approach in hematologic versus non-hematologic malignancies

Aspect	Hematologic malignancies	Non-hematologic malignancies
Disease characteristics	Heterogeneous and complex.	Degree of heterogeneity and complexity is relatively less.
Prognostication	Variable depends upon the type of malignancy, risk stratification, and molecular risk factors.	More predictable prognosis based on tumor type, stage, and grade.
Symptom management	Specific focus on anemia, bleeding, and infections.	Symptoms management tailored to tumor-specific symptoms.
Treatment approaches	Complex and individualized treatment regimens (chemotherapy, immunotherapy, stem cell transplantation, and CART-T cell therapy).	Mainly surgery, radiation, and chemotherapy.
End-of-life care	Potentially higher rates of aggressive interventions.	Greater emphasis on palliation and quality of life.
Supportive care needs	Frequent transfusion and antimicrobial requirement.	Pain control and management of tumor-related symptoms.
Referrals to palliative care	Over-dependence on hemato-oncologist and late referral to palliative care center.	Equally shared by medical, surgical, radiation, and palliative care specialists.
Access to palliative care	Tends to be lower than in solid tumors.	Greater awareness and utilization of palliative care services.
Intensive care requirements	Frequent requirement due to neutropenia, elderly age, and immunocompromised state.	Comparatively less requirement due to lower incidence of febrile neutropenia.

35.4 Symptom Burden in Hematologic Malignancies

Patients with hematologic malignancies can have varied symptoms depending upon the type of hematologic malignancies and chemotherapy received. As compared to solid tumors prevalence of pain is lower in hematologic malignancies with the notable exception of myeloma (Hung et al. 2013). Dyspnea, fatigue, drowsiness are more prevalent in hematologic malignancies as compared to their non-hematologic counterpart (Hochman et al. 2018; Tendas et al. 2009). Structured tools are available for specific hematologic malignancies like MPN to assess disease burden and should be used wherever applicable (Geyer and Mesa 2014). Due to the requirement of prolonged hospital stay in hematologic malignancies psychosocial needs are higher in that of solid tumors.

35.5 Challenges and Barriers Restricting Access to Palliative Care in Hematologic Malignancies

Hemato-oncologists often associate palliative care with end-of-life care rather than integrating early in the disease trajectory, leading to delayed symptom management and limited psychosocial support. They often struggle with prognostic uncertainty and balancing potentially aggressive and curative treatments with palliative care. Inadequate communication, counseling regarding prognosis, and stigma associated with prognosis further aggravate the situation (Howell et al. 2011). The palliative care training received by oncologists treating hematologic malignancies is inadequate for a comprehensive palliative care approach. Addressing these barriers is

Table 35.2 Indications for referral to palliative care in hematologic malignancies

Group of patients	Examples
Relapsed or refractory disease	Aggressive lymphomas or leukemias relapsing or non-responsive/ partially responsive to treatment.
Elderly patients with comorbidities	Older patients have advanced disease and other comorbidities that restrict the optimal dose of chemotherapy/immunotherapy.
End-of-life care	Patients with advanced hematologic malignancy nearing the end of life.
High-risk disease	Patients having high-risk leukemias, that is, AML, ALL OR high-grade lymphomas or myeloma.
Significant symptom burden	Patients experience significant pain, fatigue, or shortness of breath even after optimal treatment.
Patients with psychosocial needs	Patients expressing depression and emotional challenges.
Patients opting for comfort-focused care	Patients who prioritize symptom management and quality of life over aggressive or curative treatment.
Post-hematopoietic stem cell transplant	Relapse after BMT, severe graft versus host disease (GVHD), mucositis, infection, pain, or other complications related to HSCT.

essential to ensure that patients receive the highest quality of palliative care (Odejide et al. 2016; LeBlanc et al. 2015).

One of the major challenges in integrating early is the treating hemato-oncologists' reluctance to refer patients to palliative care, who perceive themselves as the sole caretaker, and patients' dependence of patients on hematologists due to the longer duration of chemotherapy protocols as compared to oncologists managing solid malignancies (Howell et al. 2011). A list of barriers to the successful integration of palliative care in hematologic malignancies is summarized in Fig. 35.2.

35.6 Integration of Palliative Care in Hematologic Malignancies and Addressing the Barriers to Integration

Evidence for integration: Studies in aggressive leukemias like acute myeloid leukemia receiving high-dose chemotherapy have reported a substantial improvement in quality of life, psychological distress, and end-of-life care with early integration of palliative care (El-Jawahri et al. 2021). In patients with hematologic malignancy receiving hematopoietic stem cell transplantation (HSCT) settings, early integration of palliative care seems to have a modest effect in decreasing the depression, anxiety, and stress associated with HSCT (El-Jawahri et al. 2015, 2017). Complications

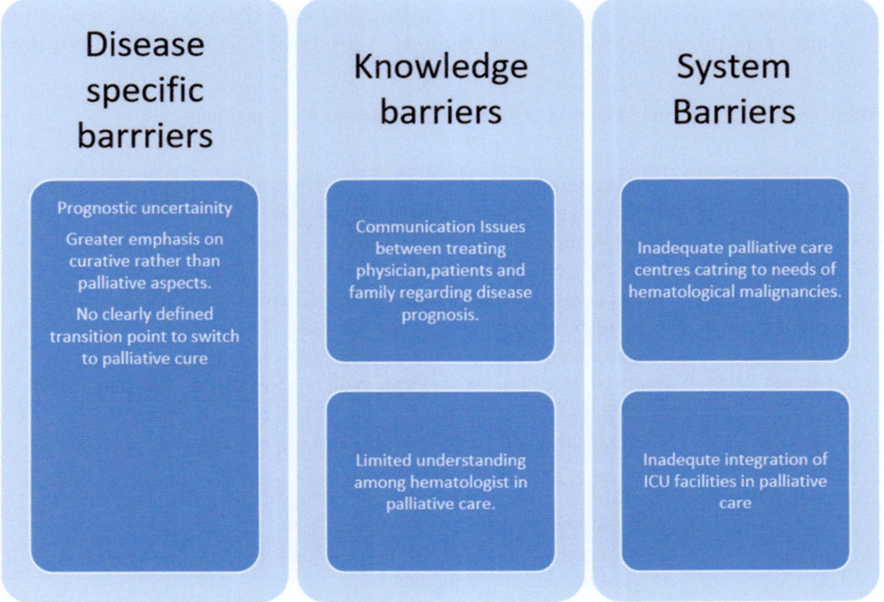

Fig. 35.2 Levels of barrier in integration of palliative care in hematologic malignancies

of BMT such as chronic GVHD should be integrated at the time of diagnosis due to the high symptom burden (El-Jawahri et al. 2018). Palliative care should be provided early in cases of relapsed/refractory/aggressive lymphomas, either at a specialty or general level (Odejide 2020). A list of studies supporting the integration of palliative care is presented in Table 35.3.

35.7 Strategies for Integration of Palliative Care in Hematology

To improve end-of-life care in patients with hematologic malignancies, it is essential to address the barriers at each level. Major areas to address for improving end-of-life care/palliative care are summarized in Table 35.4.

35.8 Disease-Specific Palliative Care for Hematologic Malignancies

Since hematologic malignancies vary greatly and are quite heterogeneous even within the same category, palliative should be tailored according to disease biology, prognosis, and progression.

(A) *Leukemia*: Classified as acute or chronic leukemias. Usually, acute leukemias are rapidly progressive and require prompt institution of high-dose

Table 35.3 Studies on integration of palliative care in hematologic malignancies

Study	Findings
El-Jawahri et al. (2017)	Palliative care improved the quality of life and mood of patients and family caregivers during hospitalization for stem cell transplantation.
Odejide et al. (2017)	Patients with hematologic malignancies are more likely to die in the absence of palliative care setting.
Odejide et al. (2020)	Factors associated with the timing of discussions among patients with hematologic malignancies were identified.
Le Blanc and El-Jawahri (2015)	Hemato-oncologists have varied perceptions highlighting the need for improved education and perception highlighting the need for improved integration.
Gautama et al. (2023)	Early palliative care improved outcomes in hematologic malignancies.
Hui et al. (2019)	Clinical factors such as knowledge and experience influence awareness about prognostication.
Morisaku et al. (2022)	Improvement in in quality of life (QOL) in the PC group in advanced relapsed refractory lymphomas.
Hui et al. (2010)	Improved discharge outcomes and survival in patients with advanced hematologic malignancies admitted to an acute palliative care unit.

Table 35.4 Major aspects to improve palliative care in hematologic malignancies (Wang et al. 2017)

Strategy	Description
Early integration	Initiate palliative care discussions early in disease trajectory as per indications.
Interdisciplinary collaborations	Foster collaboration between hematology and palliative care teams for comprehensive care.
Education and training	Provide education to health care professionals on palliative care principles and skills.
Screening and assessment	Use standardized tools to identify patients who may benefit from palliative care.
Symptom management	Focus on effective symptom management including pain control, fatigue management, and complications.
Transfusion support	RBC and platelet transfusions in emergency as well as to improve the quality of life.
Antimicrobial support	Prompt institution of antibiotics/anti-fungal in case of febrile neutropenia.
Advance care planning	Encourage decisions about goal of care, advance directives, and end-of-life preferences.
Care transitions	Ensure smooth transitions between care settings to maintain continuity of care.
Research and quality improvements	More studies in field of hematologic malignancies to refine palliative care goals.
Psychological support	Provide counseling, emotional, and spiritual support and bereavement support to patients.

chemotherapy with or without stem cell transplantation with a prolonged hospitalization and high symptom burden. In patients of acute myeloid leukemia (AML), receiving chemotherapy, palliative care integration, and optimal counseling about the prognostication of the disease has been shown to improve QOL, decrease the incidence of depression and post-traumatic stress disorder (PTSD) (El-Jawahri et al. 2021). Chronic leukemias are usually indolent unless they progress to the blastic phase or undergo aggressive transformation to high-grade tumors. Symptom burden is generally high, and since the majority of the patients have to take oral therapy for a longer period of time, adverse effects of the drugs remain a concern. There is no clear consensus for integrating palliative and end-of-life care; further studies are required in this regard.

(B) *Myeloma*: The disease course is characterized by remissions and relapses, as well as continued therapy over a long period of time. Incidence Pain experienced is greater than any other hematologic malignancy, mainly due to lytic lesions and vertebral compression fractures requiring palliative radiotherapy and opioid analgesics. Integration of palliative care is not clear, with few studies reporting benefits of early integration on quality of life (Porta-Sales et al. 2017).

(C) *Lymphoma*: Broadly classified as HL (Hodgkin's lymphoma) and NHL (Non-Hodgkin's lymphoma), later being more aggressive. NHL is further sub-classified as aggressive and indolent lymphomas. Palliative care integration should be availed in case of relapse/refractory/transformed lymphomas, worsening performance status, and organ dysfunction (Odejide 2020).

(D) *Stem cell transplantation*: Classified as autologous and allogenic, with the former experiencing fewer complications. Prolonged periods of isolation in transplant units make them predisposed to anxiety and depression (Ruiz et al. 2018). Early integration of palliative care in transplant units has been shown to improve QOL, depression, and anxiety. Chronic Graft vs Host disease cGVHD is one of the major complications in allogenic HSCT, having a high symptom burden requiring early palliative care referral.

35.9 Palliative Care in ICU Settings

Since a large number of patients with hematologic malignancy spend their end of life in the ICU. ICU protocols need to be tailored to the requirements. Individualized therapy is the way to go in ICU for hematology patients. These patients are immunocompromised and neutropenic, which increases the susceptibility to cross infections, such as strict infection control, barrier nursing, and specialized ventilation systems. Antimicrobials are used both as prophylaxis and for the management of febrile neutropenia according to hospital policy. Adequate transfusion facilities for various blood components need to be in place with awareness regarding adverse events and complications (Azoulay et al. 2009).

35.10 Future Direction

Future directions in palliative care/end-of-life care for hematologic malignancies include early integration of palliative care, tailored management strategies, psychosocial interventions, advance planning and discussion, survivorship care program, and upgrading and improving access to palliative care services for equitable care delivery.

Flowchart

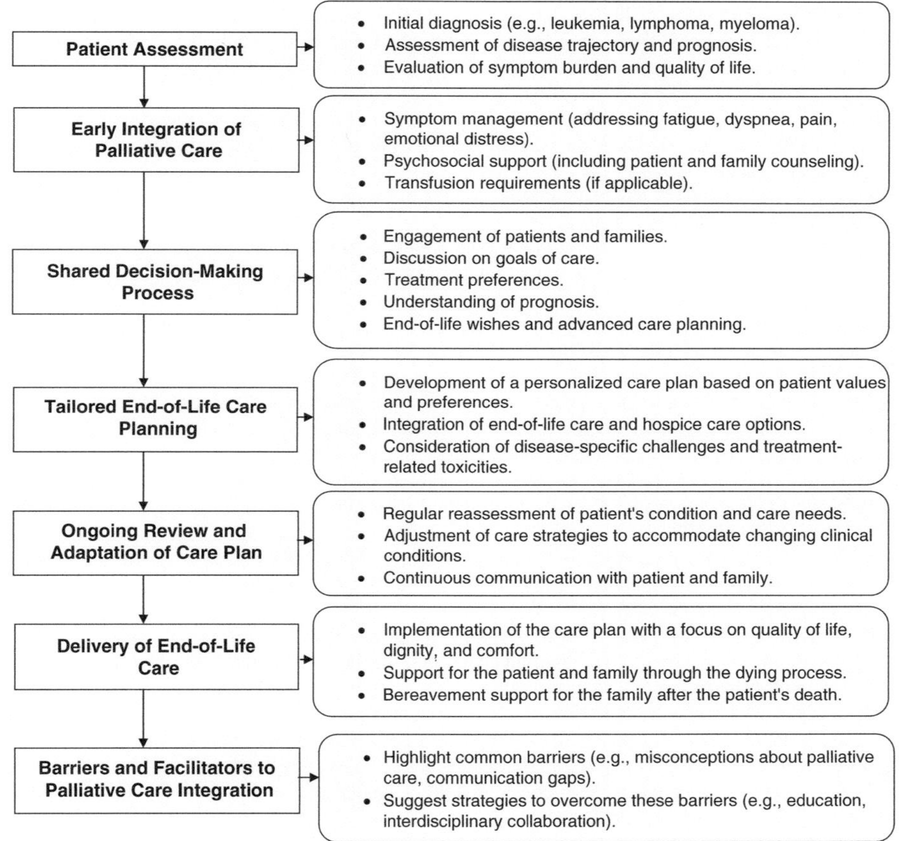

References

Azoulay É, Metnitz B, Sprung CL, Timsit JF, Lemaire F, Bauer P et al (2009) End-of-life practices in 282 intensive care units: data from the SAPS 3 database. Intensive Care Med 35:623–630

Button E, Chan RJ, Chambers S, Butler J, Yates P (2017) A systematic review of prognostic factors at the end of life for people with a hematological malignancy. BMC Cancer 17:1–15

El-Jawahri AR, Traeger LN, Kuzmuk K, Eusebio JR, Vandusen HB, Shin JA et al (2015) Quality of life and mood of patients and family caregivers during hospitalization for hematopoietic stem cell transplantation. Cancer 121(6):951–959

El-Jawahri A, Traeger L, Greer JA, VanDusen H, Fishman SR, LeBlanc TW et al (2017) Effect of inpatient palliative care during hematopoietic stem-cell transplant on psychological distress 6 months after transplant: results of a randomized clinical trial. J Clin Oncol 35(32):3714

El-Jawahri A, LeBlanc TW, Burns LJ, Denzen E, Meyer C, Mau LW et al (2018) What do transplant physicians think about palliative care? A national survey study. Cancer 124(23):4556–4566

El-Jawahri A, LeBlanc TW, Kavanaugh A, Webb JA, Jackson VA, Campbell TC et al (2021) Effectiveness of integrated palliative and oncology care for patients with acute myeloid leukemia: a randomized clinical trial. JAMA Oncol 7(2):238–245

Gautama MSN, Damayanti A, Khusnia AF (2023) Impact of early palliative care to improve quality of life of advanced cancer patients: a meta-analysis of randomised controlled trials. Indian J Palliat Care 29(1):28

Geyer H, Mesa RA (2014) Assessing disease burden in patients with classic MPNs. Best Pract Res Clin Haematol 27(2):107–119

Hochman MJ, Yu Y, Wolf SP, Samsa GP, Kamal AH, LeBlanc TW (2018) Comparing the palliative care needs of patients with hematologic and solid malignancies. J Pain Symptom Manag 55(1):82–88

Howell DA, Shellens R, Roman E, Garry AC, Patmore R, Howard MR (2011) Haematological malignancy: are patients appropriately referred for specialist palliative and hospice care? A systematic review and meta-analysis of published data. Palliat Med 25(6):630–641

Hui D, Elsayem A, Palla S, De La Cruz M, Li Z, Yennurajalingam S, Bruera E (2010) Discharge outcomes and survival of patients with advanced cancer admitted to an acute palliative care unit at a comprehensive cancer center. J Palliat Med 13(1):49–57

Hui D, Paiva CE, Del Fabbro EG, Steer C, Naberhuis J, van de Wetering M et al (2019) Prognostication in advanced cancer: update and directions for future research. Support Care Cancer 27:1973–1984

Hung YS, Wu JH, Chang H, Wang PN, Kao CY, Wang HM et al (2013) Characteristics of patients with hematologic malignancies who received palliative care consultation services in a medical center. Am J Hosp Palliat Care 30(8):773–780

Kirtane K, Downey L, Lee SJ, Curtis JR, Engelberg RA (2018) Intensity of end-of-life care for patients with hematologic malignancies and the role of race/ethnicity. J Palliat Med 21(10):1466–1471

LeBlanc TW, El-Jawahri A (2015) When and why should patients with hematologic malignancies see a palliative care specialist? Hematology Am Soc Hematol Educ Program 2015(1):471–478

LeBlanc TW, O'Donnell JD, Crowley-Matoka M, Rabow MW, Smith CB, White DB et al (2015) Perceptions of palliative care among hematologic malignancy specialists: a mixed-methods study. J Oncol Pract 11(2):e230–e238

Morisaku M, Ito K, Shimomura T, Maeda S, Mori M, Toyosato S et al (2022). Early palliative care improves overall survival in patients with lymphoma: a single-institution retrospective study. in vivo, 36(6), 2910–2917.

Odejide OO (2020) Strategies for introducing palliative care in the management of relapsed or refractory aggressive lymphomas. Hematology Am Soc Hematol Educ Program 2020(1):148–153

Odejide OO, Cronin AM, Condron NB, Fletcher SA, Earle CC, Tulsky JA, Abel GA (2016) Barriers to quality end-of-life care for patients with blood cancers. J Clin Oncol 34(26):3126–3132

Odejide OO, Cronin AM, Earle CC, Tulsky JA, Abel GA (2017) Why are patients with blood cancers more likely to die without hospice? Cancer 123(17):3377–3384

Odejide OO, Uno H, Murillo A, Tulsky JA, Abel GA (2020) Goals of care discussions for patients with blood cancers: association of person, place, and time with end-of-life care utilization. Cancer 126(3):515–522

Porta-Sales J, Guerrero-Torrelles M, Moreno-Alonso D, Sarrà-Escarré J, Clapés-Puig V, Trelis-Navarro J et al (2017) Is early palliative care feasible in patients with multiple myeloma? J Pain Symptom Manag 54(5):692–700

Ruiz M, Reynolds P, Marranzini R, Khan A, Ketterer J, Brahim A (2018) Role of early palliative care interventions in hematological malignancies and bone marrow transplant patients: barriers and potential solutions. Am J Hosp Palliat Care 35(11):1456–1460

Siegel RL, Miller KD, Jemal A (2018) Cancer statistics, 2018. CA Cancer J Clin 68(1):7–30

Tendas A, Niscola P, Cupelli L, Dentamaro T, Scaramucci L, Siniscalchi A et al (2009) Palliative sedation therapy in a bone marrow transplant unit. Support Care Cancer 17:107–108

Wang R, Zeidan AM, Halene S, Xu X, Davidoff AJ, Huntington SF et al (2017) Health care use by older adults with acute myeloid leukemia at the end of life. J Clin Oncol 35(30):3417

World Health Organization (2002) National cancer control programmes: policies and managerial guidelines. World Health Organization

MIX
Papier aus verantwortungsvollen Quellen
Paper from responsible sources
FSC® C105338

If you have any concerns about our products,
you can contact us on
ProductSafety@springernature.com

In case Publisher is established outside the EU,
the EU authorized representative is:
Springer Nature Customer Service Center GmbH
Europaplatz 3, 69115 Heidelberg, Germany

Printed by Libri Plureos GmbH
in Hamburg, Germany